COGNITIVE NEUROSCIENC

SERIES IN AFFECTIVE SCIENCE

SERIES EDITORS
Richard J. Davidson
Paul Ekman
Klaus Scherer

COGNITIVE NEUROSCIENCE OF EMOTION

Edited by
RICHARD D. LANE &
LYNN NADEL

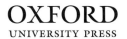

OXFORD
UNIVERSITY PRESS

OXFORD

UNIVERSITY PRESS

Oxford   New York
Auckland   Bangkok   Buenos Aires   Cape Town   Chennai
Dar es Salaam   Delhi   Hong Kong   Istanbul   Karachi   Kolkata
Kuala Lumpur   Madrid   Melbourne   Mexico City   Mumbai   Nairobi
São Paulo   Shanghai   Singapore   Taipei   Tokyo   Toronto

and an associated company in Berlin

Published by Oxford University Press, Inc.
198 Madison Avenue, New York, New York 10016

www.oup.com

First issued as an Oxford University Press paperback, 2002

Oxford is a registered trademark of Oxford University Press, Inc.

Library of Congress Cataloging-in-Publication Data
Cognitive neuroscience of emotion / edited by Richard D. Lane and Lynn
    Nadel ; and associate editors Geoffrey Ahern . . . [et al.].
        p.   cm. — (Series in affective science)
    Includes bibliographical references and index.
    ISBN 978-0-19-511888-9; 978-0-19-515592-1 (pbk.)

    1. Emotions and cognition.   2. Psychophysiology.   I. Lane,
Richard D., 1952–   .   II. Nadel, Lynn.   III. Ahern, Geoffrey
(Geoffrey L.)   IV. Series.
BF531.C55 2000
152.4—dc21   99-17111

9 8 7
Printed in the United States of America
on acid-free paper

Preface

This book provides a showcase for a remarkable assemblage of contributors who collectively are helping to shape a new approach to the study of emotion, namely harnessing the concepts and methods of cognitive neuroscience. The volume is edited by an emotion researcher and psychiatrist, Richard Lane, and by a cognitive neuroscientist, Lynn Nadel. These editors, along with their interdisciplinary team of associate editors from the University of Arizona, have assembled a stellar group of contributors in a volume that is without parallel today.

Cognitive neuroscience has enjoyed a fertile period of growth over the past decade and has been a major force in developing brain-based theories of cognitive function that honor known anatomical and functional properties of the human brain. The editors of this volume argue that emotion should properly be included within the domain of cognitive neuroscience since emotion requires cognitive operations that are indistinguishable from those essential to other processes such as attention and memory. As the editors and many of the contributors effectively illustrate, the substrates of certain cognitive and emotional processes overlap at least partially and the traditional separation between these domains is not supported when considered from the perspective of functional neuroanatomy.

The methods featured in the various contributions illustrate the power that the tools of modern neuroscience can bring to bear on the topic of emotion. Ranging from rodents to non-human primates, from normal subjects to brain-damaged patients and patients with psychiatric disorders, and from psychophysiology to brain imaging, the volume is a testament to the rapid maturity of this area, catapulting it into the forefront of biobehavioral research today.

The editors of the Series in Affective Science are delighted to include this book in the series. While this book was developed independently, the editors of this volume share our goal of promoting scholarship and research on emotion and accepted our invitation to be part of the series for that reason. The editors of this book hold that there is nothing about emotion that clearly separates it from cognition. According to this view, affective neuroscience should be viewed as a subdiscipline of cognitive neuroscience. Although it should be clear that this is not the position of the series editors, we believe that this position and its implications are worthy of serious consideration. Debates such as this, we hope, will inspire future research.

Richard J. Davidson

Contents

Contributors

JOHN P. AGGLETON, PH.D., Department of Psychology, University of Cardiff, Wales, United Kingdom

GEOFFREY L. AHERN, M.D., PH.D., Department of Neurology, University of Arizona, Tucson, Arizona

JOHN J. B. ALLEN, PH. D., Department of Psychology, University of Arizona, Tucson, Arizona

DAVID G. AMARAL, PH.D., Center for Neuroscience, University of California–Davis, Davis, California

MARGARET M. BRADLEY, PH.D., NIMH Center for the Study of Emotion and Attention, University of Florida, Gainesville, Florida

GERALD L. CLORE, PH.D., Department of Psychology, University of Illinois, Urbana-Champaign, Illinois

ANTONIO R. DAMASIO, M.D., PH.D., Department of Neurology, University of Iowa, College of Medicine, Iowa City, Iowa

RICHARD J. DAVIDSON, PH.D., Department of Psychology, University of Wisconsin-Madison, Madison, Wisconsin

RAYMOND J. DOLAN, M.D., Wellcome Department of Cognitive Neurology, Institute of Neurology, Queen Square, London, England

NATHAN J. EMERY, PH.D., Center for Neuroscience, Department of Psychiatry, California Regional Primate Research Center, University of California–Davis, Davis, California

ANDERS FLYKT, PH.D., Department of Clinical Neuroscience, Karolinska Institute, Stockholm, Sweden

BEATRICE DE GELDER, PH.D., Faculty of Social Sciences, Tilburg University, Tilburg, The Netherlands

KENNETH M. HEILMAN, M.D., Department of Neurology, University of Florida, College of Medicine, Gainesville, Florida

ALFRED W. KASZNIAK, PH.D., Department of Psychology, University of Arizona, Tucson, Arizona

BRYAN E. KOLB, PH.D., Department of Psychology, University of Lethbridge, Lethbridge, Canada

RICHARD D. LANE, M.D., PH.D, Department of Psychiatry, University of Arizona, Tucson, Arizona

PETER J. LANG, PH.D., NIMH Center for the Study of Emotion and Attention, University of Florida, Gainesville, Florida

JOSEPH E. LEDOUX, PH.D., Center for Neural Science, New York University, New York, New York

DANIEL LUNDQVIST, PH.D., Department of Clinical Neuroscience, Karolinska Institute, Stockholm, Sweden

JOHN S. MORRIS, M.B.B.S., Wellcome Department of Cognitive Neurology, Institute of Neurology, Queen Square, London, England

LYNN NADEL, PH.D., Department of Psychology, University of Arizona, Tucson, Arizona

ARNE ÖHMAN, PH.D., Department of Clinical Neuroscience, Karolinska Institute, Stockholm, Sweden

ANDREW ORTONY, PH.D., Department of Psychology, Northwestern University, Evanston, Illinois

ERIC M. REIMAN, M.D., Department of Psychiatry University of Arizona, Samaritan PET Center, Phoenix, Arizona

GARY E. SCHWARTZ, PH.D., Department of Psychology, University of Arizona, Tucson, Arizona

LAUGHLIN TAYLOR, PH.D., University of Lethbridge, Montreal Neurological Institute, Lethbridge, Canada

DANIEL TRANEL, PH.D., Psychophysiology Laboratory, Division of Cognitive Neuroscience, Department of Neurology, University of Iowa College of Medicine, Iowa City, Iowa

LAWRENCE WEISKRANTZ, PH.D., Department of Experimental Psychology, Oxford University, Oxford, England

ANDREW W. YOUNG, PH.D., Department of Psychology, University of York, Heslington, York, England

COGNITIVE NEUROSCIENCE OF EMOTION

1

The Study of Emotion from the Perspective of Cognitive Neuroscience

RICHARD D. LANE, LYNN NADEL, JOHN J. B. ALLEN,
AND ALFRED W. KASZNIAK

This book's title, and the conference upon which it was based, reflect the view within the cognitive neuroscience community at the University of Arizona that the role of cognition in emotion is an important area to pursue. The contributions in this volume were solicited with this theme in mind.

Why Emotion Might Profitably Be Studied from the Perspective of Cognitive Neuroscience

- Emotion Involves Cognitive Appraisals

Emotion may be understood as the outcome of an evaluation of the extent to which one's goals are being met in interaction with the environment (Ortony et al., 1988). Such an evaluation typically involves a cognitive process of some type; therefore, identifying what brain processes are involved in performing this evaluation and understanding how this evaluation is performed appear to fall naturally within the purview of cognitive neuroscience. Although there is controversy about the extent to which an evaluation always preceeds an emotional response, this debate hinges on how one defines cognition (see Clore and Ortony, this volume). The famous debate on this topic between Lazarus (1984) and Zajonc (1984) addressed whether complex cognition was necessary for an emotional response, not whether an evaluation of some type is performed.

- Emotion May Involve Awareness of or
  Attention to Emotional Experience

Another important aspect of emotion that appears to fall within the domain of cognitive neuroscience is conscious experience. It is questionable whether the concept of emotion would exist if emotion did not contain an element of conscious experience. Indeed, a great deal of psychological and social psychological research on emotion is founded on the belief that self-reported emotional experience provides very useful information. Current evidence, however, suggests that the process of generating and executing an emotional response can and often does proceed outside of conscious awareness (LeDoux, 1996). The field of emotion research has advanced considerably since fundamental discoveries were made regarding the neurobiological basis of emotion, discoveries that relied on manifest behavior indicative of emotion rather than emotional experience per se. The neurobiology of consciousness is an important topic within the domain of cognitive neuroscience and, as such, the neuroscience of both conscious and unconscious processes in emotion clearly is an important area of study within the domain of cognitive neuroscience as well.

- Emotion and Cognition May Involve
  Overlapping Response Systems

Explicit cognitive processes are not typically associated with specific responses. Some authors (e.g., Bradley & Lang, this volume) have argued that emotion is quintessentially about response systems (in the verbal, behavioral, and physiological domains). Even this distinction, however, breaks down upon closer scrutiny. For example, procedural knowledge is recognized as an important component of implicit cognition. There is clear overlap between such motor behavior and the action patterns thought by some to define emotion (Frijda, 1986). Another example is skin conductance, a sympathetically mediated function that has been widely used as an index of emotional arousal, and that has also become an important tool in the study of unconscious or implicit cognition. Patients with prosopagnosia manifest skin conductance responses to familiar people whom they do not consciously recognize but do not manifest skin conductance responses to unfamiliar people (Bauer, 1984; Bauer & Verfaellie, 1988; Tranel & Damasio, 1985). These skin conductance responses indicate that at some nonconscious level there is recognition of the familiar faces. A third example is classical conditioning, which inherently links stimuli with response systems (e.g., gastric acid secretion in response to a ringing bell). This type of learning is well accepted as a topic of inquiry within the field of cognitive neuroscience. It is clear that the field of cognitive neuroscience does not establish strict limits a priori regarding what is cognitive and what is not.

- Emotion Can Guide, Influence, or
  Constrain Cognition

It is also evident that emotion has important effects on mental functions that are indisputably cognitive, such as memory, attention, and perception. This important area of study clearly belongs in cognitive neuroscience as well, and, indeed, is the topic of other volumes (Christianson, 1992; Clore et al., 1994; Niedenthal and Kitayama, 1994).

- Some of the Most Productive Methods for
  Studying Emotion Are Those Shared With
  Cognitive Neuroscience

Cognitive neuroscientists use a number of well-defined and validated approaches, such as lesion studies, neuroimaging techniques, subtraction approaches, and dual-task paradigms. These approaches and others are used to dissect cognition and its neural substrates into its component elements. Investigating emotion with such approaches has been, and will continue to be, quite productive. Use of the same approaches permits direct comparisons of cognitive and emotional processes in the same metric, potentially demonstrating their distinguishing characteristics, as in the double-dissociation technique (Zola-Morgan et al., 1991), their similarity, or their interaction.

- Parsimony

Although the content of cognitive and emotional processes differs, there is at present no evidence that the neural processes subserving cognition differ in fundamental ways from those subserving emotion. General principles describing the process by which brain systems work (e.g., modularity vs. nonmodularity) may apply to both emotion and cognition. Thus, studying emotion within the field of cognitive neuroscience would appear to have many advantages.

Why Might the Neuroscience of Emotion Be Studied Independently from Cognitive Neuroscience?

An alternative view is that a cognitive approach to emotion is inherently limiting. Aristotle divided the mind into three functions: cognition, emotion, and conation (or will). Hilgard (1980) has reviewed the history of this tripartite model and its importance. To the extent that cognition and emotion are separate domains of the mind, any field called "cognitive neuroscience" would appear to be unable to do justice to the neuroscience of emotion. Indeed, a new field called "affective neuroscience" has been spawned (Davidson & Sutton, 1995; Panksepp, 1998), spurred by findings from new technologies, such as functional neuroimaging techniques and neural-tract tracing methods, that have made certain research questions amenable to empirical investigation for the first time. One of the goals of the field of affective neuroscience is to dissect emotion into its elementary mental operations and its corresponding neural substrates, a strategy comparable to that being pursued for cognition within the field of cognitive neuroscience.

Limitations to Studying Emotion Separately

If dissecting emotion into elementary mental operations and corresponding neural substrates is the agenda of affective neuroscience, the question arises whether a conceptual framework that separates emotion and cognition into different areas of research is in some ways artificial. In fact, the designation of emotion as falling outside the domain of cognitive neuroscience could be construed as an expression of antagonism between emotion and cognition that can be traced to Cartesian dualism. Descartes viewed reason as a manifestation of the soul, a phenomenon unique to human beings, while emotions were considered an expression of bodily processes, a phenomenon shared with other animals. The force of reason could oppose and control emotion, and vice versa, and thus the conceptualization of emotion and reason as antagonistic and separable appeared appropriate.

However, there has been a rapprochement between cognition and emotion. For example, Damasio (1994) showed that emotional processes are required for certain types of decision-making to occur. Other research indicates that "emotional intelligence," a particular type of socially oriented cognition (Salovey & Mayer, 1989), may be an important predictor of success in the real world independent of traditional, purely cognitive intelligence (Goleman, 1995). These findings are consistent with growing evidence that greater refinement and organizational complexity of emotion and cognition go hand in hand (Lane & Schwartz, 1987; Sommers & Scioli, 1986). Furthermore, the evidence reviewed above indicates that sensorimotor processes are part of cognition and that higher cognitive processes often play an important role in emotion. Although not intended by Davidson & Sutton (1995) or Panksepp (1998), using the term "affective neuroscience" could be construed as perpetuating a misguided antagonism between emotion and cognition.

Moreover, although the division of the mind and brain into three (or more) parts may be useful for certain conceptual purposes, there may be no such thing as pure cognition without emotion, or pure emotion without cognition. It is not likely that one can identify a structure or region of the brain that is exclusively devoted to cognition or emotion and has no interaction with the other process. Similarly, it is difficult to imagine how conation or will could be implemented in the absence of cognition or emotion. Reflexive emotional behavior involves an automatic selection of a goal-directed motor response (a type of intentionality) without the necessity of conscious choice. To the extent that consciously experienced emotion leads one to alter his or her behavior in the interest of adaptation to the social environment, that, too, is an expression of conation or intention that requires cognitive mediation.

A further consideration is the purpose of the research program of neuroscience. Ultimately we must integrate the different components of the mind to understand how they work together in daily life. Progress in a given domain may ultimately create barriers to integration if the goal of integration is not a high priority from the start. To the extent that the three components of the mind are inseparable, one must ask what is gained by separating the subcomponents of the mind from one another.

Can Noncognitive Aspects of Emotion Be Identified?

We have just argued that emotion and cognition in the intact person may be inextricably linked. As an example, a mathematical proof is an expression of pure logic that, on its surface, does not appear to inherently involve emotion. However, the inspiration and intuition involved in creating the proof, the feeling that one is on to something or is veering off course, may constitute emotional elements essential to the generation of the final product.

For conceptual purposes, however, it may be useful to consider cognition in a pure form, such as a computer program. Is it possible that emotions can be programmed into computers? Some authors argue that they can, and that doing so may be necessary for the full information processing capabilities of computers to be realized (Picard, 1997).

Similarly, the nature and content of emotional phenomena may on their surface appear to be fundamentally different from cognitive phenomena, but closer scrutiny may suggest that at their core cognitive elements of some type are involved. A key question is whether each of the different facets of emotion, such as emotion generation, emotional expression, and emotional experience, are inherently cognitive.

We would argue that any dividing line between cognition and emotion, if it exists, depends on one's definition of cognition. If one equates cognition with conscious thought, which is the traditional approach in philosophy (Griffiths, 1997), then much of emotion does not involve cognition. This brings us back to the familiar debate between Lazarus and Zajonc. Within cognitive neuroscience, however, it is now well accepted that much of cognition is implicit or outside of conscious awareness. The boundary for what is cognitive and what is not among implicit processes has not been established. If there are aspects of emotion that are not cognitive, they are to be found in the realm of implicit emotion.

To illustrate this point, consider the skin conductance (Öhman et al., this volume) and amygdala (Morris et al., 1998) responses to conditioned angry faces when they are perceived without conscious awareness in a backward masking paradigm. If one accepts that the skin conductance response in this instance is a consequence of information processing or symbolic processes of some type, it is reasonable to conclude that emotion is cognitive. If one does not accept this assumption, the challenge is to define why what transpires between stimulus and response is not cognitive.

It may also be argued that what distinguishes emotion from cognition may be its "embodiment," in that the autonomic, neuroendocrine, and musculoskeletal concomitants of emotional responses distinguish them from cognitive processes. We have discussed above, however, that such responses characterize implicit cognition. If this issue is to be resolved, it will depend on the field of cognitive neuroscience determining where cognition ends and where other noncognitive phenomena begin.

Should Cognitive Neuroscience Include Emotion?

We argue that for now the search for the location of the boundary between cognitive and noncognitive phenomena will be facilitated best by including emotion within the field of cognitive neuroscience. To the extent that this occurs, it will require an expansion of the purview of cognitive neuroscience as it is typically conceived. The textbook by Gazzaniga, Ivry, and Mangun (1998), *Cognitive Neuroscience—The Biology of the Mind*, suggests that the field of cognitive neuroscience may be open to such an expansion.

In the absence of a clear empirical foundation for separating the two fields of study, we have adopted a conservative approach. Yet, the matter has not been resolved, and certain chapters in this book discuss some of the phenomena at issue in detail. This book therefore can serve a twofold purpose: (1) to explore what is known regarding cognitive processes in emotion, and (2) to review the processes and anatomical structures involved in emotion in sufficient detail to determine whether there is something about emotion or its neural substrates that requires that they be studied as a separate domain. In our view, exclusively emotional functions that are uniquely different from cognition have not yet been demonstrated. As such, studying emotion within the field of cognitive neuroscience appears to be a reasonable strategy until new evidence indicates otherwise.

Overview of Chapter Contents

The chapters in this book can be roughly divided into four topics: the process of emotion generation, the functions of the amygdala, the conscious experience of emotion, and emotion regulation and dysregulation. We briefly review the contents of each chapter and, implicitly, the rationale for the order in which the chapters are presented.

In chapter 2, Damasio puts the current state of research on emotion and the brain in perspective. He discusses what emotion is from an evolutionary perspective, why emotion was not included in the cognitive revolution, and why emotion has been given "a second chance." He argues that the failure to distinguish between emotion and feelings (i.e., the conscious experience of emotion) can account for the previous mistrust of emotion as a suitable topic of scientific inquiry. He also contends that feelings are an important topic for future neuroscientific investigation.

The chapters on emotion generation begin with a thoughtful discussion by Clore and Ortony, who offer a detailed analysis of the role of cognition preceding emotion. Their conclusion is that one's view of the role of cognition in emotion is a function of one's definition of cognition, and that it is reasonable to hypothesize a role for cognition in all cases of emotion. This chapter, together with Damasio's, provides strong support for studying emotion from the perspective of cognitive neuroscience. In certain respects the other chapters in the book can be viewed as defining much of what is known about how emotion is instantiated in the brain.

Kolb and Taylor present a regional survey of the contribution of different brain regions to the generation and expression of emotion. Drawing on both clinical neuropsychological and animal data, they review evidence regarding the role of the frontal and temporal lobes and hemispheric asymmetries in the production and perception of facial expressions and emotional prosody.

Next, de Gelder discusses her work on a particular aspect of emotion generation: how information from different senses is brought together to create an emotional response. She presents evidence regarding the integration of visual and vocal information in the evaluation of emotional stimulus content.

Among the brain structures closely associated with emotion, the amygdala is arguably the one about which most is known. If there is to be an affective neuroscience separate from cognitive neuroscience, the amygdala must play an important role. We therefore present the views of some of the leading investigators in this area of research in the next group of chapters.

Chapters 6–8 focus on the findings from animal research. Aggleton and Young present a systematic survey of the functions of the amygdala, drawing on work performed in rats, monkeys, and, to a lesser extent, humans. They demonstrate that much is known, but it is also evident that much remains to be discovered regarding the functions of the amygdala. LeDoux takes the position that progress will be made most efficiently by studying the elementary components of what we broadly label emotion and cognition. He then presents his work on fear conditioning in the rat. He discusses the microanatomy of the amygdala and its connections with other structures and presents a model of the neural basis of conscious emotional experience. Emery and Amaral discuss the neural substrates of social cognition in the monkey, with particular emphasis on the amygdala. The social behaviors they discuss include feeding, mating, affiliation, aggression, predator avoidance, and defense.

Chapters 9 and 10 involve human research. Tranel discusses the effect of brain lesions in specific locations on skin conductance responses. He systematically examines the effect of lesions of the amygdala, anterior cingulate cortex, orbitofrontal cortex, and parietal cortex on electrodermal activity and other behavioral parameters. Dolan and Morris report their functional neuroimaging findings regarding the neural substrates of innate and acquired fear. Innate fear is evaluated by examining the brain areas activated by exposure to fearful versus happy faces. Acquired fear is evaluated by the effects of aversive conditioning. In both studies activity is observed in the amygdala as well as in other structures.

The next group of chapters deals with conscious awareness of emotion. Bradley and Lang take the position that consciousness is a hypothesis that cannot be scientifically validated by objective observations. They report their findings using the "three systems" approach of observable outputs of emotion, consisting of language, motor behavior, and physiology. Their data demonstrate that a great deal can be learned about emotion without invoking the construct of consciousness.

Drawing upon his studies of blindsight, Weiskrantz discusses the complexities of rigorously demonstrating that perception has occurred in the absence of conscious awareness. He then discusses the implications of what is known about the neural substrates of visual perception with and without awareness for the neural substrates of conscious awareness of emotion.

Öhman and colleagues, like Damasio, approach the study of unconscious emotion from an evolutionary perspective. They argue that emotionally meaningful information is automatically processed outside of conscious awareness. This information may be viewed as a signal that may or may not capture attentional mechanisms and be consciously perceived. They then review their work demonstrating that conditioned angry faces, when presented briefly followed by backward masking, are not consciously perceived but can elicit skin conductance responses nonetheless.

Heilman presents a model of emotional experience based on observations in neurological patients. His view is that a distributed network of subcortical and cortical structures mediates emotional experience, but he does not attempt to distinguish between the neural substrates of conscious and unconscious emotion. In contrast, Lane discusses how distinctions between emotional responses with and without conscious awareness can be understood from a cognitive–developmental perspective. He then draws on psychometric and functional neuroimaging data to propose a neuroanatomical model of implicit and explicit emotional processes.

The fourth group of chapters deals with affective regulation and dysregulation. Davidson discusses individual differences in normal subjects in affective style, the tendency to respond to situations with either a positively or negatively valenced emotional response. He reviews evidence that these behavioral patterns are mediated by baseline differences in the asymmetry of prefrontal activation as well as other differences in the temporal patterning of affective responses. Finally, Reiman et al. review the work they have performed on the neural substrates of normal and pathological emotion (particularly anxiety states) using positron emission tomography. This work illustrates not only what is known but helps to highlight how much remains to be learned about the neural basis of pathological emotional states.

Future Directions

This book constitutes a broad but selective survey of current knowledge about emotion and the brain. Its chapters were not written with a cognitive neuroscience focus in mind, and yet in one way or another they all address the close association between cognitive and emotional processes.

It should come as no surprise that differing viewpoints are expressed regarding the central themes of this book. For example, in discussing the cognitive antecedents of emotion, Damasio states that the stimulus causing an emotion "is processed through a variety of neural stations, but one wonders about the wisdom of calling such processing an evaluation," while Clore and Ortony are comfortable in using this term. In reviewing the functions of the amygdala, Aggleton and Young point to evidence that it participates in pleasant, unpleasant, and emotionally arousing events, Tranel emphasizes its role in aversive emotional states, and LeDoux and Dolan and Morris emphasize its role in fear. In discussing emotional experience, as alluded to above, there are major differences of opinion regarding the extent to which the conscious experience of emotion is considered a valid subject of scientific inquiry. Among those who do consider it valid, important differences exist regarding the specifics. For example, Heilman contends that the contribution of somatic feedback to emotional experience, as in the James-Lange theory, is of minor importance, while such feedback plays an important role in Damasio's somatic marker hypothesis. Other areas of disagreement will be evident also. The differing viewpoints expressed ultimately reflect the need for more research.

This book therefore has sought to bring together diverse strands of investigation with the aim of documenting our current understanding of how emotion is instantiated in the brain. Much of the work presented involves research performed during the 1990s. Although many areas of agreement exist, many points of discrepancy remain. Perhaps the findings and viewpoints discussed in this book will catalyze additional research that will ultimately resolve many of these issues.

References

Bauer, R. M. (1984). Autonomic recognition of names and faces in prosopagnosia: a neuropsychological application of the Guilty Knowledge Test. *Neuropsychologia, 22,* 457–469.

Bauer, R. M. & Verfaellie, M. (1988). Electrodermal discrimination of familiar but not unfamiliar faces in prosopagnosia. *Brain and Cognition, 8,* 240–252.

Christianson, S-Å. (Ed). (1992). *The Handbook of Emotion and Memory: Research and Theory*. Hillsdale, NJ: Lawrence Erlbaum Associates.

Clore, G. L., Schwarz, N. & Conway, M. (1994). Affective causes and consequences of social information processing. In R. S. Wyer, Jr. & T. K. Srull (Eds), *Handbook of Social Cognition*, vol. 1, *Basic Processes* (pp. 323–417). Hillsdale, NJ: Lawrence Erlbaum Associates.

Damasio, A. R. (1994). *Descartes' Error: Emotion, Reason, and the Human Brain*. New York: G. P. Putnam's Sons.

Davidson, R. J. & Sutton, S. K. (1995). Affective neuroscience: the emergence of a discipline. *Current Opinion in Neurobiology, 5*, 217–224.

Frijda, N. H. (1986). *The Emotions*. Cambridge: Cambridge University Press.

Gazzaniga, M. S., Ivry, R. B. & Mangun, G. R. (1998). *Cognitive Neuroscience—The Biology of the Mind*. New York: W. W. Norton & Co.

Goleman, D. (1995). *Emotional Intelligence*. New York: Bantam Books.

Griffiths, P. E. (1997). *What Emotions Really Are: The Problem of Psychological Categories*. Chicago: University of Chicago Press.

Hilgard, E. R. (1980). The trilogy of mind: cognition, affection, and conation. *Journal of the History of the Behavioral Sciences, 16*, 107–117.

Lane, R. D. & Schwartz, G. E. (1987). Levels of emotional awareness: a cognitive-developmental theory and its application to psychopathology. *American Journal of Psychiatry, 144*, 133–143.

Lazarus, R. (1984). On the primacy of cognition. *American Psychologist, 39*, 124–126.

LeDoux, J. E. (1996). *The Emotional Brain*. New York: Simon & Schuster.

Morris, J. S., Öhman, A. & Dolan, R. J. (1998). Unconscious processing of aversively conditioned stimuli by the human amygdala. *Nature, 393*, 467–470.

Niedenthal, P. M. & Kitayama, S. (Eds) (1994). *The Heart's Eye: Emotional Influences in Perception and Attention*. New York: Academic Press.

Ortony, A., Clore, G. L. & Collins, A. (1988). *The Cognitive Structure of Emotions*. New York: Cambridge University Press.

Panksepp, J. (1998). *Affective Neuroscience: The Foundations of Human and Animal Emotions*. New York: Oxford University Press.

Picard, R. W. (1997). *Affective Computing*. Cambridge, MA: MIT Press.

Salovey, P. & Mayer, J. D. (1989). Emotional intelligence. *Imagination, Cognition, and Personality, 9*, 185–211.

Sommers, S. & Scioli, A. (1986). Emotional range and value orientation: toward a cognitive view of emotionality. *Journal of Personality and Social Psychology, 5*, 417–422.

Tranel, D., Damasio, A. R. (1985). Knowledge without awareness: an autonomic index of facial recognition by prosopagnosics. *Science, 228*, 1453–1454.

Zajonc, R. B. (1984). On the primacy of affect. *American Psychologist, 39*, 117–123.

Zola-Morgan, S., Squire, L. R., Alvarez-Royo, P. & Clower, R. P. (1991). Independence of memory functions and emotional behavior: separate contributions of the hippocampal formation and the amygdala. *Hippocampus, 1*(2), 207–220.

2

A Second Chance for Emotion

ANTONIO R. DAMASIO

Both neuroscience and cognitive science have neglected emotion until recently. By the last quarter of the nineteenth century, Charles Darwin, William James, and Sigmund Freud had written extensively on different aspects of emotion, and Hughlings Jackson had even made a first stab at its neuroanatomy. There would have been reason to expect that the expanding brain sciences would embrace emotion and solve its riddles, just as the new century started. Unfortunately, that never happened. Emotion was left out of the scientific mainstream, and this circumstance is confirmed by the few exceptions to it—a handful of psychologists that carried out important studies on emotion; another handful of neuroanatomists interested in the limbic system; and the psychiatrists and pharmacologists that concerned themselves with the diagnosis and management of mood disorders and developed drugs which gave indirect information on the mechanisms of emotion. Emotion was not trusted, in real life or in the laboratory. Emotion was too subjective; it was too elusive and vague; it was too much at the opposite end of the finest human ability, reason. It was probably irrational to study it.

There are some curious parallels to the scientific neglect of emotion during the twentieth century. The first is the lack of an evolutionary perspective in the study of brain and mind. Neuroscience and cognitive science have proceeded almost as if Darwin never existed, although of late the situation is changing remarkably, and some might say that it is changing too much and not too well.

The second parallel concerns the disregard for the notion of homeostatic regulation. Numerous scientists, of course, were preoccupied with understanding the neurophysiology of homeostasis or with making sense of the neuroanatomy and the neurochemistry of the autonomic nervous system; or with elucidating the mechanisms of neuroendocrine regulation and of the interrelation between nervous system and immune system. But the scientific progress made in those areas had little influence in shaping prevailing views of how the brain generated mental states.

A third parallel is the noticeable absence of the notion of the organism in cognitive science and neuroscience. The mind remained linked to the brain in a somewhat equivocal relationship, and the brain remained consistently separated from the body rather than being seen as part of a complex living entity. The notion of the integrated organism, the idea of an ensemble made up of body proper and nervous system, had little or no impact in the dominant conceptions of mind and brain.

There are exceptions to all the parallels; for instance, Gerald Edelman's (1992) theoretical proposals are informed by evolutionary thinking and make use of homeostatic regulation; likewise, the "somatic marker" hypothesis is grounded on notions of evolution, homeostatic regulation, and organism (Damasio, 1994). But the theoretical assumptions according to which cognitive science and neuroscience have been conducted have not made much use of organismic and evolutionary perspectives.

This state of affairs has changed for the better in recent years, not only in general theoretical terms but also in regard to work on emotion. Both neuroscience and cognitive neuroscience seem to have embraced emotion. Important examples of this change can be found in the work of Adolphs (1995), Davidson (1993), Panksepp (1997), Davis (1992), Morris and Dolan (1996), LeDoux (1996), and others represented in this volume. Moreover, the artificial opposition between emotion and reason has been questioned and is not as easily taken for granted. For example, my work on prefrontal cortex damage has persuaded me that emotion is integral to the processes of reasoning and decision making, for worse or for better. This may sound a bit counterintuitive at first, but there is evidence to support the claim. The findings come from the study of several individuals who were patently rational in the way they governed their lives up to the time when, as a result of neurological damage in specific sites of their brains, they lost their ability to make rational decisions, and, along with that momentous defect, also lost their ability to process emotion normally. Those individuals can still use the instruments of their rationality and can still call up knowledge pertinent to the world around them. Their ability to tackle the logic of a problem remains intact. Nonetheless, many of their personal and social decisions are irrational, when considered from the common-sense perspective of a comparable individual. More often than not, those decisions are disadvantageous to them and to persons close to them. I have suggested that the delicate mechanism of reasoning is no longer affected, nonconsciously and on occasion even consciously, by signals hailing from the neural machinery that underlies emotion (Damasio, 1994, 1996).

This hypothesis is known as the "somatic marker hypothesis," and the patients who led me to propose it had damage to selected areas in the prefrontal region, especially in the ventral and medial sectors, and in the right parietal regions. Whether because of a stroke, head injury, or a tumor that required surgical resection, damage in those regions was consistently associated with the appearance of the clinical pattern I described above (i.e., a disturbance of the ability to make advantageous decisions in situations involving risk and conflict and a reduction of the ability to resonate emotionally in those same situations). Specifically, while those patients continue to exhibit what I call background emotions and primary emotions, they fail to exhibit secondary emotions, those that, for instance, are induced by a complex social situation. Before the onset of their brain damage, the individuals had shown no such impairments. Family and friends could sense a "before" and an "after," relative to the time of neurologic injury.

These findings suggest that a selective reduction of emotion is at least as prejudicial for rationality as excessive emotion. It certainly does not seem true that reason stands to gain from operating without the leverage of emotion. On the contrary, emotion probably assists reasoning, especially when it comes to personal and social matters involving risk and conflict. I suggest that emotion probably points us to the sector of the decision-making space where our reason can operate most efficiently. I do not suggest, however, that emotions are a substitute for reason, nor do I claim that emotions decide for us, nor do I deny that emotional upheavals can lead to irrational decisions. I simply state that current neurological evidence suggests that certain compromises of emotion are a problem. Well-tuned and deployed emotion, as I see it, is necessary for the edifice of reason to operate properly.

These results and hypotheses call into question the notion that emotion is an inconvenient evolutionary vestige, let alone a luxury, and bring forth a number of questions. Perhaps emotion does have some rationality built into it; perhaps it embodies a logic of survival in evolution; perhaps it does have a value in social communication; perhaps it is worth studying after all. But let us not assume the road is free and clear. Several barriers remain, the largest one being the notion that the mental representation of emotions and feelings is of a nature different from anything else studied in the broad field of mind and brain. In the discussion below, I suggest that this barrier can be overcome by adopting a provisional framework in which emotions and feelings of emotions are clearly distinguished from each other and their possible neurophysiological underpinnings are clearly specified. Naturally, I see that framework as entirely open to revision based on future empirical verification.

The Alleged Vagueness of Emotion and Feeling

The alleged vagueness of emotions and feelings is the most frequent excuse offered to justify the difficulty of studying these undesirable phenomena. A commonplace statement, from neuroscientists and cognitive scientists alike, is that somehow the representation of emotion, cognitively and neurally speaking, is of a nature different from that of other representations and that feelings are indescribable with any degree of precision. I can understand that, at first glance, the varied composition of emotions makes them difficult to capture, and it is apparent that feelings are more difficult to describe than a visual or auditory percept for which a direct provenance is immediately apparent. But greater difficulty does not mean impossibility. It is possible to produce rigorous descriptions of the mental images related to emotions and feelings. This possibility is enhanced by having some idea of the biological underpinnings of emotion and of the role that emotions are likely to play in the general scheme of living things. I suggest that most of the difficulties to which I have just alluded will dissipate when we make a principled distinction between the phenomena of emotion and feeling and when we offer a testable account of the likely substrate of the representations of feeling.

Distinguishing Emotions from Feelings of Emotions

I believe that the lack of distinction between emotions and feelings of emotions contributes greatly to these difficulties. Understanding the complex topics of emotion and feeling requires that we honor a distinction between the two. For the remainder of the chapter, I will refer to "feeling" as shorthand for "feeling of emotion." I will simply say that the term "feeling" should be reserved for the private, mental experience of an emotion. The term "emotion" should be used to designate all the responses whose perception we call feeling. In practical terms this means that you cannot observe a feeling in someone else. Likewise, no one can observe your own feelings, but some aspects of the emotions that give rise to your feelings will be patently observable to others. (Yet another distinction is important, in this regard. Feeling and knowing that you feel are separable processes. It is conceivable that some animals have emotions and feelings but are not conscious of having them, although I believe many nonhuman species are indeed conscious of their feelings.)

Emotions and feelings are part of a continuous process, but the relative publicness of emotions and the complete privacy of feelings indicate that the mechanisms along the continuum are quite different. Honoring a distinction between emotion and feeling is helpful if we are to analyze the phenomena carefully and investigate them thoroughly. Incidentally, the languages that have carried to us the heritage of Western philosophy and psychology have long had the words "feeling" and "emotion" available. The two words were probably coined because many wise thinkers, as they coped with the description of the two sets of phenomena, sensed their clear separation and saw the value of denoting them by different terms. Referring to the whole process by the single word emotion, as is now common practice among scientists and lay public, is somewhat careless.

What Are Emotions?

When we consider those conditions for which the term emotion would be applied with virtual universal agreement, I would say that emotions are specific and consistent collections of physiological responses triggered by certain brain systems when the organism represents certain objects or situations (e.g., a change in its own tissues such as that which produces pain, or an external entity such as a person seen or heard; or the representation of a person, or object, or situation, conjured up from memory into the thought process). Although the precise composition and dynamics of the responses are shaped by individual development and environment, the evidence suggests that the basics of most if not all emotional responses are preset by the genome and result from a long history of evolutionary fine tuning. Emotions, in the broad sense, are part of the bioregulatory devices with which we come equipped to maintain life and survive. Of necessity, the statement encompasses the three major kinds of emotion: background emotions, primary emotions, and secondary emotions. The view I offer here is generally compatible with that inherent in the work of authors such as Ekman (1992).

A few other traits help round out the description. First, emotions are not one single response but rather collections of responses. An emotion is always varied and complex. Second, the usual inducers of emotions are representations of objects or situations that can come either from outside an organism, as an organism interacts with the world, or are generated from the inside, either as an organism forms representations in recall or neurally represents its internal milieu states.

Third, neither kind of representation, be it external perceptual or internal re-called, need be attended to. Either can occur outside of consciousness and still induce emotional responses. Emotions can be induced in a nonconscious manner and thus appear as unmotivated to the conscious self. It is reasonable to assume that in humans most emotions are triggered in consciousness, from attended mental contents in a directed thought process, but depending on the individual and on the occasion a good number of emotions will occur without an immediately detectable inducer.

Fourth, the consistent form of the responses and their consistent link to certain inducers, indicate that, to a large extent, the biological machinery underlying emo-tion is part of the early specifications of the organism and of the nervous system in particular. The fact that emotional responses can only be triggered from certain parts of the brain rather than any part of the brain also speaks to that point.

Fifth, emotions have varied temporal profiles, although variations of profile are possible depending on circumstances and on individuals. Several emotions tend to be engaged in a "burst" pattern with fairly rapid onset, a peak of intensity and rapid decay, such as anger, fear, surprise, or disgust. Other emotions are engaged in a "wave" pattern, with gradual onset and slow decay, one pattern emerging after another without sharp boundaries (e.g., background emotions). (A brief word on terminology: when a particular emotion occurs frequently or even continuously, it is preferable to refer to the resulting state as a mood. Moods are thus distinguish-able from emotions, in general, including the background emotions with which they can easily be confounded. As for the word "affect," it should be used only to designate the entire topic of emotion and feeling, including, of necessity, the subja-cent processes of motivation and the underlying states of pain and pleasure.)

Sixth, as implied by the foregoing, the mechanisms underlying pain and plea-sure are not emotions per se, although they can evoke emotions (as happens often in instances of pain). Pain and pleasure are constituent parts of emotions and, consequently, of feelings. Much the same statement applies to the mechanisms behind drives and motivations, which are part of the basic survival equipment of an organism and often undergird emotional states.

In a typical emotion, then, certain regions of the brain, which are part of a largely preset neural system related to emotions, send commands to other regions of the brain and to most everywhere in the body proper. The commands are sent via the bloodstream, in the form of chemical molecules, or via neuronal pathways. The result of these coordinated neural and chemical commands is a global change in the state of the organism. Both the body proper and the brain are largely and profoundly affected by the set of commands, although the origin of those com-mands was circumscribed to a brain system that was responding to a particular set of sensory patterns.

Inducing Emotions

An easily apparent fact when one considers the physiology of emotions is that the kinds of stimuli that can cause emotions tend to be systematically linked to a certain kind of emotion. The classes of stimuli that cause happiness, or fear, or sadness, tend to do so fairly consistently in the same individual and in individuals who share the same social and cultural background, in spite of unique personal differences. Throughout evolution organisms have acquired the means to respond to certain stimuli, which are potentially useful or potentially dangerous from the point of view of survival, with the sort of response collection we currently call an emotion. The general purpose of emotions is the production of both a specific behavior which reacts to the inducing situation and of a change in internal state aimed at preparing the organism for that particular behavior. For certain classes of clearly dangerous or clearly valuable stimulus, evolution has prepared a matching answer in the form of an emotion. This is why, in spite of the infinite variations to be found across individuals, and across cultures, we can predict with some success that certain stimuli will produce certain emotions.

But a word of caution is needed here. When I talk about *ranges of stimuli* that constitute inducers for certain *classes of emotion*, that is really what I mean. I am allowing for a considerable variation in the type of stimuli that can induce an emotion—both across individuals and across cultures—and I am calling attention to the fact that regardless of the degree of biological presetting of the emotional machinery, unique individual development and culture probably play a role, first by influencing what constitutes an adequate inducer of a given emotion; second, by influencing some aspects of the expression of emotion; and third, by shaping the cognition and behavior that follows the deployment of an emotion. Moreover, it is important to note that although the biological machinery for emotions is likely to be largely preset, the inducers are not part of the machinery. Indeed, it is important to realize that the stimuli that cause emotions in any of us are by no means confined to the range prescribed by nature during evolution and available to our brains early in life. Organisms develop and gain factual and emotional experience with different objects and situations in the environment, and organisms thus have an opportunity to associate many objects and situations which would have been neutral from the standpoint of emotions with the objects and situations that are naturally prescribed to cause emotions. The consequence of this extension is that the range of stimuli that can produce emotions is infinite. In one way or another, most of the objects and situations we can either perceive or conjure up lead to some emotional reaction. The reaction may be weak or strong, and fortunately for us it is weak more often than not. But it is there nonetheless. Emotion is the obligate accompaniment of thinking about oneself or about one's surroundings.

I have alluded specifically to the existence of two types of stimuli capable of inducing emotion: those that are naturally prescribed do so at the outset of development and are in all likelihood the result of the fine tunings of evolution, and those that are acquired by learning in a social and cultural context and which depend on the former types of stimuli to acquire their emotional significance. We still do not know the exact limits of the former group, that of the naturally prescribed causes of emotion. Clearly, certain types of objects, because of their size, their movement, or because of the sounds they generate, induce emotions, not only in humans but in other species; fear is an example. Certain visual patterns, as, for instance, those expressed in the human face or in human body postures, also signify and can even induce emotions, and so can certain relationships among objects in certain situations; again, fear would be an example. Situations that result in certain profiles of internal conflict also give rise to specific emotions—jealousy and guilt, for instance. All of the inducers enumerated so far cause a wide range of emotions. They include the "universal" or "primary" emotions (e.g., happiness, sadness, fear, anger, surprise, disgust), as well as "social" or "secondary" emotions (e.g., jealousy, embarrassment, guilt, pride). But almost any neutral stimulus that may be associated in a powerful learning situation with any of these natural causes or the ensuing emotions can be turned into an effective inducer. Sooner or later, in any of us, almost anything can cause some emotional reaction and does. Emotions are that pervasive.

The pervasiveness of emotions would be remarkable if only the "natural" and "acquired" inducers caused them. I submit, however, that what we call emotions and moods are not only caused by these easily recognizable kinds of stimuli but are also caused by the process of regulating life itself. Certain conditions of internal state, engendered by the ongoing processes of maintaining homeostasis and by the organism's interactions with the environment that are pertinent to homeostatic regulation, induce collections of responses that are formally comparable to the conventional emotions we have been considering. I call them "background" emotions. The critical differences between the conventional emotions and background emotions lie with (1) the source of the inducer, which is usually external or representing the exterior in the case of conventional emotions, but tends to be internal in the case of background emotions, and (2) the target of the responses, whose balance is aimed at musculoskeletal and visceral sectors of the organism in the conventional emotions and at the internal milieu and viscera in "background" emotions. In short, independently of external stimuli whose representations, in the form of sensory patterns, can serve as inducers, certain states of the internal milieu and of viscera continuously induce changes that also define an emotional profile. Those changes can be traced back to the ongoing processes of homeostatic regulation, which are, in turn, consequent to a variety of antecedent events—namely, prior emotions and cognitive states. On the basis of background emotions, we feel tension or the release of tension, a sense of fatigue or of energy, a sense of well-being or of illness, and so on. A good part of the conditions we identify as moods are based on sustained background emotions, which become continuous over relatively long periods of time rather than occurring in discrete waves. These background emotional states give rise to background feelings that are the corresponding experience we have of them (see Damasio, 1994, 1999).

In conclusion, deciding what constitutes an emotion is not an easy task. Once you survey the whole range of complexity from background emotions to secondary emotions and include phenomena as diverse as well-being, on the one hand, and pride or embarrassment, on the other, one wonders if any sensible core definition of emotion can be maintained, and if a single term remains useful to describe all these states. My impression is that, for the time being, a shared core underlies all these phenomena. They all have some kind of regulatory role to play, leading in one way or another to the creation of circumstances advantageous to the organism exhibiting the phenomenon. The devices that produce all of these phenomena are preset by the genome, and they can all be engaged automatically, without conscious deliberation. The pattern of each phenomenon is fairly stereotyped in that it contains largely the same set of responses executed in largely the same manner. The considerable amount of individual variation, and the fact that culture plays a role in the shaping of some inducers of the emotions, does not deny their fundamental stereotypicity, automaticity, and regulatory purpose.

I have no problem, therefore, in lumping all of these phenomena together provided their varied complexity is acknowledged and provided one keeps an open mind for future rearrangements of the classification that new evidence may dictate. Nor do I have a problem with the use of the single word "emotion" provided we are open to possible new terms, dictated again by new evidence. In the meantime, the critical issue is to separate that which is stereotypical, automated, and directly regulatory, an emotion, from the sensing of such proceedings, the feeling of an emotion.

The Covert Nature of the Mechanisms for Inducing Emotions

Whatever the inducer, emotions are triggered by mechanisms we are not aware of and that we cannot control willfully. We can control, in part, the expression of some emotions, but most of us are not very good at it, and the result is that at any moment emotions are a fairly good index of how conducive the environment is to one's well-being. The nonconscious triggering of emotions also explains why they are not easy to mimic voluntarily.

Much of the notable debate regarding the automated or deliberated nature of emotions is difficult to follow in this perspective. Most stimuli capable of causing an emotion do so without any conscious evaluation on the part of the subject having the emotion. Processing is quite direct, from the sensory map in which the stimulus is represented (e.g., visual cortex), to the brain structure that initiates the response (e.g., the amygdala). The response is fast, but there is no "evaluation" to speak of, in the sense of a conscious and deliberated appraisal. Needless to say, the inducing stimulus is processed through a variety of neural stations, but one wonders about the wisdom of calling such processing an evaluation. True enough, certain stimuli can trigger a process of intellectual analysis in the course of which one or more particular images will come to be the inducer for an emotional response in the same automated and nonconscious manner described above. In those instances, it is perhaps more reasonable to talk about an evaluation, but even so the ultimate inducer operates as described for the nonconscious case.

I must add that by no means am I degrading emotions when I separate them from feeling and consciousness. I am simply isolating steps of a functional continuum with the aim of making the entire biological process more amenable to investigation. The full human impact of the emotions is only realized when they are sensed, when they become feelings, and when those feelings themselves are *felt*, that is, when they become known, with the assistance of consciousness. These distinctions in no way diminish the basic value of emotions (see Damasio, 1999 for a discussion on the consciousness of feelings).

The Substrate for the Representation of Emotion

There is nothing mysterious about the collection of responses I have just described, nothing vague, nothing elusive, nothing nonspecific. One can argue about the verbal labels attributed to emotional states and about the boundaries between the categories of state denoted by those labels. One can even argue about whether the term "emotion" is worth keeping. Leslie Brothers (1997) and Paul Griffiths (1997) are among those who have raised such questions, and I applaud those efforts, although I believe that the term "emotion" and the current classification can be used in a qualified manner, without much harm, as we gather additional empirical evidence and develop new theoretical frameworks. But those are different matters from considering emotions as elusive, or vague, let alone nonspecific.

The substrate for the representation of emotions is a collection of neural dispositions in a set of brain regions located in brainstem, hypothalamus, basal forebrain, amygdala, ventromedial prefrontal cortex, and cingulate cortex (see Damasio, 1994, 1999). The status of those representations is dispositional, implicit, or dormant—that is, not represented directly in consciousness. The neural basis for those representations is a collection of neural records within the neuron ensembles I designate as convergence zones (Damasio, 1989a,b; Damasio & Damasio, 1994). Once those dormant records are activated, however, they generate explicit responses that modify other neural regions (for instance, by creating a specific, explicit sensory pattern in somatosensory cortices or initiating certain behaviors) and also modify the body proper (for instance, by altering the state of viscera and internal milieu via the autonomic nervous system and the endocrine system).

Emotions are curious adaptations that are part and parcel of the machinery with which organisms regulate survival. Old as emotions are in evolution, they are a high-level component of the mechanisms of life regulation, interposed between the basic survival kit and the devices of high reason, but very much a part of the continuous loop of life regulation. For less complicated species than humans, and for absent-minded humans as well, emotions produce quite reasonable behaviors from the point of view of survival.

Emotions are always related to homeostatic regulation, always related to the processes of promoting the maintenance of life, and always poised to avoid the loss of integrity that is a harbinger of death or death itself. The emotions are inseparable from the states of pleasure or pain, from the idea of good and evil, of advantageous or disadvantageous consequences of an action, and of reward or punishment for an action.

The Substrate for the Representation of Feelings

Feelings, the feelings of emotions, that is, are the mental states that arise from the neural representation of the collection of responses that constitute an emotion within the brain structures appropriate for such a representation. The emotional states are defined by changes occurring in the chemical landscape of the body, by myriad changes occurring in viscera and in the striated muscles of the face, throat, trunk, and limbs, and by changes in the mode of processing within the brain of the many neural circuits that support cognition. What I call a feeling is the mental image we form of many, most, or even all of those changes, following swiftly on the heels of their occurrence in body and in brain. In the case of humans, feeling an emotion requires a twofold process of mental imaging: (1) imaging the kind of alterations that occur in the body proper, and (2) imaging the parallel and related alterations that occur in the mode of neural processing as expressed in certain characteristics of mental processing (e.g., speed of image generation, focus of attention). Just as a human emotion is a global change in the organism, in body and brain, a human feeling is a composite image of that global change in body and brain (Damasio, 1994, 1999).

Just as there is nothing vague, elusive, or nonspecific about emotional responses, there is nothing vague, elusive, or nonspecific about the representation of feelings. I submit that feelings have a concrete neural representation in the form of changed sensory maps in two sets of structures. The first set includes those that represent varied aspects of the body proper: the key structures are located in several nuclei of the brain stem, in the hypothalamus, in the thalamus, in the cingulate cortex, and in the somatosensory cortices of the insula and postrolandic region (SII and SI). The second set of structures, mainly located in prefrontal cortex, monitor the ongoing mode of cognitive processing. This is altered during an emotion via a host of neurotransmitter changes that originate in monoamine and acetylcholine nuclei of brainstem and basal forebrain, but target the neural circuits of the telencephalon—namely, those in the cerebral cortex. Thus, both classes of changes in organismal state that are caused by an emotional response, those in the body proper and those in the brain's own processing mode, can be mapped at several levels of the neuraxis as they occur.

It is essential to note that the substrate of feeling, the neural patterns that represent the emotional changes in body and brain, is sufficient to permit feeling to occur as a mental image, but does not allow a feeling to become conscious. In other words, I believe we can separate *having* feelings from *knowing* we have feelings. Feelings only become known when they are made conscious. The critical sequence then is (1) induction of emotion, (2) ensuing organism changes in body and brain, (3) neural patterns representing the organism changes, (4) sensing of the neural pattern in the form of images (feeling), and (5) feeling of feeling (which is part of the consciousness process).

I have argued that the collection of sensory mappings that constitute the substrate of a feeling can be achieved by a variety of mechanisms. One mechanism is entirely confined to brain structures (i.e., to the central nervous system). That mechanism is engaged, for instance, when emotion-inducing structures such as the amygdala activate, directly or indirectly, brainstem structures that cause changes in cognitive processing, that induce specific behaviors (e.g., bonding, play), or that alter the means of processing body signals.

Another mechanism involves what I have called the "body-loop," whereby through both humoral and neural routes the body landscape is changed and is subsequently represented in somatosensory structures. This latter mechanism can also be achieved by an alternate route which I have called "as-if-body loop," whereby body-related changes are enacted directly in somatosensory maps under the control of neural sites such as the prefrontal cortices. The "as-if-body-loop" mechanism bypasses the body proper.

The mechanisms I have just outlined are plausible, and a substantial part of the neuroanatomy necessary for their implementation has already been described. Evidence from experimental neuropsychology, neurophysiology, and functional neuroimaging also support their existence. The additional mechanisms I have added are a complement to the idea that feeling is a reflection of body-state changes, which is William James's seminal contribution. I must note, however, that I have not developed the idea for these additional mechanisms as a means to circumvent the classical attacks on William James's idea. In fact, as far as I can see, the anti-James evidence does not stand up to modern scrutiny. I am thinking, specifically, of evidence concerning the results of spinal cord transection in experimental animals or in natural human lesions, and of evidence from the use of peripheral adrenaline injections in normal human subjects. The evidence from such studies turns out to be irrelevant when a modern layout of the neuroanatomy and neurophysiology of emotion and feeling is carefully considered. For example, a substantial part of signals concerning the viscera and internal milieu is not transmitted through the spinal cord and is available directly to the brain stem; also, there is no reason to expect a selective action for adrenaline (a sympathetic neurotransmitter) injected in the peripheral circulation, considering that emotions are enacted by both the sympathetic and parasympathetic arms of the autonomic nervous system and that the autonomic effects related to each specific major emotion are caused by specific profiles of response originated centrally rather than by a general peripheral effect (see Damasio, 1999 for details).

We are far from solving all the questions connected to the neurobiology of emotion and feeling, although some remarkable progress is being made. That progress may be helped if some of the issues considered in this chapter receive attention in the near future.

References

Adolphs, R., Tranel, D., Damasio, H. & Damasio, A. R. (1995). Fear and the human amygdala. *Journal of Neuroscience, 15*, 5879–5892.

Brothers, L. (1997). *Friday's Footprint: How Society Shapes the Human Mind.* New York: Oxford University Press.

Damasio, A. R. (1989a). The brain binds entities and events by multiregional activation from convergence zones, *Neural Computation, 1*, 123–32.

Damasio, A. R. (1989b). Time-locked multiregional retroactivation: a systems level proposal for the neural substrates of recall and recognition. *Cognition, 33*, 25–62.

Damasio, A. R. (1994). *Descartes' Error: Emotion, Reason, and the Human Brain.* New York: G. P. Putnam's Sons.

Damasio, A. R. (1995). Toward a neurobiology of emotion and feeling: operational concepts and hypotheses. *The Neuroscientist, 1*, 19–25.

Damasio, A. R. (1996). The somatic marker hypothesis and the possible functions of the prefrontal cortex. *Proceedings of the Royal Society of London, 351*, 1413–1420.

Damasio, A. R. (1999). *The Feeling of What Happens: Body and Emotion in the Making of Consciousness.* New York: Harcourt Brace.

Damasio, A. R. & Damasio, H. (1994). Cortical systems for retrieval of concrete knowledge: the convergence zone framework. In C. Koch (Ed), *Large-Scale Neuronal Theories of the Brain* (pp. 61–74). Cambridge, MA: MIT Press.

Davidson, R. J. (1993). Parsing affective space: perspectives from neuropsychology and psychophysiology. *Neuropsychology, 7*, 464–475.

Davis, M. (1992). The role of the amygdala in fear and anxiety. *Annual Review of Neuroscience, 15,* 353–375.

Edelman, G. M. (1992). *Bright Air, Brilliant Fire.* New York: Basic Books.

Ekman, P. (1992). Facial expressions of emotion: new findings, new questions. *Psychological Science, 3,* 34–38.

Griffiths, P. E. (1997). *What Emotions Really Are.* Chicago: University of Chicago Press.

LeDoux, J. (1996). *The Emotional Brain.* New York: Simon and Schuster.

Morris, J. S., Frith, C. D., Perrett, D. I., Rowland, D., Young, A. W., Calder, A. J. & Dolan, J. R. (1996). A differential neural response in the human amygdala to fearful and happy facial expressions. *Nature, 383,* 812–815.

Panksepp, J., Nelson, E., & Bekkedal, M. (1997). Brain systems for the mediation of social separation-distress and social-reward: Evolutionary antecedents and neuropeptide intermediaries. *Annals of the New York Academy of Sciences, 80,* 78–100.

3

Cognition in Emotion: Always, Sometimes, or Never?

GERALD L. CLORE AND ANDREW ORTONY

A not uncommon reaction to claims about the role of cognition in emotions is to agree with the proverbial farmer, who, when asked for directions to the city, replied "You can't get there from here." Certainly, emotions have many characteristics that seem to justify skepticism about any involvement of cognition in them. For example, the fact that we can be surprised by our own emotions suggests that we sometimes have little insight into them, and the fact that emotions occur automatically suggests that we have little control over them. We cannot, for instance, simply decide to feel an emotion the way we can decide to think about one. Furthermore, it is not unusual for people to report emotional reactions that conflict with cognitive ones. For example, in a vivid account of his struggle with anxiety and depression, one author (Solomon, 1998) recalls lying frozen in bed, crying because he was too frightened to take a shower while at the same time knowing full well that showers are not scary. One of our goals in this chapter is to examine the implications of such observations for the idea that emotions always involve cognitive appraisal processes; we argue that a cognitive account of emotion has implications that are both more fundamental and less restrictive than the skeptical view that emotions do not necessarily involve cognition seems to imply.

We take as our starting point the idea that an emotion is one of a large set of differentiated biologically based complex conditions that are about something. Emotions in humans are normally characterized by the presence of four major components: a cognitive component, a motivational–behavioral component, a somatic component, and a subjective–experiential component. The cognitive component is the representation of the emotional meaning or personal significance of some emotionally relevant aspect(s) of the person's perceived world. These representations may be conscious or nonconscious. The motivational-behavioral component is concerned with inclinations to act on the construals of the world that these representations represent, and with their relation to what is actually done. The somatic component involves the activation of the autonomic and central nervous systems with their visceral and musculoskeletal effects. One feature of this component is changes in body-centered feelings (Damasio, 1994), but in addition a whole range of neurochemical and neuroanatomical processes are needed to make emotions possible. Finally, the subjective–experiential component is the total "subjective feeling" part of an emotion. We assume that this component is particularly elaborate in humans, that it frequently involves efforts to label the emotions, and that it typically involves an awareness of what is often an integrated whole of feelings, beliefs, desires, and bodily sensations. There is much more that we could say about what an emotion is, especially when we consider how these components interact and when we consider questions of the intensity and duration of emotions (e.g., Frijda et al., 1992). But this characterization is sufficient for our purposes here, and we suspect that most emotion theorists would not object too strongly to what we have proposed.

Not surprisingly, cognitive accounts of emotion, while certainly not denying the existence or importance of the other components, focus on the cognitive component—that is, on appraisal and appraisal processes. The central claim of such accounts is simply that emotions depend on the perceived meaning or significance of situations (Mandler, 1984), and indeed, "appraisal" simply refers to the assignment of value or emotional meaning. But, as we shall see, cognitive views need not be limited with respect to exactly how that appraisal is generated, and one of the two main themes of this chapter is that there are two fundamentally different ways in which this can happen.

Unlike sensory experiences, experiences of emotion do not represent physical features of the world, and there are no sensory receptors for emotional value. Hence, emotions require cognitive processes sufficient to generate or retrieve preferences (Zajonc, 1998) or evaluative meaning (Mandler, 1984). But no matter how modest the claim that emotions have cognitive constituents may be, it immediately confronts two problems. One concerns whether cognitive claims are testable—that is, whether they are conceptual (simply definitional) or empirical. The other has to do with how a cognitive view can handle instances in which affective feelings precede appraisals. We consider these preliminary questions before moving to our two main themes: the sources of appraisals and challenges to the cognitive view—challenges such as those posed by episodes or aspects of emotions that are unreasonable, unexpected, unconscious, uncontrollable, or linguistically inexpressible.

Definitional Issues

Some authors (e.g., Parkinson, 1997; Smedslund, 1991) have argued that the kinds of accounts of the cognitive constituents of emotions typically specified in appraisal theories are not testable. For example, in our work (Ortony et al., 1988), we characterized one emotion as "displeasure at the prospect of an undesirable event," arguing that a class of emotions that we call "fear emotions" has this appraisal as a constituent. It is true that our assertion that fear emotions arise by appraising a particular outcome as an undesirable possibility is an assumption as much as a hypothesis; if all the components of fear were present except that appraisal, we would be likely to say that it was not a proper example of fear. Yet, our claims about the eliciting conditions of fear are not vacuous. They relate to the ways we talk about emotions in everyday language, and they conform to people's experiences of emotions. Moreover, making appraisals conceptually necessary does not make the claim that emotions involve such appraisals any less consequential. Consider in this regard the concept "disease." Particular diseases are defined as conditions in which particular symptoms are caused by particular pathogens. There too, the symptoms without the relevant pathogen simply do not constitute a proper example of the disease. But the conceptual truth is still highly useful, in part because measures to alleviate the disease can target the pathogen that both defines and causes the disease. In a similar manner, measures to alleviate emotional distress can target the particular pattern of appraisal that constitutes that emotion.

We suggest that emotions are both (conceptually) defined by appraisals and (empirically) constituted by them. However, definitions of complex phenomena like emotions and black holes are subject to revision in light of new empirical data. For example, if one argued that blame was part of the definition of anger, but studies found no evidence of blame in what most people called anger, we would be wise to conclude that the definition was inadequate. The problem is that whereas the meanings of words can be specified in definitions, the same cannot be done with phenomena. The "meaning" of a phenomenon is given in theories and explanations, not definitions. If one grants these assertions, then a coherent approach to the tougher question about the meanings of terms that refer to complex phenomena becomes clearer. The meanings of terms that refer to phenomena such as emotions and black holes also cannot be given in definitions, except to say that the terms "emotions" and "black holes" refer to the phenomena encompassed by theories of emotions and black holes. This turns out to be acceptable because over time we engage in scientific negotiation (see, e.g., Boyd, 1993) about the boundaries of such phenomena (and hence the meanings of terms referring to them), and through this process the relative conceptual benefits of alternative accounts become elaborated.

The Emotion–Nonemotion Boundary

Definitional issues of the kind we have just discussed are particularly important if there really are cases of affective states that have no cognitive bases. For example, depression and chronic anxiety can presumably have purely biochemical causes, so that depressed and anxious feelings can occur without any cognitive appraisals. How does a cognitive view explain such instances? Must one assume that chronic anxiety is caused by constant thoughts about threat? Not necessarily; the claim that emotions have crucial cognitive constituents is not a claim about all affective feelings, but only a claim about emotions, and as we have demonstrated elsewhere (Clore et al., 1987; Ortony et al., 1987), not all affective states qualify as emotions.

In our definition of emotions, we noted that emotions are about something. By this we mean that they are affective (i.e., positively or negatively valenced) states that have objects (what philosophers call "intentional" states), which is why not every occurrence of an affective feeling constitutes an emotion. For example, to the extent that "fear" refers to an affective state directed toward a specific object, it qualifies as an emotion, and to the extent that "anxiety" refers to an affective state without an object, it does not qualify as an emotion. Thus, when one is afraid, the fear is crucially about something in particular, but when one feels anxious, the anxiety is not focally about anything in particular. From a biological perspective it may not matter whether a particular activation of the fear system is an emotion or a mood. But from a psychological perspective the distinction is of central importance because emotions have implications for coping that moods do not. Moods are simply feeling states, which can arise from completely physiological causes. Anxiety may feel like fear, but the information it conveys is not necessarily feedback about the current situation (Clore, 1994a).

It is important to realize, however, that moods and other objectless affective states can readily be transformed into emotions. The conversion of free-floating feelings of anxiety into an object-focused emotion of fear is illustrated by a story about a man whose obsessional concerns appear to have been driven by chronic feelings of anxiety. After the birth of his first child, this man was often concerned about his child's safety. He started worrying that when he got a little older his child might one day climb onto the garage roof, fall off the roof, and injure himself on a stone bench below. The man became so plagued by this threatening thought that he eventually hired workmen to break up the bench with sledge hammers and cart away the rubble.

Presumably, this man's free-floating feelings of anxiety guided him to his threat-filled interpretations of this and other ambiguous situations. But from a cognitive perspective, there is an important difference between the free-floating anxiety and his threat-filled perceptions, because whereas the new feelings generated by these perceptions may have been biologically indistinguishable from the free-floating anxiety that preceded them, the new feelings, having an object, both qualified as and functioned as emotions.

A specific explanation of how such preexisting affective feelings influence appraisal processes in this way is offered by the affect-as-information hypothesis (Clore, 1992; Schwarz & Clore, 1983, 1988, 1996). The hypothesis assumes that people tend to experience their affective feelings as reactions to whatever happens to be in focus at the time. As a result, chronic feelings that are present incidentally during judgment and decision making are likely to be experienced as feedback about the object of judgment or the decision alternative under consideration. This is illustrated in recent research that found that anxious feelings experienced during a risk estimation task increased the perceived likelihood of threatening events (Gasper & Clore, 1998). Hence, anxious persons may become afraid when their anxious feelings are taken as information that a threatening event is imminent.

Before leaving this topic, we note one problematic consequence of the process we have been discussing. Because they have objects, emotions motivate problem-focused coping. In the case of mildly anxious individuals, this may simply result in a tendency to worry and to display a careful personal style. But chronically anxious or depressed persons may vainly try to cope with an inexhaustible supply of plausible threats about which their feelings may seem to provide information. Moreover, failed efforts to exercise control over their affective outcomes may result in learned helplessness, a concept first used to explain the loss of motivation shown by laboratory animals that had learned they had no control over aversive experiences (Seligman & Maier, 1967). This line of research subsequently stimulated a large literature on the role of learned helplessness in causing depression (e.g., Alloy & Abrahamson, 1979). However, in this instance we are suggesting that depressed feelings may be a cause of learned helplessness and its consequent loss of coping motivation rather than solely a consequence of it.

In summary, we have argued that the definitions of terms referring to complex phenomena such as emotions inevitably implicate theories of the phenomena. Hence, in spite of criticisms to the contrary, the tenets of appraisal theories are empirical as well as definitional. We have also argued that it is not incumbent on cognitive theories of emotions to explain affective states that are not in fact emotions (see also Ortony et al., 1987). In particular, we do not need to worry about cases in which affective feelings precede cognitive appraisals. In agreement with previous treatments of emotion (e.g., Averill, 1980; Frijda, 1986), we take emotions to be affective states with objects. If one distinguishes emotions from other affective states in this way then, according to the affect-as-information hypothesis (Schwarz & Clore, 1983), the affective feelings from noncognitive sources can provide information for appraisal processes which result in genuine emotions.

Overview

The remainder of this chapter deals with how cognitive approaches can respond to challenges such as that emotions can surprise us, that they can conflict with our beliefs, be elicited by stimuli outside of awareness, and be outside of our control. To consider these questions, we shall start by briefly sketching our own account of cognition in emotion. We shall then discuss a class of cases in which emotions are reinstated rather than computed anew and discuss how these two forms of emotion generation relate to two kinds of categorization (prototype and theory based) and two forms of reasoning (associative and rule based). We then go on to show how the two routes to emotional appraisal may serve different behavioral functions (speed and flexibility). In spite of these differences, we shall demonstrate how, in the last analysis, cognition is always involved. This is true in cases of unconscious affect elicitation, which differs from conscious affect elicitation only insofar as the former is deprived of the episodic constraints on emotional meaning. It is also true for automated, conditioned, imitated, and reinstated emotions, all of which are simply manifestations of reinstated appraisals. We then discuss the often nonpropositional relation between appraisals on the one hand and motivation and behavior on the other, a relation which we think is representable linguistically as connotative meaning, before ending by summarizing our main points in 10 proposals about emotion elicitation. By way of preview, the 10 proposals are as follows:

1. Appraisals are constituents of, and therefore also necessary conditions for, emotions.
2. Emotions are affective states with objects.
3. There are two routes to emotional appraisal (reinstatement and computation).
4. These forms of appraisal parallel two kinds of categorization (prototype and theory based).
5. The two routes to emotional appraisal and the two kinds of categorization are governed by two forms of reasoning (associative and rule based).

6. The two routes to emotional appraisal or categorization may serve different behavioral functions (preparedness and flexibility).
7. The fact that some components of an emotion can be triggered before full awareness of its cause does not conflict with a cognitive view.
8. Unconscious and conscious affect elicitation differ only in the episodic constraints on emotional meaning.
9. Automated, conditioned, imitated, and reinstated emotions are all manifestations of reinstated appraisals.
10. The experiential and motivational/behavioral manifestations of appraisals, while difficult to describe in language, can be communicated through connotative meaning.

Two Routes to Appraisal

The Bottom-up Route: Situational Analysis

We start our discussion by describing the basic notion underlying appraisal theories of emotion, using our own account (Ortony et al., 1988) as the primary example. Recognizing that the terms "bottom-up" and "top-down" are relative, we can think of appraisal models as bottom-up models in the sense that the appraisals are built by assembling interpretations of data from the perceived world. According to such theories (e.g., Arnold, 1960; Lazarus, 1966; Mandler, 1984; Ortony et al., 1988; Roseman, 1984; Scherer, 1984; Smith & Ellsworth, 1985), people are continually appraising situations for personal relevance. This process involves an on-line computation of whether situations are or are likely to be good or bad for us, and, if so, in what way. For example, in a diary study of emotion that we conducted with Terence J. Turner several years ago, a young woman reported becoming angry when she learned that a friend of hers had been stealing and reselling books from a bookstore where he worked.

Analyzing that situation in terms of our model, we would say that the young woman experienced feelings of disapproval when she perceived her friend's behavior as violating an important standard. In addition, her description of the event made it clear that she was also displeased at the event because her goal of maintaining the friendship had been threatened. We would expect such perceptions to result in anger because our view is that angerlike emotions are elicited when disapproval of the action of a person (because of violated standards) is combined with being displeased at the outcome of that event (because of thwarted goals).

Our account postulates three kinds of value structures underlying perceptions of goodness and badness: goals, standards, and attitudes. Specifically, we have proposed that the outcomes of events are appraised in terms of their desirability as a function of whether they are seen as promoting or thwarting one's goals and desires. Standards, on the other hand, are relevant to appraisals of actions rather than events. Actions are appraised in terms of their praiseworthiness (or blameworthiness) depending on whether they exceed or fall short of moral, social, or behavioral standards and norms. Finally, attitudes (along with tastes) provide the basis for evaluating objects. Anything, when viewed as an object, may be experienced as appealing or unappealing, depending on whether its attributes are compatible or incompatible with one's taste and attitudes. The overall structural organization of these three sources of affect, their combinations, and the emotions based on them are illustrated in figure 3.1.

In this account, different sources of value give rise to different kinds of affective reactions. Thus, when goals are the source, one may feel pleased at outcomes that are appraised as desirable and displeased at outcomes that are appraised as undesirable. When standards are the source of value, affective reactions of approval or disapproval arise, depending on whether actions are appraised as praiseworthy or blameworthy. And when attitudes or tastes are the source of value, one likes objects (broadly construed) that are appealing and dislikes objects that are unappealing. Specific emotions are then differentiations of one or more of these three classes of affective reactions. The ways of being pleased or displeased about the outcome of events include emotions that we usually call joy, sadness, hope, fear,

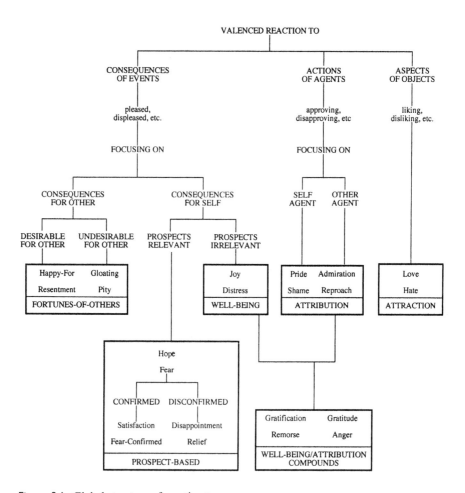

Figure 3.1. Global structure of emotion types.

disappointment, relief, gloating, and pity. Which specific emotion arises depends on whether the outcomes are past (joy, sadness) or prospective (hope, fear), and whether they concern one's own outcomes or those of another (gloating, pity). For example, a participant in one of our studies reported the goal-related emotions of fear and worry when his parents considered divorce. In this analysis, the need for security and the desire for maintaining his family would be treated as goals, threats to which, whether explicitly available to consciousness or not, produced fear.

In contrast, some emotions are based on standards rather than on goals. Pride, shame, admiration, and reproach are forms of affective reactions of approval and disapproval of someone's actions. The specific emotion depends on whether the action is one's own (pride, shame) or someone else's (admiration, reproach). For example, a different participant in our study reported the emotion of shame when he lost bladder control after drinking too much at a party. His shame is seen as a reaction to violating social standards of appropriate behavior in public.

Other emotions are based on attitudes or tastes. Emotions such as momentary (as opposed to dispositional) love, hate, and disgust are forms of the affective reactions of liking and disliking. The question of how tastes and preferences develop is a difficult one, but clearly even in this domain cognition plays a role. People's liking for food, for example, can be significantly affected by their beliefs about what it is they are eating. The sour pickle that might be so appealing with a hot dog can be quite disgusting if its taste appears when one is expecting strawberry ice cream. In other words, even something as rudimentary as whether or not we will react toward something with disgust can depend on our beliefs and expectations—paradigmatic examples of cognitions.[1] Finally, in addition to emotions based on goals, standards, or attitudes alone, some, like anger and gratitude, involve a joint focus on both goals and standards at the same time. For example, one's level of anger depends on how undesirable the outcomes of events are and how blameworthy the related actions are.

In any given situation the emotions experienced should vary as one's focus shifts among the outcomes, actions, and objects involved, so that the same event might make one feel many different emotions in a short space of time. Within this cognitive approach, each emotion type is characterized by a formal emotion specification. For example, emotions of the fear type involve being displeased at the prospect of an undesirable event. Emotions of the shame type involve disapproving of one's own blameworthy action, and emotions such as disgust involve disliking an unappealing object. The account gives such specifications for 22 common emotion types along with proposals for what cognitive variables influence the intensity of each type. For example, the perceived likelihood of an undesirable (or desirable) event is one of several cognitive variables that influences the intensity of fear (or hopefulness), whereas the degree to which one perceives oneself as having fallen short of normal expectations about one's achievements influences the intensity of shame emotions. Thus, for instance, basketball fans reported fear and concern when their team was trailing in the last five minutes of a game, whereas reports of embarrassment were saved for games in which the level of play failed to meet acceptable standards (Ortony, 1990).

It is interesting to note that this same kind of general analysis should hold for emotions in nonhuman species. It may not be unreasonable to apply such reasoning to the difference between the hang-dog expression of the family dog when he does not get to go in the car and his angry growl when someone reaches for the bone in his mouth. The former reflects a disappointmentlike state fueled by loss of an expected goal, whereas the latter appears to reflect violation of a canine standard of behavior to the effect that food (or anything else) in a dog's mouth is the rightful property of that animal, regardless of his position in the dominance hierarchy (Coren, 1994). However, as one descends the phylogenetic scale, there are limitations on the ability to interpret situations, limitations on the ability to make use of feedback from subjective experience, and limitations on the ability to respond in a flexible manner. At some point the emotion circuits simply activate fixed action patterns, and many of the cognitively mediated processes that make human emotion interesting are no longer present. Thus, although strong biological commonalities may justify the study of certain aspects of emotional processing in any mammal, it is surely not the case that all of the basic questions about emotions can be answered using animal models. For this reason, we think it is important that the scientific study of emotions not be too restricted in scope (as may happen if one investigates only emotion-related behaviors) or too restricted in range (as may happen if one investigates only the emotional reactions of lower animals). A proper account of emotions needs to do justice to the full richness and range of emotions that comprise human emotional life.

Finally, the claim that emotions have cognitive constituents does not mean that emotions are themselves cognitive events. In this regard, Reisenzein (1998) suggests that emotions are meta-cognitive or, as he says, "meta-representational." He proposes that emotion is not a reaction to a cognitive outcome of appraisal processes, but a noncognitive form of the appraisal. Rather than appraisals leading to beliefs about a situation, which then trigger emotions, the appraisals lead directly to both emotions and beliefs as alternative ways of representing the significance of the situation. Thus, emotions have cognitive constituents in the sense that appraisals are transformations of raw sensory input into psychological representations of emotional significance. However, the emotions are multifaceted, involving the simultaneous representation of emotional significance physiologically and experientially, as well as cognitively.

The Top-down Route: Appraisal Reinstatement

Not all situations seem amenable to the kind of bottom-up cognitive analysis we have just presented. Consider the case of a Vietnam veteran who reported being overcome by panic one day while working in a greenhouse. Apparently, the heat, humidity, and tropical foliage in the greenhouse triggered traumatic reactions he had felt during the war (H. Gorini, personal communication, 12 September, 1990). In such reactions, unremarkable fragments of a current experience vividly reactivate earlier experiences together with their emotional significance. The reactions surely feel strange and surprising when they first occur, and might therefore seem to provide a challenge to a cognitive account.

A similar challenge comes from experiments on emotion in which the experimental stimuli are inherently positive or negative for a given species—pictures of smiling or angry faces for human subjects, and rubber snakes for chimpanzees

(Öhman, this volume). How can a cognitive account of emotions of the sort outlined in the last section explain the efficacy of such emotionally preloaded elicitors? Surely, they require little if any cognitive analysis? They seem so different from cases in which an emotional value is computed on-line, cases that yield easily to a cognitive account. And indeed, they are different. In fact, they suggest a second source of emotional value, namely, reinstatements of prior appraisals from earlier situations, rather than the on-line appraisals of new situations in terms of current goals, standards, and attitudes. Both of these sources of emotional value were anticipated in Arnold's (1960) original treatment of appraisal, in which she proposed that new situations are often evaluated in terms of similar past experiences, as in the case of the veteran in the greenhouse.

Our response to such challenges is to show that emotions reflect cognitive appraisals with respect to the goals and concerns of the emoting individual, not only in straightforward examples of appraisal and emotion, but also in examples such as that of the fearful veteran. Fear is a reaction to appraisals of threat, and the fact that the veteran's appraisal of the greenhouse as a threat was unconscious, was pathetically mistaken, and was based on only superficial similarities to a past threat are not inconsistent with that presumption. It is still the case that a particular emotion arose when a situation took on a particular meaning. Whether emotions arise from similarity to a past situation or from a new analysis, our view is that what triggers emotion is activation of a deep structure of situational meaning. It is particular meanings that make situations occasions for anger, fear, shame, or grief. However, such meanings may arise in more than one way, and reinstatement is one of them.

- The Precedent for Reinstatement

Freud is perhaps the best example of a theorist concerned with how emotional meanings in everyday life can be traced to their origins in prior experience. He focused on how one traumatic situation can generate many subsequent instances of emotion through association, including poetic, metaphoric, and symbolic associations that are often apparent only in dreams, poetry, and humor. Though often impressing readers as bizarre, Freud's theory is interesting in the current context because it is the most thorough-going statement of a reinstatement model of emotion elicitation. Freud believed that specific emotions are rooted in pivotal traumatic situations in the experience of the child, including the birth trauma, the Oedipal situation, and so on. For example, while believing (like many after him) that anxiety is a reaction to being overwhelmed by stimuli, Freud felt the need to explain anxiety on the basis of some original experience of being overwhelmed. He concluded that, "The act of birth is the first experience of anxiety, and thus the source and prototype of the affect of anxiety" (Freud, 1900/1953).

Freud assumed that other early emotions also reoccur in analogous situations later in life. Reactions to a powerful father, for example, serve as a prototype for subsequent reactions to other authority figures. And early experiences of ambivalence toward parents and siblings were believed to transfer "to authorities, colleagues, subordinates, loved ones, friends, gods, demons, heroes, and scapegoats" (Smelser, 1998, p. 8). This theme of emotional reinstatement is also found in Freud's conception of moral emotions, with respect to which, he claimed, for example, that experiences of shame and modesty in women originate in the shame they experience as little girls when viewing their genitalia and realizing their inadequacy in comparison to the genitalia of their brothers!

Freud was obsessed with the idea that current situations could derive emotional power from symbolic connections with earlier events. For instance, falling in love—the most frequently mentioned emotion in our subjects' accounts—was for Freud a reinstatement of earlier attachments triggered by an unconscious association between the image of the parent and an exciting new person. And the jealousy, hostility, and ambivalence that sometimes emerge in loving relationships he viewed as evidence of poorly resolved conflicts with parents. Psychotherapy was intended to uncover such unconscious relationship conflicts in order to resolve them in a current relationship with a symbolic authority figure in the form of the analyst.

The idea that pivotal emotional reactions early in life form the basis of later emotions, especially in love and attachment, is also central to infant attachment theory (Bowlby, 1969). For example, Morgan and Shaver (in press, p. 1) claim that "it is impossible to understand commitments to romantic relationships unless one considers how the attachment system affects the process of falling in love and choosing a mate." They contrast cost–benefit models of relationships (Rusbult, 1980, 1983) with models based on attachment. Bowlby's theory posits an evolved tendency for infants to develop a strong bond or attachment to their primary caregiver, a bond that may be evident in vigorous emotional protests when children are separated from the caregiver.

Bowlby's ideas were amplified by Ainsworth (e.g., Ainsworth et al., 1978), who identified stable individual differences in patterns of infantile attachment. The three most studied of these are referred to as "secure," "avoidant," and "anxious." What is interesting from the current perspective is the idea that these individual differences in the emotions of attachment remain intact and are therefore ready to be reinstated in adult romantic attachments (for a review, see Shaver & Clark, 1994). The emotions associated with romantic involvement are seen as reinstated emotions occasioned by this reproduction of the original attachment situation.

The central point about the reinstatement view is not the obvious point that people learn from their prior experiences, but the idea that a current situation can bring back whole prior episodes rather than some generalization derived from them or abstract rule implicit in them. The idea is that there is a small number of pivotal, perhaps traumatic, events that serve as the reservoir from which all other affect flows—a view reminiscent of Sullivan's (1953) ideas and of Tomkins's (1979) concept of scripts. Like Freud, these reinstatement theorists anticipated the importance of a case-based approach to cognition, although their claims were less radical than Freud's.

• The Cognitive Nature of Reinstatement

We have proposed that emotions can arise through the reinstatement of prior emotional meaning, as when a current situation reminds one of (i.e., primes) a prior emotional situation, and that under certain circumstances one can be surprised by the emergence of such emotions. We believe, however, that this in no way alters the essentially cognitive nature of the eliciting conditions for the emotions so experienced. Many of the phenomena that might initially appear to challenge a cognitive account of emotion have no special relation to emotions at all. Rather, they are just general cognitive phenomena quite familiar to cognitive psychologists. In this section, we start by discussing two examples from the recent social cognition literature to substantiate this point. In both cases, innocuous manipulations lead to somewhat surprising outcomes, including in one case otherwise hidden evidence of racial prejudice, and in the other overt but unbidden behavior. These examples are intended to establish an important point—namely, that the fact that certain emotional effects may be surprising and their consequences subtle and complex is not evidence against the involvement of cognition. Such effects can be readily observed in nonemotional domains, where they clearly do have cognitive origins. Activated material, be it emotional or not, can be structurally complex and highly organized, so that accessing any part of a structurally complex representation (or schema) may have extensive implications.

Social psychological work on automaticity illustrates our point about surprisingness. Devine (1989) has shown that mere exposure to attitude objects can automatically elicit stereotypic beliefs, even in otherwise enlightened individuals. Devine reasoned that because individuals high and low in prejudice are equally knowledgeable about relevant cultural stereotypes, this knowledge may be automatically activated in anyone given the presence of a member (or some symbolic equivalent) of the stereotyped group. She proposed that individuals must engage in controlled processing to inhibit the use of the spontaneously activated prejudicial information, and that this is the case even for low-prejudiced individuals for whom the activated prejudicial information represents only part of their cultural knowledge and not their racial beliefs. In her experiments, she showed that when such racial concepts were subliminally activated so that no corrective processes were likely, high- and low-prejudiced individuals were equally likely to show their effects, a finding that would presumably be surprising to the low-prejudiced individuals.

The second point, that the results of automatically activating cognitive material can be complex as well as surprising, is clear from research reported by Bargh (1997). He showed that the subtle activation of complex cognitive structures can automatically elicit not only latent knowledge, but even overt behavior. In one such study, a stereotype of elderly people was activated by incidental exposure to such words as "Miami" and "bingo," and this activation of the old person schema was sufficient to cause subjects leaving the experiment to walk more slowly to the elevator, a finding that was also obtained in replications of the experiment. In a related experiment, subliminal exposure to the faces of individuals stereotyped as aggressive led subjects so exposed (but not others) to voice to the experimenter their complaints about difficulties in the experiment. From this line of research, it is apparent that even when unaware of the process, the material activated in memory by incoming stimuli can be extensive and complex and can produce surprising results, regardless of whether emotion is involved.

As these findings illustrate, the remarkable properties (e.g., apparently spontaneous genesis, surprisingness) that are sometimes attributed to the extracognitive nature of emotion are general characteristics of cognitive processing, albeit characteristics that are also capable of triggering the whole cascade of events that make up emotional states. Our view is that such seemingly insignificant cognitive events can have dramatic results because the elicitation of emotion is automatic when a particular configuration of activated meaning matches the eliciting conditions for a particular class of emotions (Lazarus, 1994). Because that content need not be in focal awareness, we can be surprised by our own emotions.

The fact that we can be blindsided by our emotions may make emotions seem beyond the reach of cognitive explanations, but the consequences of activating nonemotional material in memory can also be surprising. The surprise may be attributable to the structured nature of material in memory, to the involvement of procedural knowledge that is not represented as declarative knowledge, and to the fact that we may remain unaware of everything but the consequences of these processes. When a perception does have emotional implications, it may also trigger the whole range of processes involved in emotional states because the link between the perceptions that have emotional meaning and the elicitation of emotion is automatic. Although the link between appraisals and emotions may be unique to emotions, the cognitive processes that eventuate in appraisal are not. Furthermore, if cases of reinstated emotions are to be taken as serious evidence of the inadequacy of a cognitive view, it will be necessary to show that the emotional characteristics of the original situation do not have their origins in cognitive appraisals—a requirement that we suspect is, in the general case, impossible to satisfy.

Thus, although we acknowledge that there are two different ways in which emotions arise, we believe that emotions are the same regardless of which of those ways is involved in any particular case. It does not matter whether an individual case of fear or anger arises from on-line computations, from conditioning, from imitation of others, or from species-typical predispositions, fear is always a response to apparent threat and anger a response to apparent infringement. Although the same thoughts, feelings, and physiological activity do not occur in each instance of, for example, anger, our view is that all situations that trigger anger nevertheless involve general perceptions that all angry people share on all occasions of anger. Consistent with what Lazarus (1994) refers to as corelational themes, the constancy that makes a situation one of anger rather than one of fear or joy can be thought of as the deep structure of angry situations (Ketelaar & Clore, 1997). A deep structure can have many possible surface manifestations. What makes a situation one of anger is not the elicitation of angry feelings, thoughts, expressions, words, intonations, or actions, but the deep structure of angry meaning that gives these surface manifestations coherence. Particular emotions involve representations of particular kinds of psychological situations, and one of the central tasks of investigators of emotion is to characterize the structure of those psychological situations. Much progress has been made on this task by theorists including Frijda (1986), Oatley and Johnson-Laird (1987), Ortony et al. (1988), Roseman (1984), Scherer (1984), Smith and Ellsworth (1985), and Weiner (1985) (for a review, see Clore et al., 1994).

In summary, we have proposed that emotions necessarily reflect appraisals of the significance of situations, appraisals that can arise from two different processes, but we have argued that these two different routes to emotion reflect the nature of cognitive processes in general and thus are not unique to emotion. Other cognitive and perceptual processes also involve an interplay of new and old information, of bottom-up and top-down processes. At one end of this continuum are appraisals

TABLE 3.1. Dual Processes in Emotion Appraisal

	Bottom-up processes	Top-down processes
Routes to appraisal	Computed	Reinstated
Kinds of categorization	Theory based	Prototype based
Forms of reasoning	Rule based	Associative
Behavioral function	Flexibility	Preparedness

involving more computation and at the other end appraisals involving more rein-statement of previously learned significance. Table 3.1 summarizes some of the ways we elaborate this distinction in the sections that follow—for example, as kinds of theory-based or kinds of exemplar-based categorizations, which are governed by rule-based or by associative processes, and which may promote behavioral flexibility or behavioral preparedness. As table 3.1 shows, the same duality can be seen in both emotional and nonemotional processes, such as those relating to categorization and to modes of information processing, as well as those relating to adaptive behaviors. All of these dichotomies reflect a speed–accuracy trade-off, with the bottom-up processes generally slower but more accurate and the top-down ones generally faster but more error prone.

Related Dichotomies

Two Modes of Emotional Categorization

If we think of the process of emotion elicitation as involving the categorization of situations as emotionally significant, then the two routes to emotion elicitation we have discussed can be seen as equivalent to the two kinds of categorization prevalent in the cognitive literature: prototype-based (or case-based) categorization and theory-based categorization. Some emotion theorists (e.g., Fehr & Russell, 1984; Russell, 1991; Shaver et al., 1987) have maintained that, along with other concepts, emotions are best characterized as prototypes, rather than as classically defined concepts with necessary and sufficient conditions. In this view, instances are categorized on the basis of their similarity to a prototype or best example of a category (Rosch, 1973). Prototypes are held to consist of a collection of perceptually available features that tend to be found among exemplars of a category without regard to whether they are central or peripheral features. Categorization by prototype involves matching the features of potential exemplars to those of the prototype. For instance, our prototype of a grandmother might include features such as having gray hair, a kindly smile, and baking cookies. Because these are perceptually available features, they tend to be useful in helping us identify grandmothers.

Prototype-based views of categorization are in sharp contrast to theory-based views, which focuses on underlying aspects of the object, rather than on perceptually available features. Thus, in the grandmother example, the issue for theory-based approaches to categorization is not what the person *looks* like, but rather whether she is a mother of a parent, because that defines the category "grandmother." One might imagine two people searching for grandmothers, one who looks for a woman with white hair and the other who asks if anyone in the group is a mother of a parent. It is important to note that both people share the same underlying meaning of "grandmother." However, one is looking for someone who seems like a grandmother, that is, who has perceptually available features that are associated with being a grandmother, whereas the other is looking for someone who has the defining features of grandmothers. In general, the former method is faster and easier, but error prone; the latter is slower and harder to assess, but provides greater certainty.

Similarly, in the realm of emotions, people may become, for example, afraid in situations that share perceptually available features with past situations that frightened them. In such instances, they might be told, "You are just being emotional," thereby intimating that they are basing their categorization simply on the fact that a current situation reminds them of a former negative situation—that is, on how it seems, rather than on an objective analysis of the potential for harm.

We have suggested elsewhere (Clore & Ortony, 1991) that it is necessary to view emotion concepts as involving theories as well as prototypes. That is, even in the absence of shared surface features, things can be categorized together when they are believed to share deeper properties (Medin & Ortony, 1989). We proposed combining aspects of prototypes (that category membership can often be determined by similarity to a prototype or typical example) with aspects of a theory-based approach (that members of a category may also share properties that are not perceptually available). Both aspects may be useful because each serves a different information-processing function: identification and classification on the one hand, and reasoning and explanation on the other. Without a theory-based concept, people would never understand why their prototypes had the particular properties they did or how a deviant exemplar could still be in the category. But with only a theory-based concept, one might be good at reasoning but not very fast at recognizing category members because the essential features are not necessarily observable. We expressed this previously (Clore & Ortony, 1991, p. 49) by saying: "Similarity to the prototype provides a good, fast, and efficient heuristic for the identification, classification, and recognition of instances. But we also think that the prototype is of little value for reasoning and explanation. This is best accomplished by the theory-laden component of a concept, which, incidentally, can also be used as a back-up for the similarity-to-the-prototype heuristic in cases where it fails."

Two Kinds of Processing

The two kinds of emotion generation that we have discussed, as well as the two kinds of emotion categorization, are also consistent with a third cognitive processing distinction—namely, that between associative processing and rule-based processing (Sloman, 1996). In associative processing, objects are organized according to subjective similarity and temporal contiguity in experience. In rule-based processing, reasoning operates on symbolic structures. Everyday categorization appears to involve the use of both subjective similarities and rule-based reasoning. So even though young children use similarity as the basis for early categorization, they quickly come to rely on their knowledge about the unseen internal structure of things as their criteria for categorizing them (Keil, 1989). By the same token, even college students sometimes use superficial similarity as a basis for categorization (e.g., Ross, 1987). Hence, routine cognition seems to involve both associative and rule-based reasoning processes.

We concur with Smith et al. (1996), who propose that these forms of reasoning also underlie the two kinds of emotion elicitation with which this chapter is concerned. Reinstating previous emotional meanings uses similarity as a basis for emotion categorization, whereas computing new emotional values uses reasoning by rule to accomplish theory-based categorization. At this point, however, it is important to emphasize that rule-based reasoning is not necessarily conscious, explicit, or deliberative. Such reasoning can be utterly implicit, as evidenced by the fact that it can be demonstrated even in preverbal infants (e.g., Kotovsky & Baillargeon, 1994; Needham & Baillargeon, 1993).

Associative and rule-based processing can both proceed in parallel and give rise to different, even conflicting, results. We cited one such example at the outset of this chapter—the plight of the anxious and depressed person who was afraid to take a shower (associative), even as he realized that showers are not, in fact, scary (rule-based). We have also produced such a phenomenon in the laboratory. In one experiment (Weber & Clore, 1987), participants were either in an anxiety-induction group or in one of several control groups. On a series of gambles, those who had been made to feel anxious were significantly more likely to choose alternatives promising certainty and to avoid bets involving risk, even though the risky bets had clearly superior expected values. Even when they believed they would win the bets, they remained more risk averse. That is, even when rule-based reasoning suggested taking the bets, the associative reasoning dictated avoidance of risk. Despite the fact that they knew rationally that the bets were advantageous, from an experiential standpoint (because they had undergone an experimental anxiety induction) the bets felt too risky. Thus, they felt uneasy even though they knew there was nothing to fear. This experiment was conducted in the context of the affect-as-information hypothesis (Schwarz & Clore, 1983), and showed that information from feelings may be more compelling than the information from knowing (see also Bechara et al., 1994).

This same kind of conflict can occur without extraneous mood induction. A situation may be categorized as a threat either because it reminds one of a prior situation that was threatening or because a rule-based analysis shows it to involve risk. In the former instance, one need not rationally believe that the event will bring harm. But if one is reminded of a past bad outcome, then a mental representation of that bad outcome comes to mind. Because the triggers for emotions are mental representations of outcomes (rather than actual outcomes), being reminded may be sufficient to elicit an emotion, so that one can feel afraid even when one knows better.

In summary, we have proposed that a situation may elicit emotions either by reinstatement or by being perceived directly as having personal implications. In either case, the situation must be seen as having significance for one's goals, standards, or tastes/attitudes. However, that categorization may be made by case-based reasoning on the basis of similarity to a prior instance or prototype or it may be made by rule-based reasoning. In either case an emotion is automatically triggered when its eliciting conditions are satisfied. We now consider how these two processes are related to the principal behavioral functions of emotion.

Two Functions of Emotion

Two of the functions commonly attributed to (especially negative) emotions are preparation for rapid action (Toates, 1987) and flexibility of action (Scherer, 1984). But these are strange bed fellows because, while preparation is valuable for acting quickly, flexibility may often require refraining from acting quickly.

Evolutionary psychology suggests that we have innate emotion circuits that reflect the survival situations confronted by early humans during the hunter-gatherer period tens of thousands of years ago. Perhaps fear was elicited by the growls of predatory dogs or the sight of slithering snakes, anger by having someone take one's food or threaten one's kin, loneliness by being separated from one's siblings and family, sadness by losing one's mate, and so on. In this long epoch of human prehistory, individuals who responded to these recurrent situations with particular inclinations and feelings may have survived and passed on those tendencies.

To uncover the automatic and primordial aspects of emotion, many recent studies have presented affective stimuli subliminally because aspects of emotional reactions can sometimes be triggered when the individual is unaware of having seen the eliciting stimulus and before any emotional feelings are experienced (e.g., LeDoux, 1996, this volume; Öhman, this volume). Presumably, these processes prepare the organism for action and are crucial in emergencies. Set patterns of response can be prepared, ready to engage as soon as cortical processes confirm the stimulus identification. In mammals, when sensory patterns match some stored template for a threat stimulus, cardiac activity and some other autonomic nervous system processes may increase. The amount of this change may depend on the threat value of the stimulus and on how suddenly it appears. For example, in rabbits, if the threat is sufficiently strong, blood may flow to the large muscles in preparation for running away. However, although the rabbit is prepared for escape, its behavior also has some flexibility; rabbits sometimes freeze and sometimes run. Which behavior occurs apparently depends on the magnitude of the threat as indexed by the intensity of fear (Panksepp, 1998). Presumably, it makes sense for rabbits to freeze when a predator is at a distance, but as the predator gets closer, freezing becomes less advantageous. Thus, overall, the rabbit benefits from a system that triggers preparedness to run but that does not commit it to running.

On a continuum from rigidity to flexibility of response to their environment, creatures that have emotions are clearly both more complex and capable of greater flexibility. And mental health, too, is characterized by flexibility as opposed to rigidity of response (Leary, 1957). Moths that spend summer evenings banging their heads against light bulbs do not enjoy much flexibility. Higher animals, on the other hand, have emotions instead of tropisms. Humans can have very flexible reactions in emotional situations, sometimes expressing emotions directly, sometimes indirectly, and sometimes not at all.

We are suggesting that some evolutionary advantage may accrue to creatures for which emotion allows flexibility of response, in addition to automatic preparation for responding. According to Scherer (1984), the great evolutionary advantage of emotion was to allow a stimulus to be registered and reacted to without committing the organism to an overt behavior. Such protocognitive processes allowed behavior to be contingent on a stimulus, but not dictated by it. It is easy to see that it might be adaptive for emotion to facilitate a readiness to respond without committing the organism to actually doing so. Thus, it seems likely that the direct outcomes of emotion are bodily and cognitive manifestations of the significance of a stimulus, rather than behaviors themselves, even though preparation for behavior also has adaptive value. Thus there seem to be two fingers on the emotional trigger: one controlled by early perceptual processes that identify stimuli with emotional value and activate preparation for action, and a second controlled by cognitive processes that verify the stimulus, situate it in its context, and appraise its value.

Presumably, the goal of being prepared benefits from speed of processing, whereas the goal of flexibility benefits from awareness rather than from speed. We think it is no accident that the increased capacity for flexibility appears to parallel an expanded capacity for subjective experience. The subjective experience of emotion registers the urgency of a situation, provides information, and allows processing priorities to be revised. Thus, humans can entertain alternative courses of action and sample how they would feel about different outcomes, but, of course, in order to do this, they must be aware of the stimulus that occasions the processing. Much neuroscientific and cognitive research suggests that the conscious awareness of stimuli changes the process, so considerable attention has been devoted to subliminal presentations and "precognitive" emotion-related processes. The results of this line of research raise the question of whether a cognitive analysis of emotion is applicable to affective stimuli that are "precognitive" or of which we are otherwise unaware.

The Challenge of Unconscious Processes

We have already seen that some of the phenomena to which critics of cognitive accounts appeal have nothing in particular to do with emotions. In this section, we further substantiate this claim by reviewing a range of phenomena, including subliminal priming and supraliminal priming, mood and judgment effects, and the effects of trauma, with respect to their relation to conscious awareness. Our basic claim here is that the possibility of being unaware of the source of one's feelings in no way conflicts with a cognitive view of emotion elicitation. To be sure, reinstated emotions may appear to by-pass cognition, but we propose that it is simply the lack of salience of the source that makes emotions so elicited sometimes appear to be irrational and maladaptive. Likewise, the fact that emotional reactions can occur automatically and that they often seem outside of our control and beyond the reach of intentional reappraisal also seems to challenge a cognitive view of emotion. However, these facts, too, have no bearing on the cognitive view. Regardless of how appraisals are made or of people's insight into or control over the process, an emotion is elicited when one's perception of a situation matches the deep structure of situational meaning that defines that emotion. This correspondence is not affected or revealed by lack of conscious access to the elements that compose it.

Precognitive Effects

LeDoux's experiments (see LeDoux, 1996) on the role of the amygdala in the acquisition of automatic fear-related and avoidance-related phenomena in rats have become a touchstone for investigators who approach the study of emotions from the perspective of neuroscience. LeDoux's findings, as well as those of Öhman (1986, this volume), suggest not only that one need not be aware of the cause of one's emotions, but that the emotions themselves, including their behavioral consequences, may sometimes be triggered before consciousness comes into play.[2] According to this view, encountering a snake in the woods might activate avoidance behavior before one either feels fear or is even consciously aware of the snake. The explanation is that the sensory thalamus detects something with the form or movement of a snake and that this information reaches the amygdala directly a few milliseconds before it can arrive via the cortex. This direct route allows avoidance behavior to be activated and ready if the tentative identification of the stimulus is confirmed. But does this mean that cognition is not involved? We think not.

First, we would argue that in examining only the earliest part of an emotion sequence, such studies are not in fact dealing with real, full blown emotions at all. If we accept the characterization of emotion as involving cognitive, behavioral, somatic, and experiential constituents, then fascinating and important as these findings are, their incompleteness renders them degenerate instances of emotions, or at the very least, nonrepresentative ones. What these studies do show is that the initiation of avoidance behavior in response to potentially aversive stimuli, behavior that might usually be attributed to the experience of fear, can occur before fear is felt. But at the same time, they remind us that avoidance behavior does not itself constitute fear.

Second, the cognitive claim is that emotions are reactions to (or representations of) the personal meaning and significance of situations, not that emotions originate in the cerebral cortex. When neuroscientists investigate precognitive processes in emotion elicitation, they are studying early processes that occur before the cortex is involved and hence before awareness is possible, but not before meaning or significance is detected. Thus the observation that some processing of emotional meaning can occur before a stimulus is processed in the cortex indicates that cognition can be precortical, but not that emotions occur without cognitive activity. From our perspective, the detection of significance is already a cognitive process; however archetypal the representation of a snake is when it is accessed through the direct, thalamic route, the fact remains that it still is some sort of a representation of a snake,[3] and this is sufficient to qualify the process as a cognitive one. Cognition has to do with the construction, maintenance, manipulation, and use of knowledge representations (Mandler, 1984), not with consciousness. Cognition and consciousness are orthogonal constructs, and as we shall shortly see, emotions can, without contradiction, involve cognition without awareness. What is critical for the cognitive view is simply that the trigger for the cascade of events that is emotion is a representation of the value and significance of a stimulus, not the stimulus itself. The task for a cognitive theory of emotion is to describe how that value or emotional meaning arises. Thus we conclude that the fact that emotions, or at least fear (Robinson, 1998), can be elicited without awareness does not conflict with a cognitive account of emotion.[4]

More on Priming Effects

In recent years, social psychologists have become captivated by the rediscovery of subliminal exposure effects. It is now apparent that even when stimuli are available for only a few milliseconds, there is often a measurable influence on the interpretation or speed of processing of the stimuli that follow (e.g., Bargh, 1997; Greenwald et al., 1996; Murphy & Zajonc, 1993; Öhman, 1986). In a typical subliminal paradigm (e.g., Bargh, 1997), a mildly positive or negative word is presented as a prime, and then a novel or neutral stimulus (e.g., a Chinese ideograph) appears immediately, blocking awareness of the prime. The result is that the primed evaluation adheres to the subsequent stimulus so that it is then rated more positively or negatively than it would otherwise have been. Even if the task does not concern evaluation (e.g., as in pronouncing words), participants are faster at processing target items when their evaluative meaning is congruent with that of the nonconscious prime.

In contrast to these effects of unconscious primes, several investigators (e.g., Bargh, 1997; Murphy & Zajonc, 1993) have reported that the influences of affective primes disappear when respondents are aware of them. Freud was similarly impressed by such phenomena. He observed that unconscious stimuli with emotional potential could have wide-ranging effects on dreams, symptoms, and behavior that could be neutralized simply by making conscious the unconscious origin of the influence. Indeed, the point of Freud's psychoanalysis was to give patients insight into the origins of their unconscious ideas and hence to take away the power of those ideas to have far-flung effects on other beliefs and emotions.

The comparison between affective primes presented consciously and unconsciously raises questions about how such dramatic differences in effect might be explained. The explanation that we find most appealing is that there is nothing "precognitive" involved in subliminal priming, and that the meanings of masked words are processed in a perfectly ordinary way. The only difference is that the visual mask, which ensures that the image is available for only a few milliseconds, interferes with the episodic knowledge of having seen the stimulus. But it does not interfere with the semantic knowledge of what was seen. As a result, the meaning is activated, but memory for how the meaning came to mind is blocked (see Bornstein, 1992, for a related analysis). Much of the particularity of meaning of any stimulus lies in the context of its appearance. Without context, only the most general aspects of meaning are activated. Indeed, the brevity with which the stimulus is available means that even simple qualifications of meaning, such as those provided by prefixes and suffixes, are lost (Draine, 1997).

We are suggesting that the only important difference between subliminal priming and ordinary processing is that in cases of subliminal priming the presence of the visual mask interferes with episodic processing. Interference in this way ensures that all of the constraints on the primed meaning usually provided by neighboring words and by the time, place, and context of the experience are missing. Thus, unconscious priming produces semantic activation without any contextual and episodic constraints and markers (Clore & Ketelaar, 1997).

This kind of analysis of the difference between subliminal priming and routine information processing is consistent with certain neuroanatomical considerations. For example, Jacobs and Nadel (1985) distinguish two types of learning systems, each realized within separate neuroanatomical structures. One of these, the locale system, is concerned with the episodic or contextual aspects of stimuli, while the other, the taxon system, is concerned with the meaning of the stimulus free of the constraints of context. According to O'Keefe and Nadel (1978, p. 100): "Concepts and categories, the look, feel, and the sound of things, the goodness and badness of objects: All of these are represented in the taxon systems . . . what is missing is the spatio-temporal context in which this knowledge was acquired . . . this [spatio-temporal context] is provided by the locale system where representations from the taxon systems are located within a structure providing such a context."

Jacobs and Nadel (1985) go on to argue that the hippocampus serves the kinds of functions they specify for the locale system. It serves a cognitive mapping function that allows environments previously experienced to be represented and recognized. They suggest that the phenomenon of infantile amnesia can be explained by the fact that, although a great deal of enduring learning takes place in infancy, there is typically no episodic memory of it because the hippocampus, which is required to situate things in time and space, is not yet developed. In cases of damage to the hippocampus, one gets stereotyped, repetitive, and persistent behavior that is not constrained by an appropriate context in memory (O'Keefe & Nadel, 1978). Jacobs and Nadel propose that under stress, the action of the hippocampus is suppressed, leading to a similar decontextualization of traumatic memories. They report that some phobias reemerge under prolonged stress. The early learning of a fear may then lose its context specificity and become thoroughly general, resulting in a phobic attack triggered by general stress-induced dampening of hippocampal function.

Applying Jacobs and Nadel's concepts to experiments on subliminal exposure, one might think of the backward-masking procedure in experiments involving subliminal exposure also as interfering with registration in the hippocampus of the episode of seeing the priming stimulus. The result would be processing of semantic information in the taxon system, but not of the episodic information in the locale system. In any case, a variety of lines of evidence converge on the conclusion that unconscious ideas are powerful not because of anything specifically to do with affect, but simply and solely because there are no episodic constraints on the subliminally primed semantic meaning. Moreover, as we shall see in a moment, this interpretation unifies a number of phenomena that might otherwise seem unrelated.

An interesting implication of our analysis is that whether a stimulus is presented subliminally or supraliminally is not really the issue. All that is important is whether the individual is able to fully parse the stream of information. And, indeed, similar priming effects are routinely found even when the priming stimuli are clearly available for conscious inspection. For example, Srull and Wyer (1979) developed a priming procedure in which participants form a series of sentences by circling three of four alternative words for each sentence. Depending on the nature of the alternative words, a general (taxon) level of meaning (e.g., of hostility) can be activated, without focusing the attention of participants on the specific (locale) information about the source of that meaning. Under these conditions, because the number of priming instances and their embeddedness in a meaningful task prevents the priming from standing out as a separate event, the same effects occur as in unconscious priming even though the primes are conscious.

In other studies (e.g., Martin et al., 1990) the source of the primed meaning is often made obvious, but subjects are distracted by a secondary task, so that they do not focus on the priming event. It is generally understood in this literature that priming effects can be found only when participants do not focus on the source (or locale) of the meaning activated in semantic (or taxon) memory. In subliminal exposure research, the backward mask ensures this same pattern by interfering with the registration of the episodic (or locale) information. Our point, then, is that the critical element in so-called unconscious processing is not whether a stimulus is shown rapidly, but simply whether participants can parse the stream of mental events into semantic (taxon) and episodic (locale) information. This a general feature of cognitive life, and therefore not one that is in any way special to emotion.

Finally, given our explanation of "precognitive" affective effects in terms of the cognitive mechanics of backward masking, it may be a mistake for theorists to claim that research on human judgment of the kind popularized by Zajonc and his colleagues and brain-based research of the kind described by LeDoux are mutually supporting. Our caution in this regard is that the human behavioral research conducted by Zajonc always involves backward masking of the priming stimuli and therefore is amenable to an exclusively cognitive interpretation of the kind given above—an interpretation that is in no way dependent on the distinction between the direct and indirect (cortical) route to the amygdala, which is the hallmark of LeDoux's work. From this we conclude that the LeDoux research is essentially irrelevant to Zajonc's findings. By parity of reasoning, the Zajonc results, while compatible with, are not directly relevant to, those of LeDoux. LeDoux neither proposes nor has he any reason to propose that the semantic (taxon) aspects of briefly exposed stimuli get into the brain but that the episodic (locale) aspects do not. But this is precisely what we propose as the explanation of the kind of results that Zajonc presents. Furthermore, the Zajonc studies (and for that matter, the Bargh studies) concern rapid stimulus exposures, whereas the LeDoux studies concern rapid response preparation. This is another reason for suspecting that the same analysis is unlikely to apply.

Misattribution Effects

The same basic phenomenon can be seen in studies of mood and judgment. Judgments of just about anything are more positive in good moods than in bad moods. According to the affect-as-information hypothesis (Schwarz & Clore, 1983), the information on which judgments and decisions are made routinely includes information provided by affective feelings. Bechara et al. (1994) have published dramatic data that suggest that choices (made in a card game) may be mediated by feedback-produced feelings before the formation of relevant beliefs can play a role.

And other results show that feelings from an irrelevant source can influence judgments even when varied independently of beliefs about the object of judgment (Clore et al., 1994). However, this phenomenon is dependent on not experiencing (i.e., not being consciously aware of) the affective feelings as relating to the other (irrelevant) source. When the default linkage or attribution to the target stimulus is eliminated, the effect of mood on judgment also disappears. This kind of pervasive influence of affective feelings on judgment is most easily observed when the source of affect is a mood because a distinguishing feature of moods is that any situational causes are not generally salient. Unlike emotions, which are generally focused on a causal object (as when one is angry *at* someone, or afraid *of* something), moods are relatively undifferentiated feeling states with less salient cognitive content (Clore, 1994b; Ortony & Clore, 1989). As a result, mood-based feelings are easily misattributed to whatever stimulus is being processed at the time. Hence, general moods (and moodlike conditions such as depression) are much more likely than are specific emotions to result in contamination of judgments and decisions. Our explanation for this phenomenon is the same as our explanation for the influence of unconsciously primed affective meaning. The feelings associated with moods can have runaway affective meaning because they are unconstrained by any episodic harness.

The same problem is also apparent in cases of trauma in which a traumatized person ruminates about, but does not communicate about, the traumatic event (Clore, 1994a). Refusing to talk to others about emotional events does not keep one from thinking about them, and refusing to think explicitly about an event does not keep representations of it from being activated in memory and having affective consequences (Wegner, 1994). Indeed, whether one either thinks about a traumatic event constantly or tries to avoid it completely, the accompanying emotional reactions can cease to belong to a specific time, place, and circumstance. When the experience is cognitively unconstrained (i.e., when it is no longer clearly tied to a specific object), it may color the judgment of any situation to which it might appear relevant. Similar processes are seen in avoidance conditioning in rats in which the context of the original conditioned stimulus–unconditioned stimulus (CS–UCS) pairing fades in memory over time. As a result, the animal's fear (which does not fade) becomes more and more general and less and less contained (Hendersen, 1978).

A time-honored solution to this kind of problem in humans is to communicate about one's feelings. Whether expressed to professionals, friends, strangers, or simply to oneself, as in a diary (e.g., Pennebaker, 1991), organizing one's thoughts about trauma for communication appears to situate the suffering person's representations of events. This process reigns-in what can otherwise seem like runaway implications for all aspects of the person's life.

In summary, we have argued in this section that there is substantial and diverse evidence showing that when we are unable to focus on or attend to the source of primed meaning, we tend to apply that meaning indiscriminately. Thus, unconscious exposure to emotional stimuli can have surprising effects because the backward-masking procedure interferes with the episodic constraints on affective meaning that are usually available in ordinary perception or in experiments in which participants are aware of the priming event. Other than this interference with recognition provided by the mask, the processing involved in subliminal exposure does not appear to involve any processes beyond those encountered in everyday instances of perception. Evidence for this assertion includes the fact that the same kind of indiscriminate application of activated concepts can be shown without subliminal exposure, including (1) injury- or stress-induced suppression of hippocampal processes, which code memories with respect to context, as in cases of phobia or post-traumatic stress disorder (Jacobs & Nadel, 1985), (2) backward masking, which has no effect on initial processing but which interferes with the registration of stimuli in memory and hence with their later recognition, (3) ordinary conscious priming situations in which primes appear as incidental information (e.g., Higgins et al., 1977; Srull & Wyer, 1979) or in which distractions interfere with episodic registration of the priming (Martin et al., 1990), (4) mood effects on judgment, in which the nonsalience of their source allows mood-based feelings to be misattributed (Schwarz & Clore, 1983), and (5) situations in which suppression of thoughts about traumatic events interferes with situating the memories in time and place. In addition, (6) comparable phenomena appear in cases of fear conditioning, when the context of the original CS–UCS pairing fades so that fear becomes more and more generally applied (Hendersen, 1978). We suggest that all of these show the action of decontextualized semantic and affective meaning unconstrained by episodic meaning rather than the action of precognitive processing. In other words, these phenomena simply reflect ordinary cognitive processes in which there is interference with the encoding of information about time, place, and context—interference that influences the ability of perceivers to parse their momentary experience. Thus, we propose that reinstated emotions only appear to be devoid of cognition to the extent that the emotional meaning of the original situation is brought to the new situation unconstrained by the distinctive episodic and contextual knowledge that makes one situation different from another.

The Challenge of Automatic and Inaccessible Processes

In a study by Lewicki (1985), some participants had a negative affective experience when they were criticized by a person with curly hair. Much later they had a chance to choose which of two seats to sit in, one opposite a curly-haired person and the other opposite a straight-haired person. Although they were not aware of why they did so, these individuals avoided the curly-haired person. Here we have another example of a phenomenon that might seem to imply that emotion can be elicited without cognitive antecedents—that fear can be elicited by a short-cut without the activation of some threat meaning. But again, we do not think that this is the right explanation. To see why, we begin by considering instances of classical conditioning.

Conditioning and Automaticity

Classical conditioning involves a process whereby the meaning of one stimulus, the conditioned stimulus, is altered so that it comes to stand for the meaning of another, the unconditioned stimulus. After association, the conditioned response may occur automatically when the conditioned stimulus is presented, just as before conditioning it had occurred automatically when the unconditioned stimulus was presented. In other words, the conditioned stimulus acquires the capacity to elicit a response because it comes to stand for (or acquires the meaning of) the unconditioned stimulus (Hebb, 1949). As such, the response is still triggered by the same meaning, it is just that a new stimulus activates that meaning. This is known as the S-S, as opposed to the S-R, analysis of classical conditioning. The same analysis applies to learning by imitation. For example, Mineka et al. (1984) showed that when avoidance of snakes is induced in rhesus monkeys by observational learning, it is not the behavior that is learned, but the fearful meaning of the stimulus, which is then responded to with defecation, fearful expressions, and other constituents of fear itself.

A similar analysis can be applied to reinstated emotion. When a current situation triggers an emotion previously experienced in a similar situation, we assume that it can do so only if some representation of the original situation is activated. If so, then even reinstated emotions are elicited by the relevant cognitive eliciting conditions. The only change is that mental representations of those eliciting conditions have been activated when a feature of the current situation reminds one of the emotional meaning of the earlier situation. It is not that the emotion has been elicited without the usual eliciting conditions, but simply that some feature of a current situation has activated a representation of a prior situation that had those eliciting conditions. Once the eliciting conditions are in place, the emotion should follow automatically, regardless of whether those conditions are computed anew or are reinstated from a prior situation. Note that the emotion has not become automated because emotions are always automatic (rather than volitional) responses to their cognitive eliciting conditions (Lazarus, 1994). What has become conditioned, or automated, is the emotional meaning of the current situation, not the response. As before, the response follows the meaning. Indeed, this is one of the fundamental points of this chapter—that emotion elicitation is a matter of meaning, not simply of responses, whether physiological or behavioral.

Presumably, individuals can be unaware of the basis of these associations and can therefore occasionally be blindsided by their own emotions. Though fascinating, such possibilities do not contradict this analysis. The fact that emotions can be reinstated, rather than resulting from new appraisals, is important only in that the more removed an emotion is from current cognitive activity, the harder it may be to understand and to regulate.

The advantage of automatic processing is presumably a savings in time and processing resources, so that one can benefit from learning and using saved material. When a process becomes automated, something is short-circuited or a shortcut is established. This is reasonable enough, but some elaboration of what this involves may be instructive with respect to its implications for the relation between appraisals and emotions. For example, when one programs a computer to make a macro, the macro takes the place of the individual key strokes only at the conscious, motor, or user level. Representations of the key strokes are still activated, and the work of each key stroke is still done step by step.

The same is true of such automated action as playing the piano. For a beginner, the playing of every note in a piece must be a conscious and deliberate act, and each symbol on the sheet music must be mentally translated into a note on the piano and a finger on the hand. But to an experienced pianist who has learned a piece well, little conscious, deliberate self-instruction is required, except perhaps using the music as a reminder of the notes to be played. Being an experienced pianist means that far fewer deliberate or conscious mental instructions are needed to play the piano, but the pianist's fingers must still play each note. Automatization does not mean that one no longer has to play the piano; it only means that one no longer has to think about it consciously and deliberately.

To make a related point about cognitive processes, Anderson (1982, 1987) uses the analogy of interpreted versus compiled computer programs. In knowledge compilation, declarative knowledge is built into domain-specific production rules so that it is no longer necessary to hold declarative knowledge in working memory, and sequences of these productions are collapsed into single productions. Automated processes are like compiled computer programs in the sense that the individual steps that once constituted them are no longer accessible. In the skill domain, once the knowledge is encoded procedurally rather than declaratively, it is no longer in working memory. The computations are still made, but they are automated, so that changes are not as easily made.

Even automated emotional sequences triggered by nonconscious stimuli still require that contact be made with the emotional meaning of the situation. In the case of anger, for example, contact must be made with thwarted goals and violated standards—the deep structure of angry meaning. Someone whose action was angering in the past might later elicit anger quickly and automatically. But this can happen, we suggest, only to the extent that the processing of surface features activates a representation of goal thwarting and standard violations. Like cached images in a computer, frequently accessed meanings that reoccur in intimate relationships may appear quickly because they are precomputed, preloaded, and waiting. However, those meanings must still be accessed for a representation of their emotional meaning in the form of emotional feelings to occur.

So, in the paradigmatic case, a nonconscious connection between a current situation and a past one can trigger an emotional reaction automatically. If it is triggered on the basis of similarity between peripheral (and possibly irrelevant) features of the two situations, it can be hard for the person to explain, and it may be impervious to rule-based reappraisal. To observers for whom the situation does not appear to justify emotion, the reaction may seem irrational. And because the connection between the preloaded features and the reaction may not be conscious, may not be situated in time and place, and may not be open to scrutiny, attempts at rational analysis may not be helpful.

In contrast, reactions elicited by more on-line or bottom-up computation of emotional significance can often be undone by reappraising the situation. For example, if one's feelings were hurt by insulting comments from a colleague, learning that the remarks were actually about someone else would change the interpretation of the situation and eliminate hurt feelings. The emotion would go away as soon as its cognitive basis went away. Indeed, one might laugh with relief. Bandura (1973) has given a persuasive account of anger and aggression that is essentially this view. He argued for a self-arousal view of anger in which the critical variable in maintaining or eliminating anger is whether the individual focuses on the angry meaning of the situation. Similarly, he argued against a catharsis view, suggesting that whether angry behavior eliminates anger depends not on whether one uses up or drains off a pool of aggressive energy, but on whether it decreases the activation of cognitive material conducive to anger.

But once automated or compiled, meaningful changes in the appraisal of the current situation may be difficult to make. Without affecting the command that triggers the particular chunk of programming, new information may have no impact on the generation of emotional meanings that are automated and appear as wholes. A similar problem arises when a person with a strong preestablished attitude encounters new information. An attitude may be formed by many affective events that are no longer accessible once the attitude is formed because the prior experience has been compiled into one affective reaction. Although new information might end up being stored along with the prior attitude, it may not change the attitude (Wilson & Lindsey, 1998). For this reason, psychotherapy often involves an attempt to uncover the triggering condition of emotions and to relearn or reprogram the cognitive construals that support self-defeating and problematic emotional interpretations. Some therapists argue that this can only be done as the person has new experiences that compete with or replace those that are problematic.

The inference we wish to make from this discussion is that although there may be two routes to emotion elicitation, they are just that—two routes to the same emotional meaning—and it is the activation of this meaning that elicits emotion. In that sense, emotion is always a result of appraisal, even when the appraisals are automated, nonconscious, or even erroneous categorizations. For example, fear arises in response to detected or presumed threats. The fear-inducing stimulus may be linked to threat innately, by early nonverbal experience, or by extended deliberation, but without some threat meaning being activated, there can be no fear, because that is what fear is, an experiential representation of threat.

We now consider one last fact about emotion that challenges a cognitive view, namely, the fact that people are notoriously inept at describing their feelings and at explaining why they feel as they do; people are often wrong about the causes of their feelings (Nisbett & Wilson, 1977). One might assume that if emotions have cognitive origins, people should surely know about their emotions. Does our inarticulateness about our feelings serve as evidence against a cognitive view of emotion?

Linguistic Inexpressibility

One of the perspectives on emotions that we have advanced is that they involve the simultaneous manifestation of appraisals in multiple systems. So, for example, the goodness or badness of something may be manifested experientially as positive and negative feelings, and cognitively as positive or negative beliefs. When one focuses on the noncognitive modes of appraisal manifestation (e.g., affective feelings; behavioral inclinations), it is easy to lose sight of the cognitive nature of the appraisal processes. In this section, we discuss briefly the relation between appraisals and the motivational/behavioral domain.

Many of the behavioral manifestations of appraisals are the learned but often automatic strategies we use for coping with the vicissitudes of daily life. For example, people often clench their fists when receiving an injection, or raise their voices to discourage dissent. But not all of the connections between appraisals and motivations and behaviors are learned. At a more basic level there is a fundamental innate appraisal–motivation linkage—namely, the one between positive stimuli and approach and between negative stimuli and avoidance. Indeed, Davidson (1992) has argued that positive and negative affect can be reduced to approach and avoidance tendencies. An interesting experiment by Cacioppo et al. (1993) demonstrated the basicness of this connection. These investigators showed that reaction times for engaging in muscular flexion (as in pulling something toward oneself) tend to be faster for positive stimuli. Conversely, reaction times for engaging in muscular extension (as in pushing something away from oneself) are faster for negative stimuli (see also Bargh, 1997; Solarz, 1960). Interestingly, there is evidence that the connection is between appraisal and motivation rather than between appraisal and behavior because variations on this procedure produce the opposite results when arm flexion can be interpreted as withdrawing one's hand from an object (rather than as pulling an object toward oneself), and when arm extension can be interpreted as reaching for the object (rather than as pushing an object away) (M. Brendl, personal communication, 20 October 1997). Hence, it is the situated meaning of flexion and extension that is critical; the affective appraisals are manifested in the motivational realm as the desired end states of approaching or avoiding stimuli, rather than simply as triggers for distance-modulating behaviors (muscular flexion or extension) (Neumann & Strack, 1998).

We have already seen that some of the potential challenges to the cognitive basis of emotions appear to result from the apparent independence of the different constituent facets of emotions, as though the affective right hand does not always know what the cognitive left hand is doing. Indeed, Wilson and Schooler (1991) have shown that attempts to think about our reasons for gut-level decisions sometimes reduce the quality of our final decisions—a state of affairs all too familiar to relative novices (of chess, for example) who often regret second-guessing their first instincts. Many of the examples on which we have focused involve this kind of asynchrony between the experiential and conceptual aspects, which is often why we can be surprised by our feelings.

However, this apparent asynchrony between the various systems does not mean that there is no communication between them. For example, the affect-as-information model (Schwarz & Clore, 1983) is concerned with the impact of feelings in the experiential domain on judgments in the cognitive domain, and as we are about to discuss, there is often communication not just between the experiential and cognitive domains, but also between these and the motivational and behavioral domains. In addition to the idea that affective appraisals may be directly manifested as the motivation to approach or avoid something, it seems highly plausible that good and bad feelings evolved in part as ways of motivating approach or avoidance (Frank, 1988). In a similar manner, research shows that positive and negative feelings can trigger distinctive styles of cognitive processing (for a review, see Clore et al., 1994). Specifically, there is a reliable association between positive moods and inclusive, integrative, category-level processing and between negative moods and piecemeal, analytic, and item-level processing.

Yet there remains one aspect of emotional life that may still seem problematic for a cognitive approach to emotion: the difficulty we often have in being able to describe our emotional feelings and inclinations in language. However, despite the fact that feelings are often held to be notoriously difficult to describe in words, language does provide a means for achieving the communication of affect through connotative meaning. The denotative meaning of words captures the physical and descriptive attributes of objects, attributes that may assist us in discriminating one object from another. But words (and more generally utterances and texts) also have connotative meaning, meaning which allows us to communicate emotional and other experiential aspects of our perceived worlds. If we consider connotative, and not merely denotative, meaning, we realize that the problem is not that it is difficult to communicate about emotions, but only that it is difficult to describe emotions in language. This difference is especially evident in literature, poetry, drama, and the everyday use of expletives. In all of these, emotional meaning is directly expressed by choosing words with appropriate connotative meanings so that one feels the communication as well as understanding it.

Osgood et al. (1957) took this notion slightly further, making a compelling case that all words in all languages have the same three fundamental dimensions of connotative meaning: evaluation (E), potency (P), and activity (A). Moreover, Osgood (1969) argued that these dimensions evolved into universal dimensions of meaning precisely because the representations of objects that they afforded gave form and direction to behavior. Osgood explained his idea by asking what the proverbial caveman would have needed to know when encountering a completely novel stimulus. He suggested that without necessarily knowing what the novel thing was, it would have been important to know quickly whether it was good or bad, whether it was strong or weak, and whether it was moving quickly or slowly. In this way, one could discriminate saber-toothed tigers from mosquitoes, and one's coping strategy could take form by virtue of being constrained by the connotative meaning of the situation.

We suggest that although the experiential and the motivational/behavioral aspects of emotions cannot easily be conveyed propositionally, they can still be represented linguistically through the connotative meaning of words. And conversely, feeling and acting are themselves ways of realizing aspects of meaning, but the aspects of meaning they can reflect are the connotative, not the denotative aspects. In other words, feelings are one of the ways in which we can represent the affective attributes of the psychological meaning of things; we can feel goodness–badness, strength–weakness, and activity–passivity. We resonate to the emotional and connotative meaning of situations by being moved ourselves. In that sense empathy is a good example of emotional communication. However, the dynamics of connotative meaning can involve more than simply experiencing the same feeling connoted by the words used. For example, something is connotatively bad to the extent that it makes us feel bad, but it may be connotatively strong to the extent that we feel comparatively weak. These connotative dynamics have been brilliantly and formally worked out for subject–verb–object sentences by Gollob (1974). Also, Heise (1979) has taken these formulations and shown (in ingenious mathematical and computer simulations) how the connotative meanings of social roles and social actions can be represented as complementary feelings that motivate the moment-to-moment changes in behavioral interactions between people. In any case, our main point here is that this experiential aspect of meaning, which is represented in the raw in music and in the prosody of speech, is also representable in language through connotative meaning.

In summary, in this section, we have attempted to show how a cognitive account can explain emotional phenomena despite the fact that they are often surprising, irrational, and uncontrollable, and that our inability to be descriptively articulate about our emotions is to some degree offset by the affective affordances of connotative meaning. We also discussed the virtues of the view first raised by Osgood (1969), and later elaborated by Gollob (1974), Heise (1979), and others (e.g., Foa & Foa, 1974; Leary, 1957; Sullivan, 1953; Wiggins, 1980) that evaluation and the other connotative dimensions of meaning can be made manifest through feelings and action. As such, they are most naturally represented in the knower as feelings rather than as linguistically expressible propositions. Successful communication and comprehension of connotative meaning (including emotional meaning) is marked by the occurrence of complementary feelings in the other, just as successful communication and comprehension of declarative knowledge is marked by the formation in the other of relevant beliefs and propositions.

Conclusion: Ten Proposals about Emotion Elicitation

We have proposed that there are two ways in which situations may be appraised as having emotional significance, and we suggested that these are based on different categorization processes supported by different processing principles that allow emotions to modulate different and sometimes conflicting adaptive goals. However, despite the fact that there are multiple ways for situations to acquire emotional significance, emotions are elicited in only one way as a manifestation of that significance. This aspect of our discussion was summarized in table 3.1, and leads us to the first 6 of 10 proposals about the nature of emotion elicitation.

The second major theme of this chapter has been the analysis of emotional phenomena that initially seem problematic for a cognitive account of emotion. These include the precortical elicitation of emotion components, subliminal affective priming, conditioned and automated emotional responses, and the apparent inexpressibility of emotional feelings. Our general response was to argue that emotions are usefully considered either as manifestations of appraisals of emotional significance or as ways of representing such appraisals. These arguments are summarized in our last four proposals, proposals 7–10.

Taken together, we think that the arguments we have presented provide a compelling answer to the question we set out to address in this chapter: When is cognition implicated in emotion? Always, sometimes, or never? Our answer, of course, is always.

Ten Proposals

1. *Appraisals are constituents of, and therefore also necessary conditions for, emotions.* Definitions of terms referring to complex phenomena such as emotion inevitably implicate theories of the phenomena. Hence, the tenets of appraisal theories are both conceptual and empirical. Just as particular pathogens both define and

cause particular diseases, so appraisals are constituents but also causes of emotions (although not of other affective conditions). This proposal is empirical only to the extent that it offers the kind of conceptual explicitness and clarity that allows empirical progress.

2. *Emotions are affective states with objects.* Emotions are always about something, and this "aboutness" is a useful way to distinguish emotions from other affective states such as moods. Such intentional psychological states are cognitive in that the things they are about are necessarily represented, and representation is the essence of cognition. To deal with instances in which affective feelings precede cognitive appraisals, we characterized moods as feelings states without salient objects and emotions as feelings states with objects. The fact that moods lack salient objects means that moods may be experienced as information about other suitable objects, which can then contribute to appraisals that create genuine emotions.

3. *There are two routes to emotional appraisal* (reinstatement and computation). Importantly, we not only have the on-line computation of a current situation with respect to psychological sources of value, such as goals, standards, and attitudes, we also have the reinstatement of prior emotions when a current situation elicits appraisals (and hence emotions) typical of an earlier situation. The predominantly top-down, reinstatement source (together with its processing correlates) is relatively fast, but error prone. The predominantly bottom-up, "computed" source (and its correlates), tends to be slower but more reliable.

4. *These forms of appraisal parallel two kinds of categorization* (prototype and theory based). A current situation can be categorized as emotionally significant by virtue of its relation to past emotional situations. This prototype-based (case-based, examplar-based) mode of categorization can be contrasted with theory-based categorization in which the features of a current situation are (not necessarily consciously) mapped onto the defining features of particular emotions.

5. *The two routes to emotional appraisal and the two kinds of categorization are governed by two forms of reasoning* (associative and rule-based). Reinstated emotion (and prototype- or case-based emotion categorizations) may be supported by associative reasoning operating on the basis of perceptual similarity. Emotions elicited by on-line computations of appraisals (and theory-based emotion categorizations) may be supported by rule-based reasoning (which need not be conscious, explicit, or easily articulated).

6. *The two routes to emotional appraisal or categorization may serve different behavioral functions* (preparedness and flexibility). Preparedness, and the speed of action it enables, requires speed of processing. Categorization of current situations on the basis of the similarity of surface features to those of prototypic emotional situations can occur even before the identity of the stimulus has been established, its context processed, or appropriate emotional feelings generated (LeDoux, 1996). Flexibility of response is a second advantage conferred by emotion (Scherer, 1984). This is better achieved by rule-based processing. When preparation is accompanied by subjective experiences, emotions provide a mental way station. This way station provides an alternative to direct behavioral expression, allowing relevant environmental and memorial information to be entertained.

7. *The fact that some components of an emotion can be triggered before full awareness of its cause does not conflict with a cognitive view.* Recent experiments

(e.g., LeDoux, 1996) are sometimes interpreted as demonstrating that emotions can be precognitive events because the experiments show that fear-relevant behavioral activation can occur before awareness of the cause and before feelings can be generated. However, the cognitive view maintains only that the trigger for emotional processes lies in the representation of the significance of a stimulus rather than in the stimulus itself. The experiments in question simply suggest that these representations can be widely distributed in the information processing system, so that they may be partially processed in one part of the brain before being fully processed in another (sensory cortex).

8. *Unconscious and conscious affect elicitation differ only in episodic constraints on emotional meaning.* The fact that affective responses can be elicited without awareness of the eliciting stimulus is sometimes interpreted as problematic for a cognitive view of emotion. However, an analysis of the subliminal paradigm suggests that this is not the case and that the power of unconscious stimuli is simply that the visual mask interferes with episodic information about the exposure event. As a result, semantic and affective meaning is broadly activated without the constraints on its applicability usually provided by episodic information about context. Such decontextualization of meaning is also evident in phobias and infantile amnesia when the hippocampus is suppressed or undeveloped (Jacobs & Nadel, 1985), when subjects are distracted during the processing of conscious primes (Martin et al., 1990), in mood and judgment experiments (Schwarz & Clore, 1983), and when the context of avoidance conditioning is forgotten (Hendersen, 1978). Although they may have many problematic effects, none of these phenomena require an extra-cognitive explanation.

9. *Automated, conditioned, imitated, and reinstated emotions are all manifestations of reinstated appraisals.* When some (not necessarily conscious) aspect of a situation reinstates emotions from the past, it is the meaning of the prior situation, not the emotion that is activated in memory. Then, as always, emotions occur automatically when their cognitive eliciting conditions are satisfied. Once "compiled" (Anderson, 1982, 1987), however, the computations of the original appraisal program for that situation may be inaccessible, so that the emotional reaction may be difficult to explain and resistant to change.

10. *The experiential and motivational/behavioral manifestations of appraisals, although difficult to describe in language, can be communicated through connotative meaning.* Connotative meaning has a surprisingly direct relation to action (e.g., Heise, 1979) and is most naturally represented in people as feelings rather than as linguistically expressible propositions. Successful communication and comprehension of connotative meaning (including emotional meaning) is marked by the occurrence of complementary feelings in the other, just as successful communication and comprehension of declarative knowledge is marked by the formation in the other of relevant beliefs and propositions.

Acknowledgments

The authors acknowledge Judy DeLoache, James Gross, Greg Miller, Csaba Pleh, Neil Smelser, Kurt VanLehn, Dan Wegner, Michael Robinson, and Bob Wyer for helpful discussions about some of the issues raised in this chapter. Support to G.L.C. is acknowledged from NSF grant SBR 96-01298, NIMH grant MH 50074, and by a John D. & Catherine T. Macarthur Foundation grant (32005-0) to the Center for Advanced Study in the Behavioral Sciences.

Notes

1. The liking emotions also are subject to metaphorical extension as when, for example, people reported disgust at the idea of sexual relations between brothers and sisters (J. D. Haidt, personal communication, 5 November 1997).

2. This is not to say that emotions themselves can be unconscious. If, as we believe, emotions must have an experiential component, they must be felt, so one cannot be unaware of them (see also Ortony et al., 1988, pp. 176–178).

3. Interestingly, empirical research with humans (e.g., Öhman, this volume) demonstrating the activation of fear-specific physiological responses before any conscious awareness of the fear-related stimulus as yet leaves unanswered a key question: What are the boundary conditions of the aversive stimulus? For example, when in these studies, spider phobics respond with increased skin conductance to subliminally presented slides of a tarantula, we still have no idea under what conditions the effect disappears. We do not know how spiderlike the image must be, and in what respects. Experiments to address this question would provide valuable information about the nature of the unconsciously accessed representation.

4. Apart from the neurological considerations, a proponent of a noncognitive view might argue that if fear of snakes is innate, as implied by its universality among primates, then it would be an example of a noncognitive emotion. But, despite its universality among primates, fear of snakes is apparently not innate. Rather, what is innate is the readiness to learn such a fear (Mineka et al., 1984). Thus, when confronted by a snake, the trigger for fear is not merely the snake, but the threat meaning of snakes learned from others early in life.

References

Ainsworth, M. D. S., Blehar, M. C., Waters, E. & Wall, T. (1978). *Patterns of Attachment*. Hillsdale, NJ: Lawrence Erlbaum Associates.

Alloy, L. B. & Abramson, L. Y. (1979). Judgment of contingency in depressed and non-depressed students: sadder but wiser. *Journal of Experimental Psychology: General, 108*, 441–485.

Anderson, J. R. (1982). Acquisition of cognitive skill. *Psychological Review, 89*, 369–406.

Anderson, J. R. (1987). Skill acquisition: compilation of weak-method problem solutions. *Psychological Review, 94*, 192–210.

Arnold, M. B. (1960). *Emotion and Personality*. New York: Columbia University Press.

Averill, J. R. (1980). A constructivist view of emotions. In R. Plutchik & H. Kellerman (Eds), *Emotions: Theory, Research, and Experience*, vol. 1 (pp. 305–339). New York: Academic Press.

Bandura, A. (1973). *Aggression: A Social Learning Analysis*. Englewood Cliffs, NJ: Prentice-Hall.

Bargh, J. (1997). Automaticity in everyday life. In R. S. Wyer (Ed), *Advances in Social Cognition*, vol. 10 (pp. 1–61). Hillsdale, NJ: Lawrence Erlbaum Associates.

Bechara, A., Damasio, A. R., Damasio, H. & Anderson, S. (1994). Insensitivity to future consequences following damage to human prefrontal cortex. *Cognition, 50*, 7–12.

Bowlby, J. (1969). *Attachment and Loss*, vol. 1. *Attachment*. New York: Basic Books.

Bornstein, R. F. (1992). Inhibitory effects of awareness on affective responding: implications for the affect-cognition relationship. In M. Clark (Ed), *Emotion: Review of Personality and Social Psychology*, vol. 13 (pp. 235–255). Newbury Park, CA: Sage.

Boyd, R. (1993). Metaphor and theory change: what is a "metaphor" a metaphor for. In A. Ortony (Ed), *Metaphor and Thought*, 2nd ed (pp. 481–532). New York: Cambridge University Press.

Cacioppo, J. T., Priestler, J. R. & Berntson, G. G. (1993). Rudimentary determinants of attitudes II: Arm flexion and extension have differential effects on attitudes. *Journal of Personality and Social Psychology, 65*, 5–17.

Clore, G. L. (1992). Cognitive phenomenology: feelings and the construction of judgment. In L. L. Martin & A. Tesser (Eds), *The Construction of Social Judgment* (pp. 133–164). Hillsdale, NJ: Lawrence Erlbaum Associates.

Clore, G. L. (1994a). Why emotions are felt. In P. Ekman & R. J. Davidson (Eds), *The Nature of Emotion: Fundamental Questions* (pp. 103–111). New York: Oxford University Press.

Clore, G. L. (1994b). Why emotions require cognition. In P. Ekman & R. J. Davidson (Eds), *The Nature of Emotion: Fundamental Questions* (pp. 181–191). New York: Oxford University Press.

Clore, G. L. & Ketelaar, T. (1997). Minding our emotions: on the role of automatic, unconscious affect. In R. S. Wyer (Ed), *Advances in Social Cognition*, vol. 10 (pp. 105–120). Hillsdale, NJ: Lawrence Erlbaum Associates.

Clore, G. L. & Ortony, A. (1991). What more is there to emotion concepts than prototypes? *Journal of Personality and Social Psychology, 60*, 48–50.

Clore G. L., Ortony, A. & Foss, M. A. (1987). The psychological foundations of the affective lexicon. *Journal of Personality and Social Psychology, 53*, 751–766.

Clore, G. L., Schwarz, N. & Conway, M. (1994). Affective causes and consequences of social information processing. In R. S. Wyer & T. Srull (Eds), *The Handbook of Social Cognition*, 2nd ed (pp. 323–417). Hillsdale, NJ: Lawrence Erlbaum Associates.

Coren, S. (1994). *The Intelligence of Dogs*. New York: The Free Press.

Damasio, A. R. (1994). *Descartes' Error: Emotion, Reason, and the Human Brain*. New York: Putnam.

Davidson, R. J. (1992). Anterior cerebral asymmetry and the nature of emotion. *Brain and Cognition, 20*, 125–151.

Devine, P. G. (1989). Stereotypes and prejudice: their automatic and controlled components. *Journal of Personality and Social Psychology, 56*, 5–18.

Draine, S. C. (1997). Analytic limitations of unconscious language processing, (doctoral dissertation). University of Washington, Seattle.

Fehr, B. & Russell, J. A. (1984). Concept of emotion viewed from a prototype perspective. *Journal of Experimental Psychology: General, 113*, 464–486.

Foa, U. G. & Foa, E. B. (1974). *Societal Structures of the Mind*. Springfield, IL: Charles C. Thomas.

Frank, R. H. (1988). *Passions Within Reason: The Strategic Role of the Emotions*. New York: Norton.

Freud, S. (1900[1953]). The interpretation of dreams. In J. Stachey and A. Freud (Eds), *The Standard Edition of the Complete Psychological Works of Sigmund Freud*, vol. 5. London: Hogarth Press.

Frijda, N. H. (1986). *The Emotions*. New York: Cambridge University Press.

Frijda, N. H., Ortony, A., Sonnemans, J. & Clore, G. L. (1992). The complexity of intensity: issues concerning the structure of emotion intensity. In M. Clark (Ed), *Emotion: Review of Personality and Social Psychology*, vol. 13. Newbury Park, CA: Sage.

Gasper, K. & Clore, G. L. (1998). The persistent use of negative affect by anxious individuals to estimate risk. *Journal of Personality and Social Psychology, 74*, 1350–1363.

Gollob, H. F. (1974). The subject-verb-object approach to social cognition. *Psychological Review, 81*, 286–321.

Greenwald, A. G., Draine, S. C. & Abrams, R. L. (1996). Three cognitive markers of unconscious semantic activation. *Science, 273*, 1699–1702.

Hebb, D. O. (1949). *The Organization of Behavior*. New York: Wiley.

Heise, D. R. (1979). *Understanding Events: Affect and the Construction of Social Action*. New York: Cambridge University Press.

Hendersen, R. (1978). Forgetting of conditioned fear inhibition. *Learning and Motivation, 8*, 16–30.

Higgins, E. T., Rholes, W. S. & Jones, C. R. (1977). Category accessibility and impression formation. *Journal of Experimental Social Psychology, 13*, 141–154.

Jacobs, W. J. & Nadel, L. (1985). Stress-induced recovery of fears and phobias. *Psychological Review, 92*, 512–531.

Keil, F. C. (1989). *Concepts, Kinds, and Cognitive Development*. Cambridge, MA: MIT Press.

Ketelaar, T. & Clore, G. L. (1997). Emotions and reason: proximate effects and ultimate functions. In G. Matthews (Ed), *Personality, Emotion, and Cognitive Science* (pp. 355–396). Advances in Psychology Series. Amsterdam: Elsevier Science Publishers North-Holland.

Kotovsky, L. & Baillargeon, R. (1994). Calibration-based reasoning about collision events in 11-month-old infants. *Cognition, 51*, 107–129.

Lazarus, R. S. (1966). *Psychological Stress and the Coping Process*. New York: McGraw-Hill.

Lazarus, R. S. (1994). Universal antecedents of the emotions. In P. Ekman & R. J. Davidson (Eds), *The Nature of Emotion: Fundamental Questions* (pp. 163–171). New York: Oxford University Press.

Leary, T. (1957). *Interpersonal Diagnosis of Personality*. New York: Ronald Press.

LeDoux, J. E. (1996). *The Emotional Brain*. New York: Simon and Schuster.

Lewicki, P. (1985). Nonconscious biasing effects of single instances of subsequent judgments. *Journal of Personality and Social Psychology, 48*, 563–574.

Mandler, G. (1984). *Mind and Body*. New York: Norton.

Martin, L. L., Seta, J. J. & Crelia, R. A. (1990). Assimilation and contrast as a function of people's willingness and ability to expend effort in forming an impression. *Journal of Personality and Social Psychology, 59*, 27–37.

Medin, D. L. & Ortony, A. (1989). Psychological essentialism. In S. Vosniadou and A. Ortony (Eds), *Similarity and Analogical Reasoning* (pp. 175–194). New York: Cambridge University Press.

Mineka, S., Davidson, M., Cook, M. & Keir, R. (1984). Observational conditioning of snake fear in rhesus monkeys. *Journal of Abnormal Psychology, 93*, 355–372.

Morgan, H. J. & Shaver, P. R. (in press). Attachment processes and commitment to romantic relationships. In W. H. Jones & J. M. Adams (Eds), *Handbook of Interpersonal Commitment and Relationship Stability*. New York: Plenum.

Murphy, S. T. & Zajonc, R. B. (1993). Affect, cognition, and awareness: priming with optimal and suboptimal stimulus exposures. *Journal of Personality and Social Psychology, 64*, 723–739.

Needham, A. & Baillargeon, R. (1993). Intuitions about support in 4.5-month-old infants. *Cognition, 47*, 121–148.

Neumann, R. & Strack, F. (1998). Approach and avoidance: the influence of proprioceptive and exteroceptive cues on encoding of affective information. Unpublished manuscript, University of Würzburg, Germany.

Nisbett, R. E. & Wilson, T. D. (1977). Telling more than we can know: verbal reports on mental processes. *Psychological Review, 84*, 231–259.

Oatley, K. & Johnson-Laird, P. N. (1987). Towards a cognitive theory of the emotions. *Cognition and Emotion, 1*, 29–50.

Öhman, A. (1986). Face the beast and fear the face: animal and social fears as prototypes for evolutionary analyses of emotion. *Psychophysiology, 23*, 123–145.

O'Keefe, J. & Nadel, L. (1978). *The Hippocampus as a Cognitive Map*. New York: Clarendon Press.

Ortony, A. (1990). *The cognition-emotion connection*. Paper presented at the American Psychological Association, Boston, August 1990.

Ortony, A. & Clore, G. L. (1989). Emotions, moods, and conscious awareness. *Cognition & Emotion, 3*, 125–137.

Ortony, A., Clore, G. L. & Collins A. (1988). *The cognitive structure of emotions*. New York: Cambridge University Press.

Ortony, A., Clore, G. L. & Foss, M. A. (1987). The referential structure of the affective lexicon. *Cognitive Science, 11*, 341–364.

Osgood, C. E. (1969). On the whys and wherefores of E, P, and A. *Journal of Personality and Social Psychology, 12*, 194–199.

Osgood, C. E., Suci, G. J. & Tannenbaum, P. H. (1957). *The Measurement of Meaning*. Urbana, IL: University of Illinois Press.

Panksepp, J. (1998). *Affective Neuroscience: The Foundations of Human and Animal Emotions*. New York: Oxford University Press.

Parkinson, B. (1997). Untangling the appraisal-emotion connection *Personality and Social Psychology Review, 1*, 62–79.

Pennebaker, J. W. (1991). *Opening up: The Healing Power of Confiding in Others*. New York: William Morrow & Co.

Reisenzein, R. (1998). A theory of emotional feelings as meta-representational states of mind. Unpublished manuscript, University of Bielefeld, Germany.

Robinson, M. (1998). Dual processes in the cognitive elicitation of emotion. *Cognition and Emotion, 12*, 667–696.

Rosch, E. (1973). Natural categories. *Cognitive Psychology, 4*, 328–350.

Roseman, I. J. (1984). Cognitive determinants of emotion: a structural theory. In P. Shaver (Ed), *Review of Personality and Social Psychology*, vol. 5. *Emotions, Relationships, and Health* (pp. 11–36). Beverly Hills, CA: Sage.

Ross, B. H. (1987). This is like that: the use of earlier problems and the separation of similarity effects. *Journal of Experimental Psychology: Learning, Memory, and Cognition, 13*, 629–639.

Rusbult, C. E. (1980). Commitment and satisfaction in romantic associations: a test of the investment model. *Journal of Experimental Social Psychology, 16*, 172–186.

Rusbult, C. E. (1983). A longitudinal test of the investment model: the development (and deterioration) of satisfaction and commitment in heterosexual involvements. *Journal of Personality and Social Psychology, 45*, 101–117.

Russell, J. A. (1991). In defense of a prototype approach to emotion concepts. *Journal of Personality and Social Psychology, 60*, 37–47.

Scherer, K. R. (1984). On the nature and function of emotion: a component process approach. In K. R. Scherer & P. Ekman (Eds), *Approaches to Emotion* (pp. 293–317). Hillsdale, NJ: Lawrence Erlbaum Associates.

Schwarz, N. & Clore, G. L. (1983). Mood, misattribution, and judgments of well-being:

Informative and directive functions of affective states. *Journal of Personality and Social Psychology, 45*, 513–523.

Schwarz, N. & Clore, G. L. (1988). How do I feel about it? Informative functions of affective states. In K. Fiedler & J. Forgas (Eds), *Affect, Cognition, and Social Behavior* (pp. 44–62). Toronto: Hogrefe International.

Schwarz, N. & Clore, G. L. (1996). Feelings and phenomenal experiences. In E. T. Higgins & A. Kruglanski (Eds), *Social Psychology: A Handbook of Basic Principles* (pp. 433–465). New York: Guilford Press.

Seligman, M. E. P. & Maier, S. F. (1967). Failure to escape traumatic shock. *Journal of Experimental Psychology, 74*, 1–9.

Shaver, P. R. & Clark, C. L. (1994). The psychodynamics of adult romantic attachment. In J. M. Masling & R. F. Bornstein (Eds), *Empirical Perspectives on Object Relations Theories* (pp. 105–156). Washington, DC: American Psychological Association.

Shaver, P. R., Schwartz, J., Kirson, D. & O'Connor, C. (1987). Emotion knowledge: further exploration of a prototype approach. *Journal of Personality and Social Psychology, 52*, 1–11.

Sloman, S. A. (1996). The empirical case for two systems of reasoning. *Psychological Bulletin, 119*, 3–22.

Smedslund, J. (1991). The pseudoempirical in psychology and the case for psychologic. *Psychological Inquiry, 2*, 325–338.

Smelser, N. J. (1998). The rational and the ambivalent in the social sciences. *American Sociological Review, 63*, 1–16.

Smith, C. A. & Ellsworth, P. C. (1985). Patterns of cognitive appraisal. *Journal of Personality and Social Psychology, 48*, 813–838.

Smith, C. A., Griner, L. A., Kirby, L. D. & Scott, H. S. (1996). Toward a process model of appraisal in emotion. In N. Frijda (Ed) Proceedings of the Ninth Conference of the International Society for Research on Emotion (pp. 101–105). Toronto: ISRE.

Solomon, A. (1998). Anatomy of melancholy. *The New Yorker, 73*, no. 42 (Jan. 12), pp. 46–61.

Solarz, A. K. (1960). Latency of instrumental responses as a function of compatibility with the meaning of eliciting verbal signs. *Journal of Experimental Psychology, 59*, 239–245.

Srull, T. K. & Wyer, R. S., Jr. (1979). The role of category accessibility in the interpretation of information about persons: some determinants and implications. *Journal of Personality and Social Psychology, 37*, 1660–1672.

Sullivan, H. S. (1953). *The Interpersonal Theory of Psychiatry*. New York: W. W. Norton.

Toates, F. M. (1987). Motivation and emotion from a biological perspective. In V. Hamilton, G. H. Bower & N. H. Frijda (Eds), *Cognitive Perspectives on Emotion and Motivation* (pp. 3–36). Dordrecht: Kluwer Academic.

Tomkins, S. S. (1979). Script theory: differential magnification of affects. In H. E. Howe, Jr. & R. A. Dienstbier (Eds), *Nebraska Symposium on Motivation*, vol. 26 (pp. 201–236). Lincoln: University of Nebraska Press.

Weber, E. & Clore, G. L. (1987). Anxiety and risk taking. Unpublished manuscript, University of Illinois at Urbana-Champaign.

Wegner, D. M. (1994). Ironic processes of mental control. *Psychological Review, 101*, 34–52.

Weiner, B. (1985). An attributional theory of achievement motivation and emotion. *Psychological Review, 92*, 548–573.

Wiggins, J. S. (1980). Circumplex models of interpersonal behavior. In L. Wheeler (Ed), *Review of Personality and Social Psychology*, vol. 1 (pp. 265–293). Beverly Hills, CA: Sage.

Wilson, T. D. & Lindsey, S. (1998). A model of dual attitudes. Unpublished manuscript, University of Virginia, Charlottesville.

Wilson, T. D. & Schooler, J. W. (1991). Thinking too much: introspection can reduce the quality of preferences and decisions. *Journal of Personality and Social Psychology, 60*, 181–192.

Zajonc, R. B. (1998). Emotions. In D. Gilbert, S. T. Fiske & G. Lindzey (Eds), *Handbook of Social Psychology*, 4th ed, vol. 1 (pp. 591–632). New York: McGraw-Hill.

4

Facial Expression, Emotion, and Hemispheric Organization

BRYAN KOLB AND LAUGHLIN TAYLOR

Interest in the biological correlates of emotions dates back at least to Darwin's book, *The Expression of Emotions in Man and Animals*, published in 1872. There was little experimental information for another 50 years, although there were anecdotal accounts of emotional behavior in decorticated dogs, which led to the idea that emotions were not in the cortex (e.g., Goltz, 1960). By the late 1920s neurophysiologists began to examine the relationship between autonomic, endocrine, and other factors and inferred emotional states, especially rage. The physiologists continued to emphasize the role of the hypothalamic systems and to downplay the importance of forebrain structures. Psychologists became interested in emotional behavior and the brain as they began to encounter curious pathological states associated with brain injury. For example, Klüver and Bucy (1939) rediscovered an extraordinary syndrome associated with temporal lobe damage, and Goldstein (1939) described the changes in emotional behavior of people with unilateral strokes. There was little systematic study of forebrain–behavior relationships in emotion, however, until the explosion of human neuropsychological studies in the 1970s. As cognitive neuroscience has evolved and begun to study brain–behavior relationships in emotion more intensively, many approaches ranging from the study of brain-injured patients to the study of electrodermal responses or metabolic changes in response to emotion now have been developed. Each experimental approach carries assumptions about the nature of brain–behavior relationships as well as the nature of emotional experience itself. Thus, it is prudent to begin this chapter by outlining the biases and assumptions that guide our research. We then consider the likely role of frontal and temporal structures involved in emotional behavior. Next, we systematically describe the contribution of frontal and temporal lobes to social behavior, considering the production and perception of facial expression, the perception of language, and the perception of prosody. We also consider findings from a small sample of patients with parietal lobe removals in the context of the frontal and temporal patients. Finally, we address the issue of cerebral asymmetry and the production of emotional behavior.

Assumptions

First, we assume that behavioral states, including mind states, correspond to brain states. It follows that perturbations of the brain will alter behavior and mind states. Because emotion is assumed to be a behavioral and/or mind state that results from a brain state, emotion may change when the brain changes. This assumption may seem self-evident to most cognitive neuroscientists, but it has important implications for the way we study emotion. It follows from our assumption that the study of neurological patients will provide information about how the brain states are related to emotion. We must caution that we do not wish to imply that the study of neurological patients is the only method, nor even necessarily the best method, of study. We do note, however, that most of what is known about human brain function has come from studies of neurological patients.

Second, we assume that emotion is not a unitary construct but rather is a multidimensional one. Thus, emotion includes (1) physiological change, including autonomic change, (2) overt behavior ranging from facial expression to laughter to physical aggression, (3) an internal "state," which is usually referred to as "affect", and (4) cognitive behavior, which includes thoughts, perceptions, attitudes, and so on. In this chapter, and in our research, we have chosen to focus on overt behavior. From our observations we have attempted to identify the role of the frontal and temporal lobes in emotion. Because we are emphasizing only one subset of things that contribute to emotion, the generality of our observations is almost certainly limited. We hope, however, that our conclusions will be of heuristic value not only in understanding brain–behavior relations in emotion but also in understanding clinical syndromes.

Third, we assume that different emotionally relevant behaviors are controlled by dissociable neural circuits. In this sense emotion is much like memory. Until recently, it was assumed by most investigators studying the neural basis of memory that memory was a unitary phenomenon mediated by a single neural system. It is now clear that there are multiple types of memory, each mediated by different neural systems (e.g., Kolb & Whishaw, 1996). Similarly, investigators studying emotion have often assumed that a single system, such as the limbic system was responsible for controlling a multitude of behaviors ranging from love to aggression. This is unlikely; there are almost certainly multiple neural systems controlling those behaviors typically grouped by the term "emotion." Indeed, it was in 1968 that Moyer argued that there are multiple types of aggression, each of which is mediated by distinct neural structures.

Fourth, we assume that it is useful to dissociate brain–behavior relationships involved in the production of emotional behavior from those involved in the perception of emotions in others as well as the perception of emotionally relevant stimuli. In addition, we have assumed that neural circuits underlying verbal and nonverbal aspects of emotional behavior are also dissociable. These two assumptions have influenced the manner in which we have constructed our behavioral tests.

Fifth, we assume that an analysis of the neural control of facial expression provides a window on at least some of the neural systems involved in emotion.

The brain appears to have cells specialized for the analysis of faces (e.g., Perret et al., 1984), and facial expression is a powerful stimulus in human communication. Indeed, facial expression is a central feature of emotional/social behavior of most nonhuman primates and, to a lesser extent, in the behavior of other mammalian species such as canids and felids.

Sixth, it is likely that categories of emotion, such as fear, are controlled by fundamentally different neural circuits than are emotions such as happiness. Le-Doux (1995) has noted that fear is an emotion that is particularly important to human and nonhuman existence: It is a normal reaction to threatening events. Although fear is certainly influenced by experience, fear is probably easier to identify and to study in other species than other emotional states such as happiness or anger. Furthermore, there is increasing evidence for a distinct set of neural circuitry mediating fear (e.g., Davis, 1992). We have therefore paid special attention to fear in many of our studies.

Finally, like Darwin (1872), we believe that brain–behavior relationships in human emotion can only be understood in the context of the neural pathways of emotional behavior in other species, especially mammals. The organization of our emotional brain thus is determined by our evolution. Language must add a new dimension, but the basic neural systems will be found in nonspeaking animals as well. Indeed, it might be reasonable to suppose that right hemisphere functions in humans will be quite similar to those seen bilaterally in nonspeaking species.

Candidate Neural Structures

One of the consistent principles of neural organization is that there are multiple systems controlling virtually every behavior. Thus, sensory information enters the cortex through multiple channels that have distinctly different roles in sensory analysis. Once in the cortex, information travels through multiple parallel systems subserving different functions. For example, there must be systems that process significant emotionally relevant stimuli, which are presumably species specific, including olfactory stimuli (e.g., pheromones), tactile stimuli (especially to sensitive body zones), visual stimuli (e.g., facial expressions), and auditory stimuli (e.g., speech sounds, species-typical sounds such as crying or screaming). Although it is likely that the processing of these stimuli involves some of the same systems that analyze sensory inputs relevant to, say, object recognition, there is good reason to believe that at least some analysis of sensory input relevant to emotion is carried out in regions that are separable. Vision provides a good example.

The primary visual cortex of mammals sends projections to associated visual regions, which, in turn, send projections to various regions including the prefrontal cortex and amygdala. When cats encounter the "Halloween profile" (figure 4.1) of another cat they respond with a similar posture, which is followed by a slow approach to the perineal and/or head area of the stimulus cat. There is piloerection over the back and tail, slowed breathing, perspiration on the foot pads, and pupil dilation. This affective response is specific to the "Halloween" configuration; cats pay little attention to a "Picasso" cat (figure 4.1) (Kolb & Nonneman, 1975). Cats with visual cortex lesions do not respond to the stimulus, which is reasonable

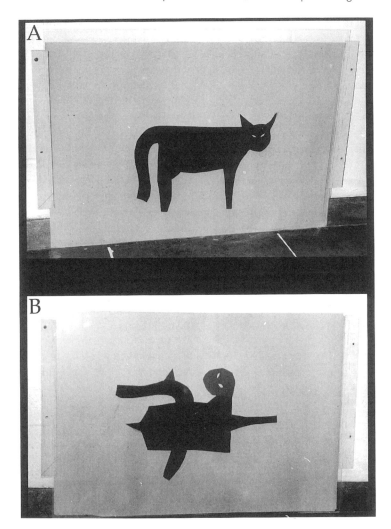

Figure 4.1. Photographs illustrating the silhouette of a cat used to elicit an affective response in cats. Top: "Halloween" cat; bottom: "Picasso" cat. Normal cats respond to the Halloween cat with a similar posture but show no response to the Picasso cat. Cats with frontal or amygdala lesions do not respond as normal cats. The cat models are mounted behind nonreflective glass.

because their pattern perception is severely compromised. Cats with amygdala lesions orient to the stimulus and approach the appropriate regions of the stimulus, but they show no affective response (that is, no piloerection or autonomic responses). Cats with frontal lesions also orient to the stimulus, but they do not approach the stimulus; rather, they actively avoid it (Nonneman & Kolb, 1974). They show no piloerection or other obvious autonomic signs that are so salient in the control animals. These results imply that there is a visual pathway to the amygdala that plays an important role in mediating fear responses to species-typical visual stimuli. Similarly, there is a visual pathway to the prefrontal cortex that plays some role in the generation of action patterns appropriate to the species-typical stimulus. The effects of amygdala and frontal lesions on the recognition of visual sign stimuli are probably not specific to the visual modality. Indeed, we have also seen parallel results with olfactory stimuli such as the recognition of conspecific urine by cats (Nonneman & Kolb, 1974).

The cat experiment illustrates the general principle that there are dissociable neural pathways involved in different aspects of social behavior. In addition to the modality-specific pathways, there are also likely to be pathways mediating cross-modal matching of visual and auditory information. An example in humans would be facial expression and prosody in speech (see de Gelder, this volume).

One prediction that follows from our cat experiment and from our assumption regarding evolutionary continuities in neural pathways for emotion is that primates with amygdala or frontal lobe injuries would be impaired at the perception of species-specific stimuli such as facial expressions or vocalizations. Indeed, there is now overwhelming evidence that damage to the frontal cortex, anterior temporal cortex, cingulate cortex, and amygdala all produce abnormalities in social interaction in both Old World and New World monkeys (for a review, see Kolb & Taylor, 1990). The close anatomical connections between the orbital prefrontal cortex and the amygdala and the emotional changes after lesions to either region suggest that these structures belong to some neural circuit regulating emotional behavior.

Patient Population

Our research has centered on patients with unilateral frontal, temporal, or parietal cortex removals either for the relief of intractable epilepsy or for the removal of well-defined tumors or cysts. The patients all had full scale IQ ratings above 80 (range of 80–146), and none of the patients were aphasic at the time of testing.On the tasks that we will discuss, there were no sex differences and there were no differences in the results relative to the age of brain injury or the age at surgery. Finally, we found no differences in the results as a function of postoperative recovery time, which ranged from 2 weeks to 20 years after surgery. Our criteria for inclusion in the experiments has been strict. Lesions must be restricted to the frontal, temporal, or parietal cortex, speech must be exclusively in the left hemisphere, and there must be no evidence of persisting epileptic foci elsewhere in the brain after surgery.

The patients in our sample include those with (1) lesions of the dorsolateral frontal lobe, including varying amounts of the medial frontal region, (2) lesions of the inferior frontal lobe, (3) lesions of the parietal cortex outside of the posterior speech zone, and (4) lesions of the anterior temporal cortex. All of the patients in the latter group also had removal of some medial temporal cortex and the amygdala. In addition, some patients had removal of some or all of the hippocampal formation.

Role of the Frontal Lobe in Social Behavior

The frontal lobes of the human comprise all the tissue in front of the central sulcus. This is a vast area, representing 30% of the neocortex, and it is made up of several functionally distinct regions that we group into three categories: motor (precentral gyrus), premotor, and prefrontal (for a review, see Kolb & Whishaw, 1996). The motor cortex is responsible for making movements of the distal musculature (tongue, fingers, toes). The premotor cortex selects movements to be made (for a detailed review, see Passingham, 1993). The prefrontal cortex controls the cognitive processes so that the appropriate movements are selected at the correct place and time (e.g., Fuster, 1989). This latter selection may be controlled by internalized information, or it may be made in response to context. There are two subdivisions of the prefrontal cortex that may function with respect to the response selection related to internal versus external information. These are the dorsolateral region and the inferior (or orbital) frontal region. The dorsolateral cortex is hypothesized to be evolved especially for the selection of behavior based on temporal memory, which is a potent form of internalized knowledge (e.g., Goldman-Rakic, 1989). People whose temporal memory is defective become dependent on environmental cues to determine their behavior. That is, behavior is not under the control of internalized knowledge but is controlled directly by environmental cues. One effect of this condition is that people with dorsolateral frontal lobe injuries can be expected to have difficulty in inhibiting behavior directed to external stimuli. They are easily distracted and tend to ignore rules that are given to them. For example, it is well documented that patients with dorsolateral frontal lesions break rules in various types of neuropsychological tests (e.g., Milner, 1964). In addition, one can easily imagine that neglecting internalized knowledge about how to behave in social situations could lead to social difficulties in people with frontal lobe injuries. For example, there are clear "rules" regarding when we speak out in social groups. Overall, these patients appear to have problems analyzing social situations, often as though they do not really comprehend what they are responding to. The end result is often that they pick the "wrong" response.

The inferior frontal region is hypothesized to have a role in the control of response selection in context. Social behavior in particular is context dependent. Behavior that is appropriate at one moment is often not appropriate if there are subtle changes in context. We can easily see the importance of social context when we reflect upon our behavior with our parents versus that with our closest friends or our children. It is a common experience that our tone of voice, the use of slang or swear words, and the content of conversations are quite different in these different contexts. People with inferior frontal lesions, which are relatively common in closed-head injuries, have difficulty with context, especially in social situations, and are notorious for making social gaffes. They also have difficulty with impulse control, although it is not so clear if this is related directly to context.

We note here parenthetically that although there are theoretical reasons for dissociating the symptoms of dorsolateral and orbital frontal lesions in humans, in real-life clinical situations the distinction is often less obvious. Both dorsolateral and orbitofrontal patients exhibit poor social/emotional behavior, and the actual observed behavior is not always helpful in determining the site of the lesion.

There is a general impression in the literature (e.g., Benson & Blumer, 1975; Kolb & Whishaw, 1996) that right frontal and left frontal lobe patients have distinctly different changes in emotional behavior. Left frontal lobe patients tend to be very quiet and display little affect, whereas right frontal lobe patients tend to be more talkative and, at times, can appear almost psychopathic in their interpersonal behaviors. In addition, there is now an extensive literature indicating that left and right frontal lobe injuries have differential effects on tests of language or working memory (for a review, see Kolb & Whishaw, 1996). We would anticipate, therefore, that we might find a left/right difference in the performance of left and right frontal lobe patients on tests of emotional behavior.

Tests of Emotional Behavior

We noted earlier that our bias has been to study emotion by focusing upon overt behavior of patients with frontal lobe injuries. In addition, we have emphasized the role of facial expression because it is a salient cue of emotional experience. Furthermore, we noted that we have chosen to distinguish between the production and perception of facial expression.

• Production of Facial Expression

We have measured the production of facial expression in various ways. First, we have measured the spontaneous facial expressions (and vocalizations) of people in various settings. This has involved using a time-sampling technique during the administration of routine neuropsychological tests or during a preoperative sodium amobarital procedure. The results show that patients with frontal lobe lesions exhibit far less spontaneous facial expression than patients with temporal or parietal lesions (see figure 4.2). It is significant that although frontal lobe lesions reduce the frequency of facial expressions, they do not effect their diversity. Thus, it is the spontaneity of the expressions that is reduced, not the ability to produce them. One striking result is that frontal lobe patients are especially unlikely to smile spontaneously during routine neuropsychological testing. Spontaneous smiling in social situations is common in other patients, and its absence can be somewhat unsettling in the novice examiner. The reduced spontaneous facial expressions of frontal lobe patients can be contrasted with their spontaneous talking. Thus, the number of spontaneous, irrelevant, comments during the performance of various tests was counted (Kolb & Taylor, 1981). Patients with left frontal lobe removals made almost no comments; those with right frontal lobe lesions made an excessive number of comments (see figure 4.2). These data show a clear dissociation between

FACING PAGE

Figure 4.2.   Relative frequencies of spontaneous facial expressions (A) and talking (B) during routine neuropsychological testing. Note that frontal lobe lesions significantly reduce the number of facial expressions. The level of spontaneous talking is significantly reduced for left frontal lesions and increased for right frontal lesions. Asterisks indicate a significant difference from other groups with same-side lesions.

A. Spontaneous Facial Expression

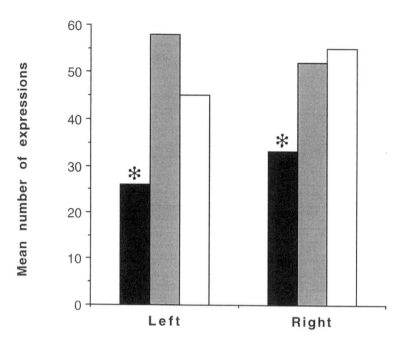

B. Spontaneous Talking

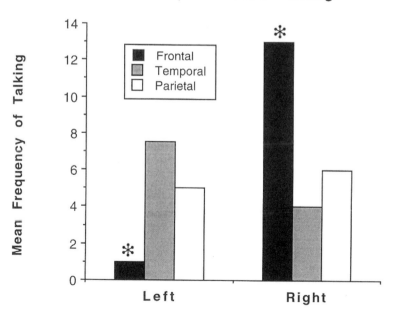

the two hemispheres for the production of spontaneous talking but not for facial expression.

Second, we have measured the ability of people to produce expressions. In one test we presented a series of photographs of real (i.e., not posed) expressions taken from old copies of *Life* magazine (happy, sad, anger, disgust, fear, surprise) and asked people to produce the same expression. In a second test we presented people with cartoons depicting a series of real-life situations and the task was to produce a facial expression that would be appropriate to the situation (see figure 4.3). In both tasks we videotaped the subjects and used Ekman's facial affect scoring system (e.g., Ekman & Friesen, 1975) to score the facial movements. In addition, we extracted still photos of the expressions produced by the subjects and asked five naive raters to judge whether the expressions were happy, sad, anger,

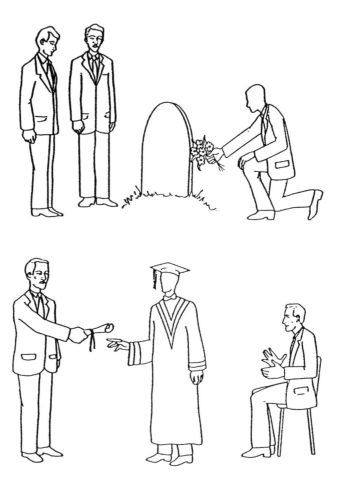

Figure 4.3. Examples of cartoon situations for which patients were asked either to produce the appropriate expression or to choose the appropriate expression from several choices for the blank face.

disgust, fear, or surprise. Finally, we separated the results for each of the different expressions (Kolb & Taylor, 1999a, 1999b). The results showed that frontal lobe patients produced less intense facial expressions and that raters had far more difficulty guessing the expression for frontal lobe patients than for others (figure 4.4). In addition, it can be seen in figure 4.4 that left frontal lobe patients were especially poor at producing expressions of fear or disgust.

To determine if there might be any localization of the movement deficit within the frontal lobe, we divided patients into those with inferior frontal damage versus those without such damage. There was a clear effect of region: the left inferior frontal lobe patients were significantly less expressive than the other groups. This result is in accord with our clinical impression that such patients show very little affect and are often considered to appear depressed (e.g., Blumer & Benson, 1975).

- Perception of Faces

Perhaps the most potent emotionally relevant stimuli that humans respond to in others are facial expression and tone of voice (prosody). To examine the ability of patients to perceive such stimuli, we devised a series of tests that parallel the tests of facial movement. First, however, it was necessary to be certain that the patients were able to perceive faces. We reasoned that if patients were unable to process faces normally, they would be expected to have difficulties in recognition of facial expression. (We were not concerned about language comprehension because none of the patients were aphasic and all had verbal IQs above 85.)

Our test of facial perception was based on a test devised by Wolff (1933) and subsequently used by many others. The test entails splitting full-face photographs (and their mirror images) down the middle, then rejoining the corresponding halves to make two symmetrical composite photographs, one created from the left side of the face, the other from the right (Kolb et al., 1983). Thus, subjects were presented with the normal face on top and the two composite faces below. The task is to indicate which of the composite pictures resembles the real face more closely. Normal right-handed subjects show a significant bias (about 70%) in favor of the right side of the normal face. In contrast, patients with either right temporal or right parietal lesions respond idiosyncratically to each photograph, presenting no overall bias in favor of either side of the face, a result suggesting that these patients process faces differently from normal subjects or from those patients with lesions elsewhere. Frontal lobe patients were indistinguishable from control subjects on this task, suggesting that they process faces normally.

- Perception of Facial Expression

To study the patients' ability to appreciate different facial expressions, we did a series of experiments in which subjects were to match different photographs of faces on the basis of emotion inferred from the facial expression or from verbal captions given to the photographs. In one test patients were given a set of six key photographs representing happiness, sadness, anger, surprise, fear, and disgust. They were then shown a series of photographs of faces from *Life* magazine and asked to choose one of the six key faces that best matched each of the *Life* faces. Again, we analyzed the responses to each expression separately. The results showed that both right and left frontal lobe patients were markedly impaired at

Expressions of Happy, Sad, Angry, Surprise for Cartoons

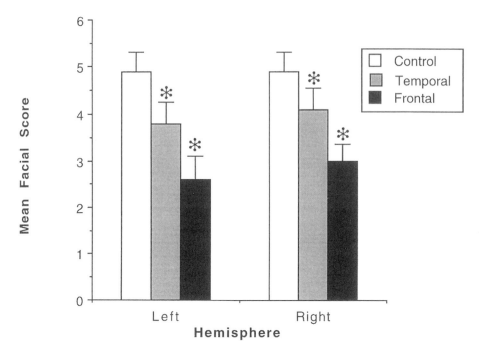

Expressions of Fear & Disgust for Cartoons

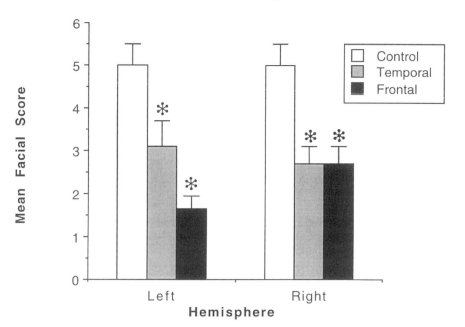

matching photographs showing fear or disgust (figure 4.5). In contrast, the frontal lobe patients performed as well as control subjects at matching the other expressions.

Finally, we asked our subjects to take the six key faces and choose the one most appropriate for the cartoon situations that we used earlier in the movement task (figure 4.3). The frontal lobe patients were impaired at this task and, in contrast to the photograph-matching task, they were impaired at all categories of emotion (figure 4.6). There were no differences between the patients with left and right hemisphere removals, nor was there any difference related to lesion locus. (We note, also, that the patients with right posterior lesions were as impaired as the frontal lobe patients on this task.)

• Perception of Language and Prosody

Our face-matching tests were intentionally constructed to avoid confounding of verbal and nonverbal descriptions of emotional state. There is evidence, however, that left hemisphere lesions might impair the ability to comprehend propositional affect (e.g., Brownell et al., 1983; Gardner et al., 1975). To investigate verbal aspects, we designed two tasks that were parallel to the facial tasks. In the first task the subjects were given a list of the six emotional states that had been depicted in the photographs. They were then read a sentence describing the events surrounding the people in the photographs from *Life* magazine that the subjects had been shown earlier; for example, "This man is at a funeral." The subjects were to choose the verbal descriptor of emotional state. Patients with left, but not right, frontal lesions were impaired at this task (Kolb & Taylor, 1981). This impairment was not related to emotional state.

In the second task we examined the recognition of prosody. Professional actors (male and female) were recruited to read sentences with different tone of voice that expressed different emotions. For example, one sentence was "what are you doing here" and it was read with different prosody to reflect either sadness, surprise, fear, or anger. The subject's task was to pick one of the six key photographs that best illustrated the emotion experienced by the speaker. Overall, both left and right frontal lobe patients were impaired at this task. It was the patients with left dorsolateral lesions who were the most impaired, however, regardless of the emotion conveyed in the voice (figure 4.7). Curiously, the patients with left inferior frontal lesions were not impaired at the task.

Localization Within the Frontal Lobe

We noted that there are strong grounds for predicting that inferior and dorsolateral frontal lesions might have dissociable effects upon emotional behavior and, in addi-

FACING PAGE
Figure 4.4. Summary of the intensity of facial expressions produced by subjects for the ambiguous cartoon task. Both the frontal and temporal patients made less intense expressions than the control subjects for situations of fear and disgust (bottom). In contrast, only the frontal lobe patients differed from control subjects for the other emotions. The low intensity of facial expressions made the expressions uninterpretable to naive observers. Asterisks indicate significant difference from control group.

Photo Matching for Fear and Disgust/Contempt

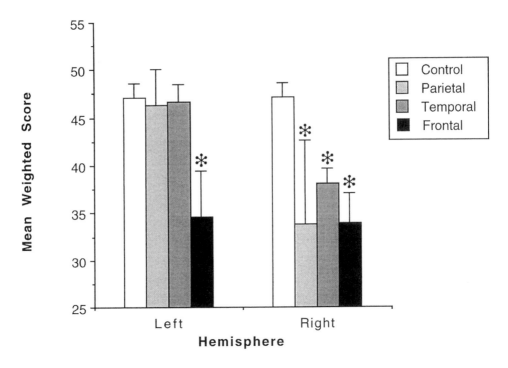

Photo Matching for Happy, Sad, Angry, Surprise

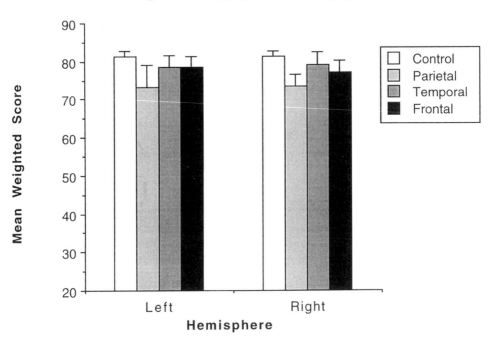

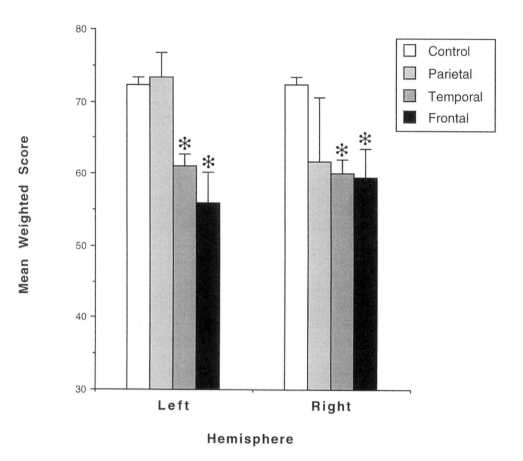

Cartoon Matching

Figure 4.6. Mean correct choices in matching photographs of key faces to the ambiguous cartoon faces. All right hemisphere patient groups were impaired. The left temporal and left frontal groups were also impaired. Asterisks indicate significant difference from control group.

FACING PAGE
Figure 4.5. Mean correct choices in matching photographs of key faces to photographs of spontaneous emotions. The right hemisphere patients all had difficulty in matching expressions of fear and disgust, whereas only the left frontal lobe patients were impaired. All groups performed as well as control subjects on the matching of the other faces. Asterisks indicate significant difference from control group.

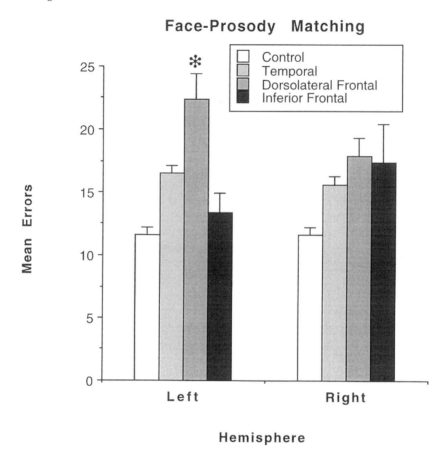

Figure 4.7. Mean errors in matching the key faces to prosody. Although temporal lobe patients had a mild deficit, the left dorsolateral frontal patients were especially impaired, whereas the left inferior frontal patients were not impaired. Right frontal lobe patients performed much like right temporal lobe patients. Asterisk indicates significant impairment compared to all other groups.

tion, that left and right frontal lobe injuries might also be dissociable. Indeed, there appear to be several dissociations. First, left inferior frontal patients have the least intense facial expressions. Second, right frontal lobe patients are more talkative than left frontal lobe patients. Third, left frontal lobe patients, but not right frontal lobe patients, were impaired at a task in which they had to match verbal descriptors of emotion with verbal descriptions of events. Finally, left dorsolateral frontal lobe patients were especially poor at matching prosody in voice with facial expression. This result is surprising because the right hemisphere has been assumed to be more central in prosody (e.g., Ross, 1981). Injury to the left inferior frontal region, however, was without effect on this task, whereas injury throughout the right frontal lobe produced a large deficit. One explanation for the poor performance of the left frontal lobe group is that the task required the subjects to listen to a sentence and then to remember the verbal prosodic information in order to match it with an appropriate face. It is possible that working memory demands for the sentences was especially difficult for the left dorsolateral patients.

It is difficult to relate these differences to the putative regional difference in the functions of the inferior and dorsolateral cortex. It would appear that both regions play a role in the production and recognition of facial expression and that their respective roles are at least partly dissociable. It is likely that the reason for the frontal involvement is not so much that the brain has evolved regions dedicated to emotion and the face, but rather that the lesions interfere with processes that result in the observed abnormalities. For instance, the frontal lobe plays a role in generating spontaneous behaviors of all types, and facial expression is simply an example. Similarly, the frontal lobe generates behavior on the basis of internal or external information. If this information is not processed appropriately, then behavior will be disrupted. We return to this point later.

Role of the Temporal Lobe in Social Behavior

The temporal lobe includes neocortical tissue as well as limbic cortex (pyriform, entorhinal) and subcortical structures (amygdala, hippocampus). The temporal neocortices are rich in connections from the sensory systems, especially vision and audition, and to and from the frontal lobe. In addition, the temporal neocortex has a major projection into the medial temporal regions, and ultimately to the amygdala and hippocampus. The amygdala has important connections to both the frontal lobe and brainstem (see Amaral, this volume) and is presumed to play a central role in emotional behavior, especially fear (e.g., LeDoux, 1995).

One obvious difference in the left and right temporal cortices is that the left is clearly involved in language processing, whereas the right is involved in processing of faces (for a review, see Kolb & Whishaw, 1996). This dissociation leads to the prediction that there will be differences in the effects of left and right temporal lobe lesions both in the perception of faces as well as language. In addition, there are clear changes in personality after temporal lobe lesions, which suggest that damage to this region is likely to have some effect on emotion (e.g., Fedio & Martin, 1983). Indeed, there can be little doubt that both amygdala and temporal cortical lesions produce significant changes in the social behavior of nonhuman primates (e.g., Dicks et al., 1969; Franzen & Myers, 1973; Klüver & Bucy, 1939).

We would be remiss if we did not emphasize at this point that our patients with temporal lobe lesions have both anterior temporal cortex and amygdala removals. Thus, we are unable to distinguish the relative roles of these structures in the behavior we recorded in our patients. In addition, many of our patients had lesions that included some or all of the hippocampal formation. There was, however, no relationship between hippocampal removal and performance on any of our tasks, which leads us to conclude that the hippocampal formation is not playing a significant role in the performance of our tasks.

Tests of Emotional Behavior

• Production of Facial Expression

Patients with temporal lobe lesions produce as many spontaneous expressions in the course of standard testing as control subjects. When these patients were given the tasks of making facial expressions in response to the photographs or cartoons, their expressions were not significantly different from control subjects for the production of happiness, sadness, anger, or surprise, but they were markedly impaired at producing expressions of fear or disgust (figure 4.4). This result is difficult to interpret. In the photograph-matching task, the temporal lobe patients may have failed to identify the facial expressions of fear and disgust, or they may have been unable to produce the expressions. Similarly, in the cartoon-matching task, they may have not understood the fear-inducing context and thus failed to make the expression, or they may again simply be unable to make the expressions. Our hunch is that the deficit is one of perception, but this remains to be proven. At any rate, whatever the deficit in the temporal lobe patients might be, it is different from that of the frontal lobe patients who made fewer spontaneous expressions and were impaired at producing all types of expressions.

• Perception of Faces

There is little doubt that right temporal lobe patients are poor at the perception of faces (e.g., Milner, 1980). It was not surprising, therefore, that right temporal lesion patients responded randomly in our split-face matching task (figure 4.3). This result implies that right temporal lobe patients are processing faces differently from other patients. In contrast, patients with left temporal lesions did not differ from control subjects on the split faces task, which is consistent with their normal performance on many other tests of facial recognition (Milner, 1980).

• Perception of Facial Expression

Patients with left temporal lobe lesions matched the six key facial expressions to the photographs of spontaneous facial expressions as well as control subjects, regardless of the facial expression. In contrast, right temporal lobe patients were impaired at the photo matching for photographs illustrating fear or disgust (figure 4.5). Furthermore, like frontal lobe patients, the right temporal lobe patients were not impaired at matching photographs of happiness, sadness, anger, or surprise. This result is somewhat surprising because it implies that right temporal lobe patients are capable of recognizing these emotions in faces, even though they have difficulty in recognizing faces. This dissociation of recognizing the entire face and a component of the face has some precedent. Campbell et al. (1986) reported a dissociation of facial recognition and lip reading in two cases of occipital injury. One patient could recognize faces but could not lip read, whereas the other could do the reverse.

We anticipated that patients with right temporal lesions would be impaired at the recognition of the appropriate facial expression in the cartoon-matching task, but we did not expect a deficit in the left temporal lobe patients.Our predictions were only partially confirmed. Right temporal lobe patients did have difficulty in selecting the correct face, but so did the left temporal lobe patients, independent of the type of emotional situation (figure 4.6).

• Perception of Language and Prosody

On the basis of evidence from other types of neuropsychological study, one would predict that patients with left temporal lesions would be impaired at the task of matching verbal descriptors of emotion with sentences describing situations, whereas right temporal lobe patients would perform as control subjects. This was confirmed (Kolb & Taylor, 1981). Similarly, we had anticipated that right temporal lobe, but not left temporal lobe, patients would be impaired at the face–prosody matching task. In fact, both groups were impaired at the task, and neither group was as poor as the left dorsolateral frontal patients. This impairment was neither large nor selective, as the patients made about 5 more errors (out of 32) than control subjects, and these errors were distributed across emotional categories.

Asymmetry of Emotional Control

The idea that the two hemispheres might have a different roles in the control of emotion goes back at least to Goldstein (1939), who suggested that left hemisphere lesions produce "catastrophic" reactions characterized by fearfulness and depression, whereas right hemisphere lesions produce "indifference." The first systematic study of these contrasting behavioral effects was done by Gainotti in 1969, who showed that catastrophic reactions occurred in 62% of his left hemisphere sample, compared with only 10% of his right hemisphere cases. In contrast, indifference was more common in the right hemisphere patients, occurring in 38%, as compared with only 11% of the left hemisphere cases. Studies of the effects of sodium amobarbital (e.g., Terzian, 1964) reinforced this view, although there were dissenting opinions (e.g., Kolb & Milner, 1981). These early studies led to considerable interest in the possibility not only of cerebral asymmetry in the control of emotional behavior, but also in the idea of lateralized abnormalities being responsible for such illnesses as schizophrenia or depression (e.g., Flor-Henry, 1979). We can now point to multiple hypotheses regarding the role of the right and left hemispheres in emotional behavior. These theories can be grouped into four general categories:

1. The right hemisphere has a general superiority (or dominance) over the left hemisphere with respect to various aspects of emotional behavior (e.g., Gainotti, 1988; Ley & Bryden, 1982).
2. The two hemispheres have a complementary specialization for the control of different aspects of mood. In particular, the left hemisphere is considered to be dominant for "positive" emotions and the right hemisphere for "negative" emotions (e.g., Sackheim et al., 1982).
3. The right hemisphere is dominant for emotional expression in a manner parallel to that of the left hemisphere dominance for language (e.g., Ross, 1984).
4. The right hemisphere is dominant for the perception of emotion-related cues such as nuances of facial expression, body posture, and prosody (e.g., Adolphs et al., 1996; Rapesak et al., 1989).

These different theoretical positions have various nuances with different theorists, but, in general, this classification can summarize most views. Unfortunately, 30 years of study has not led to a clear resolution as to which theory, if any, best fits the available data (see Gainotti and Caltagirone, 1989). One of the major difficulties in resolving the difficulties in the different theories is that there is no agreed upon definition of what may be taken as evidence of emotional behavior (e.g., Gainotti, 1989). Furthermore, the different theoretical perspectives reflect a heterogeneous set of experimental situations in which data have been gathered. Thus, we see evidence gathered from situations as diverse as the study of brain-injured patients, sodium amobarbital injections, psychiatric patients, and various measures in normal subjects (e.g., EEG, event-related potential [ERP], positron emission tomography [PET]). It is difficult, if not impossible, to reconcile the different theoretical perspectives in light of the current heterogeneous evidence.

It is unlikely that the brain evolved an asymmetrical control of emotional behavior. Rather, it seems more likely that although there may be some asymmetry in the neural control of emotion, the observed asymmetries are largely a product of the asymmetrical control of other functions such as the control of movement, language, or the processing of complex sensory information. There are clear asymmetries in the control of each of these functions, and the selective disruption of any of these processes could certainly influence both cortical and subcortical structures that directly affect emotional behavior. For example, in our own studies we have been impressed by the relative asymmetry of the perception of verbal and facial material but the relative lack of asymmetry in the overall control of production of facial expressions. We have also been struck by the symmetry in the role of the temporal lobes in our tests of comprehension of emotional context and prosody.

We noted at the beginning of this chapter that we assume an evolutionary continuum in the control of emotional behavior. It strikes us that unless there is a good reason for evolution to localize functions to one hemisphere it is unlikely to happen. It is difficult for us to identify selection pressures a priori that would lateralize the control of emotional behavior or even to lateralize complementary aspects of emotional behavior. There are, however, sound reasons for expecting that functions related to emotional behavior would be localized, either in different cortical regions or in subcortical regions such as the amygdala or hypothalamus. There is a scant literature on the effects of localized lesions on emotional behavior of people, as most naturally occuring lesions do not respect neuroanatomical boundaries. Studies of nonhuman subjects such as nonhuman primates show no evidence of asymmetry but clear evidence of dissociable roles of the dorsolateral and inferior frontal areas, the amygdala, and the limbic cortex (see Kolb & Whishaw, 1996). Unfortunately, studies of emotional behavior in nonhuman subjects with neurological interventions has gone out of fashion, with the exception of the burgeoning literature on fear (e.g., LeDoux, 1995). It is our hope that behavioral neuroscientists will once again find the study of emotion worth pursuing in laboratory animals. Meanwhile, we are hopeful that recent advances in ERP and PET technology (see Reiman et al., this volume) may allow a clearer resolution of localization of functions in the normal human brain.

Conclusions

The results of our experiments lead us to several conclusions.

1. Changes in processes and functions related to emotion can be inferred from changes in overt behavior. One of the best ways to study changes in overt behavior is to study patients with focal cerebral injuries.
2. Damage to discrete neocortical areas alters overt behavior believed to be related to emotional state (e.g., facial expression).
3. The frontal lobe plays a special role in generating spontaneous behavior, examples of which are facial expression and talking.
4. The frontal lobe is important in controlling the processes necessary to comprehend emotions in others, especially as inferred from facial expression.
5. The temporal lobe (most likely the amygdala) plays an important role in the perception of emotionally relevant stimuli, especially those related to fear.
6. There is no simple asymmetry in the control of emotional behavior. There may be an asymmetry in the neural regulation of emotion-related behavior. Alternatively, the apparent asymmetrical effects of injury, or asymmetry in electrical or metabolic activity, with respect to emotional behavior may reflect asymmetrical control of processes such as sensory perception and movement control.

References

Adolphs, R., Damasio, H., Tranel, D. & Damasio, A. R. (1996). Cortical systems for the recognition of emotion in facial expressions. *Journal of Neuroscience, 16*, 7678–7687.

Benson, D. & Blumer, D. F. (1975). Personality changes with frontal and temporal lobe lesions. In D. F. Blumer & D. Benson D. (Eds), *Psychiatric Aspects of Neurological Disease* (pp. 151–170). New York: Grune & Stratton.

Blumer, D. F. & Benson, D. (Eds) (1975). *Psychiatric Aspects of Neurological Disease.* New York: Grune & Stratton.

Brownell, H. H., Michel, D., Powelson, J. & Gardner, H. (1983). Surprise but not coherence: sensitivity to verbal humor in right-hemisphere patients. *Brain and Language, 18*, 20–27.

Campbell, R., Landis, T. & Regard, M. (1986). Face recognition and lip reading: a neurological dissociation. *Brain, 109*, 509–521.

Darwin, C. (1872). *The Expression of Emotions in Man and Animals.* London: John Murray.

Davis, M. (1992). The role of the amygdala in conditioned fear. In J. P. Eggleton (Ed), *The Amygdala: Neurobiological Aspects of Emotion, Memory, and Mental Dysfunction* (pp. 255–306). New York: Wiley-Liss.

Dicks, D., Myers, R. E. & Kling, A. (1969). Uncus and amygdala lesions: effects on social behavior in the free-ranging monkey. *Science, 165*, 69–71.

Ekman, P. & Friesen, W. V. (1975). *Unmasking the Face.* Englewood Cliffs, NJ: Prentice-Hall.

Fedio, P. & Martin, A. (1983). Ideative-emotive behavioral characteristics of patients following left or right temporal lobectomy. *Epilepsia, 254*, S117–S130.

Flor-Henry, P. (1979). Schizophrenic-like reactions and affective psychoses associated with temporal lobe epilepsy. *American Journal of Psychiatry, 126*, 400–403.

Fuster, J. M. (1989). *The Prefrontal Cortex*, 2nd ed. New York: Raven Press.

Gainotti, G. (1969). Reactions "catastrophiques" et manifestations d'indifference au cours des atteintes cerebrales. *Neuropsychologia, 7*, 195–204.

Gainotti, G. (1988). Disorders of emotions and affects in patients with unilateral brain damage. In F. Boller & J. Grafman (Eds), *Handbook of Neuropsychology*. Amsterdam: Elsevier.

Gainotti, G. (1989). The meaning of emotional disturbances resulting from unilateral brain injury. In G. Gainotti & J. C. Caltagirone (Eds), *Emotions and the Dual Brain* (pp. 147–167). New York: Springer-Verlag.

Gainotti, G. & Caltagirone, C. (Eds) (1989). *Emotions and the Dual Brain*. New York: Springer-Verlag.

Gardner, H., Ling, P. K., Flamm, L. & Silverman, J. (1975). Comprehension and appreciation of humorous material following brain damage. *Brain, 98*, 399–412.

Goldman-Rakic, P. S. (1989). Circuitry of the primate prefrontal cortex and regulation of behavior by representational memory. In F. Blum (Ed), *Handbook of Physiology, Nervous System*, vol. V. *Higher Functions of the Brain, part 1*. Bethesda, MD: American Physiological Society.

Goldstein, K. (1939). *The Organism: A Holistic Approach to Biology, Derived from Pathological Data in Man*. New York: American Book.

Goltz, F. (1960). On the functions of the hemispheres. In G. von Bonin (Ed), *The Cerebral Cortex* (pp. 118–158). Springfield, IL: Charles C. Thomas.

Klüver, H. & Bucy, P. C. (1939). Preliminary analysis of the temporal lobes in monkeys. *Archives of Neurology and Psychiatry, 42*, 979–1000.

Kolb, B. & Milner, B. (1981). Observations on spontaneous facial expression after focal cerebral excisions and after intracarotid injection of sodium Amytal. *Neuropsychologia, 19*, 505–514.

Kolb, B., Milner, B. & Taylor, L. (1983). Perception of faces by patients with localized cortical excisions. *Canadian Journal of Psychology, 37*, 8–18.

Kolb, B. & Nonneman, A. (1975). The development of social responsiveness in kittens. *Animal Behavior, 23*, 368–374.

Kolb, B. & Taylor, L. (1981). Affective behavior in patients with localized cortical excisions: role of lesion site and side. *Science, 214*, 89–91.

Kolb, B. & Taylor, L. (1990). Neocortical substrates of emotional behavior. In N. L. Stein, B. Lewenthal & T. Trabasso (Eds), *Psychological and Biological Approaches to Emotion* (pp. 115–144). Hillsdale, NJ: Lawrence Erlbaum Associates.

Kolb, B. & Taylor, L. (1999a). *The production of facial expression and prosody in patients with focal cortical lesions*. Manuscript in preparation.

Kolb, B. & Taylor, L. (1999b). *The perception of facial expression and prosody in patients with focal cortical lesions*. Manuscript in preparation.

Kolb, B. & Whishaw, I. Q. (1996). *Fundamentals of Human Neuropsychology*, 4th ed. New York: W. H. Freeman & Co.

LeDoux, J. (1995). In search of an emotional system in the brain: leaping from fear to emotion and consciousness. In M. S. Gazzaniga (Ed), *The Cognitive Neurosciences* (pp. 1049–1062). Cambridge, MA: MIT Press.

Ley, R. G. & Bryden, M. P. (1982). Hemispheric differences in processing emotions and faces. *Brain and Language, 7*, 127–138.

Milner, B. (1964). Some effects of frontal lobectomy in man. In J. M. Warren & K. Akert (Eds), *The Frontal Granular Cortex and Behavior* (pp. 313–334). New York: McGraw-Hill.

Milner, B. (1980). Complementary functional specializations of the human cerebral hemispheres. *Pontificiae Academiae Scientiarulm Scripta Varia, 45*, 601–625.

Moyer, K. E. (1968). Kinds of aggression and their physiological basis. *Communications in Behavioral Biology, 2*, 65–87.

Nonneman, A. J. & Kolb, B. (1974). Lesions of hippocampus or prefrontal cortex alter species-typical behaviors in the cat. *Behavioral Biology, 12*, 41–54.

Passingham, R. E. (1993). *The Frontal Lobes and Voluntary Action*. Oxford: Oxford University Press.

Perrett, D. I., Smith, P., Potter, D., Mistlin, A. J., Head, A. S., Milner, A. D. & Jeeves, M. A. (1984). Neurons responsive to faces in the temporal cortex: studies of functional organization, sensitivity to identity and relation to perception. *Human Neurobiology, 3*, 197–208.

Rapcsak, S. Z., Kaszniak, A. W. & Rubens, A. B. (1989). Anomia for facial expressions: evidence for a category specific visual-verbal disconnection syndrome. *Neuropsychologia, 27*, 1031–1041.

Ross, E. D. (1981). The aprosodias: functional-anatomical organization of the affective components of language in the right hemisphere. *Archives of Neurology, 38*, 561–569.

Ross, E. D. (1984). Right hemisphere's role in language, affective behavior and emotion. *Trends in Neuroscience, 7*, 343–346.

Sackheim, H. A., Greenberg, M. S., Weiman, A. L., Gur, R. C., Hungerbuhler, J. P. & Geschwind, N. (1982). Hemispheric asymmetry in the expression of positive and negative emotions. *Archives of Neurology, 39*, 210–218.

Terzian, H. (1964). Behavioral and EEG effects of intracarotid sodium Amytal injection. *Acta Neurochirugica, 12*, 230–239.

Wolff, W. (1933). The experimental study of forms of expression. *Character and Personality, 2*, 168–176.

5

Recognizing Emotions
by Ear and by Eye

BEATRICE DE GELDER

Facial expression and tone of voice occupy prominent positions in the behavioral repertoires of higher animals. The production and perception of a whole range of facial and vocal emotional behaviors constitute an essential part of the communicative competence that complex social interactions in animals and humans are based upon. A wealth of studies has already documented the instrumental role of such facial and vocal cues in regulating social behavior. The goal of this chapter is to present a new domain of investigations dealing with a novel but specific question: How does the organism deal with the perceptual problem of multiple cues when each separately contains an emotional signal and when the two are present at the same time? The specific case I will look at is that of a facial expression present together with a tone of voice.

Two major issues are involved in recognizing emotions by ear and by eye. The first concerns the question of the perceptual combination of the auditory and visual inputs: Is there evidence that the voice and the face inputs are integrated in one percept, or, alternatively, are the visual and the auditory percepts combined after each has been fully processed and each is first perceived separately? The second question relates to processing resources: Are there separate processing resources for recognizing facial and vocal emotions, or do these two recognition systems share the same functional and/or neuroanatomical resources? In the former case one would expect two more or less modality-specific systems for emotion recognition. This chapter briefly refers to historical antecedents of both the first and the second questions and subsequently presents research relevant to the first one.

In the first part of this chapter I review studies on the recognition of face and voice expressions to highlight some aspects that are relevant for understanding multimodal emotion perception and that relate to the issues of common processing resources and of multimodal perception. In the second part I present research that has specifically looked into the processing of emotional information presented in the voice and the face.

Historical Background

It is widely accepted that the voice and the face can, in principle, independently convey the same information about people's emotional states. As a consequence, for all practical purposes, seeing an angry face or hearing an angry voice leads to the same perception and these two different sensory cues conveying the same information are interchangeable. Indeed, when we view perception of emotional cues from the perspective of readiness for appropriate action, the sensory channel that provides the critical affective information, whether it is hearing the voice or seeing the face, matters very little. The notion that different sense modalities can convey the same message is part of our common sense view that to show an angry face or to sound angry means simply to be angry (Austin, 1970). The two different sensory representations carry the same content and to perceive either one of those behavioral displays is tantamount to perceiving the emotions themselves. Such a role for common sense in communication was already anticipated by Aristotle's concept of a *sensus communis*.

Nonetheless, concerns about the specificity of each sensory modality also have a long history. One notorious debate concerns the impact of the various senses on our intellectual concepts. Empiricists such as Locke wondered whether the mind has separate auditory, tactile, or visual representations, a historical debate exemplified in the literature as the "Molyneux question" (Locke, 1689). If this were the case, how does the human mind put together in a single abstract concept a representation with such different sensory origins? This question has also occupied developmental psychologists. Piaget (1952) is among the best known defenders of the view that at birth the different sensory systems or sense modalities exist in isolation and operate separately. Convergence, interaction, and integration of different sensorial inputs is the consequence of development and thus of the organisms' experience with the external world. Developmental psychology as represented by Piaget viewed abstract or intellectual representations as the products of a gradual emergence of thought processes out of sensory systems. For example, synesthesia is reputedly frequent in neonates (Lewkovicz, 1986). Its occurrence in later life is sometimes traced back to a developmental accident in the separation of the sensory channels. The entirely opposite view has also been defended. For example, Gibson (1966), Werner (1973), and Bower (1974) have argued that the neonate has a single multimodal system out of which the different senses develop over time. This question continues to interest developmental psychologists (Meltzoff, 1990).

The relevance of these long-standing epistemological and developmental concerns is now actualized by present-day scientific developments. Recent research by cognitive neuroscientists has tended to replace the notion of a unitary mind with conscious abstract representations with that of a complex architecture of interrelated modules by and large operating outside the scope of consciousness. Over the last decades, the study of the cognitive abilities of brain-damaged patients has provided us with a wealth of examples of selective loss of cognitive skills accompanied or not by loss of awareness (Weiskrantz, 1997). For example, even within the visual system there is evidence that separate representations subserve perception and action (Milner & Goodale, 1995). Such findings have challenged the idea of a single abstract concept of the visual object. More directly related to the issue of multimodality are the frequent observations made with patients suffering from visual agnosia. These patients have lost visual recognition of objects, but their tactile and/or their auditory recognition is often still intact (see Humphreys & Riddoch, 1987, for an extensive description of such a case). Other evidence is provided by studies of bimodal speech recognition. For example, in the case of representations in working memory the issue has been raised whether information about the actual input modality is also stored together with the content of the representation itself. The answer appears to be positive, as illustrated by studies of serial recall where the recency of the last auditorily presented item is reduced by a lip-read suffix—for example, a series of digits presented in the auditory modality only is followed by a digit only presented though speech reading (e.g., de Gelder & Vroomen, 1994). Thus, in the domain of bimodal speech there is increasing evidence that some degree of sensory specificity is preserved in higher cognitive processes.

Single Modality Studies of Face Emotion Recognition

Many studies on emotion recognition have used faces as stimuli to the point of suggesting that the face is the most telling bearer of an organism's emotional state. Recognition of facial expressions has been studied in its own right. It is not my goal to review these studies in any detail, except to mention some recent issues that have implications for the topic of this chapter, the relation between facial and vocal expression recognition. One such issue is the notion of basic emotion categories. Another is the question of whether it is the face as a whole or as the emergent configuration that is the bearer of the expression. Still another possibly relevant issue relates to the possible link between face and voice expressions via the production of emotional expression. Finally, I refer to questions that concern the neuroanatomical basis of emotion recognition in the face and the voice.

Basic Emotions

Empirical research on the universality of facial emotions is usually traced back to Darwin's (1872) views on the function of facial expressions. Ekman (1992) and collaborators have taken up this challenge and argued convincingly that a small set of emotions are universal. This debate is outside the scope of this chapter, except possibly for one aspect which concerns the grounds on which universality has occasionally been claimed—that is the sole link between emotion and action.

Some emotion theories have taken up Darwin's notion of a close link between emotion and action (see Frijda, 1989, for an overview). Such a view contains an intriguing suggestion about a common origin of facial and vocal expressions. The notion is that there is an intrinsic link between voice and face emotions based on the joint production of the two in one single facial gesture. A similar idea was developed in detail for the case of speech. The approach is known as the motor theory of speech perception (Liberman & Mattingley, 1985). Crudely stated, this view holds that speech sounds can be traced back to speech gestures defined as the movement patterns of the speech-producing apparatus rather than as abstract entities. The corollary of this view is particularly intriguing. It holds that the ability to recognize speech is based on the perceiver's ability to retrieve the underlying pattern of speech-production gestures upon hearing the speech sounds. The universality of human speech sounds is thus rooted in morpho-anatomical similarities across members of the species.

Facial Expressions: Parts Versus Wholes

Is the expression we spontaneously recognize in a face carried by the face as a whole or by one or more of its features perceived separately? There is little research available to answer that question. It is unclear whether the face as a whole or one or another part of the face (e.g., eyes, eyebrows, mouth) plays a more predominant role. Still, there are some indications that the eyes and the eyebrows play a relatively predominant role (Puce et al., 1996).

One means by which this issue has recently been explored is by using the well-known face inversion effect, familiar from studies that have explored identity recognition (Yin, 1969). The fact that it is much easier to match identical faces when these are presented upright than upside down is generally explained by the loss of configuration information when a face is inverted. This loss of configuration information makes it much more difficult to access information about personal identity. Does a similar situation obtain for access to expression information? Some recent findings seem to point in that direction. It is known that inverting the face makes it much harder to recognize the expression (de Gelder et al., 1997b; Searcy & Bartlett, 1996; Teunisse & de Gelder, in press). On the other hand, clear-cut categorical decisions about what expression is displayed are easier when only the upper part of the face carries the affective message and the lower part is neutral than when the full face is shown. In contrast, categorization performance is virtually random when the information critical for recognizing the expression is contained only in the lower face with the upper part of the face remaining neutral (de Gelder et al., 1998b). One should expect, though, that the relative importance of some parts over others is a function of the emotion being considered. In our study mentioned above, the importance of the upper face part was very clear for anger, sadness, and fear but did not obtain with happiness.

Whether or not recognition of facial expressions is whole face or component based is also likely to be relevant for understanding what happens when information from the face and from the voice are combined. If expression recognition results from sampling separate facial components, as argued by Ellison and Massaro (1997), it follows that each face component on its own can combine with the information about affect present in the voice and that the least informative facial feature would profit the most from the combination with a voice. But this turns out not to be the case (de Gelder et al., 1998b).

Categorical Perception

A recent approach to understanding the perception of facial expression has focused on the question of a few distinct categories, so-called basic emotions. The notion of basic categories is familiar from the speech literature, where the argument about abstract speech categories has been made for a long time (for a historic overview, see Liberman, 1996). Categorical perception of speech was originally advanced in support of the uniqueness of speech processing. The theoretical notion was that categorical perception of sounds would only be found for the specific range of speech sounds and not for auditory stimuli in general. Such findings fueled the claim that processing of linguistic information is dealt with by a specialized processor or module. The categorical perception paradigm was thus used to explore what might be the basic components of the spoken language processing ability. One might thus apply this argument to the domain of emotion perception. More specifically, the long-standing issue concerning the existence of basic emotion categories might be studied with the methodology typical of categorical perception research in order to answer the question of the existence of basic emotions.

A beginning has been made with such a research program. Recent studies have lent support to the notion of categories underlying the perception of emotions in line-drawn facial expressions (Etcoff & Magee, 1992). Using stimuli obtained by morphing between two photographs of different posed expressions, we obtained evidence for categorical perception of facial expressions in adults as well as in children (de Gelder et al., 1997b; see also Calder et al., 1996). Neuropsychological evidence about impaired categorical perception in autistic individuals (Teunisse & de Gelder, in press) and in prosopagnosia patients (de Gelder & Vroomen, 1996; de Gelder et al., 1997a) adds support to the tentative inference of basic categories of facial expressions. But some caution is in order. In some of these studies the conclusion was that findings about categorical perception of face expressions illustrate the existence of basic emotion categories. But results from those studies do not allow generalizations reaching beyond emotions in the face and do not allow inferences about abstract or supramodal emotion categories, nor can they make claims about a similar set of basic emotions that would be expressed in the voice and in the face.

Neuroanantomical Basis of Facial Emotion Recognition

A long-standing motivation of students of facial expression recognition has been to clarify the specific neuroanatomical basis of understanding facial expressions (Gainotti, 1972, 1989). The special role of the right hemisphere is well documented in studies of normal subjects. Presentation in the left visual field enhances recognition of facial expressions (Landis et al., 1979; Suberi & McKeever, 1977). This right hemisphere dominance extends as well to the production of facial expressions. The left side of the face seems to be more fluent at posing facial expressions (Bruyer, 1981; Dopson et al., 1984). Studies of unilaterally brain-damaged patients present converging evidence. However, not all authors agree on the right hemisphere privilege (e.g., Delis et al., 1988; Ekman et al., 1988), and the suggestion has been made that this claim should be restricted to negative emotions only (Ahern & Schwartz, 1985; Davidson & Tomarken, 1989).

Single Modality Studies of Voice Affect

The voice is an equally informative source for perception of a speaker's emotions as facial expression. Various authors have hinted at systematic correlation between emotions and acoustic parameters (Darwin, 1872; Ekman, 1992). But the study of how the voice conveys emotions is still in its infancy. Early studies highlighted pitch as the best cue (Williams & Stevens, 1972). Duration and intensity are also taken to play an important role (Murray & Arnott, 1993). The consensus is that there is no unique acoustic correlate for each basic emotion. Johnson and co-workers (1986) obtained good recognition rates for basic emotions expressed in a spoken sentence. Other authors have presented evidence from recognition of expression in an isolated word (Pollack et al., 1960; Scott et al., 1997). Moreover, there may also be marked individual differences in the way speakers use acoustic parameters to express one or another emotion (Lieberman & Michaels, 1962). A study by Scherer (1979) shows a fair degree of confusion between the expressions of many emotions in the voice. This evidence adds to the few data showing that vocal emotions are not always easy to distinguish. It also shows asymmetries between facial and vocal emotions that are puzzling for the common-sense view of transparent and interchangeable emotions expressions. For example, happiness is the easiest to recognize facial emotion, but when expressed in the voice only, happiness is quite hard to distinguish from a neutral expression (Scherer, 1979; Vroomen et al., 1993).

Research on affect in the voice has also been concerned with understanding the neuroanatomical basis of vocal emotions. Apparently the same situation holds for the locus of processing affective information in the voice. The bulk of the evidence supports the notion of a right hemisphere dominance (see van Lancker, 1997, for review). Evidence from dichotic studies with normal subjects (Carmon & Nachshon, 1973; Mahoney & Sainsbury, 1987) tends to favor a right hemisphere advantage for affective prosody. The role of the right hemisphere was also confirmed by recent data from a functional magnetic resonance imaging study (George et al., 1996). Researchers have used designs where the processing of affective versus propositional content was contrasted. Patients with right hemisphere damage are impaired in recognizing prosody (van Lancker & Sidtis, 1992), but process other aspects of language in the same way as normal controls.

Correspondences between Voice and Face Emotion

In the light of recent studies on the neuroanatomy of emotions and the involvement of multiple centers, concerns with hemispheric dominance may now seem a bit crude. But even if the dominant concern was the issue of laterality and whether face and voice affect were similarly localized, a companion theme is that of possibly amodal representations that would be implicated in the two sensory input systems.

A few studies represented a theoretically more ambitious approach and selected patients with either voice or face affect impairments and examined whether a symmetrical impairment was found in the other modality. Van Lancker and Sidtis (1992) investigated whether patients suffering from aprosodia or a deficit in the ability to process prosody were also impaired in facial expression recognition. A similar approach was taken in a study by Scott et al. (1997) examining perception of prosody in an amygdalectomy patient suffering from impaired recognition of facial expression. The authors report a corresponding impairment in recognition of voice expression. However, the obtained evidence is only partially convincing because it is based on correlations only. The existence of an association between deficits does not allow inferences about combined processing of affect in the face and the voice or about common processing resources or supramodal representations.

Other studies have compared the perception of voice affect with processing of propositional emotional content. Does a deficit in recognizing voice and/or face affect also manifest itself in an impaired understanding of the emotional meaning of a word or a sentence? Some studies found that these impairments were associated (Semenza et al., 1986). Others found that voice and/or face affect impairments could leave intact the ability to perceive emotion from the content of a word or sentence (Schmitt et al., 1997). The data are still too limited to allow any firm conclusions. Evidence of a clear-cut dissociation between the perceptual processes of face and voice affect and the linguistic processes of understanding propositional content would be important for a theoretical clarification of the contrast between perceptual and more cognitive aspects of emotional experience.

Are emotions expressed in the voice also perceived categorically, as has been claimed for emotions in the face? The classical methodology for the study of perceptual categories in speech can also be applied to the perception of emotion categories in the voice. Vroomen and de Gelder (1996) created a continuum between two natural tokens of semantically neutral utterances that were pronounced either in an anxious or in a happy voice. The manipulation consisted in varying the prosodic characteristics of the speech in equal physical steps. Subjects perceived the tokens categorically in the sense described above. This result suggests that there might be distinct expression categories in the voice also. It remains to be seen whether these basic voice emotion categories are the same ones argued to exist for the face.

Multimodal Perception: General Issues

The investigation of simultaneous information processing in more than one modality represents a small but fascinating field of research for cognitive psychologists and neuroscientists alike. One central phenomenon which has been explored for some decades now is ventriloquism, a situation where the perceiver attributes a voice he hears to the silent movement of the lips from another speaker (see Bertelson, 1998, for an overview). This phenomenon is mandatory, and the integration it produces is not under attentional control (Bertelson et al., in press).

A somewhat different case directly relevant here is that of speech reading or processing speech by ear and by eye. It is well known that both hearing the voice and watching the mouth movements allow one to understand spoken language. Yet in normal day-to-day circumstances the two different sensory inputs are present together and combined by the viewer/listener. The McGurk effect illustrates most dramatically the automatic and compulsory nature of this combination (McGurk & McDonald, 1976). In the McGurk effect, an experimental situation is created where a different syllable is conveyed by the information from vision and from audition. When asked to repeat what the speaker said, the viewer/listener reports a percept that is neither the heard (/ba/) nor the seen one (/ga/), but a blend, a fusion (like when a /da/ is reported) or both. Researchers agree now that understanding how spoken language competence is implemented in the two different modalities is essential for theories of spoken language competence and for understanding its neurofunctional implementation (Calvert et al., 1997).

Various models have been developed to understand audiovisual speech, and there is a rapidly increasing set of research results to test them. The two central questions reviewed above, that of sensory-specific processing routes and that of the combination in a single percept, have occupied center stage in this research over the last decade. Various explanations have been proposed for this situation: One is a complete autonomy of the input modalities; another is that independent processes take place in each modality separately. A third theory proposes audio-visual integration with or without shared processing structures (see Campbell et al., 1998; Dodd & Campbell, 1987, for overviews and Summerfield, 1992, for a discussion of different theoretical models). No single theoretical framework can at present account for the rapidly increasing mass of data. But existing models all seem to share the view that a theory that assumes the same abstract representations for the perception of both heard and seen speech must be incomplete or cannot account for the facts (see Massaro, 1998, for discussion).

Concurrent Cues and the Uses of Redundancy

The case of speech perceived by the ear as well as by the eye has an obvious parallel in the perception of emotion. In regard to vision, the organism is also often confronted with two concurrent inputs, each of them sufficient for recognizing an emotion. What would be the point of having more than just one input channel for what appears as equivalent bits of information? Such redundancy is not surprising in biological systems. But could the system actually be put together such that it can benefit from redundancy to achieve a more efficient behavioral response? Could one input system function as a backup in case of poor perceptual conditions including a breakdown of the other? Or does the organism also in normal conditions process the two inputs interactively so as to come to a more efficient response? This latter hypothesis is at the base of our research.

The first situation obtains when one of the two input channels functions as a backup system in conditions of difficult or impaired perception in the other modality. Such cases are, for example, that of noise of one channel such as difficulty hearing the speaker, but also a sensory deficit like loss of eyesight. For example, with increasing hearing loss the contribution from lip reading becomes more critical for understanding spoken language. Likewise, patients suffering from prosopagnosia that includes facial expression recognition can still tell people apart by the voice, just as loss of facial expression recognition leaves recognition of affective prosody intact and vice versa (van Lancker, 1997).

The notion that speech reading is simply available as a backup system was popular for a while among students of bimodal speech. But this hypothesis did not turn out to be satisfactory because findings showed that even in the case where one input channel was entirely nonambiguous as in normal hearing adults, the other presumably redundant channel was still processed fully.

A different possibility is that the two input systems are complementary. Such a process would be useful when there is intrinsic ambiguity in the input above and beyond the case of peripheral receptive problems just mentioned. Again, this alternative was popular for a while among students of audiovisual speech. The idea was that the visual modality complements the processing of the auditory input because it is eminently suited to provide information about place of articulation. This proposal sounded like a rational use of redundancy, but in the case of audio-visual speech it was not born out by the facts. It may be useful, though, for under-standing audiovisual emotions, at least to some extent. Complementary systems sounds like an interesting possibility, given that audition and vision differ with respect to the emotions they convey best. For example, happiness is easy to tell from the face, but when present only in the voice, it is often confused with a neutral prosody or with surprise. From the literature one gathers the impression that confusions for visible emotions would not be the same as for auditory inputs. In other words, the emotions that are more easily confused in the voice are not the same as those generating confusion in understanding facial expressions.

The research presented below was inspired by a more challenging hypothesis than that of either a secondary backup system or of two systems complement-ing each other. We set out to determine whether the best use the organism could make of redundancy would be to combine the two inputs as early as possible in the processing. Our belief was that exploiting the redundancy in all cases would lead to a faster behavioral response, whereas individual processing followed by combination should take longer. This idea was empirically testable because we could compare speed of response in the unimodal versus bimodal situation. From this perspective combination of inputs would improve the efficiency of the re-sponse.

Perceiving Emotions by Ear and by Eye

The situation where a voice and a face expression both signal an emotion is familiar from everyday life, but it has not caught the attention of laboratory researchers. The implicit assumption that information from the face and from the ear are both dealt with by the same processor and computed in an amodal representation system might partially explain this lacuna. Walker and Grolnick (1983) studied the inter-modal perception of emotions in infants by presenting faces combined with voices. Five- to seven-month-old infants looked longer at the face that carried the same expression as the voice than at the one carrying a different expression. Tartter and Braun (1994) studied the perception of the emotional meaning of syllables as a function of the facial expression the speaker had adopted in pronouncing them. They observed that a listener could gather the emotional expression of the face from listening to the syllables only. The finding that listeners can determine a speaker's emotional expression suggests that they might retrieve a production link between two separate inputs, the intonation of the voice and the expression on the face. As noted above, such an approach was defended in the earlier motor theory of speech perception. It is at the heart of some ecological approaches to understand-ing the processing of speech sounds (e.g., Fowler, 1996). Finally, the question raised in a recent study by Massaro and Egan (1996) comes close to the work described in more detail below. These authors used a synthetic face combined with a spoken word and reported evidence for the perceptual combination of both.

In our own studies we have adopted an experimental situation that is familiar from the work by McGurk and McDonald (1976) showing that concurrently presented but incompatible information provided by the lips and by the voice leads to an illusory percept (see above). The paradigm that has been extensively used to examine the combination of auditory with visual information in speech perception is a variant of the categorical perception paradigm. In a number of experiments, Massaro (1987) and collaborators have shown that adding lip-read information has an impact on the location of the auditory identification curve. In a typical experiment, a visual stimulus /da/ is combined each time with one of the stimuli of an auditory stimulus continuum obtained by stepwise synthesis between a natural spoken /ba/ and /ga/. The combination of a visual and auditory syllable changes the way the auditory syllable is perceived. One observes a displacement of the identification curve to the right or to the left depending on whether a visual /da/ or /ba/ is added. McGurk effects have also been observed for the combination of a still face and a voice (Campbell, 1996). This cross-modal bias is very robust and is obtained in a condition of integration in which subjects are asked to repeat what the speaker says, as well as in a condition of selective attention when subjects are instructed to attend to either the auditory or the visual information (see Massaro, 1987, for an overview).

Of course, the cross-modal paradigm used in the McGurk situation presents a highly artificial stimulus combination. Concurrent audition and vision are the normal situation for speech as well as for emotion expressions, and incongruent information in the two inputs is definitely not ecological. The experimental situation whereby an audiovisual conflict is generated does, however, provide a paradigm that allows us to separate the two processing streams and create conditions for observing their interaction. Of course, one may even wonder if an experimental situation of the kind presented below, where subjects are instructed to combine what they hear with what they see, actually corresponds to the normal perceptual situation. Evidence that subjects do combine the inputs might then be an artifact created by the instructions, and the data would reflect the decision strategy the subject adopts in the presence of two different inputs of which he or she is separately aware rather than a mandatory integration of both in the course of perception. Our experiments were designed to test directly these assumptions and to rule out such an explanation.

Behavioral Evidence for Cross-modal Effects between Voice and Face

In a series of recent experiments we tackled one aspect of bimodal processing concerned with the combination of the auditory and visual source and its effect on the latencies and the judgment of the displayed emotion. Our experiments used the paradigm of cross-modal bias. We first set out to examine the effect of a combination of a voice and facial expression. The faces were taken from a continuum extending between two posed tokens expressing sadness and happiness. The two tones of the voice were also sad and happy. On each bimodal trial, a still photograph of a face was presented on the screen while a voice was heard pronouncing a sentence in one of two affective tones. Subjects were instructed to judge the emotion of the person (experiment 1; de Gelder & Vroomen, 1995; submitted). We observed a huge difference in how the face was rated in the presence of either one of the two voices compared with the situation when only the face had to be recognized. Of particular interest are the bimodal trials. When the expression in the voice and that on the face are congruent, subjects are faster at judging the expression than when they only receive one input. When an ambiguous face stimulus is presented, the rating of the face is strongly affected by the concurrent voice. The result appears to provide strong evidence for the combination of voice and face information in the course of processing the emotional content.

The question prompted by such a result is whether such a combination will still take place when the subject's attention is focused only on one of the two sources. In other words, will this cross-modal effect resist an attention manipulation in which subjects are explicitly told to ignore one of the sources? It may indeed be argued that the task of judging the emotion generated by combining a still face and a spoken sentence is an artificial one and that the observed effects are due to the compelling instructions rather than presenting any evidence for how the processing system operates. The instruction might have functioned as an explicit cue to put together a voice and a face. The suspicion that the effect is due to instructions and depends on explicit attention to the two channels is reinforced by the fact that still faces were used. This method was used because of technical constraints: dubbing a face with a different voice is difficult to achieve when the auditory stimulus is a whole sentence and not just a phoneme or a short syllable as in the McGurk situation.

The same experiment was thus repeated but with different instructions (experiment 2; de Gelder & Vroomen, 1995; submitted). We now instructed the subjects to strictly judge the face only and to ignore any auditory information. The results showed that modifying the instructions did not change the basic pattern of results. We again observed a perceptual shift and noted that here also the voice has a significant effect on how the face was judged. Also, subjects are faster when they respond in the presence of two congruent inputs (happy face and happy voice) than when they are perceiving a face only (figure 5.1).

Because the recognition of a facial expression is affected by a concurrently presented voice even if the perceiver does not pay any attention to the voice, we may conclude that the combination of audition and vision is automatic. Such automatic effects or mandatory phenomena are contrasted with postperceptual effects like the ones that result from a subjective decision, as when the subject is first aware of the incongruity between the two inputs and subsequently decides using his or her judgment. Audiovisual emotion recognition thus resembles audiovisual speech and ventriloquism in this respect of being mandatory and perceptual (Bertelson et al., in press).

This finding was sufficiently promising to ask whether the reverse effect would also obtain. Is processing of voice affected by concurrently presented visual information? We examined this question by designing a situation similar to the previous one where the task was to judge the expression in the voice while ignoring the information concurrently conveyed by the face. The answer to this question is

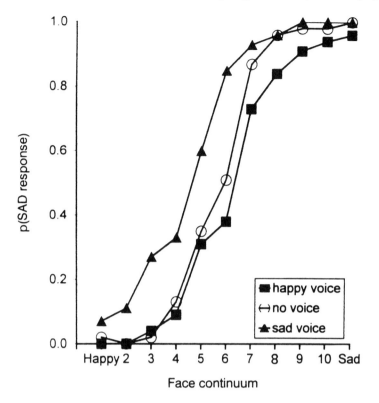

Figure 5.1. Proportion of sad responses as a function of the face continuum when combined with the happy, sad, and no voice.

clearly positive (experiment 3; de Gelder & Vroomen, submitted; see figure 5.2).
The impact of the face on the voice obtains with upright but not with inverted
faces (de Gelder et al., 1998b).

The observed phenomenon of cross-modal bias in the perception of emotion
by ear and by eye is particularly striking because it is obtained in a situation that
does not mimic the natural situation. In fact, our experimental situation only super-
ficially resembles the natural, ecological situation of concurrent inputs. Normally
the face and the voice express the same emotion. It is interesting that the system
is nevertheless strongly biased toward putting together information from voice and
face. Subjects are sometimes aware of an inconsistency between the voice and the
face expression, but this phenomenal impression of inconsistency between the two
sources seems to belong to a different, possibly higher and conscious level of
processing that does not interfere with the compelling bias of the processing system
for combining the two.

Our studies indicate that information from hearing the voice combines early
on with the processing of information from seeing the face and vice versa. But it
is important to note that this result is still compatible with the notion that processing of emotion in the face and in the voice is carried out in different, modality-

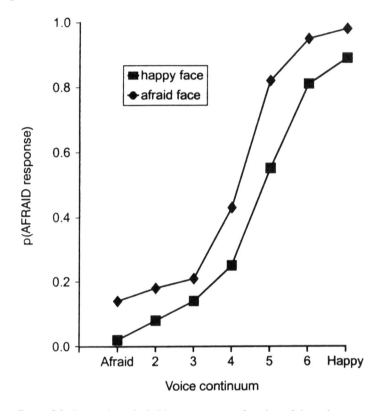

Figure 5.2. Proportion of afraid responses as a function of the voice continuum when combined with the happy and afraid face.

specific representation systems. Integration takes place after the respective sensory sources have been fully processed, as in late integration models. Such an approach has similarities with a standard late integration view of the Stroop effect (McLeod, 1991). A different approach to audiovisual theories is to postulate recoding of the input representation. Different alternatives can be considered here. Either one source is recoded into the representational system of the other (e.g., visual representations are recodded into auditory ones), or both sensory representations are recoded into a supramodal abstract representation system. A third possibility is that information in the two modalities is extracted in parallel. A version of this latter view has been defended by Massaro and collaborators. It assumes that auditory and visual features are first evaluated separately and next integrated according to a multiplicative formula before a decision is made (Massaro & Egan, 1996).

Sound theoretical preferences for one or another model require more data than are currently available. Two major issues for future research are that of the time course of the audiovisual combination at the basis of the cross-modal bias and that of the domains of information that do interact.

Regarding the time course of combination, our reaction time data as well as the robustness of the bias effect with the attention manipulation are compatible with the notion of an early integration. But a full answer to the question on the time course of integration may require evidence from other than strictly behavioral methods as argued by Stein and Meredith (1993). The question of interacting domains concerns the respective phenomena in each modality that are likely to integrate. This issue is critical for understanding the nature of the phenomenon, and it is unlikely to be settled by models that are intended to fit any situation where information from two sources is presented (Massaro & Egan, 1996). Such models deal with integration as only a quantitative issue, not considering the possibility of constraints from content specificity on bimodal pairings.

The Time Course of Audiovisual Emotion Perception: An Electrophysiological Study

When does the mind/brain put together what it hears and what it sees? An answer to this question has been pursued by cognitive psychologists applying detailed chronometric methods and results have made the case that we are dealing with truly perceptual phenomena where combination of the input streams is mandatory, not reflecting a perceptual bias or a postperceptual decision process under subjective control. The observation of shorter latencies with congruent voice–face combinations over presentations of the face only indicates that it is somehow more efficient for the system to receive bimodal input. What functional and neuroanatomical model underlies this apparent gain? One possibility is that inputs are combined early on and that the combination allows for a faster percept. But shorter latencies with congruent bimodal representations are also compatible with a race model based on the assumption that the input that is processed fastest determines the outcome.

The method of recording event-related potentials (ERPs) allows us to address issues of the time course of cognitive processes at stake in understanding language (for analysis, see Kutas & Dale, 1997). Event-related potentials have been used to study recognition of face processing and of voice expressions. But the combination of voice and face expressions has so far not been the focus of any study. Yet the tools are there to address this issue. There exists an ERP component known to be sensitive only to one modality, but it might be useful in the study of combined inputs also, the mismatch negativity (MMN), which is known to reflect processing of auditory stimuli (see Näätänen, 1992, for an overview). The MMN is elicited by a deviant stimulus in a repetitive train of standard auditory stimuli. It is an autonomous brainwave not controlled by attention, and its amplitude is larger for larger differences between the standard and deviant stimuli as well as for subjects who show a greater sensitivity to that change at the behavioral level. So far, only one study not concerned with emotion has tried to gather evidence for combined processing of auditory and visual inputs by asking whether the visual stimulus could have an impact on the processing of the auditory one. Sams et al. (1991) did record the magnetic counterpart of the MMN (MMN_m) contingent upon a change in visual stimuli using auditory presentation of a Finnish syllable, /ka/, combined with the visual presentation of face and jaw movements belonging to /ka/.

Subjects perceived either /ka/ or /ta/ (cf. the McGurk effect). They observed an MMN_m which started at 180 ms and was localized in the left supratemporal auditory cortex.

Recently we exploited the potential of the MMN for tracing the early combination of the affective tone of the voice with information provided by the expression of the face (de Gelder et al., 1999). Subjects receive concurrent voice and face stimulation, but the face sometimes carries an incongruent emotional expression (such as realized in the McGurk effect for speech). If the system is tuned to combine this dual input, as was suggested by our behavioral experiments, and if this combination consists of an early influence of the face input on the processing of the voice, this will be reflected in an MMN, or other auditory ERP components. If not, only the visual ERP components will be affected.

Our results indicate that when after a number of presentations of a voice–face pair both with the same expression, a pair is presented where the expression of the face is different, an early (100–200 ms) ERP component is elicited which strongly resembles the MMN typically associated with detection of a change in the auditory input (Näätänen, 1992). The distribution (Fz maximum) and latency (178 ms) are compatible with those of the MMN (Näätänen, 1992).

This result is the first evidence from brain-imaging techniques about the combination of auditory and visual input in the course of processing emotional messages. Besides results from behavioral studies indicating mandatory integration of face and voice information, the only suggestion so far about underlying processes has come from the observation that there is an impairment in recognizing emotions in the voice and the face in a patient with bilateral amygdala damage (Scott et al., 1997). But as we noted before, the latter evidence is only about an association of deficits and is uninformative about the question of combined processing of common representations.

The major theoretical importance of the ERP study consists in the direct evidence that face and voice input are combined early, at the latest at 178 ms after voice onset. This corroborates the conclusion based on behavioral research that supported an early combination of face and voice expressions. The behavioral data show that the identification of the voice expression is hampered by a simultaneously presented incongruous face. But the present eletrophysiological evidence that both inputs are combined at an early stage seems to rule out one of the alternatives left open by the behavioral results, that of a race model between separately processed faces and voices.

Exploring the Boundaries of a Modular Emotion Processor

I have focused on the perception of emotion by ear and by eye and summarized studies showing that the processing system combines these two input channels and does this in such a way as to arrive at an optimal behavioral response. It would, however, be counterproductive for a processing system capable of working on mutimodal combinations of inputs to do so in an unconstrained manner. So far I have not raised the issue of a selection mechanism or a gating of preliminary filter function that might be at work before input combinations are realized. The studies presented raise a host of questions having to do with the constraints on the inputs that are likely candidates for combination as well as the boundaries within which combination of inputs will be successful. Constraints might relate to spatial and temporal contiguity of the inputs, an issue I have not explored so far. A different type of constraints I anticipate will be important concern content and format. Common content is probably a critical constraint. The content condition is clearly satisfied in the audiovisual speech case where both stimuli contain speech information. But more specific constraints about the input format may also operate. For example, in the case where speech information is presented in combination with musical notes or environmental sounds, there is no interference or combination of the two input sources (Crowder & Surprenant, 1995). Will the emotion processing system also combine a face and an environmental sound other than speech, and will it combine a face expression with a written message carrying an affective content? If by module we mean a content-based system whose operations are mandatory, then audiovisual emotion seems to present us with a prime example of such a module.

A cross-modal paradigm like the one described in our studies provides a methodology for exploring the notion of a dedicated functional mechanism for affective processing. Experimental situations of bimodal stimulus presentation with either congruent or conflicting inputs are thus a good way to explore the domain of a possible specialized mechanism. Research in progress investigates whether audiovisual bias still holds across differences in gender between the voice and the face but does not occur when the auditory information is an environmental sound instead of a human voice (de Gelder and Vroomen, in preparation).

The Where of Bimodal Perception

There are a number of different aspects to the question about where in the mind/brain inputs from different modalities are combined and assimilated. What are the neural pathways relaying visual input to the auditory cortex, and what type of representations are involved? This information may be transferred via direct routes (corticocortical; for a review, see Weiskrantz, 1997) and/or indirect (relayed via subcortical structures), via neural pathways between striate and peristriate cortex, and via temporal areas which may transfer visual information about faces and facial emotions to the temporal lobe. A subcortical structure that may play a role is the amygdala, which is involved in the perception of emotions (Breitner et al., 1996; Morris et al., 1996). The amygdala sends projections to and receives input from different cortical areas including temporal and parietal cortices (Leonard et al., 1985). The amygdala also plays a role in cross-modal transfer for positively valenced situations (Nahm et al., 1993). The combination of a voice with a face may lead to a modulation of activation in the amygdala. Such a finding would suggest that affective prosody just as facial expressions is processed in the amygdala, but it may also indicate that the amygdala plays a role in combining voice and face information. It may also be the case that aside from the locus of such a modulation specific for the emotional content, other structures such as the anterior cingulate or the insula are involved in actively combining input from several sensory sources. This suggestion is tentatively supported by the particular deficits in audiovisual integration of patients suffering from Huntington disease, a degenerative brain disorder that attacks subcortical structures (de Gelder et al., 1997a).

Evidence from Neurologically Impaired Patients

Important evidence for modality-specific representation systems in the domain of speech comes from dissociations in patients suffering from neuropsychological disorders. Selective disruption of speech reading with preserved ability to process auditory speech is a prime example (Campbell et al., 1986; de Gelder et al., 1998c). Similar evidence is beginning to emerge for emotion perception. Recent data from brain-damaged subject suggests that selective impairment of facial expression perception can occur with preserved recognition of emotions in the face. More intriguingly, in some cases explicit recognition of facial expression is lost but the patient continues to process facial expressions without being aware of doing so. Such covert recognition of facial expressions was observed when faces were presented alone but also when the impact of a facial expression on the voice was studied. De Gelder et al. (1997a) studied a prosopagnosic patient who was unable to recognize any emotion from faces. We presented her with a version of the audiovisual experiments described earlier and noted that the expressions she could not recognize in isolation nevertheless had an impact on her recognition of the voice expression. The literature on preserved implicit recognition of faces offers a clue to the routes that might be involved in such implicit expression recognition (Bauer, 1984). A similar observation was made for patient suffering from blindsight. The patient could reliably distinguish two facial expressions presented to his blind field (de Gelder, Vroomen & Weiskrantz, 1999).

Emotions and Awareness

There is increasing evidence that processing of emotional messages takes place outside the scope of awareness. When subjects rate a face for gender they appear to fully process its emotional content (Morris et al., 1996). Faces that are not perceived consciously nevertheless lead to activation of the amygdala (Whalen et al., 1998). Patients that are unable to consciously report facial expressions show evidence of having processed these expressions covertly. The studies on perceiving emotions by ear and by eye summarized here are consistent with evidence that emotional messages are processed outside subjective awareness. The merging of the two input channels that convey emotional information in the case of a bimodal emotion event is thus achieved in an automatic fashion, bypassing any consciousness including awareness of incongruence between the expression in the voice and that in the face.

It appears then that our common-sense understanding about the richness and subjective accessibility of emotional experience contrasts with the evidence accumulating from the cognitive neurosciences that a significant part of emotional processes bypasses our subjective access to and our accountability for what we experience. In this final section I sketch how the notion of nonconscious emotions and that of phenomenal experience might be related.

The kind of processing of emotional meaning at stake in the studies just mentioned fits the notion of a modular process. The modular process can be viewed as perception based as well as mandatory and has sometimes been assimilated to a cognitive reflex (Fodor, 1983). But these may not be the main nor the only properties by which a process qualifies as modular. Another important aspect of modular processing concerns semantics or the representational content present at the level of modular processing of emotional messages. An example from language processing illustrates the point. In listening to a spoken sentence containing the word "bank," the language module parses the input and recognizes the word "bank." However, it does not actually select which of the different meanings of the word is used in the sentence in the context in which the sentence is spoken. At the modular stage content is shallow and not integrated within the full belief and thought systems of the subject. One way to bring out this contrast is by opposing shallow versus full processing of a stimulus (Fodor, 1983). Along these lines, one may view the representational content of emotional experience as only a matter of narrow, shallow content on the one hand and phenomenal content on the other, or to paraphrase, a contrast can be made between perceptual states of emotion and full-blown elaborate and reflexive belief states, where the meaning of an emotional stimulus is elaborated against the full richness of the subjective experience. Traditional controversies in the emotion literature related to the contrast between biological versus phenomenal and social approaches can thus each have a niche in the full picture of emotional experience and do not need to be viewed as antagonistic. Perceiving emotions in the voice, the face, or in both combined is a process that can bypass consciousness. LeDoux (1996) clearly illustrates how separate processing streams in the brain correspond to implicit and explicit emotion processes.

The concept of emotion is still intimately linked with mentalism and mind/body dualism, the notion that emotional experiences can be studied independently of their realization in body processes. From this dualistic perspective, emotional experiences still belong to the realm of subjective mental states and therefore inherit all the connotations traditionally associated with mental states such as first-person authority, accountability, access, and qualia which have weighted heavily in research on emotions and almost precluded, at least until recently, research on unconscious processing of emotions. Advances in affective neuroscience will increasingly challenge the traditional mentalist view of emotions. Questions on the specificity of the sensory channel by which emotions are produced and perceived are part of this broader non-dualistic picture.

Acknowledgments

Thanks to P. Bertelson and J. Vroomen for discussions on cross-modal perception, to R. Held for comments, and to G. Pourtois for assistance with the manuscript.

References

Ahern, G. L. & Schwartz, G. E. (1985). Differential lateralization for positive and negative emotion in the human brain: EEG spectral analysis. *Neuropsychologia, 23*, 745–755.

Austin, J. L. (1970). Other minds. In J. O. Urmson & G. J. Warnock (Eds), *Philosophical Papers*, 2nd ed. (pp. 1–45). London: Oxford University Press.

Bauer, R. M. (1984). Autonomic recognition of names and faces in prosopagnosia: a neuropsychological application of the guilty knowledge test. *Neuropsychologia, 22*, 457–469.

Baylis, G. C., Rolls, E. T. & Leonard, C. M. (1985). Selectivity between faces in the responses of a population of neurons in the cortex in the superior temporal sulcus of the monkey. *Brain Research, 342*, 91–102.

Bertelson, P. (1998). Starting from the ventriloquist: the perception of multimodal events. In M. Sabourin, F. I. M. Craik & M. Robert (Eds), *Advances in Psychological Science*, vol. 1. *Biological and Cognitive Aspects* (pp. 419–439). Hove, UK: Psychology Press.

Bertelson, P., Vroomen, J., de Gelder, B. & Driver, J. (in press). Auditory-visual spatial interaction and the orientation of visual attention. *Psychological Science*.

Bower, T. G. R. (1974). *Development in Infancy*. San Fransisco: W. H. Freeman.

Breiter, H. C., Etcoff, N. L., Whalen, P. J., Kennedy, W. A., Rauch, S. L., Buckner, R. L., Strauss, M. M., Hyman, S. E. & Rosen, B. R. (1996). Response and habituation of the human amygdala during visual processing of facial expression. *Neuron*, 1996; 17: 875–887.

Bruyer, R. (1981). Asymmetry of facial expression in brain damaged subjects. *Neuropsychologia, 19*, 615–624.

Calder, A. J., Young, A. W., Benson, P. J. & Perrett, D. L. (1996). Self priming from distinctive and caricatured faces. *British Journal of Psychology, 87*, 141–162.

Calvert, G. A., Bullmore, E. T., Brammer, M. J., Campbell, R., Williams, S. C. R., McGuire, P. K., Woodruff, P. W. R., Iversen, S. D. & David, A. S. (1997). Activation of auditory cortex during silent lipreading. *Science, 276*, 593–596.

Campbell, R. (1996). Seeing speech in space and time. In *Proceedings of the International Conference on Spoken Language Processing* (pp. 1493–1498).

Campbell, R., Landis, T. & Regard, M. (1986). Face recognition and lipreading: a neurological dissociation. *Brain, 109*, 509–21.

Campbell, R., Dodd, B. & Burnham, D. (1998). *Hearing by Eye II: Advances in the Psychology of Speechreading and Auditory-Visual Speech*. Hove, UK: Psychology Press.

Carmon, A. & Nachshon, I. (1973). Ear asymmetry in perception of emotional non-verbal stimuli. *Acta Psychologica, 37*, 351–357.

Crowder, R. & Surprenant, A. (1995). On the linguistic module in auditory memory. In B. de Gelder & J. Morais (Eds), *Speech and Reading: A Comparative Approach* (pp. 94–64). Hove, UK: Lawrence Erlbaum Associates.

Darwin, C. (1872). *The Expressions of Emotion in Man and Animals*. London: John Murray.

Davidson, R. J. & Tomarken, A. J. (1989). Laterality and emotion: an electrophysiological approach. In F. Boller & J. Grafman (Eds), *Handbook of Neuropsychology*, vol. 3 (pp. 419–441). Amsterdam: Elsevier.

de Gelder, B., Vroomen, J. & Bachoud-Levi, A. (1997a). Emotion by ear and by eye: Implicit processing of emotion using a cross-modal approach. *Fourth Annual Meeting of the Cognitive Neuroscience Society*, no. 49, p. 73.

de Gelder, B., Bocker, K. B. E., Tuomainen, J., Hensens, M. & Vroomen, J. (1999). The combined perception of emotion from voice and face: early interaction revealed by electric brain responses. *Neuroscience Letters, 260*, 133–136.

de Gelder, B., Teunisse, J-P. & Benson, P. (1997b). Categorical perception of facial expressions: categories and their internal structure. *Cognition and Emotion, 11*, 1–23.

de Gelder, B. & Vroomen, J. (1994). Memory for consonants versus vowels in heard and lipread speech. *Journal of Memory and Language, 31*, 737–756.

de Gelder, B. & Vroomen, J. (1996). Categorical perception of emotional speech. *The Journal of the Acoustical Society, 100*, 4, pt. 2: 2818.

de Gelder, B., Vroomen, J. & Bertelson, P. (1996). Aspects of modality in audio-visual processes. In D. G. Stork & M. E. Hennecke (Eds), *Speechreading by Humans and Machines*. NATO ASI Series F, vol. 150 (pp. 197–192). Berlin: Springer-Verlag.

de Gelder, B., Vroomen, J. & Bertelson, P. (1998a). Upright but not inverted faces modify the perception of emotion in the voice. *Current Psychology of Cognition, 17*, 1021–1031.

de Gelder, B., Vroomen, J. & Bertelson, P. (1998b). Cross-modal bias of voice tone on facial expression: upper versus lower halves of a face. Proceedings of the International Conference on Auditory-Visual Speech Processing (AVSP '98), (pp. 93–97), Terrigal-Sydney.

de Gelder, B., Vroomen, J. & Bachoud-Lévi, A. (1998c). Impaired speechreading and audio-visual speech integration in prosopagnosia. In R. Campbell, B. Dodd & D. Burnham (Eds), *Hearing by Eye 11, Advances in the Psychology of Speechreading and Auditory-visual Speech* (pp. 195–207). Hove, UK: Psychology Press Ltd.

de Gelder, B., Vroomen, J., & Weiskrantz, L. (1999). Covert processing of facial expressions in a blindsight patient. Annual Meeting of the Cognitive Neuroscience Society, Abstract 35A, Washington, D.C.

Delis, D. C., Kiefner, M. G. & Fridlund, A. J. (1988). Visuospatial dysfunction following unilateral brain damage: dissociations in hierarchical hemispatial analysis. *Journal of Clinical and Experimental Neuropsychology, 10*, 421–431.

Dodd, B. & Campbell, R. (1987). *Hearing by Eye: The psychology of Lip-reading*. Hove, UK: Lawrence Erlbaum Associates.

Dopson, W. G., Beckwith, B. E., Tucker, D. M. & Bullard-Bates, P. C. (1984). Asymmetry of facial expression in spontaneous emotion. *Cortex, 20*, 243–251.

Ekman, P. (1992) An argument for basic emotions. *Cognition and Emotion, 6*, 169–200.

Ekman, P., Friesen, W. V. & O'Sullivan, M. (1988). Smiles when lying. *Journal of Personality and Social Psychology, 54*, 414–420.

Ellison, J. W. & Massaro, D. W. (1997). Featural evaluation, integration and judgment of facial affect. *Journal of Experimental Psychology: Human Perception and Performance, 23*, 213–226.

Etcoff, N. & Magee, J. (1992). Categorical perception of facial expressions. *Cognition, 44*, 227–240.

Fodor, J. A. (1983). *The Modularity of Mind*. Cambridge, MA: MIT Press.

Fowler, C. A. (1996). Listeners do hear sound, tot tongues. *Journal of the Acoustical Society of America, 99*, 1730–1741.

Fried, I., Mateer, C., Ojemann, G., Wohns, R. & Fedio, P. (1982). Organization of visuospatial functions in the human cortex. *Brain, 105*, 349–371.

Frijda, N. (1989). *The Emotions*. Cambridge: Cambridge University Press.

Gainotti, G. (1972). Emotional behavior and hemispheric side of lesion. *Cortex, 8*, 41–55.

Gainotti, G. (1989). Disorders of emotions and affect in patients with unilateral brain damage. In F. Boller & J. Grafman (Eds), *Handbook of Neuropsychology*, vol. 3 (pp. 345–361). Amsterdam: Elsevier.

George, M. S., Parekh, P. I., Rosinsky, N., Ketter, T. A., Kimbrell, T. A., Heilman, K. M., Herscovitch, P. & Post, R. M. (1996). Understanding emotional prosody activates right hemisphere regions. *Archives of Neurology, 53*, 665–670.

Gianotti, M. & Pereira, N. (1972). Psychological approaches to the cerebral palsied child. *Revista Brasiliera de deficiencia mental, 7*, 5–9.

Gibson, J. J. (1966). *The Senses Considered as Perceptual Systems*. Boston, MA: Houghton Mifflin.

Humphreys, G. W. & Riddoch, J. M. (1987). *To See or Not to See*. Hove, UK: Lawrence Erlbaum Associates.

Johnson, W. F., Emde, R., Scherer, K. & Klinnert, M. D. (1986). Recognition of emotion from vocal cues. *Archives of General Psychiatry, 43*, 280–283.

Kutas, M. & Dale, A. (1997). Electrical and magnetic readings of mental functions. In M. D. Rugg (Ed.), *Cognitive Neuroscience* (pp. 197–242). Cambridge, MA: MIT Press.

Landis, T., Assal, G. & Perret, E. (1979). Opposite cerebral hemispheric superiorities for visual associative processing of emotional facial expressions and objects. *Nature, 278*, 739–740.

Lane, R. D., Reiman, E. M., Geoffrey, L. A., Schwatrz, G. E. & Davidson, R. J. (1997). Neuroanatomical correlates of happiness, sadness and disgust. *The Americam Journal of Psychiatry, 154*, 926–933.

LeDoux, J. (1996). *The Emotional Brain*. New York: Simon and Schuster.

Lewkowicz, D. J. (1986). Developmental changes in infants' bisensory response to synchronous durations. *Infant Behavior and Development, 8*, 335–353.

Leonard, C. M., Rolls, E. T., Wilson, F. A. & Baylis, G. C. (1985). Neurons in the amygdala of the monkey with responses selective for faces. *Behavioural Brain Research, 15*, 159–176.

Liberman, A. M. (1996). *Speech: A Special Code*. Cambridge, MA: MIT Press.

Liberman, A. M. & Mattingly, G. (1985). The motor theory of speech perception revised. *Cognition, 21*, 1–36.

Lieberman, P. & Michaels, S. B. (1962). Some aspects of fundamental frequency and envelope amplitude as related to emotional content of speech. *Journal of the Acoustical Society of America, 34*, 922–927.

Locke, J. (1689[1967–68]). An essay concerning human understanding. J. W. Yolton (Ed), 2 vols. London: Dent.

MacLeod, C. M. (1991). Half a century of research on the stroop effect: an integrative review. *Psychological Bulletin, 109*, 163–203.

Mahoney, A. M. & Sainsbury, R. S. (1987). Hemispheric asymmetry in the perception of emotional sounds. *Brain and Cognition, 6*, 216–233.

Massaro, D. W. (1987). *Speech Perception by Ear and Eye*. Hillsdale, NJ: Lawrence Erlbaum Associates.

Massaro, D. W. (1998). *Talking Heads*. Cambridge, MA: MIT Press.

Massaro, D. W. & Egan, P. B. (1996). Perceiving affect from the voice and the face. *Psychonomic Bulletin & Review, 3*, 215–221.

McGurk, H. & MacDonald, J. (1976). Hearing lips and seeing voices. *Nature, 264*, 746–748.

Meltzoff, A. (1990). Towards a developmental cognitive science: the implications of cross-modal matching and imitation for the development of representation and memory. *Annals of the New York Academy of Sciences, 608*, 1–37.

Milner, A. D. & Goodale, M. A. (1995). *The visual brain in action*. Oxford: Oxford University Press.

Morris, J. S., Frith, C. D., Perrett, D. I., Rowland, D., Young, A. W., Calder, A. J. & Dolan, R. J. (1996). A differential neural response in the human amygdala to fearful and happy facial expressions. *Nature, 383*, 812–815.

Murray, I. R. & Arnott, J. L. (1993). Toward the simulation of emotion in synthetic speech: a review of the literature on human vocal emotion. *Journal of the Acoustical Society of America, 93*, 1097–1108.

Näätänen, R. (1992). *Attention and Brain Function*. Hillsdale, NJ: Lawrence Erlbaum Associates.

Nahm, F. K., Tranel, D., Damasio, H. & Damasio, A. R. (1993). Cross-modal associations and the hyman amygdala. *Neurospychologia, 31*, 727–744.

Piaget, J. (1952). *The Origins of Intelligence in Children*. New York: International Universities Press.

Pollack, I., Rubenstein, H. & Horowitz, A. (1960). Communication of verbal modes of expression. *Language and Speech, 3*, 121–130.

Puce, A., Allison, T., Asgari, M., Gore, J. C. & McCarthy, G. (1996). Differential sensitivity of human visual cortex to faces, letterstrings, and textures. A functional magnetic resonance imaging study. *Journal of Neuroscience, 16*, 5205–5215.

Sams, M., Aulanko, R., Hämäläinen, M., Hari, R., Lounasmaa, O. V., Lu, S-T. & Simola, J. (1991). Seeing speech: visual information from lip movements modifies activity in the hunam auditory cortex. *Neuroscience Letters, 127*, 141–145.

Scherer, K. R. (1979). Non-linguistic vocal indicators of emotions and psychopathology. In C. E. Izard (Ed), *Emotions in Personality and Psychopathology*. New York: Plenum Press.

Schmitt, J. J. Hartje, W. & Williams, K. (1997). Hemispheric asymmetry in the recognition of conditional attitude conveyed by facial expression, prosody and propositional speech. *Cortex, 33*, 65–81.

Scott, S. K., Young, A. W., Calder, A. J., Hellawell, D. J. et al. (1997). Impaired auditory recognition of fear and anger following bilateral amygdala lesions. *Nature, 385*, 254–275.

Searcy, J. H. & Bartlett, J. C. (1996). Inversion and processing of component and spatial-relational information in faces. *Journal of Experimental Psychology: Human Perception and Performance, 22*, 904–915.

Semenza, C. Pasini, M., Zettin, M., Tonin, P., et al. Right hemisphere patients' judgements on emotions. *Acta Neurologica Scandinavia, 74*, 43–50. (1986).

Stein, B. E. & Meredith, M. A. (1993). *The Merging of the Senses*. Cambridge, MA: MIT Press.

Suberi, M. & McKeever, W. F. (1977). Differential right hemispheric memory storage of emotional and non-emotional faces. *Neuropsychologia, 15*, 757–768.

Summerfield, Q. (1991). Visual perception of phonetic gestures. In G. Mattingly & M. Studdert-Kennedy (Eds), Modularity and the Motor Theory of Speech Perception (pp. 117–137). Hillsdale, NJ: Lawrence Erlbaum Associates.

Tartter, V. & Braun, D. (1994). Hearing smiles and frowns in normal and whisper registers. *Journal of the Acoustical Society of America, 96*, 2101–2107.

Teunisse, J. P. & de Gelder, B. (in press). Impaired categorical expression of emotions in autistics. *Child Neuropsychology*.

van Lancker, D. (1997). Rags to riches: our increasing appreciation of cognitive and communicative abilities of the human right hemisphere. *Brain and Language, 57*, 1–11.

van Lancker, D. & Sidtis, J. J. (1992). The identification of affective-prosodic stimuli by left- and right-hemisphere-damaged subjects: all errors are not created equal. *Journal of Speech and Hearing Research, 35*, 963–970.

Vroomen, J., Collier, R. & Mozziconacci, S. (1993). Duration and intonation in emotional speech. In Proceedings of the Third European Conference on Speech Communication and Technology, Berlin, pp. 577–580.

Vroomen, J. & de Gelder, B. (1996). Phoneme detection in resyllabified words. *The Journal of the Acoustical Society, 100*, 4, pt. 2: 2818–2819.

Walker, A. & Grolnick, W. (1983). Discrimination of vocal expressions by young infants. *Infant Behavior and Development, 6*, 491–498.

Weiskrantz, L. (1997). *Consciousness Lost and Found*. Oxford: Oxford University Press.

Werner, H. (1973). *Comparative Psychology of Mental Development*. New York: International Universities Press.

Whalen, P. J., Rauch, S. L., Etcoff, N. L., McInerney, S. C., Lee, M. B. & Jenike, M. A. (1998). Masked presentations of emotional facial expressions modulate amygdala activity without explicit knowledge. *Journal of Neuroscience, 18*, 411–418.

Williams, C. E. & Stevens, K. N. (1972). Emotions and speech: some acoustic correlates. *Journal of the Acoustical Society of America, 52*, 1238–1250.

Yin, R. K. (1969). Looking at upside-down faces. *Journal of Experimental Psychology, 81*, 141–145.

6

The Enigma of the Amygdala: On Its Contribution to Human Emotion

JOHN P. AGGLETON AND ANDREW W. YOUNG

Although it is widely assumed that the amygdala has an important role in human emotion, the nature of that role has remained elusive. It is also assumed that this structure has an associated contribution to cognition, but, again, this has remained difficult to define (Aggleton, 1992; Anderson, 1978). These failures seem all the more surprising when it is appreciated that there is considerable evidence from studies of other primate species and from rats showing how the amygdala plays a critical role in particular aspects of emotion and cognition (Davis, 1992; Gaffan, 1992; LeDoux, 1995; McGaugh et al., 1992). The principal problem has been transferring these findings to the human amygdala. A clear example of this problem comes from descriptions of the effects of amygdala damage in humans and in other primates. While amygdala damage in monkeys produces a pronounced loss of affective behavior and a catastrophic breakdown in social interactions, comparable changes in humans are almost never reported (Aggleton, 1992). Indeed, the effects of human amygdala damage often appear unremarkable.

Trying to resolve this discrepancy is vital for our understanding of the functions of the human amygdala. This is partly because the dramatic loss of emotional behavior that is observed following amygdalectomy in monkeys has been highly influential in driving our thinking about the structure, and partly because studies with animals will be needed to address many of the questions concerning the detailed functions of the amygdala.

One explanation for these differential effects of amygdala damage on emotion is that there is a qualitative change in amygdala function across primate species, so that the contribution of the human amygdala is much diminished. In fact, this explanation runs counter to measurements showing that the overall extent of this structure has increased rather than decreased in humans (Stephan et al., 1987). Comparisons of the volume of the amygdala in different species (from Insectivora through humans) have shown that while the extent of the medial and central nuclei remain reasonably constant across species, the group of nuclei comprising the lateral, basal, and cortical nuclei actually increases in size (Stephan et al., 1987). This increase is most evident in the small-celled components such as the lateral nucleus, and this can be linked to the increased inputs from sensory association cortex to this nucleus (see Amaral, this volume). In fact, there appears to be a relatively strong association between the size of the neocortex and the extent of the basolateral-cortical nuclei group in primates (Barton & Dunbar, 1997). This is of added interest because of the positive correlation in primates between the extent of neocortex and social group size (Barton, 1996).

The gross anatomy of the amygdala thus offers no support for the view of a diminished role in emotion. Similarly, there is no reason to suppose that the principal connections of the human amygdala are markedly different from those of other primates (see Amaral, this volume), and tract analyses support this view (Klingler & Gloor, 1960). Detailed information concerning many amygdala connections in the human brain is still lacking, but the most likely species change concerns an increase in neocortical interactions (Barton & Dunbar, 1997). Although this increase may result in a shift in relative importance, it is unlikely to bring about a fundamental change in amygdala function, especially as there is much evidence indicating that the involvement of the amygdala in social/affective behavior depends on its cortical interactions (see next section).

Several new lines of research are leading to a reappraisal of amygdala function in humans and other primates, and these suggest a similarity rather than a divergence of function across species. One of these research lines arises from the important discovery that the cortical regions immediately adjacent to the amygdala are critically important for an array of cognitive functions that had previously been attributed to the amygdala. A second line of research stems from evidence that the human amygdala is important for the recognition of emotion in others, but this involvement appears to be largely restricted to a subset of basic emotions. This discovery not only offers a means by which the contribution of the amygdala to affective behavior can be systematically examined, but it also shows how descriptions of the overall state of a subject with amygdala damage could fail to detect more selective abnormalities. A third line of research stems from the rapid advances that have taken place in the analysis of the contribution of the amygdala to fear conditioning in animals. Studies using rats have revealed much about the circuitry and nature of this learning, and clinical research indicates that these findings may be directly applicable to aspects of human emotion (Bechara et al., 1995; LeDoux, 1995).

This chapter first describes how conventional surgical lesions of the monkey amygdala have consistently indicated that this region has a vital role in emotion and associated aspects of cognition. The following sections consider each of the three lines of research identified above, beginning with the ways in which the effects of conventional lesions of the monkey amygdala have had to be modified in the light of recent findings concerning adjacent cortical areas.

The Amygdala and Social/Affective Behavior in Monkeys: Effects of Conventional Surgical Lesions

The discovery that removal of the amygdala produces a striking loss of emotional behavior can be traced back to Brown and Schafer (1888), who noted that bilateral temporal lobe damage could result in an unusual tameness in the rhesus monkey. This remarkable finding was rediscovered by Klüver and Bucy (1939) in a series of studies trying to uncover the neural systems responsible for the hallucinogenic properties of the drug mescaline. They found that bilateral removal of the temporal lobes produces a highly distinctive pattern of behavioral changes (the "Klüver-Bucy syndrome"). These changes consisted of visual agnosia, a failure to identify objects visually; a loss of emotional reactivity; "orality," a tendency to examine objects with the mouth; "hypermetamorphosis," a tendency to switch rapidly from one behavior to another that is often expressed as an increase in exploratory behavior; hypersexuality; and abnormal dietary changes, most notably coprophagia (eating of feces). Subsequent studies showed that bilateral aspiration lesions of the amygdala were sufficient to induce the "tameness," the orality, the excessive exploratory behavior, and the dietary changes (Weiskrantz, 1956). It was also found that disconnecting the amygdala from sensory cortical regions results in components of the Klüver-Bucy syndrome, including the loss of emotionality (Downer, 1961; Horel et al., 1975). It has not, however, been possible to duplicate these Klüver-Bucy symptoms by damaging subcortical projection targets of the amygdala (Butter & Snyder, 1972; Stern & Passingham, 1996). These findings suggest that the dysfunctions responsible for the abnormalities lie in the cortical–amygdala interactions.

In addition to the loss of emotionality, it was discovered that removal of the amygdala could permanently disrupt the social behavior of a monkey, typically resulting in a fall in social standing (Rosvold et al., 1954). These effects, which have been recorded in a variety of monkey species, seem most apparent in adult animals. They also appear to depend on the size of the group the monkey is living in—the larger the group, the more evident the changes (Kling, 1972; Kling & Steklis, 1976). Finally, analyses of the postural and facial gestures made by animals following surgery indicates that there is a general loss of aversive and aggressive behavior (Butter & Snyder, 1972; Horel et al., 1975; Kling & Cornell, 1971; Kling & Dunne, 1976).

Removal of two other brain regions, the orbital frontal cortex and the temporal pole, has also been associated with the appearance of a partial Klüver-Bucy syndrome (Horel et al., 1975; Kling & Steklis, 1976; Myers, 1972). The deficits include changes in emotionality and a breakdown of social behavior. These findings, along with the close anatomical relationship between the three regions, led to the proposal that the amygdala, temporal pole, and orbital frontal cortex formed key components of an interlinked social-affective system that was necessary for the maintenance of social behavior (Kling & Steklis, 1976).

Studies on the effects of amygdalectomy in monkeys have also looked for possible cognitive changes. Impairments have been found on a number of related tasks including discrimination reversals (Aggleton & Passingham, 1981; Jones & Mishkin, 1972; Schwartzbaum & Poulos, 1965), learning set (Schwartzbaum & Poulos, 1965), and single trial object–reward associations (Gaffan, 1992; Spiegler & Mishkin, 1981). These impairments indicate that the amygdala enables the rapid formation of stimulus–reward associations. Because these associations may be integral in establishing the emotional significance of external events, these deficits have been linked with the loss of emotionality. Furthermore, the fact that amygdalectomized monkeys are unresponsive to stimuli that evoked emotion before surgery suggests that this impairment includes a failure to use previously learned stimulus–reward associations.

This description of amygdala function carries the clear prediction that bilateral destruction of the amygdala will retard the learning of any task involving stimulus–reward associations. In fact, it has long been accepted that amygdalectomized monkeys can show normal learning rates for some pattern and object discriminations (Aggleton & Passingham, 1981; Schwartzbaum, 1965; Zola-Morgan et al., 1989), and yet such tasks must tax stimulus–reward associations. This has led to a further refinement—namely, that the amygdala is only involved in a specific class of stimulus–reward associations (Gaffan, 1992, 1994). These involve those associations between discrete stimuli and the intrinsic, incentive value of related rewards. It is assumed that normal monkeys can solve food-rewarded discriminations in more than one way (Gaffan & Bolton, 1983). While they may choose the correct stimulus because it is associated with the intrinsic value of the reward (how good it tastes), they may select the correct item because it is linked with the external aspects of the reward (i.e., the monkey chooses the stimulus that leads to the sight of the food reward). Support for this subtle distinction comes from the apparently good visual discrimination performance found when the stimuli to be discriminated cover the rewards (i.e., a correct choice leads to the sight of the reward). In contrast, amygdalectomized monkeys show abnormal selection of novel foods (Baylis & Gaffan, 1991) and are impaired on discrimination tasks for rewards that cannot be seen (Baylis & Gaffan, 1991; Gaffan, 1992). In both situations the animal must link the sensory features of the stimulus directly with the palatability of food. A more general description of these findings is the proposal that the amygdala is involved in stimulus–affective associations.

A further effect of aspiration lesions of the amygdala is the loss of the ability to perform a tactile-to-visual cross-modal recognition task (Murray & Mishkin, 1985). The task requires the monkeys to palpate an object in the dark. The monkey is then shown the same object along with an unfamiliar object in the light. The monkey is rewarded for selecting the unfamiliar object, and to do this the monkey must now use visual cues. The possibility that the amygdala is involved in this cross-modal task has raised considerable interest because it accords with the convergence of polysensory information that occurs within this structure (Amaral, this volume) and could account for some aspects of the Klüver-Bucy syndrome, such as orality and hypermetamorphosis (Murray & Mishkin, 1985).

Reassessing the Effects of Selective Amygdala Damage: Dissociating the Contribution of the Rhinal Cortices

In all of the experiments so far described with monkeys, the amygdala lesions were made by aspiration. As a consequence, the lesions inevitably included some adjacent portions of cortex. This additional damage most often occurred in the rostral parts of the perirhinal and entorhinal cortices, as well as parts of the piriform cortex. Because the extent of this extra-amygdaloid damage is often quite restricted, it was assumed that it contributed little, if any, to the effects of amygdalectomy. There is now, however, good reason to believe that this assumption is wrong. The rhinal cortex (comprising the entorhinal cortex and perirhinal cortex) has been shown to be vital for certain aspects of learning and memory. Furthermore, even minor damage to this cortical region can disrupt performance. These contributory effects were first discovered for tests of recognition memory using the delayed nonmatching-to-sample (DNMS) procedure, but there is good reason to believe that they extend to other changes.

In a landmark study, Mishkin (1978) showed that aspiration lesions of the amygdala in rhesus monkeys could dramatically accentuate the DNMS deficit observed after hippocampal removal. It was initially assumed that this reflected the conjoint contribution of the two limbic structures to recognition memory and that the incidental damage to the adjacent cortices played no part. This interpretation had to be revised when it was found that removal of the perirhinal cortex alone was sufficient to induce a severe DNMS deficit (Meunier et al., 1993; Murray, 1992; Murray et al., 1996; Suzuki, 1996; Zola-Morgan et al., 1993). The discovery that stereotaxic lesions of the amygdala, which avoid the rhinal region, fail to potentiate the recognition deficit after hippocampectomy (Zola-Morgan et al., 1989) further indicated that it was rhinal and not amygdala damage that caused the increased impairment observed by Mishkin (1978). Confirmation of this conclusion has come with the discovery that cytotoxic lesions of the amygdala and hippocampus combined do not affect DNMS performance (Murray & Mishkin, 1998). These results all point to the fact that the apparent additive effect of amygdala removal to the DNMS deficit arises from rhinal damage and not from amygdala damage.

The discovery that even small amounts of incidental rhinal damage could have a profound effect on DNMS performance raises the question of whether such damage contributes to some of the other effects attributed to amygdalectomy. The weight of recent evidence now shows that this is so. It had been found that aspiration lesions of the amygdala, which include rostral perirhinal cortex, disrupt the learning of visual discriminations when correct choices are guided by an auditory secondary reinforcer (Gaffan & Harrison, 1987). Although it was assumed that amygdala damage was responsible for this deficit, it has been shown that bilateral excitotoxic lesions of the amygdala do not affect task performance (Malkova et al., 1997). Similarly, research into the acquisition of stimulus–stimulus associations indicates that effects previously associated with amygdala damage are probably a consequence of cortical damage. A series of studies had shown how aspiration lesions of the amygdala can disrupt learned stimulus–stimulus associations both within and between sensory modalities (Murray & Gaffan, 1994; Murray et al., 1993). For example, aspiration lesions of the amygdala impaired the postoperative retention of a visual–visual associative task in which the monkey had to learn that stimulus A goes with X but not Y, while stimulus B goes with Y but not X (Murray et al., 1993). These findings appeared to extend previous findings for cross-modal recognition (Murray & Mishkin, 1985) and point to a general role in sensory–sensory associations. But as with recognition memory, it is now emerging that the rhinal cortices are probably vital for stimulus–stimulus associative tasks (Malkova & Murray, 1996; Murray et al., 1993).

This counterevidence initially emerged from the visual–visual associative task as removal of the amygdala and hippocampus along with the adjacent rhinal cortices severely impaired task recall and acquisition (Murray et al., 1993). Thus lesions involving the length of the rhinal region produced much more severe deficits than those observed after either amygdalectomy or hippocampectomy (Murray et al., 1993). Other related evidence has come from cross-modal associations tasks. In contrast to the effects of conventional aspiration lesions, discrete neurotoxic lesions of the amygdala had no apparent effect on task performance (Malkova & Murray, 1996). Although the amygdala lesions were incomplete, leaving the possibility that extensive amygdala damage is sufficient to disrupt cross-modal matching, an alternative conclusion is that the previous amygdala lesion effects were due to damage to rhinal tissue or rhinal fibers.

These findings all indicate that although the amygdala receives an array of polysensory information, it may not be critically involved in either intramodal or cross-modal sensory–sensory interactions. This conclusion agrees with the results of a number of studies that have examined cross-modal matching performance in patients with bilateral amygdala damage. These studies, which have typically used the Nebes's Arc-Circle test, have failed to find a link between amygdala damage and performance (Lee et al., 1995; Nahm et al., 1993). Similarly, a PET study of the Nebes's Arc-Circle test failed to find any evidence for differential activation of the amygdala during the cross-modal version of the task (Banati et al., 2000). Whether the rhinal region is a critical site for this class of task remains to be determined both in monkeys and in humans, but these findings clearly cast doubt upon a wider range of findings arising from bilateral aspiration lesions of the amygdala, including those concerning emotion.

These considerations highlight the value of those studies using surgical techniques that produce more selective amygdala damage. One method is to make stereotaxic lesions, but this has only rarely been attempted with nonhuman primates. In one of the first such studies two rhesus monkeys received bilateral lesions in the basal amygdala nuclei (Turner, 1954). They displayed mild changes in affect but no other Klüver-Bucy signs (Turner, 1954). A later study (Butter & Snyder, 1972) contained an interesting comparison between two monkeys with amygdala lesions, one the result of aspiration surgery and the other following an accurate stereotaxic lesion of most of the structure. Detailed observations of their reactions to emotion-evoking stimuli showed that they displayed a similar, abnormal loss of both aggressive and aversive reactions (Butter & Snyder, 1972).

In a more extensive stereotaxic study, the effects of different-sized radiofrequency lesions of the amygdala were compared (Aggleton & Passingham, 1981). Those lesions involving most of the structure produced a clear loss of emotional responsiveness, although there was some recovery over time. The loss of emotionality was evident for most aggressive, aversive, and conflict gestures, although these same animals did show an increase in submissive gestures such as lip smacking and "presenting" (Aggleton & Passingham, 1981). These large amygdala lesions also resulted in dietary changes (e.g., the animals would now eat meat), an increased exploration of nonfood items, and some limited evidence of coprophagia. In contrast, lesions largely restricted to the lateral amygdala nucleus or the basolateral group of nuclei produced only a slight increase in exploratory behavior and no associated effects on the frequency of emotional expressions and postures. While the results of these stereotaxic surgeries indicate that bilateral amygdala damage is sufficient to produce a marked loss of emotionality, this damage must involve a considerable part of the structure. Those amygdala lesions that disrupted emotional reactivity were also those that impaired the learning of discrimination reversals, a finding that supports the idea of an association between the emotional changes and the stimulus–reward association deficit (Aggleton, 1993; Aggleton & Passingham, 1981; Weiskrantz, 1956).

The effects of stereotaxic radiofrequency lesions of the amygdala have been reexamined (Zola-Morgan et al., 1991). Monkeys with stereotaxic amygdala damage were compared directly to those with aspiration removal of the amygdala and those with removal of the perirhinal and parahippocampal cortices. Other groups included in the study had aspiration lesions of the hippocampus and of the hippocampus and amygdala combined (Zola-Morgan et al., 1991). The reactions of these monkeys to a number of object stimuli (e.g., candy, keys, a boot) and social stimuli (a monkey, a human stare, a lunging body) were then assessed. All groups with amygdala damage showed abnormal reactions to the object stimuli, reflecting a decrease in emotionality. In contrast, the perirhinal/parahippocampal lesion group showed no gross behavioral changes. Surprisingly, none of the groups showed changes in emotionality to the social stimuli. This apparent dissociation between objects and social stimuli is misleading, however, because the "emotionality" score was a joint measure that combined the willingness to explore or touch stimuli with a loss of emotional gestures. In addition, most of the amygdala lesions were incomplete. Thus these partial amygdala lesions led to an increased exploration of the objects but did not, in fact, produce a clear loss of gestures or expressions (Zola-Morgan et al., 1991). These findings therefore closely resemble those from the partial amygdala lesions described by Aggleton & Passingham (1981).

Although these stereotaxic studies are valuable, they still fail to produce a truly selective lesion of the amygdala. This is because of the likelihood of damage to white matter immediately adjacent to the lateral border of the amygdala (Aggleton & Passingham, 1981; Zola-Morgan et al., 1991) or to cortical axons that pass through the amygdala (Goulet et al., 1998). In both cases, the connections most likely to be disrupted are those from the rhinal cortical region (Murray, 1992). Evidence that compromising these connections is not sufficient to produce the hypoemotionality associated with conventional amygdala lesions comes from the finding that selective destruction of the white matter immediately lateral to the amygdala does not result in a loss of emotional responsiveness (Aggleton & Passingham, 1981). But in order to determine whether amygdala damage is sufficient, it is necessary to examine the effects of cytotoxic lesions that spare these connections.

One of the first such studies reported that bilateral ibotenic acid lesions of the amygdala can induce certain Klüver-Bucy signs (Murray et al., 1996). The lesions, which involved virtually all of the amygdala, resulted in an increased willingness to eat meat, an increased tendency to pick up and explore nonfood items, and a modest decline in emotionality (Murray et al., 1996). Informal observations indicated that these Klüver-Bucy signs were less marked than those seen after aspiration lesions (Murray et al., 1996). These impressions were supported by a study that compared the emotional reactivity of six monkeys with neurotoxic lesions of the amygdala and three with aspiration lesions (Meunier et al., 1999). The animals with neurotoxic lesions showed a loss of fearful reactions, fewer aggressive responses, and an increased tendency to examine objects, often orally. These changes were similar to those observed after aspiration lesions but did not appear as severe (Meunier et al., 1999).

The conclusion that selective amygdala damage is sufficient to disrupt social and affective behavior, is consistent with the results of single-unit recording studies. Neurons that appear to respond selectively to face stimuli were first discovered in areas of the temporal cortex (Bruce et al., 1981; Perrett et al., 1982) that project directly to the amygdala (Aggleton et al., 1980). Later studies showed that there are neurons in the amygdala that also respond to faces (Leonard et al., 1985), a finding of considerable potential significance given the importance of facial recognition for social signaling and gesturing. It was noted that some of these units responded differently to different faces, and some responded more to faces making a particular emotional expression. These face-responsive cells were most prevalent in the accessory basal nucleus (Leonard et al., 1985). It has also been found that cells in the medial amygdala, including the accessory basal nucleus, can respond selectively to more dynamic social stimuli such as approach behavior (Brothers et al., 1990). These results, which unlike many lesion studies are not contaminated by rhinal contributions, support the view that the amygdala is important for affective and social behavior.

Although selective amygdala damage is sufficient to induce changes such as hypoemotionality, increased exploration of novel stimuli, and orality, these changes often appear more pronounced when the adjacent rhinal regions are also involved. This raises the important question of whether rhinal damage on its own can produce Klüver-Bucy signs, including the loss of emotionality. As already noted, the study by Zola-Morgan et al. (1991) found no evidence of hypoemotionality after removal of the perirhinal cortex. Similarly, removal of the anterior rhinal cortex (that part adjacent to the amygdala) failed to produce other Klüver-Bucy signs such as a change in food preference or an increase in the exploration of nonfood items (Murray et al., 1996). In fact, in one report complete ablation of the rhinal cortex appeared to increase fear reactions (Meunier et al., 1991). In contrast, amygdala damage led to a reduction in fear reactions (Meunier et al., 1991).

It would appear, therefore, that selective rhinal damage does not produce a hypoemotional state. Thus the loss of recognition memory and the loss of stimulus–stimulus associations linked to rhinal cortex damage are not integral to any loss of emotion. These conclusions do not mean that rhinal tissue is not involved in processing information important for affective and social behavior, but that its contribution appears to depend on the integrity of the amygdala. This view, which derives from the more pronounced loss of emotionality after amygdala removals that include the rhinal cortex, is supported by two other lines of evidence. The first concerns the numerous direct connections between the two regions (Amaral, this volume). The second comes from the results of single-unit recording studies, as cells in the rostral rhinal cortex have been found that respond selectively to faces (Brothers & Ring, 1993). Many of these respond to stimuli of social significance such as eye contact, open mouth gestures, and the motion of conspecifics (Brothers and Ring, 1993), and they are strikingly similar to units found in the medial amygdala (Brothers & Ring, 1993; Brothers et al., 1990).

This reappraisal of the amygdala confirms that the structure is vital for social and affective behavior in monkeys, but it also emphasizes that the structure cannot be regarded in isolation. At the same time, advances in the use of neurotoxins are starting to open up new lines of inquiry, which should include an investigation into the effects of selective cytotoxic amygdala lesions on social behavior. Another area for future research concerns the relationship between the amygdala and the temporal pole. The temporal pole not only has massive interconnections with the amygdala (Aggleton et al., 1980; Stefanacci et al., 1996), but lesion studies have implicated this region in social behavior in macaques (Horel et al., 1975; Kling & Steklis, 1976). Recent anatomical studies have recharacterized much of this tissue as a rostral extension of the perirhinal cortex (Suzuki & Amaral, 1994), and it is likely that it will prove to contain many neurons that are responsive to facial and other social stimuli (Brothers & Ring, 1993). It seems likely that the addition of temporal pole damage to amygdala damage will have a far more disruptive effect on emotional responsiveness than the addition of damaged rhinal tissue adjacent to the amygdala, but this remains to be systematically investigated.

The Effects of Amygdala Damage in Humans

Selective amygdala damage is rare in humans. The majority of cases concern people who have received surgery to alleviate epilepsy, while for a smaller number it has been to alleviate behavioral disturbances, or both (Aggleton, 1992). Interpreting the outcome of these procedures is made difficult by the likely presence of temporal lobe abnormalities before and after surgery. Also, many of these surgeries used stereotaxy, with the intent to produce only partial damage within the amygdala. Furthermore, many of these surgeries have been unilateral. For these reasons the effects of many amygdala surgeries are likely to be relatively subtle. This is borne out by many of the clinical reports which comment on the lack of abnormal behavioral consequences. Thus it is generally reported that amygdala damage does not produce Klüver-Bucy signs, and it is never sufficient to induce the full amygdala syndrome observed in monkeys (Aggleton, 1992). In fact, even extensive bilateral removal of tissue in the medial temporal lobes, including the rhinal cortex, need not induce the Klüver-Bucy syndrome in humans. This is most clearly demonstrated in the famous subject H.M. who shows an unusual degree of emotional indifference but no other signs (Corkin, 1984). The full syndrome is rarely observed in humans and is only associated with much more extensive, bilateral damage that includes the rostral temporal neocortex as well as the amygdala (Marlowe et al., 1975; Terzian & Ore, 1955). It is intriguing to suppose that the rarity of the syndrome in humans may reflect an increased contribution of the temporal pole, so that this region attenuates the effect of amygdala damage and vice versa. At present this remains conjecture, but it offers a plausible explanation for a variety of findings. For instance, bilateral damage to the temporal pole (like bilateral amygdala damage) is often not sufficient to induce Klüver-Bucy signs (Hodges et al., 1992; Kapur et al., 1994). It therefore appears that damage to neither region is sufficient to disrupt emotional behavior severely as long as the other region is still able to function.

As already implied, the effects of surgical amygdala damage on emotion appear modest. In some cases there are no overt changes (Aggleton, 1992). In other cases, in which the surgery has been carried out in response to hyperaggressive behavior, the reports have tended to stress a decrease in aggression or an increase in placidity and indifference that is often seen as "normalizing" (Aggleton, 1992; Narabayashi et al., 1963; Ramanchandran et al., 1974). A problem with many of these reports, however, is that the emotional state of the subject has not been systematically examined, and the descriptions are largely anecdotal. For this reason it is difficult to tell if an increase in placidity is related to the hypoemotionality observed in monkeys.

More recently, new information has come from studies of subjects with Urbach-Wiethe disease (lipoid proteinosis). This is a rare genetic disorder that results in skin and mucosal lesions. In a significant proportion of cases it also produces bilateral calcifications in the temporal lobes. This intracranial pathology is often centered in the amygdala, but there can also be damage in adjacent, anteromedial cortex. When this intracranial damage occurs, the disorder is often accompanied by changes in emotion. In individual cases where there is confirmed amygdala involvement, these changes have been described as an increase in emotional lability and a more childlike affect (Newton et al., 1971). Others have reported an increase in agitation (Babinsky et al., 1993), or signs of social and emotional disinhibition (Tranel & Hyman, 1990). A number of Urbach-Wiethe sufferers also show evidence of paranoid delusions (Emsley & Paster, 1985; Newton et al., 1971). Epilepsy is also sometimes associated with this disorder, but is not a prerequisite for these changes in emotional responsiveness. While it is evident that these emotional changes are different from those in monkeys with amygdala damage, it must also be remembered that the pathological processes are different. In particular, the onset of Urbach-Wiethe disease is gradual and there is variable involvement of adjacent cortical regions. The reports do, however, show that pathologies in the rostral medial temporal lobe alter affective and social behavior, and this underlines the continued importance of the amygdala region.

Although descriptions of the affective state of people with amygdala damage offer a valuable first step, they fail to provide insights into the nature of the underlying disorder. A much more promising approach has come from studies examining the ability to distinguish stimuli associated with emotion. Much of this concerns evidence that amygdala damage can impair the ability to recognize different facial expressions of emotion. One of the first clues to this problem was the finding that amygdala damage can impair face recognition memory but have little effect on word recognition memory (Aggleton & Shaw, 1996; Jacobson, 1986). More specific evidence has come from single-case studies (Adolphs et al., 1994; Young et al., 1995). In one study, a woman with extensive, bilateral amygdala damage due to Urbach-Wiethe disease was found to have selective difficulty in identifying emotional expressions, yet her ability to recognize personal identity appeared normal (Adolphs et al., 1994). She was found to rate pictures of certain expressions (fear, anger, surprise) as being less intense than ratings by the control subjects, and her ratings compared to those of control subjects indicated a selective failure to recognize fear. Indeed, she seemed to lack the concept of fear, as she could not describe fear-evoking situations, nor could she draw a fearful expression (Adolphs et al.,

1995). These difficulties contrasted sharply with her performance for other emotions.

A second woman with bilateral amygdala damage was also found to have a selective impairment in the recognition of facial expressions (Young et al., 1995). This woman (D.R.) received bilateral stereotaxic amygdala lesions as part of a treatment for epilepsy. In informal conversation she shows no obvious loss of emotionality and is able to identify premorbidly familiar faces and match unfamiliar faces. She is, however, impaired at both matching and recognizing emotional facial expressions (Young et al., 1995). Follow-up studies showed that D.R. is poor at recognizing both static and moving facial expressions (Young et al., 1996) and also has difficulties in matching pictures of the same person when their expressions differ. While she could describe from memory the facial features of famous people, she was poor at imaging facial expressions of emotion (Young et al., 1996). Thus she seemed to lack knowledge concerning the facial patterning of different emotions.

When D.R. was systematically tested with tasks requiring the identification of facial expressions, she was found to have a disproportionate deficit for the recognition of fear, although she also showed some difficulty with anger and disgust (Calder et al., 1996). This task used a standard series of photographs of faces expressing different emotions. The difficulty of recognizing the emotion portrayed in some images was then increased by using computer image-manipulation techniques that "morphed" the expression of one emotion toward a second emotion. Even for these more difficult perceptual discriminations, it was primarily the recognition of fear, anger, and disgust that was impaired for D.R., while the recognition of facial expressions of happiness, sadness, and surprise was spared. When the same techniques were used to make a difficult test of identity recognition (by morphing famous faces), D.R.'s performance was completely normal (Calder et al., 1996).

A similar, selective deficit for certain emotional expressions was also found in another subject, S.E., who suffered bilateral amygdala damage following presumed viral encephalitis (Calder et al., 1996). This subject, who had extensive right temporal lobe damage combined with left temporal lobe damage apparently restricted to the region of the uncus and anteromedial amygdala area, was severely impaired in recognizing expressions of fear and showed a borderline impairment on some tests with anger. S.E. was, however, able to perform normally when required to identify expressions of happiness, surprise, sadness, and disgust (Calder et al., 1996). The finding that extensive unilateral temporal lobe damage has little if any effect on the recognition of emotional expressions (Tranel et al., 1995) adds further weight to the importance of the bilateral amygdala damage.

Both D.R. and S.E. showed particular problems with expressions of fear, and some difficulty with anger, a pattern that clearly resembles the Urbach-Wiethe subject described by Adolphs et al. (1994). This consistency is striking in view of the different etiologies in the three cases, the common feature being the bilateral amygdala pathology. Some caution is warranted, however, as there is a conflicting report of two men who displayed normal recognition of different facial expressions yet suffered complete bilateral lesions of the amygdala and surrounding temporal cortex following herpes encephalitis (Hamann et al., 1996). Both men were tested twice using the materials and procedure of Adolphs et al. (1994) but did not appear abnormal (Hamann et al., 1996). The authors suggested that the discrepancy with the study of Adolphs et al. (1994) most probably reflected the early onset of Ur-bach-Wiethe disease, which then led to a more demonstrable impairment (Hamann et al., 1996). Although this might account for subject S.M. (Adolphs et al., 1994), it does not explain the performances of D.R., who developed epilepsy in her 20s and S.E., who developed herpes encephalitis at the age of 55 (Calder et al., 1996). It was also suggested that low IQ might be a possible contributing factor (Hamann et al., 1996), but this seem unlikely as subject S.E. is of normal intelligence (Calder et al., 1996).

In view of the possible uncertainty raised by Hamann et al.'s (1996) study, the results of a recent PET study that investigated neural responses to different facial expressions are of special interest (Morris et al., 1996). Subjects viewed photo-graphs of happy or fearful faces that varied systematically in the intensity of the emotional expression. Increased levels of activation to the fearful faces were re-corded in the left medial amygdala and left periamygdaloid cortex (Morris et al., 1996; see Dolan, this volume). A recent functional magnetic resonance (fMRI) study also found increased activation, especially in the left amygdala, to the sight of fearful faces (Breiter et al., 1996). The same study also reported some increased activation to happy faces, although this was less robust. These imaging results provide direct evidence that the human amygdala is involved in the neural pro-cesses engaged by fearful facial expressions and so support the data from those subjects who were impaired at recognizing this class of expressions (Adolphs et al., 1994; Calder et al., 1996; Young et al., 1995). The medial amygdala and peria-mygdaloid cortex locations in the study of Morris et al. (1996) are of interest, as the same regions were found to contain cells that respond to stimuli of social significance in monkeys (Brothers & Ring, 1993; Brothers et al., 1990). These areas of the amygdala (the medial nucleus, the accessory basal nucleus, and the periamygdaloid cortex) are not, however, those that receive direct visual inputs from the neocortex, as the inferior temporal gyrus and the superior temporal sulcus project to the lateral nucleus (Turner et al., 1980). These medial nuclei do receive a substantial intra-amygdaloid projection from the lateral amygdala nucleus (Ag-gleton, 1985; Amaral et al., 1992) (i.e., they receive indirect visual inputs). They also receive a dense input from the temporal pole. For these reasons they are well placed to form part of system involved in gauging the affective state of others. Finally, to identify gestures and postures of conspecifics, it is often necessary to use information relating to the whole body, as suggested by positron emission tomography (PET) studies (Bonda et al., 1996).

A feature that repeatedly emerges from these studies on the amygdala is the dissociation between the processing of emotional expressions and the processing of identity. This is most evident in the finding that damage to the amygdala can impair the former but spare the latter. Other patterns of brain damage can lead to the opposite pattern of deficits and so provide double dissociations between differ-ent groups of brain-damaged subjects (Adolphs et al., 1995; Young et al., 1993). The conclusion that aspects of identity and emotion are processed separately has also been demonstrated using PET (Sergent et al., 1994). Further evidence comes from single-unit recording studies with monkeys that have uncovered populations of cells in the depths of the superior temporal sulcus that preferentially respond to expressions, whereas other populations in the inferior temporal gyrus respond to identity (Hasselmo et al., 1989). Both of these areas project to the amygdala, and both classes of units have been recorded in the amygdala (Leonard et al., 1985). In spite of this, the evidence consistently points to the conclusion that amygdala activity aids the recognition of affective expressions and that this is critical for at least one class of expressions—namely, those of fear. This evidence has largely come from clinical studies, and a persistent limitation is the lack of cases with confirmed, selective amygdala damage. For this reason there is a need to reexamine these abilities in animals. The ideal approach would be to test the ability of monkeys with cytotoxic lesions of the amygdala to distinguish or match different emotional gestures in conspecifics. This would not only help to confirm the anatomical basis of the deficit, but it would also make it possible to determine if the deficit in recognizing different expressions can be dissociated from other changes such as hypoemotionality or the breakdown of social behavior or whether these postoperative changes are interdependent.

The Amygdala and Emotional Memory

The link between the amygdala and expressions of fear is of particular interest in view of the research showing that the amygdala is involved in Pavlovian fear conditioning in animals. In studies with rats an innocuous stimulus such as a tone is paired with a noxious unconditioned stimulus (UCS) such as a footshock. After a few pairings the tone (the conditioned stimulus or CS) starts to elicit an array of conditioned responses (CR) that are indicative of fear. These include freezing, changes in heart rate, and changes in blood pressure (LeDoux, 1995, this volume). The CS is also able to potentiate the acoustic startle response (Davis, 1992). Of particular relevance has been the discovery that these processes are disrupted by a variety of amygdala manipulations, including conventional lesions, neurotoxic lesions, and the intra-amygdaloid infusion of drugs such as N-methyl-D-aspartate (NMDA) antagonists (Campeau & Davis, 1995a; Davis, 1992; LeDoux, 1995; Miserendino et al., 1990). This form of associative learning has been studied in great detail, and it now appears that different regions of the rat amygdala have distinct roles in both the acquisition and execution of the conditioned responses.

Detailed studies of auditory fear conditioning have not only highlighted the importance of the amygdala but have also revealed much about the underlying circuitry. There are two afferent routes that can mediate auditory conditioning, one a direct thalamo-amygdala pathway, the other a thalamo-cortico-amygdala pathway (LeDoux, 1995). The former direct link is thought to be sufficient to enable simple stimulus features to trigger emotions, whereas the more indirect cortical route appears to be needed when more perceptually complex auditory stimuli are involved (e.g., in differential conditioning). In the case of audition, both routes converge in the lateral nucleus. Further evidence for the involvement of the lateral nucleus has come from single-unit recording studies that have shown significant changes in responsiveness to tones in the lateral nucleus after learning, which are observed at shorter latencies than in other amygdaloid nuclei (Quirk et al., 1995). Indeed, it is now supposed that the lateral nucleus is the initial site for training-induced plasticity in auditory fear conditioning (LeDoux, 1995; Maren & Fanselow, 1996). The circuitry for visual fear conditioning is thought to be similar, with the basolateral group of nuclei (composed of the lateral, basomedial and basolateral nuclei) providing the initial site for the convergence of afferent visual information vital for fear conditioning (LeDoux, 1995).

While the lateral nucleus provides the principal input system, the central nucleus provides the output system (LeDoux, 1995; Maren & Fanselow, 1996; but see Killcross et al., 1997). The central nucleus, which receives projections from the lateral nucleus, projects to areas involved in the expression of conditioned responses. For example, projections to the central gray matter are involved in freezing responses (LeDoux, 1995), projections to the lateral hypothalamus are inolved in sympathetic autonomic responses, and projections to the reticular region are involved in the potentiation of startle responses (LeDoux, 1995). In this way different regions of the rat amygdala are involved in both the acquisition and expression of fear conditioning. The nature of the relationship between different amygdala nuclei may, however, have a further level of complexity; there is evidence that the contributions of the basolateral and central nuclei can be doubly dissociated (Killcross et al., 1997). Lesions of the central nucleus disrupt some components of fear-conditioned behavior (suppression of behavior by a conditioned fear stimulus), but not others (choice behavior leading to avoidance of a conditioned fear stimulus). The opposite pattern of behavior was found after basolateral lesions (Killcross et al., 1997). It would therefore appear that the central nucleus cannot be the output site for all of these behaviors, while the lateral nucleus cannot be the only site at which Pavlovian CS–US associations are stored. The implication of these findings is that there are multiple fear learning systems within the amygdala. This conclusion has been questioned, however (Nader & LeDoux, 1997) and awaits further testing.

It is clearly important to discover the extent to which these findings regarding the rat amygdala and fear responses extend to humans. For this reason, the recent description of a man with extensive but selective right amygdala damage (probably due to a benign tumor) is of special interest (Angrilli et al., 1996). This man showed a reduced startle response (eye blink) to a sudden burst of white noise. Furthermore, unlike the control subjects, this response failed to be potentiated by the presence of aversive slides used to provide an emotive background (Angrilli et al., 1996). These preliminary findings echo those from studies using rats and suggest a similar function across a wide range of mammals.

The involvement of the amygdala in aversive situations appears to extend to other aspects of cognition, including the modulation of memory storage. It is known that highly emotional states, such as those induced by aversive events, can alter memory formation and that an important component of this modulation occurs through the release of adrenergic stress hormones (Cahill & McGaugh, 1996). One of the critical central sites necessary for this modulation is the amygdala (McGaugh et al., 1992). One possible mechanism for these effects upon memory is via the connections from the amygdala to the hippocampus (Cahill & McGaugh, 1996). The amygdala also has direct projections to widespread regions of the temporal, frontal, and occipital cortices (Amaral et al., 1992), and it therefore seems likely that amygdala activity can modulate earlier stages of sensory processing. The amygdala also provides dense inputs to the basal forebrain region, and the projections from this area are also thought to modulate cortical processing.

These studies on aversive conditioning in rats raise inevitable questions about the functions of the human amygdala and its role in emotionally arousing events. A recent study found impaired conditioned autonomic responses in a patient with selective, bilateral amygdala damage as a result of Urbach-Wiethe disease (Bechara et al., 1995). In this study the subject was trained so that a particular colored slide (CS) and then a particular auditory signal (CS) were paired with a very loud noise (UCS). Conditioning was assessed by measuring skin conductance responses to the conditioned stimuli. The patient showed normal baseline levels of skin conductance but failed to acquire the autonomic response (Bechara et al., 1995). The same subject, however, acquired the explicit facts about the nature of the conditioned stimuli (Bechara et al., 1995). Bilateral damage to the hippocampus produced the opposite pattern of changes, whereas combined amygdala and hipppocampal damage resulted in a loss of both the autonomic conditioning and the explicit information (Bechara et al., 1995).

In a related study, an Urbach-Wiethe disease patient failed to show enhanced memory for a highly emotional section of a story, even though this was consistently observed in control subjects (Cahill et al., 1995). The selectivity of this finding has been underlined by a similar deficit in another subject with bilateral amygdala damage (Adolphs et al., 1997), which contrasted with the performance of subjects with temporal lobe amnesia (Hamann et al., 1997), who showed the expected enhancing effect of emotionally arousing elements in the story. Further support for this function of the human amygdala comes from a PET study showing that levels of glucose metabolic rate in the right amygdala correlated with the number of emotionally arousing film clips recalled by the subjects (Cahill et al., 1996). Not only was no such relationship found for neutral film clips, but the emotional sequences also led to better recall (Cahill et al., 1996). Evidence that this enhancement effect depends on β-adrenergic receptors in normal subjects (Cahill et al., 1994) further increases the similarity with findings from animals (McGaugh et al., 1992). The lack of enhancement in the Urbach-Wiethe case accorded with an earlier study, which also concerned a person with circumscribed, bilateral amygdala damage due to Urbach-Wiethe disease (Babinsky et al., 1993). This subject demonstrated intact intelligence and general memory, as is typically seen after amygdala damage (Aggleton, 1992), but did appear to have a specific affect-related disorder (Babinsky et al., 1993). This was reflected in a failure to show enhanced recognition and priming for emotional stimuli over neutral stimuli (words and pictures), deficits that might arise from the lack of amygdala projections to the cortex. Finally, there is recent evidence from a functional MRI study that increased amygdala activity occurs during exposure to affective stimuli (Irwin et al., 1996). This finding is clearly consistent with the array of evidence now indicating that the amygdala has a variety of interrelated roles concerned with the recognition of, learning about, and reaction to affective stimuli.

Conclusions

There have been a number dramatic advances in our understanding of the functions of the primate amygdala. Much of this has arisen from the need to reexamine carefully the results of conventional lesions in the region of the amygdala. New research using more selective surgical techniques has revealed that the contribution of the amygdala to processes such as recognition memory or cross-modal associations is likely to be relatively minor. At the same time, the importance of this structure for normal affective reactivity has been confirmed. There still remain, however, a number of other possible amygdala functions that require reexamination using selective neurotoxins in monkeys. These include a thorough analysis of social behavior and a systematic comparison of the animals' reactions to positive and aversive stimuli, including a reinvestigation of the performance of tasks that depend on the rapid acquisition of stimulus–reward associations.

One of the most intriguing discoveries arising from neuropsychological assessments of patients with bilateral amygdala damage is the loss of the ability to identify emotional expressions. It is important to appreciate that the deficits observed in people appear to be selective to the identification of only certain classes of expression. The most consistent deficit arises from the failure to identify fearful faces. This selectivity has been extended into the auditory domain, where again it appears that only certain types of emotive sounds are affected, most notably fear and anger (Scott et al., 1997). These and related findings suggest that the amygdala may be disproportionately involved in detecting and reacting to aversive stimuli (LeDoux, 1995).

The extent to which monkeys with selective amygdala damage fail to identify affective signals remains to be determined, although such a loss would clearly contribute to the breakdown of social behavior that is observed after amygdalectomy. Whether amygdala damage in monkeys affects all classes of affective signal or whether only specific subclasses, such as fear, are disrupted also remains to be determined. Present evidence does not help resolve this point because nearly all studies of emotional reactivity in monkeys have relied on aversive stimuli to evoke affective states. Although it is evident that amygdalectomy attenuates reactions in these circumstances, it is less certain how such monkeys would react affectively to positive stimuli. This is just one reason a thorough, systematic analysis of the social behavior of monkeys with excitotoxic amygdala lesions is required. The fact that amygdalectomized monkeys will readily approach and investigate objects, including food, and will work hard to obtain food rewards (Aggleton & Passingham, 1982) is suggestive of a normal reactivity to positive stimuli. Other support comes from a study (Malkova et al., 1997) that showed that monkeys with excitotoxic lesions of the amygdala are able to use auditory signals that had been paired with food reward to guide a series of visual discriminations. This null result is of interest because it contrasts with an earlier study that showed that aspiration lesions of the amygdala and adjacent cortex impair the same task (Gaffan & Harrison, 1987).

Taken together these results suggest that the amygdala has an especially important role in the identification of and reaction to negative (aversive) stimuli. This echoes a specific proposal by Cahill and McGaugh (1990) that the involvement of the amygdala in certain learning tasks depends on the degree of arousal evoked by the test stimuli, and, as a consequence, the effects of amygdala damage are most evident when using highly aversive stimuli. Before jumping to the conclusion that the amygdala is unimportant for positive (e.g., appetitive) conditioning, it should be remembered that excitotoxic lesions of this region in rats clearly disrupt the formation or utilization of conditioned appetitive reinforcers (Everitt & Robbins, 1992; White & McDonald, 1993). Furthermore, lesions of the central nucleus of the amygdala disrupt the appearance of conditioned orienting responses to the conditioned stimulus in an appetitive task (Gallagher & Holland, 1992). These findings underline the wide range of likely amygdala functions and help to reinforce the overall view that this structure is involved in a constellation of events related to stimulus-affective associations.

References

Adolphs, R., Cahill, L., Schul, R. & Babinsky, R. (1997). Impaired declarative memory for emotional material following bilateral amygdala damage in humans. *Learning & Memory, 4*, 291–300.

Adolphs, R., Tranel, D., Damasio, H. & Damasio, A. (1994). Impaired recognition of emotion in facial expressions following bilateral damage to the human amygdala. *Nature, 372*, 669–672.

Adolphs, R., Tranel, D., Damasio, H. & Damasio, A. R. (1995). Fear and the human amygdala. *Journal of Neuroscience, 15*, 5879–5891.

Aggleton, J. P. (1992). The functional effects of amygdala lesions in humans: a comparison with findings from monkeys. In J. P. Aggleton (Ed), *The Amygdala: Neurobiological Aspects of Emotion, Memory, and Mental Dysfunction* (pp. 485–503). New York: Wiley-Liss.

Aggleton, J. P. (1985). A description of intra-amygdaloid connections in old world monkeys. *Experimental Brain Research, 57*, 390–399.

Aggleton, J. P. (1993). The contribution of the amygdala to normal and abnormal emotional states. *Trends in Neuroscience, 16*, 328–333.

Aggleton, J. P., Burton, M. J. & Passingham, R. E. (1980). Cortical and subcortical afferents to the amygdala of the rhesus monkey. *Brain Research, 190*, 347–368.

Aggleton, J. P. & Passingham, R. E. (1981). Syndrome produced by lesions of the amygdala in monkeys (*Macaca mulatta*). *Journal of Comparative and Physiological Psychology, 95*, 961–977.

Aggleton, J. P. & Passingham, R. E. (1982). An assessment of the reinforcing properties of foods after amygdaloid lesions in rhesus monkeys. *Journal of Comparative and Physiological Psychology, 96*, 71–77.

Aggleton, J. P. & Shaw, C. (1996). Amnesia and recognition memory: a re-analysis of psychometric data. *Neuropsychologia, 34*, 51–62.

Amaral, D. G., Price, J. L., Pitkänen, A. & Thomas Carmichael, S. (1992). Anatomical organization of the primate amygdaloid complex. In J. P. Aggleton (Ed), *The Amygdala: Neurobiological Aspects of Emotion, Memory, and Mental Dysfunction* (pp. 1–66). New York: Wiley-Liss.

Andersen, R. (1978). Cognitive changes after amygdalotomy. *Neuropsychologia, 16*, 439–451.

Angrilli, A., Mauri, A., Palomba, D., Flor, H., Birbaumer, N., Sartori, G. & di Paola, F. (1996). Startle reflex and emotion modulation impairment after a right amygdala lesion. *Brain, 119*, 1991–2000.

Babinsky, R., Calabrese, P., Dunwen, H. F., Markowitsch, H. J., Brechteisbauer, D., Hauser, L. & Gehler, W. (1993). The possible contribution of the amygdala to memory. *Behavioural Neurology, 6*, 167–170.

Banati, R. B., Goerres, G. W., Tjoa, C., Aggleton, J. P. & Grasby, P. (2000). The functional anatomy of visual-tactile integration in man: a study using positron emission tomography. *Neuropsychologia, 38*, 115–124.

Barton, R. (1996). Neocortex size and behavioral ecology in primates. *Proceedings of the Royal Society of London B, 263*, 173–177.

Barton, R. & Dunbar, R. (1997). Evolution of the social brain. In A. Whiten & R. W. Byrne (Eds), *Machiavellian Intelligence*, 2nd ed. Cambridge: Cambridge University Press.

Baylis, L. L. & Gaffan, D. (1991). Amygdalectomy and ventromedial prefrontal ablation produce similar deficits in food choice and in simple object discrimination learning for an unseen reward. *Experimental Brain Research, 86*, 617–622.

Bechara, A., Tranel, D. Damasio, H. Adolphs, R., Rockland, C. & Damasio, A. R. (1995). Double dissociation of conditioning and declarative knowledge relative to the amygdala and hippocampus in humans. *Science, 269*, 1115–1118.

Bonda, E., Petrides, M. Ostry, D. & Evans, A. (1996). Specific involvement of human parietal systems and the amygdala in the perception of biological motion. *Journal of Neuroscience, 16*, 3737–3744.

Breiter, H. C., Etcoff, N. L., Whalen, P. J., Kennedy, W. A., Rauch, S. L., Buckner, R. L., Strauss, M. M., Hyman, S. E. & Rosen, B. R. (1996). Response and habituation of the human amygdala during visual processing of facial emotion. *Neuron, 17*, 875–887.

Broks, P., Young, A. W., Maratos, E. J., Coffey, P. J., Calder, A. J., Isaac, C., Mayes, A. R., Hodges, J. R., Montaldi, D., Cezayirli, E., Roberts, N. & Hadley, D. (1998). Face processing impairments after encephalitis: amygdala damage and recognition of fear. *Neuropsychologia, 36*, 59–70.

Brothers, L. (1989). A biological perspective on empathy. *American Journal of Psychiatry, 146*, 10–19.

Brothers, L. & Ring, B. (1993). Mesial temporal neurons in the macaque monkey with responses selective for aspects of social stimuli. *Behavioural Brain Research, 57*, 53–61.

Brothers, L., Ring, B. & Kling, A. (1990). Response of neurons in the macaque amygdala to complex social stimuli. *Behavioural Brain Research, 41*, 199–213.

Brown, S. & Schafer, E. A. (1888). An investigation into the functions of the occipital and temporal lobes of the monkeys brain. *Philosophical Transactions of the Royal Society of London B, 179*, 303–327.

Bruce, C., Desimone, R. & Gross, C. G. (1981). Visual properties of neurons in a polysensory area in superior temporal sulcus of the macaque. *Journal of Neurophysiology, 46*, 369–384.

Butter, C. M. & Snyder, D. R. (1972). Alterations in aversive and aggressive behaviors following orbital frontal lesions in rhesus monkeys. *Acta Neurobioligica Experimentalis, 32*, 525–565.

Cahill, L., Babinsky, R., Markowitsch, H. J. & McGaugh, J. L. (1995). The amygdala and emotional memory. *Nature, 377*, 295–296.

Cahill, L., Haier, R. J., Fallon, J., Alkire, M. T., Tang, C., Keator, D., Wu, J. & McGaugh, J. L. (1996). Amygdala activity at encoding correlated with long-term, free recall of emotional information. *Proceedings of the National Academy Science, USA, 93*, 8016–8021.

Cahill, L. & McGaugh, J. L. (1990). Amygdaloid complex lesions differentially affect retention of tasks using appetative and aversive reinforcement. *Behavioral Neuroscience, 104*, 523–543.

Cahill, L. & McGaugh, J. L. (1996). Modulation of memory storage. *Current Opinion in Neurobiology, 6*, 237–242.

Cahill, L., Prins, B., Weber, M. & McGaugh, J. L. (1994). Beta-adrenergic activation and memory for emotional events. *Nature, 371*, 702–704.

Calder, A. J., Young, A. W., Rowland, D., Perrett, I., Hodges, J. R. & Etcoff, N. L. (1996). Facial emotion recognition after bilateral amygdala damage: differentially severe impairment of fear. *Cognitive Neuropsychology, 13*, 699–745.

Campeau, S. & Davis, M. (1995a). Involvement of the central nucleus and basolateral complex of the amygdala in fear conditioning measured with fear-potentiated startle in rats trained concurrently with auditory and visual conditioned stimuli. *Journal of Neuroscience, 15*, 2301–2311.

Campeau, S. & Davis M. (1995b). Involvement of subcortical and cortical afferents to the lateral nucleus of the amygdala in fear conditioning measured with fear-potentiated startle in rats trained concurrently with auditory and visual conditioned stimuli. *Journal of Neuroscience, 15*, 2312–2327.

Corkin, S. (1984). Lasting consequences of bilateral medial temporal lobectomy: clinical course and experimental finding in H.M. *Seminars in Neurology, 4*, 249–259.

Davis, M. (1992). The role of the amygdala in conditioned fear. In J. P. Aggleton (Ed), *The Amygdala: Neurobiological Aspects of Emotion, Memory, and Mental Dysfunction* (pp. 255–305). New York: Wiley-Liss.

Downer, J. L. deC. (1961). Changes in visual gnostic functions and emotional behavior following unilateral temporal pole damage in the 'split-brain' monkey. *Nature, 191*, 50–51.

Emsley, R. A. & Paster, L. (1985). Lipoid proteinosis presenting with neuropsychiatric manifestations. *Journal of Neurology and Psychiatry, 48*, 1290–1292.

Everitt, B. J. & Robbins, T. W. (1992). Amygdala-ventral striatal interactions and reward-related processes. In J. P. Aggleton (Ed), *The Amygdala: Neurobiological Aspects of Emotion, Memory, and Mental Dysfunction* (pp. 401–429). New York: Wiley-Liss.

Gaffan, D. (1992). Amygdala and the memory of reward. In J. P. Aggleton (Ed), *The Amygdala: Neurobiological Aspects of Emotion, Memory, and Mental Dysfunction* (pp. 471–483). New York: Wiley-Liss.

Gaffan, D. (1994). Role of the amygdala in picture discrimination learning with 24-h intertrial intervals. *Experimental Brain Research, 99*, 423–430.

Gaffan, D. & Bolton, J. (1983). Learning of object-object associations by monkeys. *Quarterly Journal of Experimental Psychology (B), 35*, 149–155.

Gaffan, D. & Harrison, S. (1987). Amygdalectomy and disconnection in visual learning for auditory secondary reinforcement by monkeys. *Journal of Neuroscience, 7*, 2285–2292.

Gallagher, M. & Holland, P. C. (1992). Understanding the function of the central nucleus: Is simple conditioning enough? In J. P. Aggleton (Ed), *The Amygdala: Neurobiological Aspects of Emotion, Memory, and Mental Dysfunction* (pp. 307–321). New York: Wiley-Liss.

Goulet, S., Doré, F. Y. & Murray, E. A. (1998). Aspiration lesions of the amygdala disrupt the rhinal corticothalamic projection system in rhesus monkeys. *Experimental Brain Research, 119*, 131–140.

Hamann, S. B., Cahill, L., McGaugh, J. L. & Squire, L. R. (1997). Intact enhancement of declarative memory for emotional material in amnesia. *Learning & Memory, 4*, 301–309.

Hamann, S. B., Stefanacci, L., Squire, L. R., Adolphs, R., Tranel, D., Damasio, H. & Damasio, A. (1996). Recognizing facial emotion. *Nature, 379*, 497.

Hasselmo, M. E., Rolls, E. T. & Baylis, G. C. (1989). The role of expression and identity in the face-selective responses of neurons in the temporal visual cortex of the monkey. *Behavioural Brain Research, 32*, 203–218.

Hodges, J. R., Patterson, K., Oxbury, S. & Funnell, E. (1992). Progressive fluent aphasia with temporal lobe atrophy. *Brain, 115*, 1783–1806.

Horel, J. A., Keating, E. G. & Misantone, L. J. (1975). Partial Klüver-Bucy syndrome produced by destroying temporal neocortex or amygdala. *Brain Research, 94*, 347–359.

Irwin, W., Davidson, R. J., Lowe, M. J., Mock, B. J., Sorenson, J. A. & Turski, P. A. (1996). Human amygdala activation detected with echo-planar functional magnetic resonance imaging. *NeuroReport, 7*, 1765–1769.

Jacobson, R. (1986). Disorders of facial recognition, social behavior and affect after combined bilateral amygdalotomy and subcaudate tractotomy—a clinical and experimental study. *Psychological Medicine, 16*, 439–450.

Jones, B. & Mishkin, M. (1972). Limbic lesions and the problem of stimulus-reinforcement associations. *Experimental Neurology, 36*, 362–377.

Kapur, N., Ellison, D., Parkin, A. J., Hunkin N., Burrows, E., Sampson, S. A. & Morrison, E. A. (1994). Bilateral temporal lobe pathology with sparing of medial temporal lobe structures: lesion profile and pattern of memory disorder. *Neuropsychologia, 32*, 23–38.

Killcross, S., Robbins, T. W. & Everitt, B. J. (1997). Different types of fear-conditioned behaviour mediated by separate nuclei within amygdala. *Nature, 388*, 377–380.

Kling, A. (1972). Effects of amygdalectomy on social-affective behaviour in non-human primates. In B. E. Eleftheriou (Ed), *The Neurobiology of the Amygdala* (pp. 511–536). New York: Plenum Press.

Kling, A. & Dunne, K. (1976). Social-environmental factors affecting behavior and plasma testosterone in normal and amygdala lesions *M. speciosa. Primate, 17*, 23–42.

Kling, A. & Cornell, P. (1971). Amygdalectomy and social behavior in the caged stump-tailed macaque. *Folia Primatology, 14*, 91–103.

Kling, A. & Dunne, K. (1976). Social-environmental factors affecting behavior and plasma testosterone in normal and amygdala lesioned *M. speciosa. Primate, 17*, 23–42.

Kling, A. & Steklis, H. D. (1976). A neural substrate for affiliative behavior in nonhuman primates. *Brain Behavior and Evolution, 13*, 216–238.

Klingler, J. & Gloor, P. (1960). The connections of the amygdala and of the anterior temporal cortex in the human brain. *Journal of Comparative Neurology, 115*, 333–369.

Klüver, H. & Bucy, P. C. (1939). Preliminary analysis of functions of the temporal lobes in monkeys. *Archives of Neurology and Psychiatry, 42*, 979–1000.

LeDoux, J. E. (1995). Emotion: Clues from the brain. *Annual Review of Psychology, 46*, 209–35.

Lee, G. P., Reed, M. F., Meador, K. J., Smith, J. R. & Loring, D. W. (1995). Is the amygdala crucial for cross-modal association in humans? *Neuropsychology, 9*, 236–245.

Leonard, C. M., Rolls, E. T., Wilson, F. A. W. & Baylis, G. C. (1985). Neurons in the amygdala of the monkey with responses selective for faces. *Behavioural Brain Research, 15*, 159–176.

Malkova, L., Gaffan, D. & Murray, E. A. (1997). Excitotoxic lesions of the amygdala fail to produce impairment in visual learning for auditory secondary reinforcement but interfere with reinforcer devaluation effects in rhesus monkeys. *Journal of Neuroscience, 17*, 6011–6020.

Malkova, L. & Murray, E. A. (1996). Effects of partial versus complete lesions of the amygdala on crossmodal associations in cynomolgus monkeys. *Psychobiology, 24*, 255–264.

Maren, S. & Fanselow, M. S. (1996). The amygdala and fear conditioning: has the nut been cracked? *Neuron, 16*, 237–240.

Marlowe, W. B., Mancall, E. L. & Thomas, J. J. (1975). Complete Klüver-Bucy syndrome in man. *Cortex, 11*, 53–59.

McGaugh, J. L., Introini-Collison, I. B., Cahill, L., Kim, M. & Liang, K. C. (1992). Involvement of the amygdala in neuromodulatory influences on memory storage. In J. P. Aggleton (Ed), *The Amygdala: Neurobiological Aspects of Emotion, Memory, and Mental Dysfunction* (pp. 431–451). New York: Wiley-Liss.

Meunier, M., Bachevalier, J., Murray, E. A., Malkova, L. & Mishkin, M. (1999). Effects of aspiration vs neurotoxic lesions of the amygdala on emotional reactivity in rhesus monkeys. *European Journal of Neuroscience, 11*, 4408–4418.

Meunier, M., Bachevalier, J., Mishkin, M. & Murray, E. A. (1993). Effects on visual recognition of combined and separate ablations of the entorhinal and perirhinal cortex in rhesus monkeys. *Journal of Neuroscience, 13*, 5418–5432.

Meunier, M., Bachevalier, J., Murray, E. A., Merjanian, P. M. & Richardson, R. (1991). Effects of rhinal cortical or limbic lesions on fear reaction in rhesus monkeys. *Society for Neuroscience Abstract, 17*, 337.

Miserendino, M. J. D., Sananes, C. B., Melia, K. R. & Davis, M. (1990). Blocking of acquisition but not expression of conditioned fear-potentiated startle by NMDA antagonists in the amygdala. *Nature, 345*, 716–718.

Mishkin, M. (1978). Memory in monkeys severely impaired by combined but not by separate removal of amygdala and hippocampus. *Nature, 273*, 297–298.

Morris, J. S., Frith, C. D., Perrett, D. I., Rowland, D., Young, A. W., Calder, A. J. & Dolan, R. J. (1996). A differential neural response in the human amygdala to fearful and happy facial expressions. *Nature, 383*, 812–815.

Murray, E. A. (1992). Medial temporal lobe structures contributing to recognition memory: The amygdaloid complex versus the rhinal cortex. In J. P. Aggleton (Ed), *The Amygdala: Neurobiological Aspects of Emotion, Memory, and Mental Dysfunction* (pp. 453–470). New York: Wiley-Liss.

Murray, E. A. & Gaffan, D. (1994). Removal of the amygdala plus subjacent cortex disrupts the retention of both intramodal and crossmodal associative memories in monkeys. *Behavioural Neuroscience, 108*, 494–500.

Murray, E. A., Gaffan, E. A. & Flint, R. W. (1996). Anterior rhinal cortex and amygdala: dissociation of their contributions to memory and food preference in rhesus monkeys. *Behavioural Neuroscience, 110*, 30–42.

Murray, E. A., Gaffan, D. & Mishkin, M. (1993). Neural substrates of visual stimulus-stimulus association in rhesus monkeys. *Journal of Neuroscience, 13*, 4559–4561.

Murray, E. A. & Mishkin, M. (1985). Amygdalectomy impairs crossmodal association in monkeys. *Science, 228*, 604–606.

Murray, E. A. & Mishkin, M. (1998). Object recognition and location memory in monkeys with excitotoxic lesions of the amygdala and hippocampus. *Journal of Neuroscience, 18*, 6568–6582.

Murray, E. A. & Wise, S. P. (1996). Role of the hippocampus plus subjacent cortex but not amygdala in visuomotor conditional learning in rhesus monkeys. *Behavioural Neuroscience, 110*, 1261–1270.

Myers, R. E. (1972). Role of prefrontal and anterior temporal cortex in social behavior and affect in monkeys. *Acta Neurobiologica Experimentalis, 32*, 567–579.

Nader, K. & LeDoux, J. E. (1997). Is it time to invoke multiple fear learning systems in the amygdala? *Trends in Cognitive Sciences, 1*, 241–244.

Nahm, F. K. D., Tranel, D., Damasio, H. & Damasio, A. R. (1993). Cross-modal associations and the human amygdala. *Neuropsychologia, 31*, 727–744.

Narabayashi, H., Nagao, T. Saito, Y., Yoshida, M. & Nagahata, M. (1963). Stereotoxic amygdalotomy for behavior disorders. *Archives of Neurology, 9*, 1–16.

Newton, F. H., Rosenberg, R. N., Lampert, P. W., & O'Brien, J. S. (1971). Neurologic involvement in Urbach-Wiethe's disease (lipoid proteinosis). *Neurology, 21*, 1205–1213.

Perrett, D. I., Rolls, E. T. & Caan, W. (1982). Visual neurones responsive to faces in the monkey temporal cortex. *Experimental Brain Research, 47*, 329–342.

Quirk, G. J., Repa, C. & LeDoux, J. (1995). Fear conditioning enhances short-latency auditory responses of lateral amygdala neurons—parallel recordings in the freely behaivng rat. *Neuron, 15*, 1029–1039.

Ramachandran, V., Balasubramaniam, V. & Kanaka, T. S. (1974). Follow-up of patients treated with stereotaxic amygdalotomy. *Indian Journal Psychiatry, 16*, 299–306.

Rosvold, H. E., Mirsky, A. F. & Pribram, K. H. (1954). Influence of amygdalectomy on social behaviours in monkeys. *Journal of Comparative and Physiological Psychology, 47*, 133–178.

Schwartzbaum, J. S. (1965). Discrimination behavior after amygdalectomy in monkeys. *Journal of Comparative and Physiological Psychology, 60*, 314–319.

Schwartzbaum, J. S. & Poulos, D. A. (1965). Discrimination behavior after amygdalectomy in monkeys. *Journal of Comparative and Physiological Psychology, 60*, 320–328.

Scott, S., Young, A. W., Calder, A. J., Hellawell, D. J., Aggleton, J. P. & Johnson, M. (1997). Auditory recognition of emotion after amygdalotomy: impairment of fear and anger. *Nature, 385*, 254–257.

Sergent, J., Ohta, S., MacDonald, B. & Zuck, E. (1994). Segregated processing of facial identity and emotion in the human brain: a PET study. *Visual Cognition, 1*, 349–369.

Spiegler, B. J. & Mishkin, M. (1981). Evidence for the sequential participation of inferior temporal cortex and amygdala in the acquisition of stimulus-reward associations. *Behavioural Brain Research, 3*, 303–317.

Stefanacci, L., Suzuki, W. A. & Amaral, D. G. (1996). Organization of connections between the amygdaloid complex and perirhinal and parahippocampal cortices in macaque monkeys. *Journal of Comparative Neurology, 375*, 552–582.

Stephan, H., Frahm, H. D. & Baron, G. (1987). Comparison of brain structure volumes in insectivora and primates VII. Amygdaloid components. *Journal für Hirnforschung, 28*, 571–584.

Stern, C. E. & Passingham, R. E. (1996). The nucleus accumbens in monkeys (*Macaca fascicularis*): II. Emotion and motivation. *Behavioural Brain Research, 75*, 179–193.

Suzuki, W. A. (1996). The anatomy, physiology and functions of the perirhinal cortex. *Current Opinion in Neurobiology, 6*, 179–186.

Suzuki, W. A. & Amaral, D. G. (1994). Perirhinal and parahippocampal cortices of the macaque monkey: cortical afferents. *Journal of Comparative Neurology, 350*, 497–533.

Terzian, H. & Ore, G. D. (1955). Syndrome of Klüver-Bucy. Reproduced in man by bilateral removal of temporal lobes. *Neurology, 5*, 373–380.

Tranel, D. & Hyman, B. T. (1990). Neuropsychological correlates of bilateral amygdala damage. *Archives of Neurology, 47*, 349–355.

Turner, B. H., Mishkin, M. & Knapp, M. (1980). Organization of the amygdalopetal projections from modality-specific cortical association areas in the monkey. *Journal of Comparative Neurology, 191*, 515–543.

Turner, E. A. (1954). Cerebral control of respiration. *Brain, 77*, 448–486.

Weiskrantz, L. (1956). Behavioral changes associated with ablations of the amygdaloid complex in monkeys. *Journal of Comparative Physiological Psychology, 49*, 381–391.

White, N. M. & McDonald, R. J. (1993). Acquisition of a spatial conditioned place preference is impaired by amygdala lesions and improved by fornix lesions. *Behavioural Brain Research, 55*, 269–281.

Young, A. W., Aggleton, J. P., Hellawell, D. J., Johnson, M., Broks, P. & Hanley, J. R. (1995). Face processing impairments after amygdalotomy. *Brain, 118*, 15–24.

Young, A. W., Hellawell, D. J., Van de Wal, C. & Johnson, M. (1996). Facial expression processing after amygdalotomy. *Neuropsychologia, 34*, 31–39.

Young, A. W., Newcombe, F., de Haan, E. H. F., Small, M. & Hay, D. C. (1993). Face perception after brain injury. *Brain, 116*, 941–959.

Zola-Morgan, S., Squire, L. R., Alvarez-Royo, P. & Clower, R. P. (1991). Independence of memory functions and emotional behavior: separate contributions of the hippocampal formation and the amygdala. *Hippocampus, 1*, 207–220.

Zola-Morgan, S., Squire, L. R. & Amaral, D. G. (1989). Lesions of the amygdala that spare adjacent cortical regions do not impair memory or exacerbate the impairment following lesions of the hippocampal formation. *Journal of Neuroscience, 9*, 1922–1936.

Zola-Morgan, S., Squire, L. R., Clower, R. P. & Rempel, N. L. (1993). Damage to the perirhinal cortex exacerbates memory impairment following lesions to the hippocampal formation. *Journal of Neuroscience, 13*, 251–265.

7

Cognitive–Emotional Interactions: Listen to the Brain

JOSEPH LEDOUX

Through the ages, cognition and emotion have been viewed as separate but equal aspects of the mind. The goal of a theory of mind was traditionally to understand how cognition, emotion, and other mental processes contribute to and interact in the making of the mind. But around the middle of the twentieth century, an intellectual hegemony, now called cognitive science, began that ultimately led to an approach to the mind that intentionally left the study of emotion out (see LeDoux, 1996). Recently, there have been a number of attempts to reunite emotion and cognition in the mind, usually by inserting emotion into the cognitive view of the mind (see Ekman & Davidson, 1994). These have not succeeded, as there is still more confusion than consensus about the relation between emotion and cognition and the place of these two concepts in a theory of mind.

The source of the confusion, I believe, is that the terms "cognition" and "emotion" do not refer to real functions performed by the brain but instead to collections of disparate brain processes. For example, on the cognitive side we have perception, memory, attention, action, and so on. But each of these turns out to be shorthand terms for more fundamental processes—vision versus touch, implicit versus explicit memory, attention versus preattentive processes, etc. And each can also be broken down into more fundamental processes—for example, visual perception is not a single process but is made up of a variety of component functions (e.g., form, color, motion processes). Similarly, emotions are made up of component functions (subjective experience, stimulus evaluation, physiological responses, feedback, elicited behaviors, voluntary behaviors, and so on), and it is likely that the brain representations of at least some of these functions are unique for different emotions. Thus, the true nature of the relation between cognition and emotion will not be understood until the interaction rules that relate component processes on both sides of the cognitive–emotional equation are specified.

How, then, should we figure out the interaction rules? Emotion and cognition have usually been studied independent of the way the brain works. While this purely psychological approach is valuable, a far more powerful approach results when we use the brain as a source of information about psychological processes.

The brain can, on the one hand, constrain psychological theories and, on the other, can suggest new insights that were not obvious from psychological theory and experimentation alone. Thus, by studying how an emotion, such as fear, is represented in the brain, we can see exactly what the neural components of the system are. We can then ask how the component processes in that neural system relate to components of systems that mediate various cognitive processes. A similar approach can be taken for other emotion systems.

In this chapter, I outline an approach like this for the emotion of fear. I first discuss why I think fear is a good emotion to start with and then lay out what we have learned about the fear system by studying a particular model of fear—namely, classical fear conditioning. I show how we might then begin to understand the relation between cognition and emotion by examining neural interactions between the fear system and systems involved in specific aspects of perception, memory, and other cognitive processes.

What Is Fear and Why Do We Care about It?

Fear is a normal reaction to threatening situations and is a common occurrence in daily life. When fear becomes greater than that warranted by the situation or begins to occur in inappropriate situations, a fear or anxiety disorder exists (e.g., Marks, 1987; Öhman, 1992). Excluding substance abuse problems, anxiety disorders account for about half of all the conditions that people see mental health professionals for each year (Manderscheid & Sonnenschein, 1994). It seems likely that the fear system of the brain is involved in at least some anxiety disorders, and it is thus important that we understand in as much detail as possible how the fear system works. This information may lead to a better understanding of how anxiety disorders arise and how they might be prevented or controlled. If through studies of fear we were only to learn about fear-related processes, we would still have accomplished quite a lot.

William James said that nothing marks the difference between humans and other animals more than the reduction of conditions under which humans experience fear (James, 1890). Although predation by other species is fairly rare for humans, we face other dangers that require us to be ready to defend ourselves on short notice. Psychological stress, for example, can be harmful to physical and psychological well being (McEwen & Sapolsky, 1995), and modern life is full of physical dangers (injuries and death from automobile or airplane accidents, health risks from tobacco and radiation, sports injuries, electric shocks from misuse of household appliances) that occur as by-products of activities introduced by humans. Furthermore, our capacities for thinking, remembering, and imagining greatly expand the range of real and imagined objects and events that can activate the fear system.

When we use the term "fear," we are naturally inclined to think of the feeling of being afraid. As important as subjective feelings like fear are to our lives, it seems likely that these were not the functions that were selected for in the evolution of the fear system or other emotion systems. Fearful feelings, for example, occur when a more basic neural system (the system that evolved to detect and respond to danger) functions in a brain that also has the capacity to be conscious of its own activities (LeDoux, 1996). All animals (from bugs and worms to birds, lizards, pigeons, rats, monkeys, and people) are able to detect and respond to danger. Most animals in fact exist on both sides of the food chain, and their daily lives consist, in large part, of activities involved in finding food and avoiding becoming someone else's lunch. The ability to detect and respond to danger, then, is the function that the fear system evolved to perform, and the feelings of fear that occur when this system is active in a human brain (and perhaps some others) is a consequence of having this system plus a system for conscious awareness.

The implications of this situation are enormous for a science of emotion. It is entirely possible that the basic fear system is the same in animals that do and do not have robust conscious awareness and experience robust feelings of fear. If so, we can study how the fear system functions independent of any contribution this system makes to subjective feelings of fear. And we can study the fear system in animals, even if we cannot prove that they experience feelings of fear. This is key because only through such studies can the detailed biology of a brain system be understood. That the neural system underlying fear is similar in humans and other animals is supported by experimental studies that have used a common behavioral tool for studying fear—namely, fear conditioning—as described below.

How Do We Study Fear?

There are a number of experimental tools for studying fear and anxiety in animals (including humans), but one of the simplest and most straightforward is fear conditioning. With this procedure, meaningless stimuli acquire affective properties when they occur in conjunction with a biologically significant event. The initially neutral stimulus is called a conditional (or conditioned) stimulus (CS) and the biologically significant one an unconditional (or unconditioned) stimulus (US). Through CS–US associations, innate physiological and behavioral responses come under the control of the CS (figure 7.1). For example, if a rat hears a tone (CS) followed by an electric shock (US), after a few tone–shock pairings it will exhibit a complex set of conditioned fear responses to the tone (Blanchard & Blanchard, 1969; Bolles & Fanselow, 1980; Bouton & Bolles, 1980; Estes & Skinner, 1941; Mason et al., 1961; McAllister & McAllister, 1971; Schneidermann et al., 1974). Included are direct alterations in the activity of autonomic (e.g., heart rate, blood pressure), endocrine (hormone release), and skeletal (conditioned immobility, or "freezing") systems, as well as modulations of pain sensitivity (analgesia) and somatic reflexes (fear-potentiated startle, fear-potentiated eyeblink responses). These responses represent evolutionarily programmed activities that are expressed involuntarily in the presence of danger. Fear conditioning works throughout the phyla, having been studied experimentally in flies, worms, snails, fish, pigeons, rabbits, rats, cats, dogs, monkeys, baboons, and humans (see LeDoux, 1996).

Fear conditioning may not tell us all we need to know about all aspects of fear or all aspects of fear or anxiety disorders, but it is an excellent starting point. Furthermore, many of the other fear assessment procedures, such as the various forms of avoidance conditioning, crucially involve an initial phase of fear conditioning that then provides motivational impetus for the later stages of instrumental

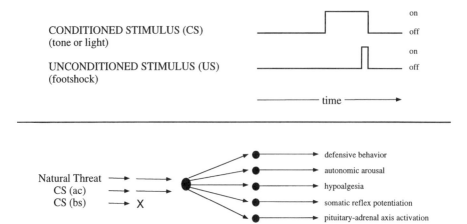

Figure 7.1. Classical fear conditioning.

avoidance learning (e.g., Dollard & Miller, 1950; Mowrer, 1939, 1960; Mowrer & Lamoreaux, 1946). There are some fear assessment procedures that do not require learning (e.g., open field, the elevated maze, or light-avoidance tasks), but these are somewhat less amenable to a neural systems analysis than fear conditioning, due mainly to the fact that the stimulus situation is often poorly defined in these procedures.

Neural System Underlying Fear Conditioning

The neural networks underlying fear conditioning have been elucidated (for reviews, see Davis, 1992a, 1992b, Davis et al., 1994; Kapp et al., 1992, 1994; Le-Doux, 1994, 1996; Maren & Fanselow, 1996; Rogan & LeDoux, 1996). The pathways involved differ somewhat depending on the sensory modality and other properties of the CS. Below, I focus on the pathways involved when a simple auditory CS (a pure tone) is used, as these pathways have been characterized in the most detail (see fig. 7.2). In addition, I focus on studies of rats, as most of the findings are from this species. However, the auditory findings, except for the sensory afferent components of the pathway, apply to other modalities, and the rat findings are relevant to other mammals, including humans, as well as a variety of other vertebrates (see LeDoux, 1996). The neural organization of the fear system, in other words, seems to be conserved throughout much of vertebrate, including mammalian, evolution.

   Conditioning to a single tone paired with footshock involves transmission through the auditory pathways of the brainstem to the level of the auditory relay nucleus in the thalamus, the medial geniculate body (MGB) (LeDoux et al., 1984). The signal is then transmitted from all regions of the auditory thalamus to the auditory cortex, and from a subset of thalamic nuclei to the amygdala. The thalamo-amygdala pathway originates primarily in the medial division of the MGB

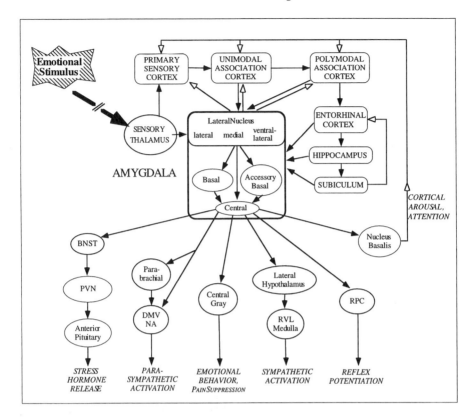

Figure 7.2. Neural pathways of conditional fear.

and the associated posterior intralaminar nucleus, collectively referred to as MGm/ PIN (LeDoux et al., 1990b). The auditory association cortex also gives rise to a projection to the amygdala (Mascagni et al., 1993; Romanski & LeDoux, 1993a,b). Both the thalamo-amygdala and thalamo-cortico-amygdala pathways terminate in the sensory input region of the amygdala, the lateral nucleus (LA) (see LeDoux et al., 1990b; Mascagni et al., 1993; Romanski & LeDoux, 1993; Turner & Herkenham, 1991). In fact, the two pathways converge onto single neurons in the LA (Li et al., 1996b). Damage to the LA interferes with fear conditioning (LeDoux et al., 1990a), which can be mediated by either the thalmao-amygdala or thalamo-cortico-amygdala pathways (for discussion, see Campeau & Davis, 1995; Corodimas & LeDoux, 1995; Romanski & LeDoux, 1992). Temporary inactivation of the LA and the adjacent basal nucleus (Helmstetter & Bellgowan, 1994; Muller et al., 1997) or pharmacological blockade of excitatory amino acid receptors in this region (Gerwitz & Davis, 1997a; Kim & Fanselow, 1992; Maren & Fanselow, 1996; Miserendino et al., 1991) also disrupts the acquisition of conditioned fear, and facilitation of excitatory amino acid transmission enhances the rate of fear learning (Rogan et al., 1997).

The auditory cortex is not required for the acquisition of conditioned fear, but the processing capacities of cells in auditory cortex are modified during fear conditioning (Weinberger, 1995). However, the auditory cortex (and its connection to the amygdala) is probably involved in conditioning to more complex stimuli (Gentile et al., 1986; Jarrel et al., 1987; McCabe et al., 1992), though the exact nature of its role remains unclear (Armony et al., 1997a,b).

What are the advantages of the parallel processing capabilities of this system? First, the existence of a subcortical pathway allows the amygdala to detect threatening stimuli in the environment quickly, in the absence of a complete and time-consuming analysis of the stimulus. This "quick-and-dirty" processing route may confer an evolutionary advantage to the species. Second, the rapid subcortical pathway may function to prime the amygdala to evaluate subsequent information received along the cortical pathway (LeDoux, 1986; Li et al., 1996b). For example, a loud noise may be sufficient to alert the amygdala, at the cellular level, to prepare a response to a dangerous predator lurking nearby, but defensive reactions may not be fully mobilized until the auditory cortex analyzes the location, frequency, and intensity of the noise to determine specifically the nature and extent of this potentially threatening signal. The convergence of the subcortical and cortical pathways onto single neurons in the LA (Li et al., 1996b) provides a means by which the integration could take place. Third, recent computational modeling studies show that the subcortical pathway can function as an interrupt device (Simon, 1967) that enables the cortex, by way of amygdalo-cortical projections, to shift attention to dangerous stimuli that occur outside the focus of attention (see Armony et al., 1997a, 1996,).

Once sensory information is processed in the LA, it is transmitted via intra-amygdala connections (see Pitkänen et al., 1995, 1997; Savander et al., 1995, 1996a,b,c) to the basal and accessory basal nuclei, where it is integrated with other incoming inputs, and to the central nucleus, which serves as the main output station of the amygdala. The basal and accessory basal nuclei also project to the central nucleus, giving rise to multiple parallel links from the LA to the central nucleus. The efferent projections from the central nucleus orchestrate brain stem systems involved in various aspects of emotional reactivity.

Damage to the various regions of the amygdala described above interferes with fear conditioning, regardless of how fear conditioning is measured. However, damage to areas to which the central amygdala projects interferes with the expression of conditioned fear in individual response modalities. For example, lesions of the central gray selectively disrupt conditioned defensive motor activity, such as freezing behavior (Fanselow, 1991; LeDoux et al., 1988; Wilson & Kapp, 1994). In contrast, lesions of the lateral hypothalamus disrupt conditioned sympathetic responses, such as blood pressure elevation, leaving conditioned freezing intact (Iwata et al., 1986; LeDoux et al., 1988; Smith et al., 1980). Other brain stem nuclei appear to be important for the mediation of other specific responses in conditioned fear networks (for summary, see Davis, 1992b; LeDoux, 1995a,b).

Humans with damage to the temporal lobe restricted to or including the amygdala have deficits in fear conditioning (Bechera et al., 1995; LaBar et al., 1995). Furthermore, functional imaging studies have shown activation of the amygdala during fear conditioning (LaBar et al., 1998). The role of the human amygdala in fear is also supported by a several studies showing activation by fear-related facial expressions (Breiter et al., 1996; Morris et al., 1996) and interference of detection of fear by amygdala damage (Adolphs et al., 1994, 1995; Young et al., 1995; but see Hamann et al., 1996). Other studies suggest a role for the human amygdala in mediating the effects of emotional arousal on cognitive memory (Cahill et al., 1995, 1996).

Single- and multiple-unit electrophysiological recording studies, mostly in rats and rabbits, have provided important insights into the kinds of stimulus processing that occur in the LA and other amygdala areas during fear conditioning. Populations of neurons within the lateral, basal, and central nuclei (Applegate et al., 1982; Maren et al., 1991; Muramoto et al., 1993; Pascoe & Kapp, 1985; Quirk et al., 1995; Uwano et al., 1995) exhibit conditioned-induced changes in firing patterns and sensory responsivity. Recent work has focused extensively on the LA because it is the entry point of sensory processing (Quirk et al., 1995, 1997a,b). Examples of cellular modifications in the LA are illustrated in figure 7.3. Several key points should be noted. First, the most prominent increases in firing rates in the LA occur at the earliest response latency (less than 15 msec after CS onset), reflecting changes in efficacy of signal processing in the direct thalamo-amygdala pathway (Quirk et al., 1995). The conditioned modifications seen in other subnuclei, in contrast, occur at later intervals (e.g., 30–50 msec after CS onset in the central nucleus; Pascoe & Kapp, 1985). The implications of these latency differences and the relationship among conditioned alterations observed at each of these sites suggest that significant processing occurs within amygdala circuits between input and output stages.

Second, there is evidence for altered functional coupling among local neurons in the LA during conditioning (figure 7.4; Quirk et al., 1995). The synchrony of spontaneous firing found in this region is maintained long after conditioning has

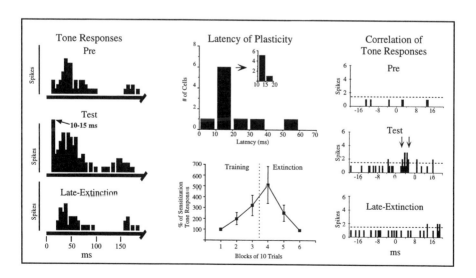

Figure 7.3. Conditioned unit responses in the amygdala.

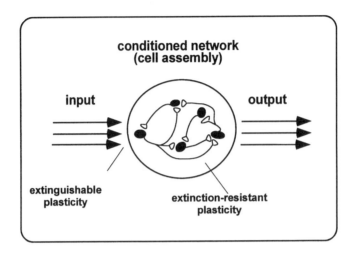

Figure 7.4. Conditioned cell assemblies in the amygdala.

taken place, suggesting that the amygdala may be involved in the long-term encoding and maintenance of emotional memories (LeDoux, 1996; Fanselow and Le-
Doux, 1999; LeDoux, 1992a,b; but see McGaugh et al., 1992, 1995; Cahill &
McGaugh, 1998). Third, neuronal populations within the LA exhibit conditioning-
induced modifications of receptive field properties, as evidenced by shifts in auditory tuning curves favoring the tuning frequency of the auditory cue used as a CS
(Bordi & LeDoux, 1993). Adaptive frequency tuning is also found in the auditory
thalamus and auditory cortex in fear conditioning tasks and may reflect different
aspects of stimulus processing in each of these brain regions (for review, see Weinberger, 1995). Fourth, although other areas in the circuit, such as the auditory cortex,
exhibit conditioned plasticity, the changes require more trials to be established, the
response latencies are longer than in the LA, and amygdala lesions prevent some of
the cortical changes from taking place (Quirk et al., 1997a,b; Armony et al., 1998).
There thus seems to be a primacy of LA plasticity in the circuitry.

Plasticity in the LA has also been studied by inducing long-term potentiation
(LTP) in the thalamo-amygdala pathway (Clugnet & LeDoux, 1990; Rogan & Le-
Doux, 1995), which results in enhanced processing of auditory stimuli through the
pathway (figure 7.5; Rogan & LeDoux, 1995). This shows that natural stimuli can
make use of artificially induced plasticity. Most important, though, natural learning
(fear conditioning) enhances the processing of auditory stimuli in the same way
(Rogan et al., 1997). Fear conditioning, in other words, induces an LTP-like neural
change in the lateral amygdala (fig. 7.6). Together with the unit recording studies,
these findings point toward synaptic changes in the input pathways to the amygdala
as being important in the learning experience.

In other brain areas, LTP is mediated by calcium influx through N-methyl-D-
asparate (NMDA) receptors and a host of subsequent molecular changes (e.g.,
Lynch, 1986; Bliss & Collingridge, 1993; Huang et al., 1996; Madison et al., 1991;
Malenka & Nicoll, 1993; Staubli, 1995). Intra-amygdala blockade of NMDA recep-

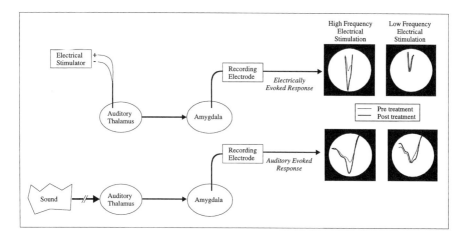

Figure 7.5. Long-term potentiation in the lateral nucleus of the amygdala.

tor function disrupts the acquisition of conditioned fear responses but does not affect the expression of those responses once acquired (Fanselow & Kim, 1994; Gerwitz & Davis, 1997a; Maren et al., 1996a; Miserendino et al., 1990). These results are consistent with the notion that conditioning depends on NMDA receptor activation in the amygdala. However, there is also evidence that NMDA receptors are involved in routine synaptic transmission in the amygdala (Li et al., 1995, 1996b; Maren et al., 1996a), which complicates the interpretation of the behavioral studies. Recent studies have used drugs (ampakines) that facilitate rather than disrupt excitatory transmission (Rogan et al., 1997). These studies show that the rate of fear conditioning, but not the amount, is enhanced when AMPA receptors are facilitated. This result mirrors the effects of these drugs on hippocampal LTP (Staubli et al., 1994) and suggests that common NMDA-dependent mechanisms may be involved.

Studies using genetically altered mice have begun to suggest some of the intracellular mechanisms that might be triggered by calcium influx through NMDA receptors during fear conditioning. Work to date has implicated cAMP signaling pathways as well as calcium-calmodulin kinase (CaMK) pathways (Bourtchuladze et al., 1994; Mayford et al., 1996). Because the same second messengers are involved in hippocampal-dependent spatial learning in mammals and in conditioning in invertebrates, it seems likely that different forms of learning are distinguished not so much by the underlying molecular machinery of learning as by the circuits within which those molecules act.

In summary, the amygdala is a major site of fear plasticity in the brain. Neural modification there allow novel stimuli associated with danger to gain access to evolutionarily old defense-response networks. The key pathways involve transmission of sensory information into the amygdala. The amygdala is involved in fear conditioning in all vertebrates that have been studied. Some progress has been made in elucidating the molecular basis of fear conditioning, and this is likely to be an area where significant breakthroughs will come in the next few years.

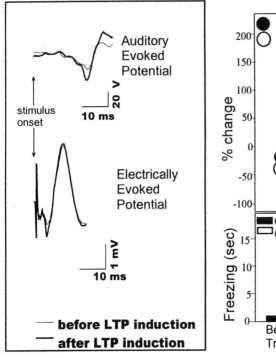

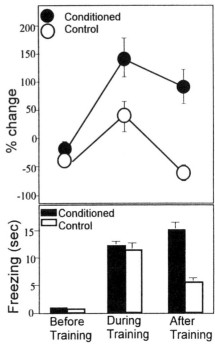

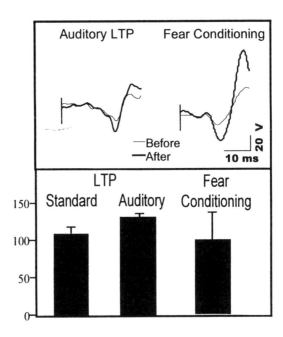

Figure 7.6. Fear conditioning induces long-term potentiation in the lateral nucleus of the amygdala.

Cognition and Emotion: What Does the Brain Say?

The amygdala is key to the basic organization of the fear network. Its job is two-fold. It must first determine whether immediately present stimuli pose a threat to well-being, and if potential threat is present, the amygdala must then orchestrate behavioral responses and associated autonomic and endocrine reactions that increase the likelihood of surviving the danger.

Armed with an understanding of the neural architecture of fear conditioning, we can now turn to the question of how this particular emotional processing network interacts with cognitive processes. We will examine the relation between certain cortical regions involved in specific cognitive processes and the amygdala. The processes mediated by these cortical regions, and the manner in which they interact with the amygdala in fear conditioning, suggest some principles that account for cognitive emotional interactions involving the fear system.

Sensory Cortex and Amygdala: Perception of and Attention Toward Dangerous Stimuli

The amygdala receives inputs from cortical sensory processing regions of each sensory modality (Amaral et al., 1992; Price et al., 1987; Turner et al., 1980) and can, as for fear conditioning, determine whether stimuli processed through those channels are sources of potential danger. However, the amygdala also projects back to cortical sensory processing areas (Amaral et al., 1992). This anatomical arrangement suggests that in addition to processing the emotional significance of external stimuli transmitted to the amygdala from cortical areas, the amygdala might also influence the processing that occurs in these areas. And although the amygdala also receives and processes the significance of sensory stimuli from sensory areas in the thalamus, it does not project back to these areas (see LeDoux et al., 1985, 1990b).

The amygdala only receives inputs from the late stages of cortical sensory processing, but it projects back to the earliest stages (Amaral et al., 1992). This means that once the amygdala is activated by a sensory event from the thalamus or cortex, it can begin to regulate the cortical areas that project to it, controlling the kinds of inputs it receives. This may be a way the amygdala could participate in focusing attention toward emotionally relevant stimuli in the environment. Given that the cortex and amygdala are simultaneously activated by thalamic sensory inputs (Quirk et al., 1997b), it is possible that thalamic activation of the amygdala might begin to regulate cortical processing before cortical representations are fully built up. Amygdala regulation of the cortex could involve facilitating processing of stimuli that signal danger even if such stimuli occur outside of the attentional field (Armony et al., 1996, 1997a, 1998), but might also involve the inhibition of select stimuli along the lines suggested by the controversial field of research called "perceptual defense" (for a summary, see Erdelyi, 1985; LeDoux, 1996).

The amygdala can also influence the cortical sensory processes indirectly by way of projections to various arousal networks, including the basal forebrain cholinergic system, the brainstem cholinergic system, and the locus ceruleus noradrenergic system, each of which innervates widespread areas of the cortex (Saper,

1987). Thus, once the amygdala detects danger, it can activate these arousal systems, which could then influence sensory processing, perhaps by regulating cortical attention (e.g., Aston-Jones et al., 1996; Gallagher & Holland, 1992; Kapp et al., 1992; Weinberger, 1995).

Two lines of evidence support the view that the amygdala regulates cortical attentional/perceptual processing. First, stimulation of the amygdala results in a desynchronization of cortical EEG, which typically occurs when attention is directed to some stimulus (Kapp et al., 1994). Second, during fear conditioning some cells in the auditory cortex exhibit an increase in neural activity during the CS that anticipates the occurrence of the US (Quirk et al., 1997b). These cells may be involved in the direction of attention to the spatio-temporal aspects of the US. Damage to the amygdala prevents the emergence of this conditioned neural response (Armony et al., 1998). This does not imply that the amygdala is involved in all aspects of cortical attention, but instead that it may be involved in the direction and focusing of attention toward dangerous stimuli or stimuli that predict danger (Armony et al., 1996, 1997a).

Hippocampal Cortex and Amygdala:
Contextual Constraints on Fear

A stimulus can be dangerous in one situation (context) and benign, or perhaps interesting, in another. A rattlesnake behind a glass in the zoo poses little threat, but the same snake, encountered while on a walk through the woods, would elicit fear in most of us. Furthermore, environmental contexts may acquire affective properties through prior experiences. If snakes are repeatedly confronted on a particular path through the woods, that path will itself become threatening.

Animals, including humans, thus have to be able to evaluate implications of environmental contexts and situations, including social situations. This has been investigated in the laboratory through studies of contextual fear conditioning. For example, if a rat is conditioned to expect a footshock in the presence of a tone in a conditioning chamber, when the rat is placed back into the chamber, it will exhibit fear reactions not only to the tone CS but also to the conditioning chamber itself, even in the absence of the tone (Kim & Fanselow, 1992; Phillips & LeDoux, 1992). In fact, fear reactions may develop to an environmental context in which shock is administered without the presentation of an explicit CS (Blanchard & Blanchard, 1972; Helmstetter, 1992; Phillips & LeDoux, 1994). The role of context in conditioned associations has been increasingly recognized as an important factor contributing to this form of emotional learning and memory (Bouton, 1993).

Recent studies have shown that the hippocampus contributes to the formation and retention of contextual fear associations. Hippocampal lesions made before training interfere with the acquisition of conditioned responses to the experimental context but do not prevent conditioning to an explicit CS such as a tone (Phillips & LeDoux, 1992, 1994, 1995; Selden et al., 1991). In addition, lesions made after training impair the retention of contextual fear associations but have no effect on conditioned responses to an explicit, unimodal CS (Kim & Fanselow, 1992). This selective retrograde amnesia for contextual fear is temporally graded because lesions made more than two weeks after training do not have an effect (Kim &

Fanselow, 1992). These observations are consistent with current cognitive theories of contextual/relational processing in the hippocampus (Cohen & Eichenbaum, 1993; Nadel & Willner, 1980; O'Keefe & Nadel, 1978; Sutherland & Rudy, 1989), as well as with network models specifying a time-limited hippocampal contribution to the formation of explicit memory (Gluck & Myers, 1997; McClelland et al., 1995). The perirhinal cortex (Corodimas & LeDoux, 1995) and septum (Sparks & LeDoux, 1995) may also contribute to contextual processing.

Although it is not yet clear how contextual information coded in the hippocampus interacts with emotional expression systems, there is bidirectional neural communication between the hippocampal formation and the amygdala (Amaral et al., 1992; Canteras & Swanson, 1992; Ottersen, 1982). These pathways may provide one avenue for the initial engagement of emotional reactions to contextual cues and the imparting of emotional meanings to contexts.

Recently, the role of the hippocampus in contextual conditioning has been questioned on two grounds. First, hippocampal damage does not always impair context conditioning (Gisquet-Verier & Doyere, 1997; Maren et al., 1997; Phillips & LeDoux, 1995). This most likely is due to the use of conditions that bias the animal towards being conditioned to specific cues in the environment rather than to the context per se, thus allowing conditioning to proceed independently of the hippocampus (see Phillips & LeDoux, 1995). If lesions are made before training, animals are more likely to condition to elemental cues because they are unable to condition to the context itself (Frankland et al., 1998). The inconsistency resulting from pretraining lesions may be due to inconsistency in the degree to which individual animals condition to elemental cues in the context or background when the hippocampus is damaged before learning.

The second point of contention comes from studies suggesting that hippocampal effects on context conditioning, as measured by freezing behavior, are secondary to changes in activity levels produced by the lesions—more activity competes with freezing and drives down the scores, leading to a false result with respect to context (Good & Honey, 1997; McNish et al., 1997). However, there are number of problems with this interpretation (for a discussion, see Maren et al., 1998; McNish et al., 1998). One problem is that hippocampal lesions have no effect on freezing to a tone CS measured by freezing. McNish et al. argued that tone conditioning is stronger, and therefore resistant to competition by activity. However, during the early phase of training when tone conditioning is weak, hippocampal lesions still are ineffective. Another problem is that for indiviudal animals, the amount of general activity in a novel environment does not correlate inversely with the amount of freezing. In other words, hippocampal lesions can lead to an increase in activity; the degree of increased activity does not predict the amount of freezing and cannot be the explanation for the freezing deficit. In sum, the arguments against a role of the hippocampus in context are not convincing.

Medial Temporal Lobe and Amygdala:
Explicit Memories about Dangerous Stimuli

It is now widely recognized that there are a variety of memory systems in the brain, some of which work in parallel (see Cohen & Eichenbaum, 1993; O'Keefe &

Nadel, 1978; Squire, 1993). For example, information about stimuli associated with painful or otherwise unpleasant experiences is, as we have seen, stored through the amygdala and related brain regions. This system mediates the emotional reactions elicited when these stimuli are reencountered. It operates at an implicit or unconscious level (LeDoux, 1996). However, we obviously also have explicit or conscious memories about emotional situations. These, like other explicit memories, are mediated by the medial temporal lobe memory system involving the hippocampus, rhinal cortex, and related cortical areas (Cohen & Eichenbaum, 1993; Murray, 1992; Squire, 1995). The implicit memories of emotional events have been called "emotional memories," and the explicit memories have been called "memories about emotions" (LeDoux, 1996). Implicit emotional memories are automatically elicited in the presence of trigger stimuli and do not require conscious retrieval or recall, whereas explicit memories of emotion are retrieved consciously. In humans, damage to the amygdala interferes with implicit emotional memories but not explicit memories about emotions, whereas damage to the medial temporal lobe memory system interferes with explicit memories about emotions but not with implicit emotional memories (Bechera et al., 1995; LaBar et al., 1995). For example, patients with amygdala lesions do not exhibit conditioned fear responses to a CS but remember that a CS was related to a US, while patients with hippocampal damage exhibit conditioned responses but have no memory of a CS–US pairing experience.

Explicit memories with and without emotional content are mediated by the medial temporal lobe system, but those with emotional content differ from those without such content. The former tend to be longer lasting and more vivid (see Christianson, 1992). What accounts for this? The amygdala is the key.

Studies by McGaugh and colleagues (see Cahill et al., 1995, 1996) have shown that stories with emotional content are remembered better than similar stories lacking emotional implications. Further, lesions of the amygdala or systemic administration of a β-adrenergic antagonist prevents this effect. In animal studies, they showed that the effects of beta blockers on memory are due to antagonism of epinephrine released from the adrenal gland (see Packard et al., 1995). One model that accounts for some of these effects is that once the amygdala detects an emotionally significant stimulus, it initiates the release of epinephrine by way of the sympathetic innervation of the adrenal gland. Although the mechanism of action is not fully understood, epinephrine circulating in the blood then influences memory storage in the medial temporal lobe memory system (possibly by way of the vagus nerve and its connections with the locus coeruleus, which innervates the amygdala and hippocampus and many other forebrain areas). Thus, peripheral feedback from responses controlled by the amygdala is yet another way that the amygdala can influence cortical areas, albeit indirectly. The feedback amplifies explicit memories, making them more vivid and enduring.

Medial Prefrontal Cortex and Amygdala:
Changing Stimulus Meaning on the Fly

Fear responses tend to be stubbornly persistent. This is extremely useful. If we survive danger once and can keep an enduring record of the events that led up to the danger, we can use that information to protect ourselves in the future. However, this highly adaptive feature of fear learning can turn into a liability in certain situations. For example, people have all sorts of fears and worries that interfere with routine life. In addition to plain anxiety, fear enters into a variety of mental disorders, including panic, post-traumatic stress disorder, obsessive–compulsive disorder, and phobias. A large part of the mental health community's job is to help people rid themselves of unwanted fears.

Laboratory established fears can be reduced (extinguished) by giving the CS without the US. Although it can take some time for extinction to occur, eventually the CS, if given alone enough times, will lose its potency as an elicitor of fear. This is much less true of clinical fears, which are not easily disposed of by exposure to the fear-eliciting stimuli (see Jacobs & Nadel, 1985). As a result, it has been proposed that some clinical fears (especially phobias) involve a special kind of learning, so-called prepared learning, that involves stimuli that were dangerous to our ancestors (Öhman, 1992; Seligman, 1971). Although there appears to be support for this view, it is also possible that the kind of learning that takes place is the same for laboratory and clinical fears, and what differs is the kind of brain that does the learning.

We found that following lesions of the ventromedial prefrontal cortex, the extinction of conditioned fear is greatly prolonged (Morgan & LeDoux, 1995; Morgan et al., 1993; but see Gewirtz et al., 1997a). Extinguishable fear is thus converted into extinction-resistant fear by altering the integrity of the medial prefrontal cortex. These results suggest that the medial prefrontal region is involved in regulating the amygdala on the basis of the current meaning of stimuli. When this region is damaged, the amygdala continues to respond on the basis of past learning rather than new information. These results complement findings from electrophysiological studies showing that neurons within the orbite-frontal cortex are particularly sensitive to changes in stimulus-reward associations (Rolls, 1996; Thorpe et al., 1983). Thus, it is possible that the medial prefrontal cortex is somehow altered in patients with clinical fears, making it difficult for them to extinguish the fears they learn.

Gewirtz et al. (1997b) failed to replicate these findings. However, we have repeated the study several times (Morgan & LeDoux, 1995; Morgan et al., 1993) and are confident in the results. While the difference might be explained in terms of different procedures used, one would hope that the effects are sufficiently general to apply beyond specific paradigms. Additional studies will be required to fully understand the contribution of the medial cortex to fear extinction.

Cortico-Striatal-Amygdala Interactions:
From Fear Reaction to Action

The defensive responses considered so far are hard-wired reactions to danger signals. These are evolution's gifts to us. They provide a first line of defense against danger. Some animals rely mainly on these. But mammals, especially humans, are able to make the transition from reaction to action. This is one of the benefits of the forebrain expansion that characterizes mammalian evolution.

Considerably less is understood about the brain mechanisms of emotion action than reaction, due in part to the fact that emotional actions come in many varieties and are limited only by the ingenuity of the actor. For example, once we are freezing and expressing physiological responses to a dangerous stimulus, the rest is up to us. On the basis of our expectations about what is likely to happen next and our past experiences in similar situations, we make a plan about what to do. We become instruments of action.

Instrumental responses in situations of danger are often studied using avoidance-conditioning procedures. Avoidance is a multistage learning process (Mowrer, 1960). First, conditioned fear responses are acquired. Then, the CS becomes a signal used to initiate responses that prevent encounters with the US. Finally, once avoidance responses are learned, animals no longer show the characteristic signs of fear (Linden, 1969; Solomon & Wynne, 1954). The involvement of an instrumental component to some aversive learning tasks may explain why these are not dependent on the amygdala for long-term storage (McGaugh et al., 1995; Packard et al., 1995).

Because avoidance learning involves fear conditioning, at least initially, it will be subject to all the factors that influence fear conditioning and conditioned fear responding. However, because avoidance learning involves more than simple fear conditioning, it is to be expected that avoidance will be subject to influences that have little or no effect on conditioned fear. Much more work is needed to understand how fear and avoidance interact and thus how emotional actions emerge out of emotional reactions. However, it seems, from what we know so far, that like other habit systems (Petri & Mishkin, 1994), interactions between the amygdala, basal ganglia, and neocortex are important in avoidance (Everitt & Robbins, 1992; Killcross et al., 1997).

Lateral Prefrontal Cortex: Working Memory,
Consciousness, and Subjective Feelings

Ever since James (1890) asked whether we are afraid of a bear because we run or whether we run because we are afraid, the study of emotion has been focused on the question of where fear and other subjective emotional states come from. Defined this way, progress in understanding emotion hinges on a solution to the problem of consciousness. In other areas of psychology, progress has been made in treating mental functions as processes. For example, we know quite a lot about how the brain processes color, but almost nothing about how color is experienced. Throughout this chapter, I have tried to deal with the emotion fear from a processing point of view and have sidestepped the problem of consciousness. This approach allows us to study fundamental emotional mechanisms in animals with and without consciousness (also, it eliminates the necessity of deciding what consciousness is and who has it).

Nevertheless, consciousness is an important part of the study of emotion and other mental processes. The mechanisms of consciousness are probably the same for emotional and nonemotional subjective states and what distinguishes these states is the brain system that consciousness is aware of at the time.

We are far from solving what consciousness is, but a decent working hypothesis is that it has something to do with working memory, a serially organized mental workspace where things can be compared and contrasted and mentally manipulated

(Baars, 1988; Johnson-Laird, 1988; Kihlstrom, 1987; Kosslyn & Koenig, 1992; Shallice, 1988). Working memory allows us, for example, to compare an immediately present visual stimulus with information stored in long-term (explicit) memory about similar stimuli or stimuli found in similar locations.

A variety of studies of humans and nonhuman primates point to the prefrontal cortex, especially the dorsolateral prefrontal areas, as being involved in working memory processes (Cohen et al., 1997; D'Espisito et al., 1995; Fuster, 1989; Goldman-Rakic, 1988). Immediately present stimuli and stored representations are integrated in working memory by way of interactions between working memory systems, sensory processing systems, which serve as short-term memory buffers as well as perceptual processors, and the medial temporal lobe memory system. Recently, the notion has arisen that working memory may involve interactions between several prefrontal areas, including the anterior cingulate and orbital cortical regions, as well as dorsolateral prefrontal cortex (for summary, see LeDoux, 1996).

Now suppose that the stimulus is affectively charged, say, a trigger of fear. The same sorts of processes will be called upon as for stimuli without emotional implications, but in addition, working memory will become aware of the fact that the fear system of the brain has been activated. This additional information, when added to perceptual and mnemonic information about the object or event, may be the condition for the subjective experience of an emotional state of fear (figure 7.7).

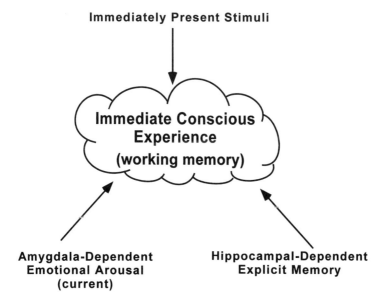

Figure 7.7. Working memory and emotional experience.

But what is the additional information added to working memory when the fear system is activated? As noted above, the amygdala projects to many cortical areas, even some that it does not receive inputs from. It can thus influence the operation of perceptual and short-term memory processes, as well as processes in higher order areas. Although the amygdala does not have extensive connections with the dorsolateral prefrontal cortex, it does communicate with the anterior cingualte and orbital cortex, two other components of the working memory network. But in addition, the amygdala projects to nonspecific systems involved in the regulation of cortical arousal, such as the noradrengergic, cholinergic, serotonergic, or dopaminergic systems. And the amygdala controls bodily responses (behavioral, autonomic, endocrine), which then provide feedback that can influence cortical processing indirectly. Thus, working memory receives a greater number of inputs and receives inputs of a greater variety, in the presence of an emotional stimulus than in the presence of other stimuli. These extra inputs may just be what is required to add affective charge to working memory representations and thus to turn subjective experiences into emotional experiences.

Conclusions

Information about how the brain is organized can constrain the way we think about emotional and other psychological functions. By studying an emotion such as fear and its neural representation, we identify the neural components of the system. This then allows us to ask how the component processes in that neural system relate to components of systems that mediate cognitive processes. In this way, we can let the brain guide us in our attempt to understand cognitive–emotional interactions. The success of this approach within the area of fear should pave the way for similar explorations for other emotions and their relation to cognitive processes.

References

Adolphs, R., Tranel, D., Damasio, H. & Damasio, A. R. (1994). Impaired recognition of emotion in facial expressions following bilateral damage to the human amygdala. *Nature, 372*, 669–672.

Adolphs, R., Tranel, D., Damasio, H. & Damasio, A. R. (1995). Fear and the human amygdala. *Journal of Neuroscience, 15*, 5879–5891.

Amaral, D. G., Price, J. L., Pitkanen, A. & Carmichael, S. T. (1992). Anatomical organization of the primate amygdaloid complex. In J. P. Aggleton (Ed), *The Amygdala: Neurobiological Aspects of Emotion, Memory, and Mental Dysfunction* (pp. 1–66). New York: Wiley-Liss.

Applegate, C. D., Frysinger, R. C., Kapp, B. S. & Gallagher, M. (1982). Multiple unit activity recorded from amygdala central nucleus during Pavlovian heart rate conditioning in rabbit. *Brain Research, 238*, 457–462.

Armony, J. L., Quirk, G. J. & LeDoux, J. E. (1998). Differential effects of amygdala lesions on early and late plastic components of auditory cortex spiketrains during fear conditioning. *Journal of Neuroscience, 18*, 2592–2601.

Armony, J. L., Servan-Schreiber, D., Cohen, J. C. & LeDoux, J. E. (1996). Emotion and cognition interactions in the thalalmo-cortico-amygdala network: theory and model. *Cognitive Neuroscience Society Abstracts, 3*, 76.

Armony, J. L., Servan-Schreiber, D., Cohen, J. D. & LeDoux, J. E. (1997a). Computational modeling of emotion: Explorations through the anatomy and physiology of fear conditioning. *Trends in Cognitive Sciences, 1*, 28–34.

Armony, J. L., Servan-Schreiber, D., Romanski, L. M., Cohen, J. D. & LeDoux, J. E. (1997b). Stimulus generalization of fear responses: effects of auditory cortex lesions in a computational model and in rats. *Cerebral Cortex, 7*, 157–165.

Aston-Jones, G., Rajkowski, J., Kubiak, P., Valentino, R. & Shipley, M. (1996). Role of the locus coeruleus in emotional activation. *Progress Brain Research, 107*, 379–402.

Baars, B. J. (1988). *A Cognitive Theory of Consciousness*. New York: Cambridge University Press.

Bechara, A., Tranel, D., Damasio, H., Adolphs, R., Rockland, C. & Damasio, A. R. (1995). Double dissociation of conditioning and declarative knowledge relative to the amygdala and hippocampus in humans. *Science, 269*, 1115–1118.

Blanchard, R. J. & Blanchard, D. C. (1969). Crouching as an index of fear. *Journal of Comparative Physiological Psychology, 67*, 370–375.

Blanchard, C. D. & Blanchard, R. J. (1972). Innate and conditioned reactions to threat in rats with amygdaloid lesions. *Journal of Comparative Physiological Psychology, 81*, 281–290.

Bliss, T. V. P. & Collingridge, G. L. (1993). A synaptic model of memory: long-term potentiation in the hippocampus. *Nature, 361*, 31–39.

Bolles, R. C. & Fanselow, M. S. (1980). A perceptual-defensive-recuperative model of fear and pain. *Behavioral and Brain Sciences, 3*, 291–323.

Bordi, F. & LeDoux, J. E. (1993). Sensory-specific conditioned plasticity in lateral amygdala neurons. *Society for Neuroscience Abstracts, 19*, 1227.

Bourtchuladze, R., Frenguelli, B., Blendy, J., Cioffi, D., Shutz, G., Silva, A. J. (1994). Deficient long-term memory in mice with a targeted mutation of the cAMP-responsive element binding protein. *Cell, 79*, 59–68.

Bouton, M. E. & Bolles, R. C. (1980). Conditioned fear assessed by freezing and by the suppression of three different baselines. *Animal Learning and Behavior, 8*, 429–434.

Bouton, M. E. (1993). Context, time, and memory retrieval in the interference paradigms of Pavlovian learning. *Psychological Bulletin, 114*, 80–99.

Breiter, H. C., Etcoff, N. C., Whalen, P. J., Kennedy, W. A., Rausch, S. L., Buchner, R. L., Strauss, M. M., Hyman, S. E., Rosen, B. R. (1996). Response and habituation of the human amygdala during visual processing of facial expression. *Neuron, 17*, 875–87.

Cahill, L., Babinsky, R., Markowitsch, H. J. & McGaugh, J. L. (1995). The amygdala and emotional memory. *Nature, 377*, 295–296.

Cahill, L., Haier, R. J., Fallon, J., Alkire, M. T., Tang, C., Keater, J., Wu, J., McGaugh, J. L. (1996). Amygdala activity at encoding correlated with long-term, free recall of emotional information. *Proceedings of the National Academy of Sciences, USA, 93*, 8016.

Cahill, L. & McGaugh, J. L. (1998). Mechanisms of emotional arousal and lasting declarative memory. *Trends in Neurosciences, 21*, 294–299.

Campeau, S. & Davis, M. (1995a). Involvement of the central nucleus and basolateral complex of the amygdala in fear conditioning measured with fear-potentiated startle in rats trained concurrently with auditory and visual conditioned stimuli. *Journal of Neuroscience, 15*, 2301–2311.

Campeau, S. & Davis, M. (1995b). Involvement of subcortical and cortical afferents to the lateral nucleus of the amygdala in fear conditioning measured with fear-potentiated startle in rats trained concurrently with auditory and visual conditioned stimuli. *Journal of Neuroscience, 15*, 2312–2327.

Canteras, N. S. & Swanson, L. W. (1992). Projections of the ventral subiculum to the amygdala, septum, and hypothalamus: a PHAL anterograde tract-tracing study in the rat. *Journal of Comparative Neurology, 324*, 180–194.

Christianson, S.-A. (1992). *Handbook of Emotion and Memory: Research and Theory.* Hillsdale, NJ: Lawrence Erlbaum Associates.

Clugnet, M. C. & LeDoux, J. E. (1990). Synaptic plasticity in fear conditioning circuits: induction of LTP in the lateral nucleus of the amygdala by stimulation of the medial geniculate body. *Journal of Neuroscience, 10*, 2818–2824.

Cohen, N. J. & Eichenbaum, H. (1993). *Memory, Amnesia, and the Hippocampal System.* Cambridge: MIT Press.

Cohen, J. D., Perlstein, M. W., Braver, T. S., Nystrom, L. E., Noll, D. C., Jonides, J. C. & Smith, E. E. (1997). Temporal dynamics of brain activation during a working memory task. *Nature, 386*, 604–608.

Corodimas, K. P. & LeDoux, J. E. (1995). Disruptive effects of posttraining perihinal cortex lesions on conditioned fear: contributions of contextual cues. *Behavioral Neuroscience, 109*, 613–619.

Davis, M. (1992a). The role of the amygdala in fear-potentiated startle: implications for animal models of anxiety. *Trends in Pharmacological Science, 13*, 35–41.

Davis, M. (1992b). The role of the amygdala in conditioned fear. In J. P. Aggleton (Ed), *The Amygdala: Neurobiological Aspects of Emotion, Memory, and Mental Dysfunction* (pp. 255–306). New York: Wiley-Liss.

Davis, M., Falls, W. A., Campeau, S. & Kim, M. (1994). Fear potentiated startle: a neural and pharmacological analysis. *Behavioral Brain Research, 58*, 175–198.

D'Esposito, M., Detre, J., Alsop, D., Shin, R., Atlas, S., & Grossman, M. (1995). The neural basis of the central executive sytem of working memory. *Nature, 378*, 279–281.

Dollard, J. C. & Miller, N. E. (1950). *Personality and Psychotherapy.* New York: McGraw-Hill.

Ekman, P. & Davidson, R. (1994). *The Nature of Emotion: Fundamental Questions.* New York: Oxford University Press.

Erdelyi, M. H. (1985). *Psychoanalysis: Freud's Cognitive Psychology.* New York: Freeman.

Estes, W. K. & Skinner, B. F. (1941). Some quantitative properties of anxiety. *Journal of Experimental Psychology, 29*, 390–400.

Everitt, B. J. & Robbins, T. W. (1992). Amygdala-ventral striatal interactions and reward-related processes. In J. P. Aggleton (Ed), *The Amygdala: Neurobiological Aspects of Emotion, Memory, and Mental Dysfunction* (pp. 401–429). New York: Wiley-Liss.

Fanselow, M. S. & Kim, J. J. (1994). Acquisition of contextual Pavlovian fear conditioning is blocked by application of an NMDA receptor antagonist D,L-2-amino-5-phosphonovaleric acid to the basolateral amygdala. *Behavioral Neuroscience, 108*, 210–212.

Frankland, P. W., Cestari, V., Filipkowski, R. K., McDonald, R. J. & Silva, A. J. (1998). The dorsal hippocampus is essential for context discrimination but not for contextual conditioning. *Behavioral Neuroscience, 112*, 863–874.

Fuster, J. M. (1989). *The Prefrontal Cortex.* New York: Raven Press.

Gallagher, M. & Holland, P. C. (1992). Understanding the function of the central nucleus: is simple conditioning enough? In J. P. Aggleton (Ed), *The Amygdala: Neurobiological Aspects of Emotion, Memory, and Mental Dysfunction* (pp. 307–321). New York: Wiley-Liss.

Gentile, C. G., Jarrell, T. W., Teich, A., McCabe, P. M. & Schneiderman, N. (1986). The role of amygdaloid central nucleus in the retention of differential Pavlovian conditioning of bradycardia in rabbits. *Behavioural Brain Research, 20*, 263–273.

Gewirtz, J. C. & Davis, M. (1997a). Second-order fear conditioning prevented by blocking NMDA receptors in amygdala. *Nature, 388*, 471–473.

Gewirtz, J. C., Falls, W. A. & Davis, M. (1997b). Normal conditioned inhibition and extinction of freezing and fear potentiated startle following electrolytic lesions of medial prefrontal cortex in rats. *Behavioral Neuroscience, 111*, 1–15.

Gisquet-Verrier, P. & Doyere, V. (1997). Lesions of the hippocampus in rats do not affect conditioning to context cues in classical fear conditioning. *Social Neuroscience, 23*, 1609.

Gluck, M. A. & Myers, C. E. (1997). Psychobiological models of hippocampal function in learning and memory. *Annual Review of Psychology, 48*, 481–514.

Goldman-Rakic, P. S. (1988). Topography of cognition: parallel distributed networks in primate association cortex. *Annual Review of Neuroscience, 11*, 137–156.

Good, M. & Honey, R. C. (1997). Dissociable effects of selecgtive lesions to hippocampal subsystems on exploratory behavior, contextual learning, and spatial learning. *Behavioral Neuroscience, 111*, 487–493.

Hamann, S. B., Stefanacci, L. & Squire, L. R. (1996). Recognizing facial emotion. *Nature, 379*, 497.

Helmstetter, F. (1992). Contribution of the amygdala to learning and performance of conditional fear. *Physiology and Behavior 51*, 1271–1276.

Helmstetter, F. J. & Bellgowan, P. S. (1994). Effects of muscimol applied to the basolateral amygdala on acquisition and expression of contextual fear conditioning in rats. *Behavioral Neuroscience, 108*, 1005–1009.

Huang, Y.-Y., Nguyen, P. V., Abel, T. & Kandel, E. R. (1996). Long-lasting forms of synaptic potentiation in the mammalian hippocampus. *Learning and Memory, 3*, 74–85.

Iwata, J., LeDoux, J. E., Meeley, M. P., Arneric, S. & Reis, D. J. (1986). Intrinsic neurons in the amygdaloid field projected to by the medial geniculate body mediate emotional responses conditioned to acoustic stimuli. *Brain Research, 383*, 195–214.

Jacobs, W. J. & Nadel, L. (1985). Stress-induced recovery of fears and phobias. *Psychological Review, 92*, 512–531.

James, W. (1890). *Principles of Psychology*. New York: Holt.

Jarrell, T. W., Gentile, C. G., Romanski, L. M., McCabe, P. M. & Schneiderman, N. (1987). Involvement of cortical and thalamic auditory regions in retention of differential bradycardia conditioning to acoustic conditioned stimulii in rabbits. *Brain Research, 412*, 285–294.

Johnson-Laird, P. N. (1988). *The Computer and the Mind: An Introduction to Cognitive Science*. Cambridge, MA: Harvard University Press.

Kapp, B. S., Supple, W. F. & Whalen, P. J. (1994). Effects of electrical stimulation of the amygdaloid central nucleus on neocortical arousal in the rabbit. *Behavioral Neuroscience, 108*, 81–93.

Kapp, B. S., Whalen, P. J., Supple, W. F. & Pascoe, J. P. (1992). Amygdaloid contributions to conditioned arousal and sensory information processing. In J. P. Aggleton (Ed), *The Amygdala: Neurobiological Aspects of Emotion, Memory, and Mental Dysfunction* (pp. 229–254). New York: Wiley-Liss.

Kihlstrom, J. F. (1987). The cognitive unconscious. *Science, 237*, 1445–1452.

Killcross, S., Robbins, T. W. & Everitt, B. J. (1997). Different types of fear-conditioned behavior mediated by separate nuclei within amygdala. *Nature, 388*, 377–380.

Kim, J. J. & Fanselow, M. S. (1992). Modality-specific retrograde amnesia of fear. *Science, 256*, 675–677.

Kosslyn, S. M. & Koenig, O. (1992). *Wet Mind: The New Cognitive Neuroscience*. New York: Macmillan.

LaBar, K. S., LeDoux, J. E., Spencer, D. D. & Phelps, E. A. (1995). Impaired fear conditioning following unilateral temporal lobectomy in humans. *Journal of Neuroscience, 15*, 6846–6855.

LaBar, K., Gatenby, J. C., Gore, J. C, LeDoux, J. E., & Phelps, E. A. (1998). Human amygdala activation during conditioned fear acquisition and extinction: a mixed trials fMRI study. *Neuron, 20*, 937–945.

LeDoux, J. E. (1986). Sensory systems and emotion. *Integrative Psychiatry, 4*, 237–248.

LeDoux, J. E. (1992a). Emotion and the amygdala. In J. P. Aggleton (Ed), *The Amygdala: Neurobiological Aspects of Emotion, Memory, and Mental Dysfunction* (pp. 339–351). New York: Wiley-Liss.

LeDoux, J. E. (1992b). Brain mechanisms of emotion and emotional learning. *Current Opinion in Neurobiology, 2*, 191–198.

LeDoux, J. E. (1994). Emotion, memory and the brain. *Scientific American, 270*, 32–39.

LeDoux, J. E. (1995a). In search of an emotional system in the brain: leaping from fear to emotion and consciousness. In M. S. Gazzaniga (Ed), *The Cognitive Neurosciences* (pp. 1049–1062). Cambridge, MA: MIT Press.

LeDoux, J. E. (1995b). Emotion: Clues from the brain. *Annual Review of Psychology, 46*, 209–235.

LeDoux, J. E. (1996). *The Emotional Brain.* New York: Simon and Schuster.

LeDoux, J. E., Cicchetti, P., Xagoraris, A. & Romanski, L. M. (1990a). The lateral amygdaloid nucleus: sensory interface of the amygdala in fear conditioning. *Journal of Neuroscience, 10*, 1062–1069.

LeDoux, J. E., Farb, C. F. & Ruggiero, D. A. (1990b). Topographic organization of neurons in the acoustic thalamus that project to the amygdala. *Journal of Neuroscience, 10*, 1043–1054.

LeDoux, J. E., Iwata, J., Cicchetti, P. & Reis, D. J. (1988). Different projections of the central amygdaloid nculeus mediate autonomic and behavioral correlates of conditioned fear. *Journal of Neuroscience, 8*, 2517–2529.

LeDoux, J. E., Ruggiero, D. A. & Reis, D. J. (1985). Projections to the subcortical forebrain from anatomically defined regions of the medial geniculate body in the rat. *Journal of Comparative Neurology, 242*, 182–213.

LeDoux, J. E., Sakaguchi, A. & Reis, D. J. (1984). Subcortical efferent projections of the medial geniculate nucleus mediate emotional responses conditioned by acoustic stimuli. *Journal of Neuroscience, 4*, 683–698.

Li, X. F., Armony, J. L. & LeDoux, J. E. (1996a). GABA$_a$ and GABA$_b$ receptors differentially regulate synaptic transmission in the auditory thalamo-amygdala pathway: an in vivo microiontophoretic study and a model. *Synapse, 24*, 115–124.

Li, X. F., Stutzmann, G. E. & LeDoux, J. L. (1996b). Convergent but temporally separated inputs to lateral amygdala neurons from the auditory thalamus and auditory cortex use different postsynaptic receptors: in vivo, intracellular and extracellular recordings in fear conditioning pathways. *Learning & Memory, 3*, 229–242.

Li, X., Phillips, R. G. & LeDoux, J. E. (1995). NMDA and non-NMDA receptors contribute to synaptic transmission between the medial geniculate body and the lateral nucleus of the amygdala. *Experimental Brain Research, 105*, 87–100.

Linden, D. R. (1969). Attenuation and reestablishment of the DER by discriminated avoidance conditioning in rats. *Journal of Comparative Physiology and Psychology, 69*, 573.

Lynch, G. (1986). *Synapses, Circuits, and the Beginnings of Memory.* Cambridge, MA: MIT Press.

Madison, D. V., Malenka, R. C. & Nicoll, R. A. (1991). Mechanisms underlying long-term potentiation of synaptic transmission. *Annual Review of Neuroscience, 14*, 379–397.

Malenka, R. C. & Nicoll, R. A. (1993). NMDA-receptor-dependent synaptic plasticity: multiple forms and mechanisms. *Trends in Neuroscience, 16*, 521–527.

Manderscheid, R. W. & Sonnenschein, M. A. (1994). *Mental Health, United States 1994.* Rockville, MD: U.S. Dept. of Health and Human Services.

Maren, S., Poremba, A. & Gabriel, M. (1991). Basolateral amygdaloid multi-unit neuronal correlates of discriminative avoidance learning in rabbits. *Brain Research, 549,* 311–316.

Maren, S., Aharonov, G. & Fanselow, M. S. (1997). Neurotoxic lesions of the dorsal hippocampus and Pavlovian fear conditioning in rats. *Behavioural Brain Research, 88,* 261–274.

Maren, S., Anagnostaras, S. G. & Fanselow, M. S. (1998). The startled seahorse: is the hippocampus necessary for contextual fear conditioning? *Trends in Cognitive Sciences, 2,* 39–41.

Maren, S., Aharonov, G. & Fanselow, M. S. (1996b). Retrograde abolition of conditional fear after excitotoxic lesions in the basolateral amygdala of rats. *Behavioral Neuroscience, 110,* 718–726.

Maren, S., Aharonov, G., Stote, D. L. & Fanselow, M. S. (1996a). N-Methyl-d-aspartate receptors in the basolateral amygdala are required for both acqusition and expression of the conditional fear in rats. *Behavioral Neuroscience, 110,* 1365–1374.

Maren, S. & Fanselow, M. S. (1996). The amygdala and fear conditioning: has the nut been cracked? *Neuron, 16,* 237–240.

Marks, I. (1987). *Fears, Phobias, and Rituals: Panic, Anxiety and Their Disorders.* New York: Oxford University Press.

Mascagni, F., McDonald, A. J. & Coleman, J. R. (1993). Corticoamygdaloid and corticocortical projections of the rat temporal cortex: *A phaseolus vulgaris* leucoagglutinin study. *Neuroscience, 57,* 697–715.

Mason, J. W., Mangan, G., Brady, J. V., Conrad, D. & Rioch, D. M. (1961). Concurrent plasma epinephrine, norepinephrine and 17-hydroxycorticosteroid levels during conditioned emotional disturbances in monkeys. *Psychosomatic Medicine, 23,* 344–353.

Mayford, M., Bach, M. E., Huang, Y.-Y., Wang, L. & Hawkins, R. D. (1996). Control of memory formation through regulated expression of a CaMKII transgene. *Science, 274,* 1678–1683.

McAllister, W. R. & McAllister, D. E. (1971). Behavioral measurement of conditioned fear. In F. R. Bush (Ed), *Aversive Conditioning and Learning* (pp. 105–179). New York: Academic Press.

McCabe, P. M., Schneiderman, N., Jarrell, T. W., Gentile, C. G., Teich, A. H., Winters, R. W., & Liskowsky, D. R. (1972). Central pathways involved in differential classical conditioning of heart rate responses. In I. Gormezano (Ed), *Learning and Memory: The Behavioral and Biological Substrates* (pp. 321–346). Hillsdale, NJ: Lawrence Erlbaum Associates.

McClelland, J. L., McNaughton, B. L. & O'Reilly, R. C. (1995). Why there are complementary learning systems in the hippocampus and neocortex: insights from the successes and failures of connectionist models of learning and memory. *Psychological Review, 102,* 419–457.

McEwen, B. & Sapolsky, R. (1995). Stress and cognitive functioning. *Current Opinion in Neurobiology, 5,* 205–216.

McGaugh, J. L., Introini-Collison, I. B., Cahill, L., Kim, M. & Liang, K. C. (1992). Involvement of the amygdala in neuromodulatory influences on memory storage. In J. P. Aggleton (Ed), *The Amygdala: Neurobiological Aspects of Emotion, Memory, and Mental Dysfunction* (pp. 431–451). New York: Wiley-Liss.

McGaugh, J. L., Mesches, M. H., Cahill, L., Parent, M. B., Coleman-Mesches, K., & Salinas, J. A. (1995). Involvement of the amygdala in the regulation of memory storage.

In J. L. McGaugh, F. Bermudez-Rattoni & R. A. Prado-Alcala (Eds), *Plasticity in the Central Nervous System* (pp. 18–39). Hillsdale, NJ: Lawrence Erlbaum Associates.

McNish, K. A., Gewirtz, J. C. & Davis, M. (1997). Evidence of contextual fear after lesions of the hippocampus: a disruption of freezing but not fear-potentiated startle. *The Journal of Neuroscience, 17,* 9353–9360.

Miserendino, M. J. D., Sananes, C. B., Melia, K. R. & Davis, M. (1990). Blocking of acquisition but not expression of conditioned fear-potentiated startle by NMDA antagonists in the amygdala. *Nature, 345,* 716–718.

Morgan, M. & LeDoux, J. E. (1995). Differential contribution of dorsal and ventral medial prefrontal cortex to the acquisition and extinction of conditioned fear. *Behavioral Neuroscience, 109,* 681–688.

Morgan, M. A., Romanski, L. M. & LeDoux, J. E. (1993). Extinction of emotional learning: contribution of medial prefrontal cortex. *Neuroscience Letters, 163,* 109–113.

Morris, J. S., Frith, C. D., Perret, D. I., Rowland, D., Young, A. W., Calder, A. J., & Dolan, R. J. (1996). A differential neural response in the human amygdala to fearful and happy facial expressions. *Nature, 383,* 812–815.

Mowrer, O. H. (1939). A stimulus-response analysis of anxiety and its role as a reinforcing agent. *Psychological Review, 46,* 553–565.

Mowrer, O. H. (1960). *Learning Theory and Behavior.* New York: Wiley.

Mowrer, O. H. & Lamoreaux, R. R. (1946). Fear as an intervening variable in avoidance conditioning. *Journal of Comparative Psychology, 39,* 29–50.

Muller, J., Corodimas, K. P., Fridel, Z. & LeDoux, J. E. (1997). Functional inactivation of the lateral and basal nuclei of the amygdala by muscimol infusion prevents fear conditioning to an explicit CS and to contextual stimuli. *Behavioral Neuroscience, 111,* 683–691.

Muramoto, K., Ono, T., Nishijo, H. & Fukuda, M. (1993). Rat amygdaloid neuron responses during auditory discrimination. *Neuroscience, 52,* 621–636.

Murray, E. A. (1992). Medial temporal lobe structures contributing to recognition memory: the amygdaloid complex versus the rhinal cortex. In J. P. Aggleton (Ed), *The Amygdala: Neurobiological Aspects of Emotion, Memory, and Mental Dysfunction* (pp. 453–470). New York: Wiley-Liss.

Myers, C. E. & Gluck, M. A. (1994). Context, conditioning, and hippocampal rerepresentation in animal learning. *Behavioral Neuroscience, 108,* 835–847.

Nadel, L. & Willner, J. (1980). Context and conditioning: a place for space. *Physiological Psychology, 8,* 218–228.

Öhman, A. (1992). Fear and anxiety as emotional phenomena: clinical, phenomenological, evolutionary perspectives, and information-processing mechanisms. In M. Lewis & J. M. Haviland (Eds), *Handbook of the Emotions* (pp. 511–536). New York: Guilford.

O'Keefe, J. & Nadel, L. (1978). *The Hippocampus as a Cognitive Map.* Oxford: Clarendon Press.

Ottersen, O. P. (1982). Connections of the amygdala of the rat. IV: Corticoamygdaloid and intraamygdaloid connections as studied with axonal transport of horseradish peroxidase. *Journal of Comparative Neurology, 205,* 30–48.

Packard, M. G., Cahill, L. & McGaugh, J. L. (1994). Amygdala modulation of hippocampal-dependent and caudate nucleus-dependent memory processes. *Proceedings of the National Academy of Science, USA, 91,* 8477–8481.

Packard, M. G., Williams, C. L., Cahill, L. & McGaugh, J. L. (1995). The anatomy of a memory modulatory system: from periphery to brain. In N. E. Spear, L. P. Spear & M. L. Woodruff (Eds), *Neurobehavioral Plasticity: Learning, Development, and Response to Brain Insults* (pp. 149–150). Hillsdale, NJ: Lawrence Erlbaum Associates.

Pascoe, J. P. & Kapp, B. S. (1985). Electrophysiological characteristics of amygdaloid central nucleus neurons during Pavlovian fear conditioning in the rabbit. *Behavioral Brain Research, 16*, 117–133.

Petri, H. L. & Mishkin, M. (1994). Behaviorism, cognitivism and the neuropsychology of memory. *American Scientist, 82*, 30–37.

Phillips, R. G. & LeDoux, J. E. (1992a). Overlapping and divergent projections of CA1 and the ventral subiculum to the amygdala. *Society for Neuroscience Abstracts, 18*, 518.

Phillips, R. G. & LeDoux, J. E. (1992b). Differential contribution of amygdala and hippocampus to cued and contextual fear conditioning. *Behavioral Neuroscience, 106*, 274–285.

Phillips, R. G. & LeDoux, J. E. (1994). Lesions of the dorsal hippocampal formation interfere with background but not foreground contextual fear conditioning. *Learning and Memory, 1*, 34–44.

Phillips, R. G. & LeDoux, J. E. (1995). Lesions of the fornix but not the entorhinal or perirhinal cortex interfere with contextual fear conditioning. *Journal of Neuroscience, 15*, 5308–5315.

Pitkänen, A., Savander, V. & LeDoux, J. L. (1997). Organization of intra-amygdaloid circuitries: an emerging framework for understanding functions of the amygdala. *Trends in Neurosciences, 20*, 517–523.

Pitkänen, A., Stefanacci, L., Farb, C. R., Go, C. G., LeDoux, J. E., & Amaral, D. G. (1995). Intrinsic connections of the rat amygdaloid complex: projections originating in the lateral nucleus. *Journal of Comparative Neurology, 356*, 288–310.

Price, J. L., Russchen, F. T. & Amaral, D. G. (1987). The limbic region. II: The amygdaloid complex. In A. Bjorklund, T. Hokfelt & L. W. Swanson (Eds), *Handbook of Chemical Neuroanatomy*, vol. 5. *Integrated Systems of the CNS*, pt. 1 (pp. 279–388). Amsterdam: Elsevier.

Quirk, G. J., Armony, J. L. & LeDoux, J. E. (1997b). Fear conditioning enhances different temporal components of toned-evoked spike trains in auditory cortex and lateral amygdala. *Neuron, 19*.

Quirk, G. J., Repa, J. C. & LeDoux, J. E. (1995). Fear conditioning enhances short-latency auditory responses of lateral amygdala neurons: parallel recordings in the freely behaving rat. *Neuron, 15*, 1029–1039.

Quirk, G. J., Armony, J. L., Repa, J. C., Li, X.-F. & LeDoux, J. E. (1997a). Emotional memory: a search for sites of plasticity. *Cold Spring Harbor Symposia on Biology, 61*, 247–257.

Rogan, M. T. & LeDoux, J. E. (1995). LTP is accompanied by commensurate enhancement of auditory-evoked responses in a fear conditioning circuit. *Neuron, 15*, 127–136.

Rogan, M. T. & LeDoux, J. E. (1996). Emotion: systems, cells, synaptic plasticity. *Cell, 85*, 469–475.

Rogan, M., Staubli, U. & LeDoux, J. E. (1997). AMPA-receptor facilitation accelerates fear learning without altering the level of conditioned fear aquired. *Journal of Neuroscience, 17*, 5928–5935.

Romanski, L. M. & LeDoux, J. E. (1993a). Organization of rodent auditory cortex: anterograde transport of PHA-L from MGv to temporal neocortex. *Cerebral Cortex, 3*, 499–514.

Romanski, L. M. & LeDoux, J. E. (1993b). Information cascade from primary auditory cortex to the amygdala: corticocortical and corticoamygdaloid projections of temporal cortex in the rat. *Cerebral Cortex, 3*, 515–532.

Romanski, L. M. & LeDoux, J. E. (1992). Equipotentiality of thalamo-amygdala and thalamo-cortico-amygdala projections as auditory conditioned stimulus pathways. *Journal of Neuroscience, 12*, 4501–4509.

Saper, C. B. (1987). Diffuse cortical projection systems: anatomical organization and role in cortical function. In V. B. Mountcastle, F. Plum & S. R. Geiger (Eds), *Handbook of Physiology. 1: The Nervous System*, vol. V. *Higher Functions of the Brain* (pp. 169–210). Bethesda, MD: American Physiological Society.

Savander, V., Go, C. G., LeDoux, J. E. & Pitkanen, A. (1995). Intrinsic connections of the rat amygdaloid complex: projections originating in the basal nucleus. *Journal of Comparative Neurology, 361*, 345–368.

Savander, V., Go, C.-G., LeDoux, J. E. & Pitkanen, A. (1996a). Intrinsic connections of the rat amygdaloid complex: projections originating in the accessory basal nucleus. *Journal of Comparative Neurology, 374*, 291–313.

Savander, V., LeDoux, J. E. & Pitkanen, A. (1996b). Interamygdala projections of the basal and accessory basal nucleus of the rat amygdaloid complex. *Neuroscience, 76*, 725–735.

Savander, V., LeDoux, J. E. & Pitkanen, A. (1996c). Topographic projections from the periamygdaloid cortex to select subregions of the lateral nucleus of the amygdala in the rat. *Neuroscience Letters, 211*, 167–170.

Schneiderman, N., Francis, J., Sampson, L. D. & Schwaber, J. S. (1974). CNS integration of learned cardiovascular behavior. In L. V. DiCara (Ed), *Limbic and Autonomic Nervous System Research* (pp. 77–309). New York: Plenum Press.

Selden, N. R. W., Everitt, B. J. & Robbins, T. W. (1991a). Telencephalic but not diencephalic noradrenaline depletion enhances behavioural but not endocrine measures of fear conditioning to contextual stimuli. *Behavioural Brain Research, 43*, 139–154.

Selden, N. R. W., Everitt, B. J., Jarrard, L. E. & Robbins, T. W. (1991b). Complementary roles for the amygdala and hippocampus in aversive conditioning to explicit and contextual cues. *Neuroscience, 42*, 335–350.

Seligman, M. E. P. (1971). Phobias and preparedness. *Behavior Therapy, 2*, 307–320.

Shallice, T. (1988). Information processing models of consiousness. In A. Marcel & E. Bisiach (Eds), *Consciousness in Contemporary Science* (pp. 305–333). Oxford: Oxford University Press.

Simon, H. A. (1967). Motivational and emotional controls of cognition. *Psychological Review, 74*, 29–39.

Smith, O. A., Astley, C. A., Devito, J. L., Stein, J. M. & Walsh, R. E. (1980). Functional analysis of hypothalamic control of the cardiovascular responses accompanying emotional behavior. *Federation Proceedings, 39*, 2487–2494.

Solomon, R. L. & Wynne, L. C. (1954). Traumatic avoidance learning: the principles of anxiety conservation and partial irreversibility. *Psychology Review, 61*, 353.

Sparks, P. D. & LeDoux, J. E. (1995). Septal lesions potentiate freezing behavior to contextual but not to phasic conditioned stimuli in rats. *Behavioral Neuroscience, 109*, 184–188.

Squire, L. R., Knowlton, B. & Musen, G. (1993). The structure and organization of memory. *Annual Review in Psychology, 44*, 453–495.

Staubli, U. (1994). In *Parallel properties of LTP and memory* (Ed) J. L. McGaugh. New York: Oxford University Press.

Staubli, U. V. (1995). Parallel properties of long-term potentiation and memory. In J. L. McGaugh, N. M. Weinberger & G. Lynch (Eds), *Brain and Memory: Modulation and Mediation of Neuroplasticity* (pp. 303–318). New York: Oxford University Press.

Sutherland, R. J. & Rudy, J. W. (1989). Configural association theory: the role of the hippocampal formation in learning, memory, and amnesia. *Psychobiology, 17*, 129–144.

Thorpe, S. J., Rolls, E. T. & Maddison, S. (1983). The orbitofrontal cortex: neuronal activity in the behaving monkey. *Experimental Brain Research, 49*, 93–115.

Turner, B. & Herkenham, M. (1991). Thalamoamygdaloid projections in the rat: a test of the amygdala's role in sensory processing. *Journal of Comparative Neurology, 313*, 295–325.

Turner, B. H., Mishkin, M. & Knapp, M. (1980). Organization of the amygdalopetal projections from modality-specific cortical association areas in the monkey. *Journal of Comparative Neurology, 191*, 515–543.

Uwano, T., Nishijo, H., Ono, T. & Tamura, R. (1995). Neuronal responsiveness to various sensory atimuli, and associative learning in the rat amygdala. *Neuroscience, 68*, 339–361.

Weinberger, N. M. (1995). Parallel properties of long-term potentiation and memory. In M. S. Gazzaniga (Ed), *The Cognitive Neurosciences* (pp. 1071–1090). Cambridge, MA: MIT Press.

Wilson, A. & Kapp, B. S. (1994). Effect of lesions of the ventrolateral periaqueductal gray on the Pavlovian conditioned heart rate response in the rabbit. *Behavioral and Neural Biology, 62*, 73–76.

Young, A. W., Aggleton, J. P., Hellawell, D. J., Johnson, M., Broks, P., & Hanley, J. R. (1995). Face processing impairments after amygdalotomy. *Brain, 118*, 15–24.

8

The Role of the Amygdala in Primate Social Cognition

NATHAN J. EMERY AND DAVID G. AMARAL

Studying the neural basis of primate social cognition is a relatively recent enterprise which has been facilitated by expansive growths in the fields of neuroscience and primatology (Brothers, 1990). A major focus of this research in nonhuman and human primates has been the amygdaloid complex, a prominent telencephalic region located in the anteromedial temporal lobe. In this chapter, we briefly review the anatomical connectivity of the primate amygdaloid complex and initial studies which looked at the effect of amygdala lesions on social behavior in monkeys. We then propose a hypothesis of amygdala function based on its anatomy that specifically addresses how the amygdala might interpret social information (such as facial expressions) and initiate appropriate behavioral responses. We then apply this hypothesis to the everyday behaviors of a macaque monkey, in the neuroethological tradition, and discuss the importance of the amygdala to these behaviors.

Overview of the Neuroanatomy of the Primate Amygdala

The amygdaloid complex is a heterogeneous region located just anterior to the hippocampus in the medial temporal lobe. The use of the term "amygdaloid complex" emphasizes that this region is composed of a group of at least 13 nuclei and cortical areas. Each of these major subdivisions is typically further partitioned into two or more subdivisions. Having said this, we will use the terms "amygdaloid complex" and "amygdala" synonymously in this chapter. It is beyond the scope of this chapter to provide a detailed review of the cytoarchitectonic organization and intrinsic and extrinsic connectivity of the primate amygdala. A summary of this type can be found in Amaral et al. (1992). Rather, we provide an overview of the features of amygdala neuroanatomy that are relevant to our proposal concerning its role in social cognition.

The major nuclei of the primate amygdala are illustrated in figure 8.1. These are typically grouped into deep nuclei (lateral, basal, accessory basal, and paralaminar), superficial regions (medial, anterior, and posterior cortical nuclei, nucleus of

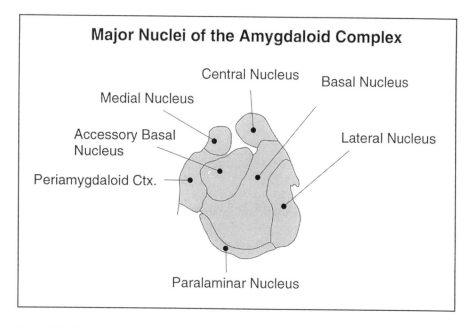

Figure 8.1. Schematic drawing of a coronal section of the monkey amygdaloid complex, displaying the major nuclei and borders between nuclei.

the lateral olfactory tract, periamygdaloid cortex), and other nuclei (central, anterior amygdaloid area, amygdalohippocampal area and intercalated nuclei). The deep nuclei have the greatest interaction with the neocortex and hippocampal formation and presumably are most intimately involved in sensory processing. The medial nuclei are more closely associated with olfactory regions and with the hypothalamus and may play a regulatory role in maternal, sexual, and other species-specific homeostatic mechanisms. Of the other nuclei, only the central nucleus has been studied functionally. It appears to have widespread influence over many of the visceral and autonomic effector regions of the brainstem. For example, it mediates, in part, the cardiovascular and respiratory alterations associated with fear (LeDoux, 1996).

Although the intrinsic connections of the primate amygdala have been influently studied over the last two decades (Aggleton, 1985), many of the details of information flow within and between the various amygdaloid nuclei are not known. We have evaluated the intrinsic connections of the lateral nucleus, and the resulting paper (Pitkanen & Amaral, 1998) provides an indication of the organization and complexity of these local pathways. A schematic summary of the amygdala's intrinsic connections is portrayed in figure 8.2. The lateral nucleus receives much of the sensory information from the neocortex and in this way functions much like the entorhinal cortex of the hippocampal formation. The lateral nucleus gives rise to projections to the basal, accessory basal, and periamygdaloid cortex (Pitkanen & Amaral, 1991). These projections are mostly unidirectional because the basal, accessory basal, and periamygdaloid cortex do not significantly project

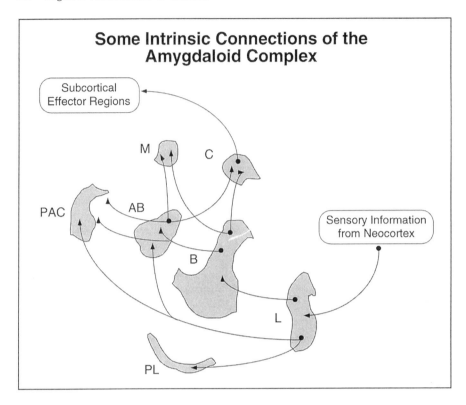

Figure 8.2. Schematic drawing displaying the major nuclei of the amygdaloid complex and their interconnections. Sensory information enters the lateral nucleus, which projects to the basal nuclei and the periamygdaloid cortex. There are no projections back to the lateral nucleus. The basal nuclei project to the central and medial nuclei, which in turn project to subcortical effector regions.

back to the lateral nucleus. The basal nucleus also projects to more medially situated areas of the amygdala, and both the basal and the accessory basal nucleus projects to the medial and central nuclei. Again, these projections are largely unreciprocated. Thus, the general principle of intrinsic amygdala circuitry is that there is a lateral-to-medial unidirectional flow of information.

Perhaps the major change in modern thinking concerning the neuroanatomy of the primate amygdala deals with the extensiveness and diversity of both its efferent and afferent connections. Even as recently as the early 1970s, the amygdala was thought mainly to be interconnected with the hypothalamus. But, as indicated in figure 8.3, the amygdala is involved in a variety of interconnections with many other brain regions. The amygdala is, indeed, interconnected with a variety of brainstem structures. Although a number of nuclei are interconnected with the diencephalon, the most extensive subcortical connections arise from the central nucleus (figure 8.4). The projections of the central nucleus innervate many of the visceral and autonomic effector regions of the brainstem. There are, for example, direct

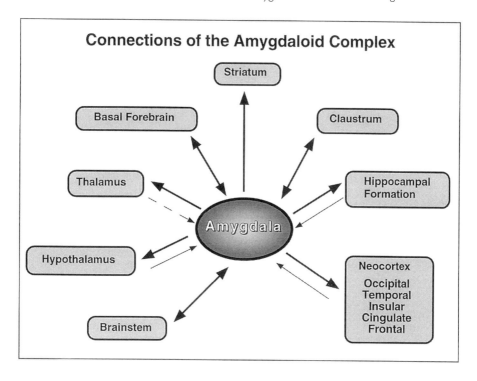

Figure 8.3. All the major connections of the amygdaloid complex.

projections to the parabrachial nuclei that are involved in respiratory control and to the dorsal motor nucleus of the vagus that is involved in cardiovascular control. Projections from the central nucleus have been mapped even into the intermedio-lateral cell column of the spinal cord. We have demonstrated that a large portion of this descending central nucleus projection arises from γ-aminobutyric acid (GABA)ergic neurons (Jongen-Relo & Amaral, 1998).

The amygdala also has extensive interconnections with the basal forebrain. In addition to the well-known connections to the bed nucleus of the stria terminalis (which is often portrayed as a rostral extension of the central nucleus), several amygdaloid nuclei also project heavily to the cholinergic neurons of the basal nucleus of Meynert. In fact, it appears that the amygdala may provide one of the largest inputs to these cholinergic cell groups (Russchen et al., 1985a). Thus, even if the amygdala had no direct projections to the neocortex (which it does), it might exert substantial control over cortical excitability by modulating the output of the cholinergic basal forebrain neurons which innervate vast territories of the neo-cortex.

The amygdala does not have direct interconnections either with the primary motor cortex or with the cerebellum. However, it is possible for the amygdala to affect motor functioning via its extensive interconnections with the striatum. Not only does the amygdala project to the so-called limbic striatum, made up of the nucleus accumbens and the ventral pallidum, but it also projects heavily to neostria-

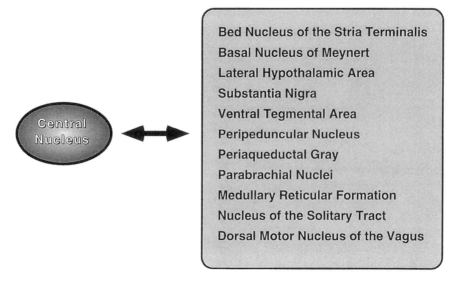

Figure 8.4. All the major connections between the central nucleus and subcortical structures. The central nucleus receives limited neocortical input (mainly from the insular cortex) and gives rise to no connections to the neocortex.

tal structures such as the head and tail of the caudate nucleus and to the putamen (Russchen et al., 1985b). It is worth mentioning that the amygdala also has extensive reciprocal connections with the claustrum, although the functional significance of these is entirely unknown.

The monkey amygdala is also intimately interconnected with many portions of the hippocampal formation. Although some of these projections are reciprocal, our studies indicate that the projections from the amygdala to the hippocampal formation are substantially stronger than those from the hippocampal formation to the amygdala. One interpretation of this anatomy is that the amygdala is providing an additional type of sensory information to the hippocampal formation, perhaps the emotional or species-specific significance of an event, which is used in conjunction with other information to build an episodic memory. The lateral nucleus provides a substantial input to the entorhinal cortex. The basal and accessory basal nuclei, moreover, give rise to projections that terminate in the hippocampus proper and in the subiculum. The subiculum is the main source of return projections to the amygdala, and these terminate mainly in the basal nucleus.

One of the more surprising findings concerning the neuroanatomy of the primate amygdala in the last two decades is the extensive interconnections with the neocortex (Amaral & Price, 1984; Amaral et al., 1992). The monkey amygdala receives inputs from the frontal lobe, primarily from the medial and orbitofrontal regions, from the temporal lobe, primarily from anterior portions of inferotemporal cortex (IT), and from the superior temporal gyrus, the perirhinal cortex, and the anterior cingulate gyrus. The amygdala does not appear to receive inputs from the dorsolateral frontal cortex, from posterior portions of the temporal lobe, from the occipital cortex, or from posterior regions of the cingulate gyrus. Unlike the hippo-campal formation, which receives sensory input primarily from polysensory con-vergence areas, the amygdala receives both higher order unimodal sensory informa-tion as well as polysensory input.

The monkey amygdala also gives rise to extensive projections back to the neocortex. And the clear but surprising finding is that the amygdala projects to a much greater region of the neocortex than it receives input from. This is perhaps best illustrated with respect to the visual system (figure 8.5). As indicated pre-viously, the amygdala receives an input from unimodal visual areas located in the anterior portion of IT, area TE. This region comes at the end of the "ventral stream" of hierarchical visual processing. Neurons in area TE are most responsive to com-plex visual objects such as faces. The projections from area TE terminate preferen-tially in the dorsal portion of the lateral nucleus. The lateral nucleus does not project back to the visual cortex, but it does project to the adjacent basal nucleus. And the basal nucleus gives rise to extensive projections that innervate essentially all portions of the ventral visual stream and even extend into primary visual cortex (area V1). These return projections terminate primarily at the border between layers I and II and in layer VI, which is the typical termination pattern for a feedback projection. Although other modalities have not been studied as thoroughly, it ap-

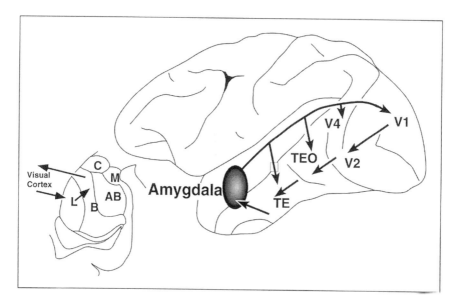

Figure 8.5. Schematic representation of the amygdala's relationship with the cortical areas of the so-called ventral visual processing stream. The lateral nucleus of the amygdala re-ceives projections from area TE and the superior temporal sulcus in the anterior temporal lobe. This visual information is conveyed to the basal nucleus, which projects back to ar-eas in the ventral processing stream, including primary visual cortex (V1). It is suggested that the back projections function in modulating visual input into the amygdala or in focus-ing attention to behaviorally significant stimuli.

pears that essentially the same type of situation occurs at least for auditory and somatosensory information. The function of these return projections remains a mystery, but they would have the potential of modulating sensory information flow at early stages of perceptual processing perhaps on the basis of the "mood" or emotional state of the animal.

By way of closing this section on the neuroanatomy of the amygdala, we would also like to highlight the point that the amygdala is extremely heterogeneous in its neurochemical organization. In fact, the amygdala has a rich intrinsic and extrinsic chemical neuroanatomy. It has, for example, the highest density of benzo-diazepine/$GABA_A$ receptors in the brain and also has a rich distribution of opiate receptors. Neurons in the amygdala express all of the neurotransmitter candidates, peptides, calcium binding proteins, and so on, as neurons in the neocortex. Given this richness of connections and chemical mediators, we now move to a survey of the potential functions of the primate amygdala.

History of the Primate Amygdala and Social Behavior

The role of the amygdala in primate social behavior has been studied indirectly since Brown and Shafer (1888) lesioned the temporal cortex of a rhesus monkey and discovered profound deficits in its emotional and social behavior. This experiment remained undiscovered and unmentioned in the history of neuroscience until Heinrich Klüver and Paul Bucy (1937) lesioned the anterior temporal lobe of a number of rhesus monkeys. The lesions they performed were very extensive, consisting of (in some extreme cases) the temporal pole, perirhinal and entorhinal cortices, IT and subcortical structures; the amygdala, hippocampus, septal nuclei, and the striatum. The behavioral deficits they reported were as dramatic as the extent of the lesions. The monkeys displayed a number of behavioral abnormalities which were consistent across animals. First, the animals displayed "psychic blindness," a term they used to refer to the approach of animate and inanimate objects without hesitation or fear. Second, the monkeys displayed excessive oral tendencies; they investigated objects with their mouth instead of their hands, independent of whether the object was edible or inedible. In this regard, the monkeys tended to eat meat, a food which is not typically tolerated by normal rhesus monkeys. Third, the monkeys would react and attend to all visual stimuli, or so-called hypermeta-morphosis, independent of the stimulus's biological significance. This may be attributed to the visual agnosia (or inability to recognize objects), which was displayed in some of the animals. Fourth, the monkeys showed profound emotional disturbances, such as a dramatic reduction in fear reactions to the presence of the human experimenters, and a massive blunting of aggression. Finally, the monkeys showed signs of hypersexuality, such as a display of excessive masturbation, copulation with any object, and fellatio; either with opposite or same sex monkeys.

Weiskrantz (1956) found that the behavioral abnormalities displayed in the "Klüver-Bucy syndrome" could be produced by lesions of the amygdala alone. Lesions of the amygdala in rhesus monkeys produced a large reduction in motor activity and the subjects approached all presented objects (including previously aversive objects such as the experimenters, sticks, and gloves), and they were generally tame and unexcitable. This result has been replicated many times (Horel & Keating, 1972; Horel et al., 1975), and the importance of a visual input to the amygdala has been stressed in these studies. Downer (1961), for example, made a unilateral lesion of the amygdala in a monkey and sutured the eye on the contralateral side of the lesion. Downer also cut the corpus callosum, thereby blocking any visual information from reaching the amygdala from the contralateral side. He then threatened the monkey, which in normal circumstances elicited an aggressive response from the monkey, but this subject was unresponsive to the threatening gestures of the experimenter. Threatening auditory and somatosensory stimulation elicited normal aggressive responses from the subject. Downer then removed the suture from the contralateral eye and sutured the ipsilateral eye. In this instance, the monkey threatened the experimenter as normal.

Although total lesions of the amygdala have been shown to produce the full symptoms of the Klüver-Bucy syndrome, the amygdala, as discussed previously, is a collection of multiple nuclei, with different and diverse afferents and efferents from the cortex and the subcortical nuclei. Aggleton and Passingham (1981) made selective radio-frequency lesions of the whole amygdala, the basal and lateral nuclei, the lateral nucleus alone, the dorsal nuclei, and the white matter that borders the amygdala laterally and dorsally (the temporal stem). They found that only lesions of the whole amygdala produced the entire Klüver-Bucy syndrome.

Although the Klüver-Bucy syndrome displays a dramatic group of abnormal behaviors (including emotional behaviors), it does not specifically address the question of the role of the amygdala in primate social behavior. The subjects in the studies described above were either studied alone or in pairs. Rosvold et al. (1954) were the first to describe the effects of amygdala lesions on monkey social behavior (i.e., the subjects were tested in social groups). They found that social hierarchies were disrupted; the most dominant animal who received a bilateral amygdala lesion fell in dominance.

One name synonymous with the effects of amygdala lesions on monkey social behavior is Arthur Kling (Steklis, 1998). Kling and colleagues lesioned the amygdala of rhesus macaques in seminatural settings, such as at the Caribbean Regional Primate Center on Cayo Santiago (Dicks et al., 1969). They also carried out similar lesions in caged vervets (Kling et al., 1969), free-ranging vervets (Kling et al., 1970) and stumptailed macaques in different-sized social groups (Kling & Cornell, 1971). The environment in which the subjects were observed appeared to have interesting influences on their social behavior. For example, caged vervets who received amygdalectomies displayed all the symptoms of the Klüver-Bucy syndrome. But when the lesioned animals were released into the wild, they were unresponsive to group members and failed to display appropriate social signals (affiliative or aggressive; Kling & Carpenter, 1968; Kling et al., 1970). All subjects withdrew from other animals and were often found killed or never reentered their original social groups. A similar pattern of results was displayed by rhesus macaques with amygdalectomies released into their original social groups on Cayo Santiago (an island containing many hundreds of macaque monkeys; food provisioned by experimenters; Dicks et al., 1969).

One unusual aspect of the amygdala's presumed function is the opposing roles it plays in positive and negative types of behavior. The function of the amygdala in negative behaviors, such as fear and aggression, will be described in later sections. The role of the amygdala in positive behaviors (feeding and sexual behavior) represents special cases and is described next. The role of the amygdala in primate sexual behavior is rather controversial (Spies et al., 1976). As mentioned earlier, one of the symptoms of the Klüver-Bucy syndrome is hypersexuality. The singly housed monkeys with temporal lobe lesions frequently had erections, masturbated or manipulated their genitals, engaged in autofellatio, rubbed themselves against the cage bars and often presented their anogenital region to the observers (Klüver & Bucy, 1939). Therefore, although no sexual stimuli in the form of females in estrus were present, the subjects displayed many forms of sexual behavior which would be associated with these forms of stimuli in normal social situations. When the subjects were paired with a female, long copulations ensued (>30 min), and they often engaged in multiple copulations during a short period of time. When the subjects were paired with another male, multiple instances of homosexual copulation and masturbation were observed. These results, however, have not been replicated to the same level of intensity when the lesions were confined to the amygdala.

In socially housed monkeys with amygdala lesions, Kling and Cornell (1971) described a small increase in mounting and copulation by one adult male from prelesion levels and an increase in mounting, erections, and mount solicitations by juvenile males (Kling, 1968). Kling and Dunne (1976) described the sexual behavior of males and females housed either in a small enclosure or a larger half-acre corral. In the small enclosure, there was an increase in homosexual masturbation and heterosexual copulation and masturbation, whereas in the larger corral, there was hardly any sexual behavior recorded. This last result highlights the differences between behavioral effects due to differences in social environment.

One interesting aspect of the effects of amygdala lesions on sexual behavior are the differences between males and females. In Klüver and Bucy's initial studies, only males were lesioned. However, Kling's studies have examined sex differences in social and sexual behavior. For example, Kling (1974) studied one female who displayed an increase in aggression, coupled with male mounting. The female displayed inappropriate sexual behavior, such as male copulatory positions and pelvic thrusting and frequently masturbated by rubbing against the cage bars. Therefore, the amygdala appears to be either involved in the discrimination of appropriate sexual signals and initiating appropriate sexual responses (at appropriate times) or in a restraining mechanism for male sexual behavior (a sexual switch; i.e., in males without an amygdala, the switch would constantly be on).

A second positive behavior affected by amygdala lesions in monkeys is feeding behavior. In a number of studies, monkeys with amygdala lesions have displayed abnormal preferences for different foods (Aggleton & Passingham, 1981, 1982; Baylis & Gaffan, 1991; Murray et al., 1996; Ursin et al., 1969; Weiskrantz, 1956). In the original Klüver-Bucy studies (1939), the temporal lobe lesioned animal could not discriminate between different objects based on physical properties. Amygdala-lesioned monkeys did not appear to be able to discriminate between different types of foods, such as raisins, peanuts, banana, and meat. In their natural environment, macaques do not typically eat meat. However, amygdala-lesioned monkeys readily choose meat when presented with a choice between a normally eaten food and meat (Aggleton & Passingham, 1981, 1982; Ursin et al., 1969). Amygdala-lesioned monkey also do not appear to associate significance to foods. Malkova et al. (1997) tested control and lesioned animals for preferences between two foods using a visual discrimination task. The subjects were then satiated on the preferred food before being presented with a visual discrimination task with both objects rewarded (preferred [satiated] food versus nonpreferred food). The monkeys with amygdala lesions indiscriminately chose both foods, whereas the control animals consistently chose the unsatiated food. This result suggests that the amygdala is required to attach affective significance to objects, such as foods which had led to satiation.

As can be deemed from the previous studies, the role of the amygdala in primate social behavior and cognition is still tentative. A large number of technical problems are associated with the earlier literature, problems which can now be solved using new technologies. What are the main problems with the studies performed to date?

1. Lesion technique: Up to the late 1980s and early 1990s, all lesions were made either by aspiration or radio-frequency techniques which not only damage fibers of passage but also tend to damage surrounding cortical areas. Recent lesion techniques, using excitotoxic substances such as ibotenic acid, spare fibers of passage and therefore only lesion the structure of interest. This method increases the reliability of interpretations of behavioral deficits. It also reduces the possibility of removing overlying cortical and subcortical areas during surgical procedures.

2. Histological analysis: Many studies either did not verify that their lesions targeted the amygdala or histology was not performed because the subject animals could not be recovered from their free-ranging situation (Dick et al., 1969; Kling et al., 1970). The brain surgeries on the free-ranging vervets were performed on a kitchen table in the middle of the African savannah (Steklis, 1998). A number of the animals in these studies died after release. This has been attributed to heightened aggression toward the amygdala-lesioned monkeys by the normal members of the troop, but postsurgical complications could have also played a role.

3. Behavioral analysis: Although previous studies did record alterations in social behavior, few quantitative data were collected in a systematic manner. Anecdotal evidence was presented for many aspects of the monkeys' social behavior. This was due mainly to the state of primate behavioral research at the time of these studies, many of which occurred before Altmann's (1974) paper reviewing precise methods for recording behavioral data.

Hypothesis of Amygdala Function

A detailed understanding of the anatomical connections of the amygdala is essential for formulating a hypothesis of its specific function in social behavior. This hypothesis can then be used to discuss how the amygdala may be engaged in different types of behavior such as feeding, aggression, affiliation, and sexual behavior. One underlying problem with the studies described above is that they lacked a specific hypothesis that explained the function of the amygdala during social behavior. For example, does the amygdala process sensory information integral to the communication of social signals? Is it involved in the evaluation of sensory information within a specific behavioral context? Is it required for the initiation of social and associated physiological responses? Or is it involved in all of these functions? We suggest that the amygdala is, indeed, fundamentally involved in all of these functions. Moreover, we suggest that different nuclei of the amygdala are preferentially involved in each of these functions.

The anatomy of the amygdaloid complex suggests that it may be integral for a number of different functions important for normal social behavior. A general framework/hypothesis for viewing the role of the amygdala in social cognition would include the following considerations. First, the amygdala receives highly processed sensory information (including multimodal information), which terminates in highly specific locations within the lateral nucleus. The initial processing stage within the amygdala may therefore be important for the perception of species-specific signals and objects (not limited to social signals, and may include the perception of food or predators, see below).

Second, sensory information from the lateral nucleus passes to the basal nucleus. This transfer of information undoubtedly involves another level of information processing that may correspond to the transfer from perception to cognition (socio-affective cognition). It is not known what form this conversion takes or which structures are involved. It is likely, however, that the socio-affective evaluation of the salience of sensory stimuli within the appropriate behavioral context occurs within the basal nucleus of the amygdala. Again, the neuroanatomy of the basal nucleus is consistent with this idea. Because the basal nucleus is the major recipient of input from the orbitofrontal cortex and the orbitofrontal cortex is involved in some aspect of social awareness (Myers et al., 1973), it is the ideal location for a coincidence detector that attempts to match a particular social signal with a particular social context.

Finally, the basal nucleus gives rise to a prominent projection to the central nucleus (whereas the lateral nucleus has little or no direct projections to the central nucleus). Once a social signal is perceived and interpreted to occur in a valid social context, the central nucleus (and other amygdala nuclei) are in a significant position to influence appropriate behavioral responses to the perception of social signals. This influence would be exerted via the amygdala's many connections with subcortical areas, such as the hippocampus, brainstem, hypothalamus, striatum, and basal forebrain. The amygdala also projects to the orbitofrontal cortex and the premotor cortex (Avendano et al., 1983), which may function to influence cognitive decision making and motor output, respectively.

An example of how this circuitry might mediate the behavioral response to a facial expression is outlined in figure 8.6. In this scenario, basic sensory information concerning the perception of faces as a distinct class of objects enters the amygdala via the lateral nucleus. Faces, for example, are processed as a class of objects in the polysensory region of the superior temporal sulcus (STS), IT, and prefrontal cortex, but it is not known which brain region converts the complex sensory signal "face" into the socially significant signal "facial expression X,"

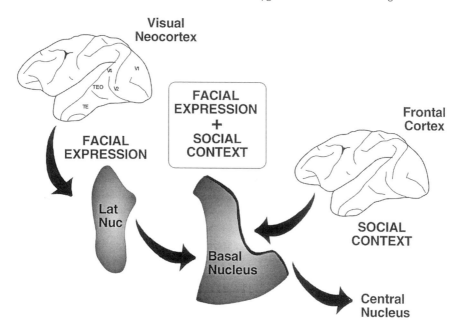

Figure 8.6. The hypothesis of amygdala function in primate social cognition suggests that social stimuli, such as facial expressions, enter the lateral nucleus of the amygdala from visual neocortex (areas TE and the superior temporal sulcus). Facial expressions are usually communicated within a particular social context (i.e., during an aggressive encounter by a particular individual). The basal nucleus receives a projection from the lateral nucleus (expression) and projections from the orbitofrontal cortex. Information concerning social context (based on stored social knowledge of group members) is conveyed to the basal nucleus from the orbitofrontal cortex, where an appropriate response (physiological and behavioral) is evaluated. The appropriate response is then initiated via basal nuclei projections back to neocortex and via central nucleus projections to effector structures, such as the brainstem and hypothalamus.

which is important for the communication of characteristic emotional states or intentions. We hypothesize that this categorization of facial expressions occurs in the lateral nucleus. Information about the category of facial expression is then conveyed to the basal nucleus. The basal nucleus also receives information concerning the social context in which the facial expression is made. The response to the face might be entirely different if it is produced by a dominant alpha male as opposed to an immature juvenile. If the basal nucleus detects the coincidence of a threatening posture produced by a dominant animal, then a fear response (for appeasement) or an escape response (to escape injury) should be generated. A fear response may be elicited by directing motor cortex (and probably the striatum) to produce a fear grimace (by manipulating the correct facial musculature), to produce a cowering posture, to release cortisol (the stress-related hormone) via the hypothalamic-pituitary-adrenal (HPA) axis and to control the different visceral, respiratory, and cardiac centers in the brainstem to initiate appropriate responses to a fearful stimulus (increased blood flow and cardiac output, increased rate of breathing, and reductions in visceral functions). The latter components of the fear response would be mediated by the central nucleus. The response to a rattlesnake may be entirely different in the context of a walk in the dessert or in the herpetarium of the San Diego Zoo.

Although the hypothesis presented above is consistent with available neuroanatomical, behavioral, and electrophysiological data on the primate amygdala, the precise mechanism and location of these functions is speculative. Only more refined lesion studies, and particularly electrophysiological analyses, will provide the data on which these speculations will rise or fall. Given, however, that this scenario of amygdala function was correct in broad strokes, we now investigate how it may come into play in a variety of daily activities of macaque monkeys in a normal social setting.

Neuroethology of Amygdala and Monkey Behavior

A normal day in the life of a macaque monkey presents a number of distinct challenges that require efficient neural systems to manage them. For example, monkeys need to analyze whether a situation is dangerous, such as facing a predator compared to interacting with an affiliative conspecific. In this section, we describe some of the routine behaviors present during a normal monkey's day-to-day life, describe the perceptual, motor, hormonal, and visceral functions devoted to each behavior, and describe how the input–output connections of the amygdala are important for each type of behavior. We argue that the normal functioning of these behaviors depends on the presence of the amygdala and that the behaviors are not displayed or are changed if the amygdala is lesioned or dysfunctional.

During its everyday behavior, a monkey encounters a number of different potentially dangerous and challenging social and dietary scenarios that require perceptual and cognitive abilities that have not developed in other mammals such as rodents, ungulates, or carnivores. The majority of Old World monkeys, such as macaques and baboons, are diurnal and live mainly a terrestrial existence (Clutton-Brock & Harvey, 1980). Primates, therefore, rely substantially on visual forms of communication (Zeller, 1987). Conversely, prosimians such as lemurs are nocturnal and are therefore inhibited against using vision as the primary means of communication.

Macaque monkeys use a large variety of facial expressions to communicate (presumably) their emotional state and their intentions (Bertrand, 1969; Redican, 1975; Zeller, 1987; Hinde & Rowell, 1962; van Hoof, 1962). A well-developed facial musculature system allows such forms of expression to be used within a communicative context (Huber, 1961). Some expressions have been described as expressions of dominance, such as the "open-mouth threat face," whereas others are indicative of a submissive temperament, such as the "fear grimace." Further expressions are used in affiliative encounters, such as during grooming, copulation, and infant–mother contact ("lip-smacking," "yawn," and "pucker-face"). Neurophysiological studies of face processing in macaques has revealed that particular facial expressions may elicit selective responses from single neurons in IT, STS, rostral entorhinal cortex, and amygdala (Brothers & Ring 1993; Brothers et al., 1990; Hasselmo et al., 1989; Nahm et al., 1996; Perrett & Mistlin, 1990; Perrett et al., 1984). Simian primates also use a large number of auditory signals during normal social interaction (such as affiliative coos and grunts) and to warn conspecifics of predators (alarm calls; Cheney & Seyfarth, 1990). Auditory communication is unrestrained by time of day or environment and can be an important means of communication whether in a darkened forest canopy or an open savanna during daylight.

Communication via the somatosensory channel is also important for a large number of primates (Dunbar, 1991). Grooming, for example, plays a significant role in the communication of affiliation and submission to dominant animals, and it may secure bonds between mating partners or between mother and infant (Jolly, 1985). Communication by touch may also be important for defining the subtle differences between a playful slap and a slap as part of an aggressive encounter, for example. Determining these differences and the positive effects of grooming may be processed by a particular neural pathway. Friedman et al. (1986) proposed that the somatosensory pathway from the primary and secondary somatosensory cortices (S1 and S2) to the tertiary somatosensory areas (A5, A7b) and insular cortex (Ig and Id), and finally the amygdala and hippocampus, is a possible route by which the limbic system (e.g., amygdala and hippocampus) can learn about and place into memory somatosensory stimuli. This pathway may also function in the attribution of socio-emotional significance to somatosensory stimuli, such as grooming or aggressive contact.

Information can also be transmitted via the olfactory channel. It is a controversial issue whether Old World monkeys, apes, and humans use chemical signals during social interaction. Recent studies in humans have suggested that pheromones are important for human social communication (Stern & McClintock, 1998). Pheromones may also be important components of macaques' sexual behavior (Michael & Keverne, 1968; Michael et al., 1976). Early studies (largely in rats) placed the amygdala as an olfactory structure. The primate amygdala has a large number of connections with olfactory cortex (Carmichael et al., 1994) and the olfactory bulb (Turner et al., 1978), and these connections may function in attributing socio-emotional significance to olfactory stimuli such as pheromones. This is more likely in prosimians and New World monkeys where olfactory communication is used (Klopfer, 1977) and where the ancient olfactory nucleus of the amygdala, the lateral nucleus of the olfactory tract, is more prominent than in the macaque monkey (Stephan et al., 1987).

In discussing the relationship of the anatomical connectivity of the amygdala to normal macaque behavior, we have assigned behaviors to distinct groups. An average day in the life of a macaque monkey may include all or some of the following categories of behaviors. Macaque monkeys spend the majority of their time trying to find and then process food (Clutton-Brock & Harvey, 1980). They also mate, groom, and form affiliative relationships (with kin, "friends," and sexual partners), fight, play, and defend territory and themselves from rival conspecifics and from predators.

Feeding Behavior

The greatest part of a normal macaque's day is spent in finding and processing food (45%; Goldstein & Richard, 1989). Different types of foods require different methods of processing, which in turn require specific neural systems to recognize, remember the location of, and extract the nutrients from different food types. The majority of diurnal (day-living) primates eat fruit, which requires high-level color vision (Allman, 1982). Fruit eaters are usually highly social, depending on the form of fruit they eat (Milton, 1981). The majority of fruit-eating primates eat green or bitter fruits, which are plentiful and clumped in large resources, thereby enabling many animals to feed in one tree (Jolly, 1985). Other primates, such as spider monkeys, eat ripe fruits which are rare and widely distributed, so large social groups are required to split into smaller foraging parties to find food (fission-fusion groups). Macaques eat abundant types of fruit, such as figs, which are easy to process. Eating abundant foods which can sustain a large number of animals on one tree provides increased opportunities for social interaction.

Eating fruit is a relatively simple task for most primates. Good color vision is required to locate specific types of fruit and to assess the level of ripeness or toxins that may be present. Olfaction and taste are also important indicators of the palatability of food. Highly distributed resources such as ripe fruit require a highly developed spatial memory system to remember where a previously encountered desirable or plentiful food source is located within a forest environment. A fine level of dexterity may be required to reach fruits in the high branches of trees, and fine manipulative ability may be required for removing the skin and seeds of some fruits.

Fruit color is probably processed before fruit type, as the brain region primarily concerned with color processing, area V4 (Heywood & Cowey, 1992) is located in the visual processing pathway before the IT, which codes the recognition of objects (including food items). The sight of different foods elicits neural responses from single neurons within the IT and the amygdala (Nishijo et al., 1988; Ono et al., 1983; Ono et al., 1989). Amygdala neurons receive direct inputs from the IT (Iwai & Yukie 1987), and the cooling of the IT reduces the activity of neurons responsive to foods (Ono & Nishijo, 1992), and the latency of neural responses to foods is longer in the amygdala neurons. Neurons within the lateral hypothalamus were also found to be responsive to similar food stimuli, with even longer response latencies (Fukuda et al., 1987; Fukuda & Ono, 1993, Ono et al., 1980, 1989). The amygdala projects directly to the lateral hypothalamus (Amaral et al., 1982), and it is suggested that the amygdala attributes valence to particular foods and the lateral hypothalamic area contributes to the visceral "feeling of satisfaction" after eating. The neurons in the amygdala and hypothalamus may also be responsive to the rewarding or aversive nature of the food stimuli (Rolls et al., 1976; Rolls, 1992). For example, the response to a slice of watermelon was reduced dramatically when the fruit was made aversive by adding salt to it (Ono & Nishijo, 1992). This response was diminished first for gustatory, then subsequently for visual responses (even though the appearance of the food had not changed). A number of gustatory neurons (responsive to the four basic taste groups, sweet, salt, sour, bitter) have been reported in the monkey amygdala (Scott et al., 1993). It is suggested that the neurons may not be responding to the perceptual attributes of the taste stimuli, but to the emotional or hedonic appreciation of the different taste types.

Larger, solitary, or sedentary primates tend to be folivorous. Foliage is an abundant resource, which requires special dietary adaptations to process (Aiello & Wheeler, 1995). Larger amounts of foliage are required to provide the same energy levels as fruit or meat. Folivorous primates tend to be less social than frugivorous (fruit-eating) primates, due to the high abundance of a widely distributed food resource. Highly functioning color vision is less important for foliage eaters than fruit eaters; however, the levels of toxins present in leaves may be determined by other modalities such as olfaction.

The final category of food processors are those primates which catch and eat different types of prey, such as insects, frogs, snakes, birds, and rodents. Macaques do not hunt large animals, but their diet does include insects. The capture of insects requires a complex motion processing system and a sophisticated and efficient sensorimotor system used to transfer the recognition of prey, a determination of their motion, and a prediction of their motion into a motor program which directs the limbs and extremities to catch the insect.

Although there have been no studies on the neural basis of predatory behavior in primates, the amygdala may be implicated due to its circuitry and the effect of amygdala lesions on predatory behavior in cats and rodents. Lesions of the amygdala in wild rats and cats causes a profound loss in forms of predatory aggression (Karli et al., 1972). Motion is processed primarily by neurons within extrastriate cortical visual areas, MT and MST (Maunsell & Newsome, 1987). This initial form of processing may enable the primate to locate the prey and predict their next possible movements. Recognition of the prey's species and subsequent motion would most likely be processed by IT and/or the STS. A population of neurons within the STS respond to different types of biological movement, such as a person walking in one particular direction (Emery 1997; Oram & Perrett, 1996; Perrett et al., 1985). It is probable that other categories of animal motion (quadrupedal running, jumping, flying, swimming, etc.) would also elicit neural responses within this cortical region. The preys' species would also be likely to be coded within this region, as responses to the faces of other animal species (Emery, 1997) have been recorded from single cells in the dorsal bank of the STS. The specific attributes of the recognized animal related to feeding, such as, is this animal edible, is this animal poisonous, is this animal nutritious, does this animal taste good, may be determined by the amygdaloid complex (Ono & Nishijo, 1992).

Once the animal has been identified as a nutritious, tasty source of nutrients and the direction of its motion has been predicted, the primate can attempt to catch the animal. As described earlier, the amygdala sends output projections to different parts of the striatum (see Amaral et al., 1992, for review). The primate striatum has been implicated in the initiation of movement sequences (Parent & Hazrati, 1993) and thereby may be one route by which the amygdala may influence the motor system for catching insects. Another possible route may be via premotor cortex, which receives a direct projection from the amygdala (Avendano et al., 1983). And, of course, the direct connections between the basal nucleus and widespread regions of visual and other sensory cortices may be involved in directing the attention of the sensory cortex to the vigilant pursuit of the prey.

Mating Behavior

For male macaque monkeys, mating is wholly dependent on the hormonal status of the females. If females are not experiencing estrus, males will not be permitted to mate. Estrus is the hormonally induced period when female nonhuman primates facilitate mating. Although female macaques do not accommodate a specific mating posture or lordosis seen in female rodents, they do adopt other receptive postures, which either allow a male to proceed with intromission or not. Before any form of sexual behavior can be initiated, both sexes must recognize members of the opposite sex. Males must target their sexual advances toward healthy, receptive females, and females must direct their proceptivity to mate to healthy, strong (high-ranking) males. The signals which macaques use during sexual behavior are dependent on the gender of the animal projecting and receiving the signals and are primarily visual in nature. (The role of olfactory signals or pheromones in the sexual behavior of monkeys, apes, and humans is not known, but it is suggested that their role is minor compared to their use by nonprimate animals and prosimians; Michael et al., 1976.)

The clearest indicator of female receptiveness for mating is the change in size and color of the anogenital region during estrus. In female rhesus macaques, the genital and perineal region turn bright red and increase in size. This sexual swelling is produced by an increase in estrogen (at the beginning of estrus), and dilation of blood vessels and increased water retention in the hindquarters (Dixson, 1983). The sexual swelling is the primary indicator of female receptivity to male mounting. Females initiate sexual contacts with males (proceptivity) by directing ("presenting") their hindquarters to attractive, prospective partners. Sexual presentation consists of lifting the tail to reveal the sexual swelling and associated coloration changes, directing the hindquarters toward the prospective mate and looking directly at the male, usually with associated eye contact (Wickler, 1967; Koyama et al., 1988). Eye contact from a female also has been shown to be a sufficient stimulus to elicit erection and ejaculation in male long-tailed macaques (Linnankoski et al., 1993). Male reactions to the presentation of a female in estrus include gazing at them, gazing while manipulating the female genital region (with lip-smacking), mounting (with or without erection), or coitus (friction movements).

The neural basis of sexual behavior in macaques will undoubtedly be different in males and females due to differences in their behavior. As stated above, females only mate during precise, hormonally controlled times during their menstrual cycle. Therefore, a male can only mate with a female when her neural and endocrine system provide the opportunity to mate. The sexual neurophysiology of the males is dependent on the behavior of the females, such as recognition of sexual signals signifying that the female is in estrus (e.g., sexual swellings). The females' sexual neurophysiology is controlled internally and, therefore, is to a major extent independent of the behavior of the males. Different neural mechanisms, therefore, should dominate the neurophysiology of each sex (Aou et al., 1984, 1988; Okada et al., 1991; Oomura et al., 1988; Slimp et al., 1981).

In males, neurons within the IT and STS may provide basic visual information concerning the gender of individuals. This mechanism must be highly developed in macaques and all primates with low sexual dimorphism. When the size difference between males and females is small, the ability to differentiate between the sexes is either determined via other methods (such as olfaction), or via subtle visual/auditory cues. As stated earlier, a small population of neurons within the anterior ventral temporal cortex are sensitive to the sight of faces and bodies. Although gender differences in cell responses have not been explicitly studied, it is possible that cell responses are specific at this level of processing. Some cells within the IT are identity specific (Hasselmo et al., 1989; Perrett et al., 1984a), and some cells differentiate between male and female human experimenters. Neurons with similar responses have been reported in the amygdala (Brothers et al., 1990; Leonard et al., 1985; Rolls, 1984).

Female macaques in estrus display striking visual indications of their disposition for mating. It is probable that such signals are coded within the anterior temporal cortex and amygdala. Good color vision (supported by neurons within area V4 in the ventral visual pathway) is required to recognize the level of reddening of the anogenital region. (A particular intensity of red may be associated with a certain stage of estrus.) Proceptive females also present their hindquarters to prospective mates. Neurons within the STS respond to bodies and body parts directed to different views, respective to the viewer (Wachsmuth et al., 1994). Similar neurons may be used to respond appropriately to a sexual presentation. Although the olfactory brain structures of the macaque are less developed than in New World monkeys and prosimian primates, olfactory information does enter the amygdala from the piriform cortices and the main and accessory olfactory bulbs (Amaral et al., 1992; Turner et al., 1978). There is some evidence that females transmit chemical signals from the vagina, which is used as an indicator of hormonal status (Michael et al., 1976).

Once information concerning the sexual status and proclivity of females to mate has entered the amygdala via the lateral nucleus, an appropriate behavioral action in response to these specific sexual signals must be initiated. The amygdala is in a unique anatomical position to respond to sexual signals and to influence appropriate male sexual responses. The accessory basal and medial nuclei project to the ventromedial hypothalamus, the central nucleus projects to the lateral hypothalamic area, and the basal (magnocellular division) and central nuclei project to the lateral tuberal nucleus (Amaral et al., 1992; Price, 1986; Price & Amaral, 1981). In rats, the amygdala can effect the preoptic area via the lateral nucleus which projects to the amygdalo-hippocampal area (AHA), which in turn projects to the preoptic area (Simerly & Swanson, 1986). It is not known how the amygdala can effect the preoptic area in monkeys, although a similar mechanism may be proposed.

The projection from the amygdala to the hypothalamus may be involved in the initiation of penile erection and eventually ejaculation, as electrical stimulation of the amygdala (MacLean & Ploog, 1962; Robinson & Mishkin, 1968) causes penile erection, and stimulation of the preoptic area (hypothalamus) causes erection and ejaculation with repeated stimulation (Robinson & Mishkin, 1966). Stimulation of the rostral putamen also causes erection, but if stimulated in the presence of females, causes mounting, intromission, and thrusting (Perachio et al., 1979). Presumably, the control of male genitalia is affected by neural feedback from the basal ganglia (and possibly the motor cortex) and hormonal feedback from the hypothalamic-pituitary-gonadal (HPG) axis. During copulation there is an increase in cardiac output and respiration and a decrease in nonessential visceral functions (Masters & Johnson, 1966). This may be controlled by output projections from the central nucleus of the amygdala to the brainstem autonomic regions (Jongen-Relo & Amaral, 1998; Price & Amaral, 1981).

Various facial and vocal signals are produced during copulation. The rhesus macaque copulation call, produced during sex, may be used as an indicator of health and genetic status to other females (Hauser, 1993). It is possible that the amygdala is involved in the production of this call, as information concerning the presence of other females near to the copulating couple (visual, olfactory, or auditory) is transferred into an outward signal (sensorimotor transformation). There is indirect evidence from brain stimulation and recording experiments in the squirrel monkey that the amygdala controls the expression of emotional vocalizations (as would be associated with copulation), directly (Jurgens, 1982; Lloyd & Kling, 1988), via the cortex (Jurgens, 1986), or via the brainstem (Jurgens & Pratt, 1979). Males and female monkeys also lip-smack during copulation, which may be a response to orgasm (Goldfoot et al., 1980). This may be controlled by the amygdala in similar ways to the copulation call.

Auditory information reaches the amygdala in a highly processed form. Mating calls are used by some male primates as courtship displays, possibly to advertise their health and genetic status (Hauser, 1993). Rhesus macaque males produce calls during copulation only when the competition for females in estrus is low, and they may be a method to signal to other females the genetic viability of the signaling macaque (Hauser, 1996). Females may therefore use such forms of auditory information (in addition to visual cues) via the primary auditory areas of the superior temporal gyrus to the lateral nucleus of the amygdala to make choices of possible sexual partners.

The neural control of sexual behavior in female monkeys is likely to be different from males. As stated earlier, the hormonal state of the female is the best predictor of subsequent sexual interaction. A rise in estrogen from the ovaries causes an enlargement and reddening of the anogenital area (probably via the hypothalamus and brainstem). Estrogen levels are kept high by a positive feedback loop, receiving sensory information from the amygdala which is passed on to the HPG axis.

The female's sexual signals incite interest from males. Females either tolerate mating (receptivity) or actively seek mating (proceptivity). Receptive females will permit males to mount them, but do not overtly accommodate intromission. The amygdala may initiate motor responses (such as the mounting posture) via interactions with the basal ganglia and premotor cortex. Females that actively encourage mating may be demonstrating preferences about the genetic makeup of their prospective partner. Visual information concerning the sex, physical health, direction of attention (interest), and social status of males enters the amygdala via the lateral nucleus from the cortex of the STS. An evaluation of the genetic fitness and the appropriate action may be made via the orbitofrontal cortex, although it is unknown whether any decisions made by female monkeys concerning mate choice are intentional (although there is some evidence that they are; Small, 1993).

Affiliative Behavior

Affiliative behaviors can be defined as "those behaviors that promote the development of, and serve to maintain, social bonds within primate society" (Steklis & Kling, 1985, p. 94). In humans, affiliative behavior is the guiding force behind the majority of human social interactions. Family and friends are extremely important stabilizing factors in relationships with others, and the default for all human interaction is altruistic behavior: courtesy, kindness, and consideration to others (Ridley, 1996). The situation is different in nonhuman primates. Two types of behavior form the backbone of stable social systems: aggression and affiliation. Aggression is discussed in the next section.

Many nonhuman primates, including macaques, have demonstrated their ability to form long-term alliances and "friendships" and perform acts of reconciliation after aggressive encounters (Cords, 1997; de Waal, 1989; Smuts, 1985). Specific components of affiliative behavior such as grooming are used to cement alliances and to diffuse agonistic encounters. Affiliative behavior is also an essential component of behaviors directed from a mother to her infant, as discussed at the end of this section. Two forms of affiliative behavior and their possible neural mechanisms will be discussed here: spatial proximity and grooming. Animals that tolerate one another are more likely to spend time in close proximity than other animals. Neural mechanisms within the anterior temporal cortex, especially the STS, may evaluate another individual's position in the world relative to the viewer (Perrett et al., 1995). If the individual is a potential threat (either a dominant male, a female favored by the alpha male, or previously aggressive individual), the behavioral significance of the individual may be evaluated by the basal nucleus of the amygdala using inputs from the orbitofrontal cortex and the hippocampal formation.

Grooming is an important method for cleaning the body surface (auto-grooming), but social or allogrooming has been suggested to play a more important role in affiliative behaviors such as the formation of social relationships and the maintenance of coalitions (Dunbar, 1991; Spruijt et al., 1992; Tomasello & Call, 1997). Allogrooming is an important tension reducer in monkeys (Schino et al., 1988). Somatosensory stimulation in the form of grooming from a "friend" may be interpreted by the amygdala (lateral and basal nuclei), which initiates a physiological response—a decrease in heart rate. This may be controlled by the central nucleus of the amygdala (Reis & Oliphant, 1964). This, in effect, relaxes the monkey being groomed, which produces a condition in which the groomed monkey is less likely to initiate aggressive behavior toward the grooming monkey.

Grooming, and affiliative behavior in general, have been related to the opiate system (Peffer et al., 1986). For example, Meller et al. (1980) found that blocking opiate receptors with the opioid antagonist naltrexone caused an increase in allogrooming in socially housed male talapoin monkeys. Fabre-Nys et al. (1982) also found an increase in grooming and groom invitations in naltrexone- and naloxone-treated talapoin monkeys in pairs. Finally, Martel et al. (1995) found that administration of naloxone to young rhesus monkeys increased their affiliative behaviors (contact with mother, contact vocalizations, and attempts to suckle). Opiate receptor blockade appears to enhance the requirement for social contact as expressed through grooming relationships. Endogenous opiate systems may also be related to grooming and affiliation. Keverne et al. (1989) measured cerebrospinal fluid β-endorphin in talapoin monkeys and found an increase in the opioid after social contact (grooming and groom solicitation), but only in previously isolated monkeys. There are large numbers of opiate receptors in the amygdala (LaMotte et al., 1978). There are also a large number of μ-opiate receptors in the periamygdaloid cortex and the sensory neocortical areas receiving projections from and projecting to the amygdala (Lewis et al., 1981). It remains to be determined whether the endogenous amygdaloid opioid systems are involved in the mediation of antagonist-increased grooming or whether this modulation occurs in one of the regions interconnected with the amygdala.

Although many forms of sociality are displayed by different primate species (solitary, monogamy, multifemale harems, fission-fusion groups, heterosexual bands, etc.), one form of affiliative behavior is common to all primate species: the bond between a mother and infant. Infants show typical reactions when separated from their mother, such as protest and despair (Harlow, 1974). Infants also display various forms of affiliative behavior toward their mothers with the effect of receiving comfort, food, protection, and vigilance from the mother; close proximity, extensive body contact, suckling, grooming, huddling, clinging, and embracing. The neural basis of primate maternal behavior has received little research effort and has concentrated, not surprisingly, on the three areas of the affiliative processing circuit proposed by Kling and Steklis (1976): the amygdala, orbitofrontal cortex, and anterior temporal pole. Lesions of these areas lead to similar behavioral abnormalities in monkey mothers. The lesioned mothers either physically abuse their infants, occasionally leading to death, or neglect them, either by refusing to suckle them or by failing to retrieve or protect them when they move away (Bucher et al., 1970; Franzen & Myers, 1973; Kling, 1972; Masserman et al., 1958; Myers et al., 1973).

Similar lesions in infant monkeys, however, did not disrupt the infants' mother-directed behaviors, such as reaching and suckling the nipple, clinging, grasping, and becoming distressed when separated from their mothers (Steklis & Kling, 1985). Neonatal lesions of the amygdala have profound effects on peer social interaction (Bachevalier, 1994; Thompson et al., 1977), such as responding to social invitation and initiating contact. This appears at odds with the data described above for mothers and infants. It is possible that brain systems other than the amygdala, temporal pole, and prefrontal cortex control mother-directed behavior in infant monkeys, although this seems unlikely. Further research on mother–infant interaction and brain lesions is required.

Maternal behavior (and infant mother-directed behavior) is actually a complex of myriad behaviors, the neural basis of which is likely to be as complex. Once an infant is born, the mother recognizes the infant as an infant and must recognize that it is her own and that she has to afford nurturing, protective and vigilant behavior toward the infant. Visual recognition of the infant may occur within the STS. It can be assumed from previous neurophysiological studies (e.g., Desimone et al., 1984; Perrett et al., 1982) that neurons in the STS respond primarily to different classes of monkey faces—males, females, infants, juveniles, adults, and so on. Therefore, some mechanism within the anterior temporal cortex responds to the physical features of an infant. A mother may learn that a newly born infant is hers from other signals, in particular, olfactory signals (Kaplan & Cubicciotti, 1980). A young mother may have experienced other females giving birth and the subsequent nurturing of the resultant infant. Possibly through social learning and visual or olfactory recognition, the new mother may direct its attention to the new infant which is clinging and suckling.

After birth, the mother's hormonal and neural systems (hypothalamus) will control the release of oxytocin, which in turn stimulates lactation for suckling. These systems may ultimately be controlled by the amygdala, which receives sensory input concerning the eminent birth (contractions, then sensory cues of the newborn infant). The mother then initiates a program of nurturing behaviors, such as grooming, feeding, and protection, which allows development of the infant and development of the attachment relationship between mother and infant (Lee, 1983). Mother-initiated behaviors directed to the infant may be under the hormonal control of oxytocin, although there are few data at present to suggest this in nonhuman primates (see Nelson & Panksepp, 1998, for a review of nonprimate species).

Infant monkeys appear to discriminate their mothers from other adult females using visual cues alone (Nakamichi & Yoshida, 1986). Rodman et al. (1993) found neurons responsive to different faces within IT and STS of four-month-old rhesus macaque infants. Visual responses were absent in infants younger than four months, but the response profile of the visually responsive neurons in four-month-old infants was the same as in adults (Desimone et al., 1984; Perrett et al., 1982). The ability to perceive social stimuli appears to develop earlier than four months. Mendelson et al. (1982) found that infants during the first week of life can discriminate faces from other objects (i.e., they show particular interest in faces), and at three weeks old they can discriminate whether a face is directed toward them or away and also appear to appreciate the significance of a threat (i.e., turning away when presented with a face with staring eyes). These results suggest that the infant forms an early attachment to its mother and can use specific neural systems to recognize its mother from other individuals.

It is not known whether the infant macaque brain, in particular the amygdala, contains templates for certain social stimuli such as faces, olfactory cues, or a mother's touch. As we have described earlier, perception of biologically significant stimuli occurs in the sensory cortex (such as the STS and insula), at the level of components or objects without biological significance. For example, a threat face can be perceived as two staring eyes, open mouth, ears back, and so on, without its biological function (aggression) being processed. We have suggested that the basal nucleus determines the social significance of these stimuli, such as a threat face for aggression. It would therefore be useful for innate templates of social stimuli to be present in the basal nucleus at birth, so that a newborn infant can perceive its mother and orient toward a source of food (i.e., the nipple). The context in which particular social stimuli are used develops with experience based on this innate template. This may be why infant monkeys can perceive faces as a distinct class of objects during the first week of life, but cannot perceive changes in gaze direction or appreciate the significance of threatening facial expressions until they are three weeks old. The amygdala develops relatively early in gestation (embryonic day E30–E50), but the separate nuclei do not differentiate until later in development (Kordower et al., 1992). This suggests a level of plasticity that may function in learning particular social contexts after birth.

Aggressive Behavior

"Aggression" is the encompassing term associated with a wide variety of different agonistic behaviors seen in many primate species, particularly in monkeys and apes. Aggression is a complex topic that can only be briefly summarized in this review. Aggression takes many different forms. Three forms of aggressive encounter will be discussed within the context of primate social interaction and the role of the amygdala; competitive aggression, intergroup aggression, and play aggression, each requiring a dedicated neural machinery to perform its function, a component of which is the amygdaloid complex.

Competitive aggression includes agonistic behavior during encounters that affect rankings in a dominance hierarchy (Bernstein, 1981), and agonistic behavior displayed during competition over resources, such as food and mating partners. Intergroup aggression occurs when two or more social groups encounter one another, either at a shared resource, such as a fruit tree, or a water pool, or when the groups' territories overlap. Intergroup aggression, however, rarely leads to physical contact aggression (Bernstein & Ehardt, 1985), suggesting that either different neural pathways control this form of agonistic behavior or that the neural pathways employed can differentiate between familiar (group member) versus unfamiliar animals (different group member) and appropriate inhibition can be brought to bear. Intergroup aggression probably does not manifest into physical contact aggression, as the potential losses from physical aggression can be great (if another individual is unknown to you, so are their strengths and weaknesses). Playful aggression occurs during infant and juvenile development and is seen as a precursor of adult agonistic behavior. It may also function as a method by which aggressive skills required in adulthood are learned without paying the costs of injury or death (Symons, 1978). As such, playful aggression requires a different perspective or, in other words, it is aggressive acts conducted in a benign social context.

For monkeys, aggression is too costly in Darwinian terms to be used without advantages to the initiator of the aggression. It therefore occurs for a specific purpose and only when other courses of action are unavailable. For example, a subordinate animal may fail to display an appropriate submissive gesture after stealing a dominant animal's food or engage in an illicit copulation with a female in estrus. To exert its status, the dominant animal must respond with a threat and be prepared to engage in physical aggression.

For a brain region to be considered a neural center for aggression, two criteria must be established. First, complex sensory information concerning social signals (such as facial expressions, vocalizations, postures, etc.) must directly enter the proposed neural center. Second, the neural center must have extensive output connections to brain regions. One of the functions of these connections is to initiate aggressive behavior (via motor response patterns, hormonal systems, and autonomic nervous system).

As for the other behaviors described in this chapter, the amygdala may be important for aggressive behavior by interpreting social signals as threatening and initiating appropriate neural, hormonal and behavioral actions (figure 8.7). Before a potential aggressive encounter, the dominant animal issues a threat. The threat is usually followed by a submissive gesture from a subordinate animal, but may lead to physical contact aggression if displayed to a dominant or equally ranked animal (Bernstein et al., 1983). The visual appearance of different facial expressions has been described for neurons within the STS (Hasselmo et al., 1988; Perrett et al., 1990, 1995) and the amygdala (Brothers & Ring, 1993; Brothers et al., 1990; Nahm et al., 1991, in preparation). As we have described, the STS projects heavily to the lateral nucleus of the amygdala (Aggleton et al., 1980; Stefanacci & Amaral, in preparation). The individual components of a threatening facial expression are processed in the STS (open mouth, staring eyes, ears pushed back) and conveyed to the lateral nucleus. The lateral nucleus attributes a particular "expression label" to these facial components (e.g., threat versus yawn). The identity of the individual producing the facial expression may also be processed by the lateral nucleus via connections from IT (Iwai & Yukie, 1987; Iwai et al., 1987). Information concerning the particular facial expression being viewed is conveyed to the basal nuclei. The particular social context in which the face is viewed (i.e., displayed by a dominant animal compared to a subordinate juvenile) may be provided by projections from the orbitofrontal cortex to the basal nuclei. The appropriate behavioral response is then initiated via projections from the basal nuclei to sensory and association areas of the cortex. Distinct physiological responses may be initiated via projections of the central nucleus to subcortical structures, such as the brainstem and hypothalamus.

Information about the potential for aggressive confrontation can also be transferred via postures and gestures. A macaque usually threatens another by directing its whole body rigidly toward an individual, with piloerection of fur, head bobbing toward the potential protagonist, and occasional lunges of the entire body. Cells within the STS respond to movements of different body parts (Oram et al., submitted; Perrett et al., 1989), including the extremities and the head. Exaggerated body movements may also be important indicators of an indivdual's propensity to attack. The STS also contains neurons that respond to the speed of another's motion (Emery, Oram, & Perrett, unpublished observations), and the direction of their motion in relation to the viewer (Oram & Perrett, 1996; Perrett & Emery, 1994; Perrett et al., 1985, 1990). As with facial expressions, the perceptual components of postures and gestures are processed in the STS, but the socio-affective significance of the postures and gestures to the viewing animal in a particular context is completely dependent on the lateral and basal nuclei of the amygdala (in conjunction with the orbitofrontal cortex).

Vocalizations, such as a "bark" (Hauser et al., 1993), usually accompany a threatening gesture. Specific vocalizations elicit neuronal responses within the auditory cortex of monkeys (Rauschecker et al., 1995). These auditory areas also project to the amygdala and terminate within the lateral nucleus (Amaral et al., 1992).

In some species of nonhuman primates (particularly prosimians and New World monkeys), olfactory signals are used for aggressive purposes, such as territory boundaries (Klopfer, 1977). As macaques do not appear to use olfactory sig-

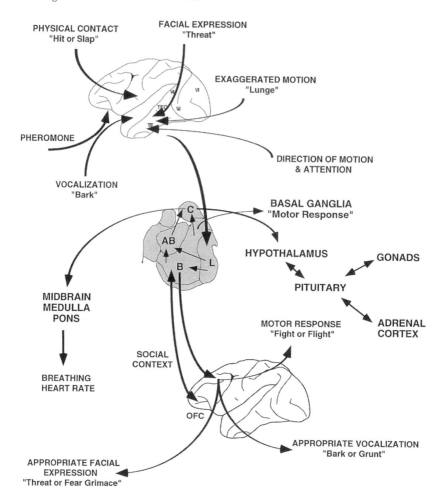

PHYSICAL CONTACT
"Hit or Slap"

FACIAL EXPRESSION
"Threat"

EXAGGERATED MOTION
"Lunge"

PHEROMONE

DIRECTION OF MOTION
& ATTENTION

VOCALIZATION
"Bark"

BASAL GANGLIA
"Motor Response"

C

AB

B   L

HYPOTHALAMUS   GONADS

PITUITARY

MIDBRAIN
MEDULLA
PONS

MOTOR RESPONSE
"Fight or Flight"

ADRENAL
CORTEX

BREATHING
HEART RATE

SOCIAL
CONTEXT

OFC

APPROPRIATE VOCALIZATION
"Bark or Grunt"

APPROPRIATE FACIAL
EXPRESSION
"Threat or Fear Grimace"

Figure 8.7. Sensory information conveying potentially aggressive signals and the identity of a potential participant, is processed by different areas of the neocortex. This sensory information is then conveyed to different sensory regions of the lateral nucleus of the amygdala. Polysensory information (possibly converged from the unimodal sectors of the lateral nucleus) is passed from the ventral lateral nucleus to the basal nucleus. Socio-emotional significance of the aggressive stimuli in relation to the social context of the aggressive signal (i.e., from a dominant animal) is determined by the basal nuclei and connections with the OFC. This information may be retrieved by the amygdala and used to produce an appropriate behavioral response (e.g., fear grimace to a dominant animal). Increases in *testosterone and cortisol* may be initiated via connections between the amygdala and the hypothalamus (via the hypothalamic-pituitary-adrenal and hypothalamic-pituitary-gonadal axes). Once an appropriate behavioral response has been determined, the correct physiological responses are initiated through projections from the central nucleus to the brainstem to control respiration and heart rate. The appropriate behavioral response is initiated via projections from the basal nuclei to the basal ganglia and (pre)motor cortex, which produces appropriate facial expressions, vocalizations, and motor responses (fight or flight).

nals in this manner, this will not be discussed further here. However, it is likely that the amygdala would be used for this form of communication in other primates, due to the large number of connections between the olfactory bulb (Turner et al., 1978), olfactory cortex (Carmichael et al., 1994), and the amygdala.

The somatosensory system may play an important role in determining whether a certain form of contact—for example, a slap—is either an aggressive act or part of normal play. As stated earlier, the amygdala receives highly processed (i.e., has passed through many processing stages) somatosensory information from the insula (Friedman et al., 1986; Mufson et al., 1981). Highly processed somatosensory information may also be received from the polysensory region of the STS (Mistlin, 1988). Similarly to the specific neural coding of different individual faces or facial expressions in the STS and the attachment of affective significance based on social context by nuclei in the amygdala, different complex tactile patterns, such as a stroke versus a hit versus a groom, may be coded in different areas of the tactile processing pathway. The perceptual characteristics of a somatosensory event such as a slap would be processed in the somatosensory cortex and insula before entering the lateral nucleus of the amygdala (i.e., a slap is a sharp blow of the hand on the body). The lateral nucleus would then determine that this particular somatosensory stimulus (slap) is usually performed during an aggressive encounter (although often performed during aggressive play by infant and juvenile macaques). The basal nuclei would process the effect of the somatosensory stimulus within a particular social context via its inputs from the orbitofrontal cortex. For example, a slap from a large, unknown animal during a battle for territory may require overt physical retaliation or appeasement dependent on the social context in relation to the monkey being aggressed against. If the attacking animal is much larger than the attacked animal and has won many previous aggressive encounters and has a large coalition base, a retaliatory attack will be more likely to result in further harmful aggression. In this context, appeasement and retreat may be a safer form of behavioral response. If the attacker is smaller with no history of aggression, a more appropriate behavioral response would be to attack in retaliation.

The amygdala projects to the hypothalamus and therefore has potential control over the HPA and HPG axes. As discussed in the section on sexual behavior, the amygdala's influence on the hypothalamus may be either via a direct route from the accessory basal and medial nuclei to the ventromedial hypothalamus, the central nucleus to the lateral hypothalamic area and the basal (magnocellular division) and central nuclei to the lateral tuberal nucleus (Amaral et al., 1992; Price, 1986; Price & Amaral, 1981). The amygdala may also influence the hypothalamus via an indirect route from the lateral nucleus to the amygdalo-hippocampal area (AHA) to the preoptic area (Simmerly & Swanson, 1986).

The HPA axis is primarily associated with the stress response and the release of cortisol from the adrenal gland. The cortisol is then released into the bloodstream. Social stress (such as occurs in relation to aggression) increases peripheral cortisol levels (Sapolsky, 1995), and long-term social stress can affect the morphology of the hippocampus, destroying neurons (Uno et al., 1989), induce arteriosclerosis (Kaplan et al., 1982), increase heart rate (Kaplan et al., 1990) and reduce the viability of the immune system (Coe, 1993; Cohen et al., 1992). The amygdala may influence an increase in cortisol in response to aggressive encounters via the hypothalamus, but the amygdala is also in an anatomical position to influence the response of visceral structures via the autonomic nervous system (Amaral et al., 1992). The central nucleus projects to the brainstem structures that control vital life functions, such as heart rate and blood pressure, breathing, gastrointestinal function, and homeostatic functions such as sweating and piloerection. Increases in heart rate and breathing are associated with aggression to target increased blood flow to the muscles and oxygen to the lungs for use either in retaliatory attack or a flight response.

Predator Avoidance and Defense

Although foraging for food or interacting with conspecifics are important components of the daily routine of monkeys, the avoidance of predators is paramount to their survival. A number of different animals hunt and feed on monkeys: leopards, tigers and other large felines, eagles, snakes, crocodiles, and also other primates such as baboons and chimpanzees (Cheney & Seyfarth, 1990). Monkeys, therefore, must have the ability to distinguish between these different types of predators using visual, auditory, and olfactory cues. The signals indicating the presence of a predator appear in two forms. During the physical presence of a predator, a monkey must recognize the species of predator (from visual, auditory, and olfactory cues) and evaluate the possible associated dangers. For example, snakes present less of a physical danger to monkeys than leopards (snakes can be mobbed by a small group of monkeys; Cheney & Seyfarth, 1990), so greater fear responses are associated with the presence of leopards than snakes. Signs of a predator's recent presence, such as the carcasses of previous prey, tracks, and movement in the undergrowth, are also important signals of the possible presence of a predator and the species of that animal (although recent evidence in vervet monkeys suggests that they cannot interpret these secondary signals, Cheney & Seyfarth, 1990).

The perception of predators, either directly via visual signals (body shape, motion) or tracks, vocalizations (alarm calls from conspecifics or noises produced by predators themselves, such as cats purring or roaring or eagles shrieking) or olfactory signals, is likely to occur within the STS and IT and the auditory areas of the superior temporal gyrus (STG). Neurons responsive to the sight of different animals have been found within the polysensory region of the STS (Emery, 1997), and direction of another's motion also elicits cell responses in this region of cortex (Oram & Perrett, 1996; Perrett et al., 1985). Although a predator or predator-related signal is perceived in the sensory areas of cortex, the label "animal or predator" would be attached to the stimulus in the lateral nucleus. Whether the perceived animal is dangerous to the observing monkey is again dependent on a particular context (i.e., whether the animal has been experienced previously or what the outcomes of this encounter were). As with social context, this information is likely to be provided by inputs to the basal nuclei from the orbitofrontal cortex. If the animal was encountered previously and the monkey survived or the animal was observed eating a conspecific, an appropriate physiological and behavioral response may be initiated via the basal nuclei's projections to cortex and the central nucleus' projections to effector brain structures. Signals such as alarm calls would also be sufficient to elicit a response, based again on experience of the previous outcomes of different alarm calls. This enables a vervet monkey, for example, to respond appropriately to an eagle alarm call (look into the air and hide in the trees) compared to a leopard alarm call (run into the bush; Cheney & Seyfarth, 1990).

Summary

We have provided a short overview of the major neuroantomical features of the monkey amygdala. The hallmark of this connectivity is that the amygdaloid complex is privy to high-level sensory information from all modalities. This information is further processed within the complex intrinsic circuitry of the amygdala, where other sources of information, such as social context from the orbitofrontal cortex, are added. Using all available sources of perceptual and social information, the amygdala may determine the species-specific relevance of a perceived complex stimulus such as a facial expression. Based on the significance of the stimulus, the amygdala may participate in the generation of an appropriate behavioral response. Modern neuroanatomical studies have demonstrated that the primate amygdala gives rise to widespread neural connections by which many brain systems can be engaged to produce a behavior. We have summarized a series of behaviors in the daily life of a typical macaque monkey and described how the amygdala may be important in bringing them about. Although much of this chapter has been speculative, it may provide a heuristic perspective from which to design future behavioral and electrophysiological analyses of the monkey amygdala.

References

Aggleton, J. P. (1985). A description of intra-amygdaloid connections in Old World monkeys. *Experimental Brain Research, 57,* 390–399.

Aggleton, J. P., Burton, M. J. & Passingham, R. E. (1980). Cortical and subcortical afferents to the amygdala of the rhesus monkey (*Macaca mulatta*). *Brain Research, 190,* 347–368.

Aggleton, J. P. & Passingham, R. E. (1981). Syndrome produced by lesions of the amygdala in monkeys (*Macaca mulatta*). *Journal of Comparative and Physiological Psychology, 95,* 961–977.

Aggleton, J. P. & Passingham, R. E. (1982). An assessment of the reinforcing properties of foods after amygdaloid lesions in rhesus monkeys. *Journal of Comparative and Physiological Psychology, 96,* 71–77.

Aiello, L. C. & Wheeler, P. (1995). The expensive tissue hypothesis: the brain and the digestive system in human and primate evolution. *Current Anthropology, 36,* 199–221.

Allman, J. (1982). Reconstructing the evolution of the brain in primates through the use of comparative neurophysiological and neuroanatomical data. In E. Armstrong & D. Falk (Eds), *Primate Brain Evolution: Methods and Concepts* (pp. 13–28). New York: Plenum Press.

Altmann, J. (1974). Observational study of behavior: sampling methods. *Behaviour, 49,* 227–266.

Amaral, D. G., Veazey, R. B. & Cowan, W. M. (1982). Some observations on hypothalamo-amygdaloid connections in the monkey. *Brain Research, 252,* 13–27.

Amaral, D. G. & Price, J. L. (1984). Amygdalo-cortical projections in the monkey (*Macaca fasicularis*). *Journal of Comparative Neurology, 230*, 465–496.

Amaral, D. G., Price, J. L., Pitkanen, A. & Carmichael, S. T. (1992). Anatomical organization of the primate amygdaloid complex. In J. P. Aggleton (Ed), *The Amygdala, Neurobiological Aspects of Emotion, Memory and Mental Dysfunction* (pp. 1–66). New York: Wiley-Liss.

Aou, S., Oomura, Y. & Yoshimatsu, H. (1988). Neuron activity of the ventromedial hypothalamus and the medial preoptic area of the female monkey during sexual behavior. *Brain Research, 455*, 65–71.

Aou, S., Yoshimatsu, H. & Oomura, Y. (1984). Medial preoptic neuronal responses to connatural females in sexually inactive male monkeys (*Macaca fuscata*). *Neuroscience Letters, 44*, 217–221.

Avendano, C., Price, J. L. & Amaral, D. G. (1983). Evidence for an amygdaloid projection to premotor cortex, but not to motor cortex in the monkey. *Brain Research, 264*, 111–117.

Bachevalier, J. (1994). Medial temporal lobe structures and autism: a review of clinical and experimental findings. *Neuropsychologia, 32*, 627–648.

Baylis, L. L. & Gaffan, D. (1991). Amygdalectomy and ventromedial prefrontal ablation produce similar deficits in food choice and in simple object discrimination learning for an unseen reward. *Experimental Brain Research, 86*, 617–622.

Bernstein, I. S. (1981). Dominance: the baby and the bath water. *Behavioral and Brain Sciences, 4*, 419–457.

Bernstein, I. S. & Ehardt, C. L. (1985). Intragroup agonistic behavior in rhesus monkeys (*Macaca mulatta*). *International Journal of Primatology, 6*, 209–226.

Bernstein, I, Williams, L. & Ramsay, M. (1983). The expression of aggression in Old World monkeys. *International Journal of Primatology, 4*, 113–125.

Bertrand, M. (1969). The behavioural repertoire of the stumptail macaque: a descriptive and comparative study. *Bibliotheca Primatologia, 11*, 1–273.

Brothers, L. (1990). The social brain: a project for integrating primate behavior and neurophysiology in a new domain. *Concepts in Neuroscience, 1*, 27–51.

Brothers, L. & Ring, B. (1993). Mesial temporal neurons in the macaque monkey with responses selective for aspects of social stimuli. *Behavioural Brain Research, 57*, 53–61.

Brothers, L., Ring, B. & Kling, A. (1990). Response of neurons in the macaque amygdala to complex social stimuli. *Behavioural Brain Research, 41*, 199–213.

Brown, S. & Shafer, E. A. (1888). An investigation into the functions of the occipital and temporal lobes of the monkey's brain. *Philosophical Transactions of the Royal Society of London: Biological Sciences, 179*, 303–327.

Bucher, K., Myers, R. E. & Southwick, C. (1970). Anterior temporal cortex and maternal behavior in monkey. *Neurology, 20*, 415.

Carmichael, S. T., Clugnet, M.-C. & Price, J. L. (1994). Central olfactory connections in the macaque monkey. *Journal of Comparative Neurology, 346*, 403–434.

Cheney, D. L. & Seyfarth, R. M. (1990). *How Monkeys See the World*. Chicago: University of Chicago Press.

Clutton-Brock, T. H. & Harvey, P. H. (1980). Primates, brains and ecology. *Journal of Zoology, 190*, 309–323.

Coe, C. L. (1993). Psychosocial factors and immunity in nonhuman primates: a review. *Psychosomatic Medicine, 55*, 298–308.

Cohen, S., Kaplan, J. R., Cunnick, J. E., Manuck, S. B. & Rabin, B. S. (1992). Chronic social stress, affiliation and cellular immune response in nonhuman primates. *Psychological Science, 3*, 301–304.

Cords, M. (1997). Friendships, alliances, reciprocity and repair. In A. Whiten & R. W. Byrne (Eds), *Machiavellian Intelligence 2: Extensions and Evaluations* (pp. 24–49). Cambridge: Cambridge University Press.

Desimone, R., Albright, T. D., Gross, C. G. & Bruce, C. (1984). Stimulus-selective properties of inferior temporal neurons in the macaque. *Journal of Neuroscience, 4*, 2051–2062.

de Waal, F. (1989). *Peacemaking among Primates*. Cambridge, MA: Harvard University Press.

Dicks, D., Myers, R. E. & Kling, A. (1969). Uncus and amygdala lesions: effects on social behavior in the free ranging rhesus monkey. *Science, 165*, 69–71.

Dixson, A. F. (1983). Observations on the evolution and behavioral significance of "sexual skin" in female primates. *Advances in the Study of Behavior, 13*, 63–106.

Downer, J. L. (1961). Changes in visual gnostic functions and emotional behaviour following unilateral temporal pole damage in the 'split-brain' monkey. *Nature, 191*, 50–51.

Dunbar, R. I. M. (1991). Functional significance of social grooming in primates. *Folia Primatologia, 57*, 121–131.

Emery, N. J. (1997). Neuroethological studies of primate social perception (doctoral dissertation). University of St. Andrews.

Fabre-Nys, C., Meller, R. E. & Keverne, E. B. (1982). Opiate antagonists stimulate affiliative behavior in monkeys. *Pharmacology, Biochemistry and Behavior, 16*, 653–659.

Franzen, E. A. & Myers, R. E. (1973). Neural control of social behavior: prefrontal and anterior temporal cortex. *Neuropsychologia, 11*, 141–157.

Friedman, D. P., Murray, E. A., O'Neill, B. & Mishkin, M. (1986). Cortical connections of the somatosensory fields of the lateral sulcus of macaques: evidence for a corticolimbic pathway for touch. *Journal of Comparative Neurology, 252*, 323–347.

Fukuda, M. & Ono, T. (1993). Amygdala-hypothalamic control of feeding behaviour in monkey: single cell responses before and after reversible blockade of temporal cortex or amygdala projections. *Behavioural Brain Research, 55*, 233–241.

Fukuda, M., Ono, T. & Nakamura, K. (1987). Functional relations among inferotemporal cortex, amygdala, and lateral hypothalamus in monkey operant feeding behavior. *Journal of Neurophysiology, 57*, 1060–1077.

Goldfoot, D. A., Westerborg-Van Loon, H., Groeneveld, W. & Koos Slob, A. (1980). Behavioral and physiological evidence of sexual climax in the female stump-tailed macaque (*Macaca arctoides*). *Science, 280*, 1477–1478.

Goldstein, S. J. & Richard, A. F. (1989). Ecology of rhesus macaques (*Macaca mulatta*) in northwest Pakistan. *International Journal of Primatology, 10*, 531–567.

Harlow, H. F. (1974). *Learning to Love*. San Francisco: Jason Aronson.

Hasselmo, M. E., Rolls, E. T. & Bayliss, G. C. (1989). The role of expression and identity in the face selective responses of neurons in the temporal visual cortex of the monkey. *Behavioural Brain Research, 32*, 203–218.

Hauser, M. D. (1993). Rhesus monkey copulation calls: honest signals for female choice? *Proceedings of the Royal Society of London: Biological Sciences, 254*, 93–96.

Hauser, M. D, (1996) *The Evolution of Communication*. Cambridge, MA: MIT Press.

Hauser, M. D., Evans, C. S. & Marler, P. (1993). The role of articulation in the production of rhesus monkey, *Macaca mulatta*, vocalizations. *Animal Behaviour, 45*, 423–433.

Heywood, C. A. & Cowey, A. (1992a). Cortical area V4 and its role in the perception of color. *Journal of Neuroscience, 12*, 4056–4065.

Hinde, R. A. & Rowell, T. E. (1962). Communication by postures and facial expressions in the rhesus monkey. *Symposium of the Zoological Society of London, 8*, 1–21.

Horel, J. A. & Keating, E. G. (1972). Recovery from a partial Klüver-Bucy syndrome in the monkey produced by disconnection. *Journal of Comparative and Physiological Psychology, 79*, 105–114.

Horel, J. A., Keating, E. G. & Misantone, L. J. (1975). Partial Klüver-Bucy syndrome produced by destroying temporal neocortex or amygdala. *Brain Research, 94*, 347–359.

Huber, E. (1961). The facial musculature and its innervation. In C. G. Hartman & W. L. Straus (Eds), *Anatomy of the Rhesus Monkey (Macaca mulatta)* (pp. 176–188). New York: Hafner.

Iwai, E. & Yukie, M. (1987). Amygdalofugal and amygdalopetal connections with modality-specific visual cortical areas in macaques (*Macaca fuscata, M. mulatta, and M. fascicularis*). *Journal of Comparative Neurology, 261*, 362–387.

Iwai, E., Yukie, M., Suyama, H. & Shirakawa, S. (1987). Amygdalar connections with middle and inferior temporal gyri of the monkey. *Neuroscience Letters, 83*, 25–29.

Jolly, A. (1985). *The Evolution of Primate Behavior*. New York: Macmillan.

Jongen-Relo, A. & Amaral, D. G. (1998). Evidence for a GABAergic projection from the central nucleus of the amygdala to the brainstem of the macaque monkey: a combined retrograde tracing and in situ hybridization study. *European Journal of Neuroscience, 10*, 2924–2933.

Jurgens, U. (1982). Amygdalar vocalization pathways in the squirrel monkey. *Brain Research, 241*, 189–196.

Jurgens, U. (1986). The squirrel monkey as an experimental model in the study of cerebral organization of emotional vocal utterances. *European Archives of Psychiatry and Neurological Sciences, 1*, 40–43.

Jurgens, U. & Pratt, R. (1979). Role of the periaqueductal gray in vocal expression of emotion. *Brain Research, 167*, 367–378.

Kaplan, J. N. & Cubicciotti, D. D. (1980). Early perceptual experience and the development of social preferences in squirrel monkeys. In R. W. Bell & W. P. Smotherman (Eds), *Maternal Influences and Early Behavior* (pp. 253–270). New York: Spectrum.

Kaplan, J. R., Manuck, S. B., Clarkson, T. B., Lusso, F. M. & Taub, D. M. (1982). Social status, environment and atherosclerosis in cynomolgus monkeys. *Arteriosclerosis, 2*, 359–368.

Kaplan, J. R., Manuck, S. B. & Gatsonis, C. (1990). Heart rate and social status among male cynomolgus monkeys (*Macaca fascicularis*) housed in disrupted social groupings. *American Journal of Primatology, 21*, 175–181.

Karli, P., Vergnes, M., Eclancher, F., Schmitt, P. & Chaurand, J. P. (1972). Role of the amygdala in the control of "mouse-killing" behavior in the rat. In B. E. Eleftheriou (Ed), *The Neurobiology of the Amygdala* (pp. 553–580). New York: Plenum Press.

Keverne, E. B., Martensz, N. D. & Tuite, B. (1989). Beta-endorphin concentrations in cerebrospinal fluid of monkeys are influenced by grooming relationships. *Psychoneuroendocrinology, 14*, 155–161.

Kling, A. (1968). Effects of amygdalectomy and testosterone on sexual behavior of male juvenile macaques. *Journal of Comparative and Physiological Psychology, 65*, 466–471.

Kling, A. (1972). Effects of amygdalectomy on socio-affective behavior in non-human primates. In B. E. Eleftheriou (Ed), *Neurobiology of the Amygdala* (pp. 511–536). New York: Plenum Press.

Kling, A. (1974). Differential effects of amygdalectomy in male and female nonhuman primates. *Archives of Sexual Behavior, 3*, 129–134.

Kling, A. & Cornell, R. (1971). Amygdalectomy and social behaviour in the caged stump-tailed macaque. *Folia Primatologia, 14*, 91–103.

Kling, A., Dicks, D. & Gurowitz, E. M. (1969). Amygdalectomy and social behavior in a caged group of vervets. In R. Carpenter (Ed), *Proceedings of the Second International Congress of Primatology* (pp. 232–241). New York: Karger.

Kling, A. & Dunne, K. (1976). Social-environmental factors affecting behavior and serum testosterone in normal and amygdala lesioned *M. speciosa*. *Primates, 17*, 23–42.

Kling, A., Lancaster, J. & Benitone, J. (1970). Amygdalectomy in the free-ranging vervet. *Journal of Psychiatric Research, 7*, 191–199.

Kling, A. & Steklis, H. D. (1976). A neural substrate for affiliative behaviour in non-human primates. *Brain, Behavior and Evolution, 13*, 216–238.

Klopfer, P. H. (1977). Communication in prosimians. In T. A. Sebeok (Ed), *How Animals Communicate* (pp. 841–850). Bloomington: Indiana University Press.

Klüver, H. & Bucy, P. C. (1937). "Psychic blindness" and other symptoms following bilateral temporal lobectomy in rhesus monkeys. *American Journal of Physiology, 119*, 352–353.

Klüver, H. & Bucy, P. C. (1939). Preliminary analysis of functions of the temporal lobes in monkeys. *Archives of Neurology and Psychiatry, 42*, 979–1000.

Koyama, Y., Fujita, I, Aou, S. & Oomura, Y. (1988). Proceptive presenting elicited by electrical stimulation of the female monkey hypothalamus. *Brain Research, 446*, 199–203.

Kordower, J. H., Piecinski, P. & Rakic, P. (1992). Neurogenesis of the amygdaloid nuclear complex in the rhesus monkey. *Developmental Brain Research, 68*, 9–15.

LaMotte, C. C., Snowman, A., Pert, C. B. & Snyder, S. H. (1978). Opiate receptor binding in rhesus monkey brain: association with limbic structures. *Brain Research, 155*, 374–379.

LeDoux, J. E. (1996). *The Emotional Brain: The Mysterious Underpinnings of Emotional Life*. New York: Simon and Schuster.

Lee, P. C. (1983). Caretaking of infants and mother-infant relationships. In R. A. Hinde (Ed), *Primate Social Relationships: An Integrated Approach* (pp. 146–151). Oxford: Blackwell.

Leonard, C. M., Rolls, E. T., Wilson, F. A. W. & Baylis, G. C. (1985). Neurons in the amygdala of the monkey with responses selective for faces. *Behavioural Brain Research, 15*, 159–176.

Lewis, W. E., Mishkin, M., Bragin, E., Brown, R. M., Pert, C. B. & Pert, A. (1981). Opiate receptor gradients in monkey cerebral cortex: correspondence with sensory processing hierarchies. *Science, 211*, 1166–1169.

Linnankoski, I, Gronroos, M. & Pertovaara, A. (1993). Eye contact as a trigger of male sexual arousal in stump-tailed macaques (*Macaca arctoides*). *Folia Primatologia, 60*, 181–184.

Lloyd, R. L. & Kling, A. S. (1988). Amygdaloid electrical activity in response to conspecific calls in squirrel monkey (*Saimiri sciureus*): influence of environmental setting, cortical inputs and recording site. In J. D. Newman (Ed), *The Physiological Control of Mammalian Vocalizations* (pp. 137–151). New York: Plenum Press.

MacLean, P. D. & Ploog, D. W. (1962). Cerebral representation of penile erection. *Journal of Neurophysiology, 25*, 29 55.

Malkova, L., Gaffan, D. & Murray, E. A. (1997). Excitotoxic lesions of the amygdala fail to produce impairment in visual learning for auditory secondary reinforcement but interfere with reinforcer devaluation effects in rhesus monkeys. *Journal of Neuroscience, 17*, 6011–6020.

Martel, F. L., Nevison, C. M., Simpson, M. J. A. & Keverne, E. B. (1995). Effects of opioid receptor blockade on the social behavior of rhesus monkeys living in large family groups. *Developmental Psychobiology, 28*, 71–84.

Masserman, J. H., Levitt, M., McAvoy, T., Kling, A. & Pechtel, C. (1958). The amygdalae and behavior. *American Journal of Psychiatry, 115*, 14–17.

Masters, W. & Johnson, V. (1966). *Human Sexual Response.* Boston: Little Brown.

Maunsell, J. H. & Newsome, W. T. (1987). Visual processing in monkey extrastriate cortex. *Annual Review of Neuroscience, 10*, 363–401.

Meller, R. E., Keverne, E. B. & Herbert, J. (1980). Behavioral and endocrine effects of naltrexone in male talapoin monkeys. *Pharmacology, Biochemistry and Behavior, 13*, 663–672.

Mendelson, M. J., Haith, M. M. & Goldman-Rakic, P. S. (1982). Face scanning and responsiveness to social cues in infant rhesus monkeys. *Developmental Psychology, 18*, 222–228.

Michael, R. P., Bonsall, R. W. & Zumpe, D. (1976). Evidence for chemical communication in primates. *Vitamins and Hormones, 34*, 137–186.

Michael, R. P. & Keverne, E. B. (1968). Pheromones in the communication of sexual status in primates. *Nature, 218*, 746–749.

Milton, K. (1981). Distribution patterns of tropical plant foods as an evolutionary stimulus to primate mental development. *American Anthropologist, 83*, 534–548.

Mistlin, A. J. (1988). Neural mechanisms underlying the perception of socially relevent stimuli in the macaque monkey (doctoral dissertation). University of St. Andrews.

Mufson, E. J., Mesulam, M. M. & Pandya, D. N. (1981). Insular interconnections with the amygdala in the rhesus monkey. *Neuroscience, 6*, 1231–1248.

Murray, E. A., Gaffan, E. A. & Flint, R. W. (1996). Anterior rhinal cortex and amygdala, dissociation of their contributions to memory and food preference in rhesus monkeys. *Behavioural Neuroscience, 110*, 30–42.

Myers, R. E., Swett, C. & Miller, M. (1973). Loss of social group affinity following prefrontal lesions in free-ranging macaques. *Brain Research, 64*, 257–269.

Nahm, F. K., Albright, T. D. & Amaral, D. G. (1991). Neuronal responses of the monkey amygdaloid complex to dynamic visual stimuli. *Society for Neuroscience Abstracts, 17*, 473.

Nakamichi, M. & Yoshida, A. (1986). Discrimination of mother by infant among Japanese macaques (*Macaca fuscata*). *International Journal of Primatology, 7*, 481–489.

Nishijo, H., Ono, T. & Nishino, H. (1988). Single neuron responses in amygdala of alert monkey during complex sensory stimulation with affective significance. *Journal of Neuroscience, 8*, 3570–3583.

Okada, E., Aou, S., Takaki, A., Oomura, Y. & Hori, T. (1991). Electrical stimulation of male monkey's midbrain elicits components of sexual behavior. *Physiology and Behaviour, 50*, 229–236.

Ono, T., Fukuda, M., Nishijo, H., Sasaki, K. & Muramoto, K. I. (1983). Amygdaloid neuronal responses to complex visual stimuli in an operant feeding situation in the monkey. *Brain Research Bulletin, 11*, 515–518.

Ono, T. & Nishijo, H. (1992). Neurophysiological basis of the Klüver-Bucy syndrome: responses of monkey amygdaloid neurons to biologically significant objects. In J. P. Aggleton (Ed), *The Amygdala: Neurobiological Aspects of Emotion, Memory, and Mental Dysfunction* (pp. 167–190). New York: Wiley-Liss.

Ono, T., Nishino, H., Sasaki, K., Fukuda, M. & Muramoto, K. (1980). Role of the lateral hypothalamus in feeding behavior. *Brain Research Bulletin, 5*, 143–149.

Ono, T., Tamura, R., Nishijo, H., Nakamura, K. & Tabuchi, E. (1989). Contribution of amygdalar and lateral hypothalamic neurons to visual information processing of food and nonfood in monkey. *Physiology and Behaviour, 45*, 411–421.

Oomura, Y., Aou, S., Koyama, Y., Fujita, I. & Yoshimatsu, H. (1988). Central control of sexual behavior. *Brain Research Bulletin, 20*, 863–870.

Oram, M. W. & Perrett, D. I. (1996). Integration of form and motion in the anterior superior temporal polysensory area (STPa) of the macaque monkey. *Journal of Neurophysiology, 76*, 109–129.

Nelson, E. E. & Panksepp, J. (1998). Brain substrates of infant-mother attachment: contributions of opioids, oxytocin and norepinephrine. *Neuroscience and Biobehavioral Reviews, 22*, 437–452.

Parent, A. & Hazrati, L. (1993). Anatomical aspects of information processing in primate basal ganglia. *Trends in Neurosciences, 16*, 111–116.

Peffer, P. G., Byrd, L. D. & Smith, E. O. (1986). Effects of d-amphetamine on grooming and proximity in stumptail macaques: differential effects on social bonds. *Pharmacology, Biochemistry and Behavior, 24*, 1025–1030.

Perachio, A. A., Marr, L. D. & Alexander, M. (1979). Sexual behavior in male rhesus monkeys elicited by electrical stimulation of preoptic and hypothalamic areas. *Brain Research, 177*, 127–144.

Perrett, D. I. & Emery, N. J. (1994). Understanding the intentions of others from visual signals: neurophysiological evidence. *Current Psychology of Cognition, 13*, 683–694.

Perrett, D. I., Harries, M. H., Mistlin, A. J., Hietanen, J. K., Bevan, R., Thomas, S., Ortega, J. O., Oram, M. W. & Brierly, K. (1990). Social signals analysed at the single cell level: someone's looking at me, something touched me, something moved! *International Journal of Comparative Psychology, 4*, 25–55.

Perrett, D. I. & Mistlin, A. J. (1990). Perception of facial characteristics by monkeys. In W. C. Stebbins & M. A. Berkley (Eds), *Comparative Perception II* (pp. 187–215). New York: John Wiley.

Perrett, D. I., Mistlin, A. J., Harries, M. H. & Chitty, A. J. (1989). Understanding the visual appearance and consequence of hand actions. In M. A. Goodale (Ed), *Vision and Action: The Control of Grasping* (pp. 163–180).

Perrett, D. I., Oram, M. W., Wachsmuth, E. & Emery, N. J. (1995). Understanding the behaviour and "minds" of others from their facial and body signals: studies of visual processing within the temporal cortex. In T. Nakajima & T. Ono (Eds), *Emotion, Memory and Behavior: Studies on human and Non-human Primates* (pp. 155–167). Tokyo: Japan Scientific Societies Press.

Perrett, D. I., Rolls, E. T. & Caan, W. (1982). Visual neurons responsive to faces in the monkey temporal cortex. *Experimental Brain Research, 47*, 329–342.

Perrett, D. I., Smith, P. A. J., Potter, D. D., Mistlin, A. J., Head, A. S. M. & Jeeves, M. A. (1984a). Neurons responsive to faces in the temporal cortex: studies of functional organization, sensitivity to identity and relation to perception. *Human Neurobiology, 3*, 197–208.

Perrett, D. I., Smith, P. A. J., Potter, D. D., Mistlin, A. J., Head, A. S., Milner, A. D. & Jeeves, M. A. (1984b). Visual cells in the temporal cortex sensitive to face view and gaze direction. *Proceedings of the Royal Society of London: Biological Sciences, 223*, 293–317.

Perrett, D. I., Smith, P. A. J., Mistlin, A. J., Chitty, A. J., Head, A. S. P., Broennimann, R., Milner, A. D. & Jeeves, M. A. (1985). Visual analysis of body movements by neurons in the temporal cortex of the macaque monkey: a preliminary report. *Behavioural Brain Research, 16*, 153–170.

Pitkanen, A. & Amaral, D. G. (1991). Demonstrations of projections from the lateral nucleus to the basal nucleus of the amygdala: a PHA-L study in the monkey. *Experimental Brain Research, 83*, 465–470.

Pitkanen, A. & Amaral, D. G. (1998). Organization of the intrinsic connections of the monkey amygdaloid complex: projections originating in the lateral nucleus. *Journal of Comparative Neurology, 398*, 431–458.

Price, J. L. (1986). Subcortical projections from the amygdaloid complex. *Advances in Experimental Medicine and Biology, 203,* 19–33.

Price, J. L. & Amaral, D. G. (1981). An autoradiographic study of the projections of the central nucleus of the monkey amygdala. *Journal of Neuroscience, 1,* 1242–1259.

Rauschecker, J. P., Tian, B. & Hauser, M. D. (1995). Processing of complex sounds in the macaque non-primary auditory cortex. *Science, 268,* 111–114.

Redican, W. K. (1975). Facial expressions in nonhuman primates. In L. A. Rosenblum (Ed), *Primate Behavior: Developments in Field and Laboratory Research* (pp. 104–194). New York: Academic Press.

Reis, D. J. & Oliphant, M. C. (1964). Bradycardia and tachycardia following electrical stimulation of the amygdaloid region in monkey. *Journal of Neurophysiology, 27,* 893–912.

Ridley, M. (1996). *The Origins of Virtue.* London: Penguin Books.

Robinson, B. W. & Mishkin, M. (1966). Ejaculation evoked by stimulation of the preoptic area in monkey. *Physiology and Behaviour, 1,* 269–272.

Robinson, B. W. & Mishkin, M. (1968). Penile erection evoked from forebrain structures in *Macaca mulatta. Archives of Neurololgy, 19,* 184–198.

Rodman, H. R., Scalaidhe, P. O. & Gross, C. G. (1993). Response properties of neurons in temporal cortical visual areas of infant monkeys. *Journal of Neurophysiology, 70,* 1115–1136.

Rolls, E. T. (1984). Neurons in the cortex of the temporal lobe and in the amygdala of the monkey with responses selective for faces. *Human Neurobiology, 3,* 209–222.

Rolls, E. T. (1992). Neurophysiology and functions of the primate amygdala. In J. P. Aggleton (Ed), *The Amygdala: Neurobiological Aspects of Emotion, Memory and Mental Dysfunction* (pp. 143–166). New York: Wiley-Liss.

Rolls, E. T., Burton, M. J. & Mora, F. (1976). Hypothalamic neuronal responses associated with the sight of food. *Brain Research, 111,* 53–66.

Rosvold, H. E., Mirsky, A. F. & Pribram, K. H. (1954). Influence of amygdalectomy on social behaviour in monkeys. *Journal of Comparative and Physiological Psychology, 47,* 173–178.

Russchen, F. T., Amaral, D. G. & Price, J. L. (1985a). The afferent connections of the substantia innominata in the monkey, *Macaca fascicularis. Journal of Comparative Neurology, 242,* 1–27.

Russchen, F. T., Bakst, I, Amaral, D. G. & Price, J. L. (1985b). The amygdalostriatal projections in the monkey. An anterograde tracing study. *Brain Research, 329,* 241–257.

Sapolsky, R. M. (1995). Social subordinance as a marker of hypercortisolism: some unexpected subtleties. *Annals of the New York Academy of Sciences, 771,* 626–639.

Schino, G., Scucchi, S., Maestripieri, D. & Turillazzi, P. G. (1988). Allogrooming as a tension-reduction mechanism: a behavioral approach. *American Journal of Primatology, 16,* 43–50.

Scott, T. R., Karadi, Z., Oomura, Y., Nishino, H., Plata-Salaman, C. R., Lenard, L., Giza, B. K. & Aou, S. (1993). Gustatory neural coding in the amygdala of the alert macaque monkey. *Journal of Neurophysiology, 69,* 1810–1820.

Simerly, R. B. & Swanson, L. W. (1986). The organization of neural inputs to the medial preoptic nucleus of the rat. *Journal of Comparative Neurology, 246,* 312–342.

Slimp, J. C., Hart, B. L. & Goy, R. W. (1978). Heterosexual, autosexual and social behavior of adult male rhesus monkeys with medial preoptic-anterior hypothalamic lesions. *Brain Research, 142,* 105–122.

Small, M. F. (1993). *Female Choices: Sexual Behavior of Female Primates.* New York: Cornell University Press.

Smuts, B. B. (1985). *Sex and Friendship in Baboons.* New York: Aldine de Gruyter.

Spies, H. G., Norman, R. L., Clifton, D. K., Ochsner, A. J., Jensen, J. N. & Phoenix, C. H. (1976). Effects of bilateral amygdaloid lesions on gonadal and pituitary hormones in serum and on sexual behavior in female rhesus monkeys. *Physiology and Behaviour, 17*, 985–992.

Spruijt, B. M., Van Hoff, J. A. R. A. M. & Gispen, W. H. (1992). Ethology and neurobiology of grooming behaviour. *Physiological Reviews, 72*, 825–851.

Steklis, H. D. (1998). Arthur S. Kling: pioneer of the primate social brain. *American Journal of Primatology, 44*, 227–230.

Steklis, H. D. & Kling, A. (1985). Neurobiology of affiliative behavior in nonhuman primates. In M. Reite & T. Field (Eds), *The Psychobiology of Attachment and Separation* (pp. 93–134). Orlando, FL: Academic Press.

Stephan, H., Frahm, H. D. & Baron, G. (1987). Comparison of brain structure volumes in insectivora and primates VII: amygdaloid components. *Journal of Hirnforsch, 5*, 571–584.

Stern, K. & McClintock, M. K. (1998). Regulation of ovulation by human pheromones. *Nature, 392*, 177–179.

Symons, D. (1978). *Play and Aggression: A Study of Rhesus Monkeys.* New York: Columbia University Press.

Thompson, C. I., Bergland, R. M. & Towfighi, J. T. (1977). Social and nonsocial behaviours of adult rhesus monkeys after amygdalectomy in infancy or adulthood. *Journal of Comparative and Physiological Psychology, 91*, 533–548.

Tomasello, M. & Call, J. (1997). *Primate Cognition.* Oxford: Oxford University Press.

Turner, B. H., Gupta, K. C. & Mishkin, M. (1978). The locus and cytoarchitecture of the projection areas of the olfactory bulb in *Macaca mulatta. Journal of Comparative Neurology, 177*, 381–396.

Uno, H., Tarara, R., Else, J. G., Suleman, M. A. & Sapolsky, R. M. (1989). Hippocampal damage associated with prolonged and fatal stress in primates. *Journal of Neuroscience, 9*, 1705–1711.

Ursin, H., Rosvold, H. E. & Vest, B. (1969). Food preference in brain lesioned monkeys. *Physiology and Behaviour, 4*, 609–612.

van Hoof, J. A. R. A. M. (1962). Facial expressions in higher primates. *Symposium of the Zoological Society of London, 8*, 97–125.

Wachsmuth, E., Oram, M. W. & Perrett, D. I. (1994). Recognition of objects and their component parts: responses of single units in the temporal cortex of the macaque. *Cerebral Cortex, 5*, 509–522.

Weiskrantz, L. (1956). Behavioral changes associated with ablations of the amygdaloid complex in monkeys. *Journal of Comparative and Physiological Psychology, 49*, 381–391.

Wickler, W. (1967). Socio-sexual signals and their intra-specific imitation among primates. In D. Morris (Ed), *Primate Ethology* (pp. 89–189). London: Weidenfeld and Nicolson.

Zeller, A. C. (1987). Communication by sight and smell. In B. B. Smuts, D. L. Cheney, R. M. Seyfarth, R. W. Wrangham & T. T. Struhsaker (Eds), *Primate Societies* (pp. 433–439). Chicago: University of Chicago Press.

9

Electrodermal Activity in Cognitive Neuroscience: Neuroanatomical and Neuropsychological Correlates

DANIEL TRANEL

Electrodermal activity (EDA) is arguably the most popular, and in many respects the most informative, psychophysiological measure that has been used to study cognition, particularly emotion. This chapter begins with a review of recent evidence that has shed light on neural substrates of EDA. I then summarize several of our recent investigations which have used EDA to study emotion and other higher order cognitive processes in a variety of lesion-based neuropsychological studies. Our work, and that of a number of other contributors to this book (Bradley, Lang, Öhman; see also Hugdahl, 1995), illustrates how the integration of psychophysiology and cognitive neuroscience has allowed important new insights into emotion and memory.

Central Control of Electrodermal Activity

The neuroanatomical substrates of EDA in humans are not well understood (for reviews, see Boucsein, 1992; Edelberg, 1972; Fowles, 1986; Venables & Christie, 1973, 1980). Most of the direct anatomical evidence comes from work done in cats, which may not generalize well to humans (cf. Wang, 1964). A few studies of EDA in brain-damaged subjects (Heilman et al., 1978; Holloway & Parsons, 1969; Morrow et al., 1981; Oscar-Berman & Gade, 1979; Zoccolotti et al., 1982) led to a general consensus that right hemisphere lesions tended to reduce or abolish electrodermal responses, whereas left hemisphere lesions did not seem to produce a consistent pattern of abnormality. Also, work in humans (Luria, 1973; Luria & Homskaya, 1970; Luria et al., 1964; Raine et al., 1991) and nonhuman primates (Grueninger et al., 1965; Kimble et al., 1965) has indicated that the dorsolateral frontal and orbitofrontal regions may be important in the central control of EDA.

We recently studied the EDA of subjects with focal lesions to various regions of the telencephalon in an effort to gain more detailed knowledge about the neural substrates of EDA (Tranel & H. Damasio, 1994).

Methods

• Subjects

Thirty-six brain-damaged subjects (21 men, 15 women) were selected from the Patient Registry of the University of Iowa's Division of Cognitive Neuroscience, on the basis of the following considerations: (1) All subjects were right handed. (2) Subjects had focal, stable lesions that could be clearly demarcated on the basis of neuroimaging information derived from magnetic resonance imaging (MRI) (or in a few cases, computer tomography), using our standard method (Damasio & Damasio, 1989; H. Damasio & Frank, 1992). Neuroimaging studies were conducted at least 3 months after the onset of brain damage. (3) A variety of different lesion loci in both left and right hemisphere were included, and left and right hemisphere lesions were selected so as to have some comparability in terms of size and location. (4) Subjects had to have normal attention and sufficient comprehension and visual perception to cooperate with the experiments, as determined from standard neuropsychological methods (Tranel, 1996). Twenty normal control subjects (13 men, 7 women), matched to the brain-damaged population on age and education, were also studied.

• Stimuli

There were 2 types of stimuli: (1) physical, 2 basic, unconditioned stimuli, a deep breath and loud noise, (2) psychological, 10 highly charged, affectively laden pictures (nudes, mutilated bodies), prepared as slides.

• Skin Conductance Recording and Procedure

Psychophysiological experiments were conducted at least 6 months after onset of brain injury. Skin conductance was recorded from the thenar and hypothenar eminences of the right and left hands, using standard methods (Tranel & H. Damasio, 1989, 1994).

A 5-min rest period followed attachment of the electrodes. During the final 30 sec of the rest period, the two physical stimuli were administered. The 10 affectively charged pictures were randomly mixed with 30 neutral, nonemotional pictures, and these 40 stimuli were presented one at a time for 2 sec each.

• Data Quantification and Analysis

For each of the 2 physical stimuli and the 10 psychological stimuli, a latency window of 1–4 sec after stimulus onset was specified, and the amplitude of the largest skin conductance response (SCR) having onset within the window was measured (the criterion for smallest scorable SCR was set at 0.01 µS). Then, for each subject and for each hand, two variables were calculated: (1) physical SCR, the average SCR to the 2 physical stimuli, (2) psychological SCR, the average SCR to the 10 highly charged pictures. These averages are referred to as magnitudes because they were based on all available stimulus presentations. It should be noted that nonresponses were fairly common in the defective subjects, and occurred for the majority of the stimulus presentations.

Two approaches to data analysis were used. First, we conducted a case-by-case analysis of the neuroanatomical and psychophysiological findings in each of the 36 brain-damaged subjects. We defined as defective all SCR values that fell below the lower limit of the range of control subject performance and considered each subject in terms of whether the SCRs were normal or not and in terms of the lesion location. For the physical stimuli, the cut-off score was 0.38 µS (control range = 0.39–3.04 µS); for the psychological stimuli, the cut-off score was 0.46 µS (control range = 0.47–1.37 µS). This approach allowed us to form several groups, in which certain lesion loci were associated with consistent defects in skin conductance responding. Second, we conducted statistical comparisons to determine the reliability of the groupings arrived at from the case-by-case approach, using non-parametric techniques (Mann-Whitney U test).

Results

- Group 1: Damage Centered in the
  Ventromedial Prefrontal Region

Ten subjects had damage centered in the ventromedial prefrontal region, including orbitofrontal and lower mesial frontal cortices. In 8 of the 10, the damage was bilateral. Six subjects in this group had defective SCRs to psychological stimuli, but not to physical ones (table 9.1). Detailed inspection of the lesions in the six defective responders indicates that involvement of the anterior cingulate gyrus and the dorsolateral prefrontal region was another common feature. Two subjects with unilateral ventromedial prefrontal lesions produced SCRs that were within the range of normal controls. The psychological SCRs of the eight subjects with bilateral ventromedial frontal damage were compared to those of the controls, and the

TABLE 9.1. Skin Conductance Response Magnitudes (µS) in Brain-Damaged Subjects (defective scores are underlined)

Group[a]	Average (SD)	Range
Ventromedial ($n = 6$)		
Physical	1.08 (0.36)	0.65–1.54
Psychological	0.11 (0.15)	0.00–0.35
Right inferior parietal ($n = 4$)		
Physical	0.34 (0.18)	0.08–0.50
Psychological	0.11 (0.07)	0.03–0.18
Anterior cingulate gyrus ($n = 5$)		
Physical	0.36 (0.57)	0.03–1.37
Psychological	0.11 (0.16)	0.00–0.40

[a]In each group, data are presented for subjects who had defective skin conductance responses for either physical or psychological stimuli or both. Brain-damaged subjects with normal skin conductance responses are not included here.

significant result ($p < .01$) indicates that as a group, the bilateral ventromedial subjects produced smaller psychological SCRs than did the controls.

- Group 2: Right Inferior Parietal Damage

Another lesion location that appeared frequently in subjects who were defective on one or both of the SCR indices was the right inferior parietal region. Four subjects had damage in this region, and all had SCR defects (table 9.1). When damage included both the anterior (supramarginal gyrus) and posterior (angular gyrus) parts of the region, and when the lesion destroyed most of the angular gyrus, the SCR deficiency was more pervasive. The same lesion pattern on the left was not associated consistently with SCR deficiency.

The statistical comparison of the four right parietal subjects to controls was significant ($p < .001$); in contrast, the comparison of the six left parietal subjects to controls was not significant ($p > .05$). A comparison of the four right parietal subjects to the six left parietal subjects was significant ($p < .05$). These outcomes support the conclusion that defective SCR responding was consistently associated with damage to the right inferior parietal region, but not with comparable damage on the left.

- Group 3: Anterior Cingulate Gyrus Damage

The anterior cingulate gyrus was another frequent site of damage associated with defective skin conductance responding. Five subjects with severely impaired SCRs had damage to the anterior cingulate gyrus (table 9.1), and in three, anterior cingulate damage was extensive. Statistical comparison of the group 3 subjects with controls was significant ($p < .025$), supporting the conclusion that the anterior cingulate gyrus is an important neural correlate of skin conductance responding. The results from group 3 suggest that defective SCRs occur with extensive anterior cingulate gyrus damage, especially when the damage involves the anteriormost portion of the region.

Summary

We obtained several consistent findings that point to particular neural regions as important anatomical correlates of electrodermal activity. Figure 9.1 shows the approximate locations of these regions.

The ventromedial frontal region includes the orbitofrontal and lower mesial frontal cortices. Bilateral damage to this region, especially when combined with damage to the anterior cingulate gyrus and dorsolateral prefrontal region, was associated consistently with impaired skin conductance responding. Another intriguing feature of this group is that SCRs tended to be impaired for psychological stimuli, but not for physical ones. The results suggest that the ventromedial frontal region may play an especially important role in the modulation of electrodermal responses to stimuli that derive their "signal value" from psychological, as opposed to physical, properties (A. R. Damasio et al., 1990, 1991).

Extensive damage to the right inferior parietal region region tended to abolish SCRs; more limited damage was associated with defects for psychological, but not for physical, stimuli.

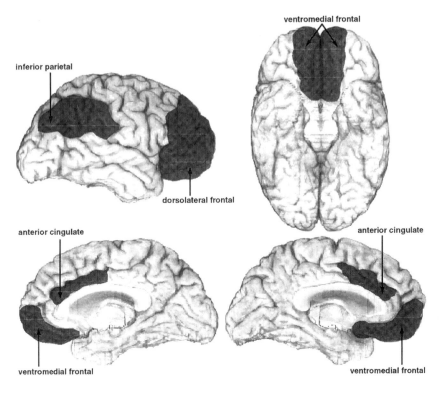

Figure 9.1. Lateral (upper left) and mesial (lower left) views of the right hemisphere; mesial (lower right) and inferrior (upper right) view of the left hemisphere. The regions that we found to be important for electrodermal activity are shaded in gray, and include the right inferior parietal and dorsolateral frontal regions, the anterior cingulate bilaterally, and the ventromedial frontal region. (Adapted with permission from Cambridge University Press [Tranel & H. Damasio, 1994].)

Damage to the anterior cingulate gyrus was associated with impairments in SCRs to both physical and psychological stimuli, particularly when the damage was extensive. This was true for both unilateral (right or left) and bilateral lesions.

Other results from this study hinted at the possibility that the anterior portion of the right dorsolateral prefrontal region may also play a role in the neural modulation of electrodermal responding.

The Role of the Amygdala in Electrodermal Activity

Several lines of investigation have implicated the amygdala as an important modulator of EDA (Bagshaw & Benzies, 1968; Dallakyan et al., 1970; Lang et al., 1964; Mangina & Beuzeron-Mangina, 1996), particularly with regard to emotional behavior (e.g., Aggleton, 1992; Halgren, 1992; LeDoux, 1992; Rolls, 1992). Studies in humans, however, have yielded somewhat mixed results (Davidson et al.,

1992; Lee et al., 1989, 1995; Toone et al., 1979). Our studies of EDA and the amygdala have suggested an important, but not necessary, role for the amygdala in skin conductance responding (Bechara et al., 1995; Tranel & A. R. Damasio, 1993; Tranel & H. Damasio, 1989; Tranel & Hyman, 1990). We have found that bilateral amygdala damage interferes with autonomic fear conditioning, but not with SCRs to basic orienting stimuli (Bechara et al., 1995), a result that is consistent with animal work along these lines (Kim & Fanselow, 1992; Phillips & LeDoux, 1992).

It has been shown that patients with bilateral amygdala damage can generate normal SCRs to visual and auditory stimuli (Kiloh et al., 1974; Lee et al., 1989; Tranel & A. Damasio, 1993; Tranel & H. Damasio, 1989; Tranel & Hyman, 1990). Also, unilateral amygdala lesions, such as those produced in patients with unilateral temporal lobectomies, do not affect electrodermal responses, at least in some paradigms (Toone et al., 1979; see Davidson et al., 1992, for a possible exception). These findings suggest that even if the amygdala is normally involved in autonomic modulation, which appears likely in light of work in nonhuman primates (Bagshaw & Benzies, 1968; Bagshaw et al., 1965) and in humans (Dallakyan et al., 1970; see also Lee et al., 1989), it is not a necessary neuroanatomical substrate of electrodermal responses.

It seems unlikely that the amygdala would turn out to have no consistent role in the higher modulation of EDA, given its key position as an autonomic effector and its salient role in much emotional behavior (LeDoux, 1996). The amygdala is a link in the anatomical route that joins sensory association cortices to preganglionic elements in the sympathetic nervous system, which innervate the dermal eccrine glands responsible for generation of electrodermal activity (Aggleton, 1985; Herzog & Van Hoesen, 1976; Price & Amaral, 1981; Saper et al., 1978; Venables & Christie, 1980). Nonetheless, available evidence suggests that at least under some circumstances, normal EDA is possible in patients with bilateral amygdala lesions (Bechara et al., 1995; Tranel & H. Damasio, 1989; Tranel & Hyman, 1990). Our recent work on this issue is summarized below.

Skin Conductance Responses After Bilateral Amygdala Damage

We measured the skin conductance responses to visual and auditory stimuli in two subjects with bilateral destruction of the amygdala (Tranel & H. Damasio, 1989; Tranel & Hyman, 1990).

Methods

SUBJECTS   One of the subjects was the patient known as Boswell, who was 60 years old at the time of the psychophysiological investigations. Boswell is a right-handed man who sustained extensive bilateral destruction of the limbic system following herpes simplex encephalitis at the age of 48. He has no basic neurological deficits other than anosmia. He has a profound amnesic syndrome that has been extensively characterized elsewhere (Damasio et al., 1989). A detailed anatomical analysis has indicated that Boswell has bilateral mesial temporal lobe damage that includes all of the amygdala and hippocampus. All of the amygdaloid nuclei are destroyed, and, in addition, all of the white matter in which amygdala afferents and efferents would course is destroyed bilaterally (figure 9.2). However, both basal ganglia complexes are intact, and there is no damage to the thalamus or hypothalamus.

The other subject with bilateral amygdala damage is SM-046. She was 23 years old at the time of the psychophysiological investigations. As a result of Urbach-Wiethe disease, SM-046 sustained bilateral mineralization of the amygdala. Extensive neuroanatomical analyses have indicated that amygdala damage is complete but highly circumscribed, with essentially no involvement of other structures (Adolphs et al., 1994, 1995; Bechara et al., 1995; Nahm et al., 1993; Tranel & Hyman, 1990). A positron emission tomography (PET) study has confirmed the dysfunctional status of the amygdala, bilaterally, in SM-046 (Adolphs et al., 1995).

For the baseline condition and experiments 1 and 2 described below, the skin conductance responses of Boswell and SM-046 were compared to seven normal

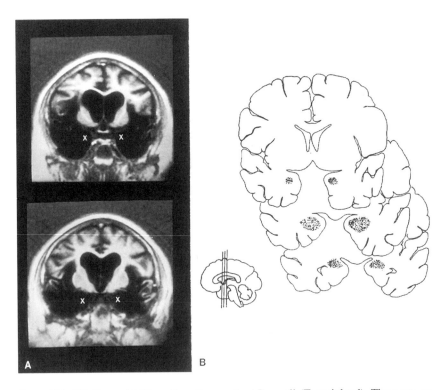

Figure 9.2. (A) Coronal MR sections from patient Boswell (T_1 weighted). The more anterior cut is on top. Note the entire bilateral destruction of the region of the amygdala (x). (B) Line drawings of three brain sections corresponding to the area encompassed by the MR cuts shown in panel 2A. The site of the normal amygdala is marked (dotted areas). (Reprinted with permission from Pergamon Press [Tranel & H. Damasio, 1989].)

control subjects (see Tranel & H. Damasio, 1989). For experiments 3 and 4, other relevant control data were used, as indicated below.

PROCEDURES AND DATA QUANTIFICATION   Skin conductance was recorded during a baseline condition and during four experimental situations, using standard methods (Tranel & H. Damasio, 1989, 1994). For the baseline condition, subjects were instructed to sit quietly and relax and to refrain from movement. There ensued 5 min of continuous recording of skin conductance. The data were analyzed qualitatively.

In experiment 1, skin conductance was recorded for 10 min. A stimulus with known "signal value," the subject's first name (Leiblich, 1969), was presented approximately once per minute during this session. For each stimulus presentation, a latency window of from 1–5 sec after stimulus onset was specified,[1] and the SCR with the largest amplitude that had its onset within this latency window was measured.

In experiment 2, the stimuli were slides depicting various visual items with which the subject had a high degree of familiarity, including faces, places, and personal effects. The slides were presented one at a time, and for each, the subject was asked to provide a brief description. Skin conductance responses were scored as in experiment 1, except that the latency window was extended from 1 to 10 sec to accommodate the increased processing time necessary for the more complex stimuli used in this experiment.

In experiment 3, the subjects were shown 22 pictures (as slides), one at a time in random order. In the set, six pictures were targets (i.e., pictures with high emotional value (such as nudes and mutilation), and 16 were nontargets (i.e., neutral pictures (such as farm scenes). The pictures were presented for 2 sec each, with about 20 sec between stimuli. The SCR data were scored in the same manner as for experiment 1, and then an average SCR was calculated for the target stimuli and for the nontarget stimuli.

Experiment 4 was similar to experiment 3, except that the stimuli were words. The subjects were shown 23 words (on slides), one at a time in random order. In the set, 7 words were targets (i.e., words with high emotional value such as "masturbation"), and 16 were nontargets (i.e., neutral words such as "science"). The procedure and scoring for this experiment were the same as for experiment 3.

• Results

Boswell and SM-046 generated normal skin conductance records during the baseline recording condition (figure 9.3). The records depict several characteristic features: a downward drifting baseline, several nonspecific fluctuations of normal amplitude (Mefferd et al., 1969), and typical recovery limbs (Venables & Christie, 1980).

In experiment 1, Boswell and SM-046 produced normal SCRs to their first names (table 9.2). Both subjects produced SCRs to every stimulus presentation. When viewing familiar visual stimuli in experiment 2, Boswell and SM-046 produced SCRs that were similar to those generated by normal control subjects (table 9.3). For experiment 3, the skin conductance results from the two brain-damaged

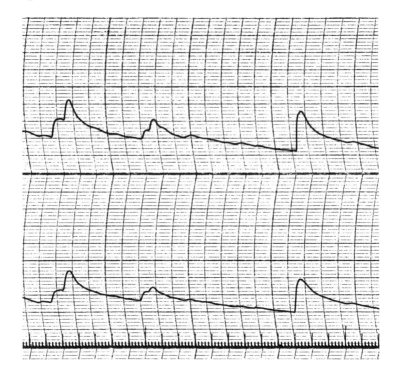

Figure 9.3. Samples of polygraph records from Boswell (left panel) and
SM-046 (right panel), obtained during baseline condition. Top tracing =
right hand; bottom tracing = left hand.

subjects were compared with data from 20 control subjects studied with a similar
paradigm (Schrandt et al., 1989; Tranel & H. Damasio, 1994). Boswell and SM-
046 generated large-amplitude SCRs to the target pictures (table 9.3), demonstrating the same target–nontarget electrodermal discrimination as was evident in the
controls.

Control data for experiment 4 were derived from previous studies using a
similar paradigm (Schrandt et al., 1989; Trigoboff, 1979). Comparing Boswell and
SM-046 to the controls, it is evident that both subjects were normal and produced
large-amplitude responses to the target, but not the nontarget, words (table 9.3).

• Comment

The results of these studies show that two subjects with complete bilateral destruction of the amygdala were capable of generating normal phasic and tonic patterns
of skin conductance, at least under the conditions in our studies. This suggests that
the amygdala is not a necessary component of the neural substrate of these responses and that there are alternate neural units and pathways that link sensory
cortices to autonomic effectors. Such alternate routes might involve direct visual
and auditory projections to autonomic stations such as the hypothalamus, perhaps

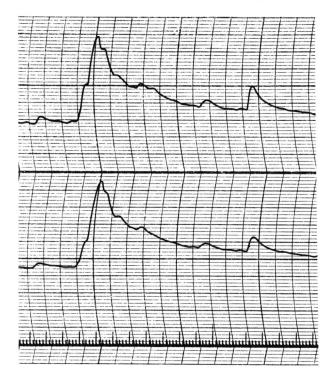

Figure 9.3. *Continued.*

by way of the thalamus, as was postulated by Luria and Homskaya (1970); or there could be indirect connections using prefrontal cortices.

The Role of the Amygdala in Conditioning and Declarative Knowledge

Studies in animals have indicated that the amygdala is important for emotional conditioning and, in particular, for the acquisition of conditioned responses to aversive or fear-producing stimuli (Davis, 1992; LeDoux, 1994, 1996). The role of the amygdala in the acquisition of declarative knowledge, however, is less clear. Some

TABLE 9.2. Skin Conductance Responses to First Name Stimulus

Subject	Average amplitude (µS) (SD)	% of stimuli responded to	Range
Boswell	0.39 (0.20)	100	0.10–0.70
SM-046	0.36 (0.36)	100	0.04–1.08
Controls ($n = 7$)	0.40 (0.16)	100	0.05–1.67

TABLE 9.3. Skin Conductance Responses (μS) to Various Stimuli

	Boswell	SM-046	Controls
Familiar visual stimuli	0.15	0.19	0.16
Emotional pictures			
Target	0.59	0.52	0.77
Nontarget	0.03	0.01	0.08
Emotional words			
Target	0.43	0.60	0.54
Nontarget	0.01	0.02	0.04

work in nonhuman primates has indicated that the amygdala is critical for normal learning (e.g., Mishkin, 1978; Murray, 1990), but other studies have suggested that the amygdala may not play a crucial role, or at least that its role is not independent from subjacent cortex (e.g., Mishkin & Murray, 1994; Murray & Gaffan, 1994; Zola-Morgan et al., 1989). Results in the few human cases available are also inconclusive (Lee et al., 1988, 1995; Nahm et al., 1993; Tranel & Hyman, 1990). Several recent studies have shed additional light on this issue, indicating, for example, that the amygdala has a role in learning information that has significant emotional valence (Bechara et al., 1995; Cahill et al., 1995, 1996; Davis, 1992; LaBar et al., 1995; LeDoux et al., 1990; Markowitsch et al., 1994).

We recently conducted a study in which we contrasted the learning of declarative knowledge and the acquisition of conditioned responses in subjects with focal bilateral damage to the amygdala, the hippocampus, or both (Bechara et al., 1995).

• Methods

SUBJECTS   Three subjects with distinct brain lesions were studied. The first was SM-046, whose neuropsychological and neuroanatomical profiles were referenced above. She has focal bilateral amygdala lesions, but no damage to the hippocampus. In most respects, she has normal anterograde memory, and her other cognitive abilities are largely intact. The second subject was WC-1606. He is a 47-year-old, right-handed man who, 4 years before the conditioning studies described below, sustained bilateral damage to the hippocampus (specifically, CA1 neurons) as a consequence of severe ischemia-anoxia. His amygdalae, however, are intact bilaterally. WC-1606 has anterograde amnesia for both verbal and nonverbal material, in keeping with his lesion, but his basic intellectual abilities are normal, and he has normal attention, speech, language, and perception. The third subject was RH-1951, a 42-year-old, right-handed man who suffered herpes simplex encephalitis at the age of 28. He sustained extensive bilateral damage to both amygdala and hippocampus as a consequence. RH-1951 has severe anterograde amnesia for verbal and nonverbal material and significant retrograde amnesia for nonverbal information. However, he has normal intellect, speech, language, perception, and attentional capacities.

In sum, these three subjects provide key anatomical contrasts: bilateral amygdala lesions without hippocampal involvement (SM-046), bilateral hippocampal lesions without amygdala involvement (WC-1606), and bilateral amgydala and hippocampal damage (RH-1951). We also studied four normal control subjects, who were of comparable age and education as the brain-damaged subjects.

PROCEDURES   Two conditioning experiments were conducted, one visual–auditory and one auditory–auditory. In the visual–auditory experiment, four monochrome slides (green, blue, yellow, blue) were the conditioned stimuli; in the auditory–auditory experiment, four computer-generated tones (of different frequencies) were the conditioned stimuli (CS). In both experiments, a sudden loud noise (boat horn) served as the unconditioned stimulus (UCS). Each conditioning experiment was performed three times in SM-046 and twice in WC-1606 and RH-1951. The dependent measure was the SCR, which was recorded using standard methods (Tranel & H. Damasio, 1994).

The conditioning protocol was composed of three phases. (The protocol was identical for the visual–auditory and auditory–auditory experiments, with the exception that the CS were color slides in the former and tones in the latter.) The first was a habituation phase, where the subject was presented the CS (slides or tones) repeatedly, in random order, until the stimuli no longer elicited orienting SCRs from the subject (defined as SCRs <0.05 μS).[2] In the conditioning phase, the four color slides (or tones) were presented in irregular order, one at a time. There were 26 presentations, of the following nature: 6 were blue slides followed by the UCS (horn); 6 were blue slides without the UCS; 14 were red, green, or yellow slides, none of which was ever followed by the UCS. Thus, the blue slide was the paired CS. (This arrangement was the same for the tones; i.e., one tone served as the paired CS, and the other three were nonpaired CS.) In the extinction phase, the paired CS was presented repeatedly until it no longer elicited SCRs from the subject.

The stimuli in the conditioning experiments were presented for 2 sec each, with 10–20 sec between stimuli. Subjects were requested to sit quietly, pay attention to each stimulus, and refrain from moving or talking. Five minutes after completion of the conditioning experiment, the subject was administered a questionnaire to determine the subject's acquisition of declarative knowledge of the experiment (i.e., whether the subject has learned factual information about the procedures). Questions were asked about the nature of the CS and about the nature of the CS–UCS relationship. There were four questions, and a total of four points was possible if all questions were answered correctly.

- Results

AUTONOMIC CONDITIONING   As shown by the SCR data (figure 9.4), the four control subjects (averaged in the figure) produced large-amplitude SCRs to the paired CS in both the visual–auditory (black) and auditory–auditory (gray) experiments. These SCRs were significantly larger than the SCRs produced to the unpaired CS. In contrast, subject SM-046 failed to produce discriminatory SCRs to the paired CS, and this absence of autonomic conditioning obtained for both the visual and auditory experiments. Subject WC-1606 did acquire conditioned autonomic responses, as evidenced by his large-amplitude SCRs to the paired CS and

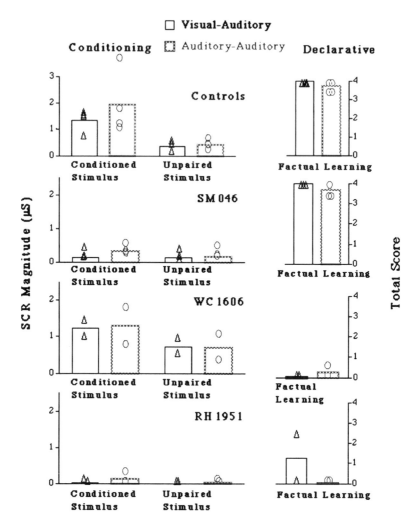

Figure 9.4. Magnitudes of skin conductance responses (SCRs) and total factual learning scores from the visual–auditory (black) and auditory–auditory (gray) conditioning experiments, from normal controls ($n = 4$), patient SM-046 (three trials), patient WC-1606 (two trials), and patient RH-1951 (two trials). For the controls, each triangle or circle denotes data from one participant; for the patients, the symbols denote one trial. The bars represent the mean SCR magnitudes for the conditioned stimulus (left column) and unpaired stimulus (middle column), and factual learning scores (right column). (Reprinted with permission from The American Association for the Advancement of Science [Bechara et al., 1995].)

the relatively smaller SCRs to the unpaired CS. In RH-1951, there was no indication of autonomic conditioning; like SM-046, he failed to generate discriminatory SCRs to the paired CS in either the visual or auditory experiment.

The conditioning defects of SM-046 and RH-1951 cannot be explained by a basic impairment of skin conductance responding. The capacity of SM-046 to generate SCRs under certain conditions has been amply demonstrated (e.g., Tranel & Hyman, 1990; see above). RH-1951 is also capable of generating SCRs under certain conditions. In fact, all of the subjects in the current study had normal SCRs to the UCS (figure 9.5), and as far as SM-046 and RH-1951 are concerned, this result replicates and extends our previous work indicating that the amygdala is not a necessary component of the neural substrate of SCRs to basic orienting stimuli.

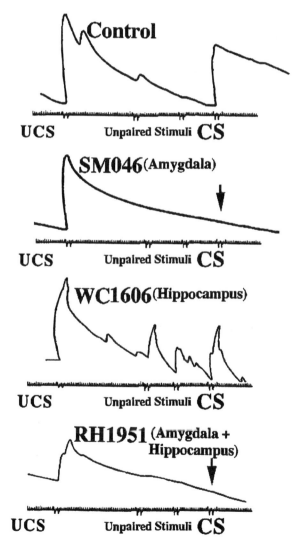

Figure 9.5. Samples of the polygraph records from a control subject and patients SM-046, WC-1606, and RH-1951, showing skin conductance response (SCR) recording from the left hand during the visual–auditory conditioning experiment. In all subjects, the unconditioned stimulus (US; boat horn) elicited a large-amplitude SCR (about 2.0 μS). A large-amplitude SCR (about 1.8 μS) to the conditioned stimulus (CS) is evident in the control and in WC-1606, but is entirely absent in SM-046 and RH-1951 (arrows). (Reprinted with permission from The American Association for the Advancement of Science [Bechara et al., 1995].)

DECLARATIVE LEARNING   The four control subjects attained nearly perfect scores on the factual learning questionnaire (figure 9.4). SM-046's performance was similar; she had excellent recall of the experiments, and answered accurately nearly all of the factual questions. In contrast, WC-1606 was severely impaired in his factual learning. RH-1951 was also severely impaired on the factual learning questionnaire.

• Comment

This study demonstrates a clear double dissociation, neuroanatomically and neuropsychologically. Bilateral amygdala damage (SM-046) precluded the acquisition of conditioned SCRs, but spared the ability to acquire declarative knowledge about the same situation. Bilateral hippocampal damage (WC-1606) had the opposite effect—autonomic conditioning was normal, but declarative learning was impaired. The outcome in RH-1951 is consistent with both effects, insofar as his bilateral amygdala and hippocampal lesions impaired autonomic conditioning and declarative learning.

We have interpreted these results as indicating that the human amygdala is critical for emotional conditioning and for the coupling of exteroceptive sensory information with interoceptive information concerning somatic states (Bechara et al., 1995; A. R. Damasio, 1994; Nahm et al., 1993; also see Furmark et al., 1997). The hippocampus, on the other hand, has a well-known role in learning declarative knowledge, but appears to be unnecessary for the acquisition of conditioned autonomic responses. This double dissociation between emotional and declarative learning offers insights on how different forms of knowledge come together in the human brain.

Electrodermal Activity and Somatic Marker Activation

It is well established that stimuli with strong affective valence produce large-amplitude SCRs in normal subjects (e.g., Bradley et al., 1992). Some brain-damaged subjects, particularly those with bilateral ventromedial prefrontal lesions, fail to generate SCRs to such stimuli (A. R. Damasio et al., 1990, 1991). We have interpreted this outcome as reflecting an impairment of somatic marker activation (see Damasio, 1994, 1996) (i.e., defective activation of bodily states that would normally accompany the perception of emotionally arousing stimuli). The somatic marker framework has been elaborated in detail elsewhere (see A. R. Damasio, 1996), but in brief, the theory posits that "marker" signals arising in bioregulatory processes (including those expressed in emotions and feelings) are key influences guiding responses to various stimuli and situations. The markers can be overt or covert, but in either case, they are critical for normal reasoning and decision-making (see Bechara et al., 1997; Öhman & Soares, 1997).

Covert Face Recognition and the
Somatic Marker Hypothesis

We posited that somatic marker activation (indexed by EDA) should occur in relationship to perceiving highly familiar faces, given that such stimuli have a high degree of personal relevance, familiarity, and overall "signal value" (Tranel & A. R. Damasio, 1985, 1988; Tranel et al., 1985). Following this rationale, we predicted that subjects with ventromedial prefrontal lesions would show defective electrodermal responses to familiar faces, as they do for other emotionally laden visual stimuli. This prediction has received empirical support (Tranel et al., 1995). Specifically, we found that four subjects with bilateral ventromedial prefrontal lesions failed to generate SCRs to pictures of familiar faces derived from either the retrograde or anterograde compartments. This outcome contrasted with that obtained in five prosopagnosic patients, where there was clear electrodermal discrimination of familiar faces in the retrograde and even in the anterograde compartments (figure 9.6). Given that the ventromedial subjects have normal overt recognition of the

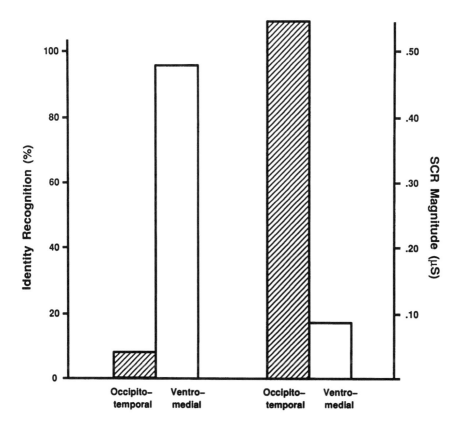

Figure 9.6. The double dissociation between overt and covert face recognition. Average identity recognition scores (left ordinate) and skin conductance response (SCR) magnitudes (right ordinate) for four ventromedial prefrontal and five occipitotemporal subjects, averaged across both retrograde and the anterograde stimulus sets, are depicted. For overt recognition, indexed by identity recognition, the occipitotemporal subjects were severely impaired, whereas the ventromedial subjects were normal. The reverse outcome obtained for the covert index (SCRs). (Reprinted with permission from MIT Press [Tranel et al., 1995].)

faces, while the prosopagnosics do not, the results constitute a double dissociation between overt and covert face recognition. This experiment indicates that the neural systems that process the somatic-based valence (emotional significance) of stimuli are separate from and parallel to the neural systems that process the factual information associated with those same stimuli.

Defective Somatic Marker Activation to Auditory Stimuli

A question so far unanswered is whether the somatic marker impairment would occur in relationship to sensory modalities other than the visual. For example, would a subject with bilateral ventromedial prefrontal lesions fail to generate SCRs to target stimuli presented in the auditory modality, in a manner analogous to the impairment evident for visual stimuli? We explored this question in the experiment described below.

- Subject

The subject was EVR-318, who has been extensively described in previous publications (Eslinger & Damasio, 1985; A. R. Damasio et al., 1990; Tranel, 1994). Briefly, he developed profoundly impaired social conduct and decision making following bilateral ventromedial prefrontal lesions. He is otherwise quite intact and has superior intellectual abilities, memory, language, and perception. His severely defective autonomic responding to target visual stimuli has been extensivley documented (A. R. Damasio et al., 1990, 1991; Tranel, 1994). The impairment covers face stimuli in addition to emotionally laden pictures (Tranel et al., 1995) and covers verbal as well as nonverbal stimuli presented visually (Tranel & A. R. Damasio, 1990).

- Auditory Experiments

We designed a set of experiments that provided a direct parallel in the auditory modality to the visual experiments we conducted previously. Both nonverbal and verbal conditions were investigated. For the nonverbal condition, we selected a variety of target nonverbal sounds (e.g., siren, screaming, sex sounds), and various nontarget sounds (birds chirping, water running). For the verbal condition, we presented target words auditorily (e.g., "masturbation," "penis"), mixed with nontarget words (e.g., "philosophy," "frog"). In both conditions, there were 8 targets and 32 nontargets. For both conditions, the stimuli were presented one at a time, in random order, and skin conductance was recorded and quantified according to standard methods (Tranel & H. Damasio, 1994).

The results are summarized in table 9.4. EVR-318 failed to generate discriminatory SCRs to the target sounds or to the target words (there was a hint of responsiveness to the words, but the difference between the target and nontarget averages was not statistically significant). This outcome is parallel to his performance with visual stimuli, where he showed a similiar impairment in responding autonomically to emotionally laden nonverbal and verbal stimuli.

TABLE 9.4. Mean Skin Conductance Responses (μS) in Subject
EVR-318 as a Function of Modality and Stimulus Type

Stimulus type	Auditory modality (SD)		Visual modality (SD)	
	Target	Nontarget	Target	Nontarget
Nonverbal	0.00	0.00	0.00	0.00
	(0.00)	(0.01)	(0.01)	(0.01)
Verbal (words)	0.11	0.01	0.01	0.02
	(0.23)	(0.02)	(0.01)	(0.01)

• Comment

The results from these experiments extend our previous work showing that impaired somatic state activation occurs as a multimodal defect in a patient with
ventromedial prefrontal damage. The multimodal nature of the impairment is consistent with predictions derived from the theoretical framework alluded to earlier
(A. R. Damasio, 1996). Specifically, given that the key neural region supporting
the activation of somatic markers is the ventromedial prefrontal region, and given
the amodal nature of this cortex, we would expect a multimodal impairment in
autonomic responses to emotional stimuli, given a lesion in the ventromedial prefrontal region. The current results provide empirical support for this prediction.

Other Cognitive and Neural Correlates of Electrodermal Activity

Material-specific Autonomic Responses

Based on investigation of a large number of normal control subjects, we have
observed that, in general, it is easier to obtain large SCRs with nonverbal stimuli
as compared to verbal ones. Words, even when they are rated as extremely "shock-
ing," usually produce lower amplitude SCRs than pictures of comparable semantic
content, and this is true of target words that are considered vulgar (e.g., "piss") as
well as those that are acceptable (e.g., "urine").

In patient EVR-318, the loss of autonomic responses to emotionally charged
stimuli occurred for both nonverbal and verbal stimuli. This raises an interesting
question: Is it possible to find material-specific SCR impairments (i.e., impairments
that develop for nonverbal material but not verbal, or vice versa)? Recently, we
had an opportunity to explore this question in preliminary fashion in a patient with
a right prefrontal lesion. In collaboration with Julie Wilson, several experiments
were designed and conducted that showed that the patient had normal autonomic
responses to verbal material, but impaired responses to nonverbal material (J. Wilson, unpublished data). This effect covered both passive responses to emotionally
charged stimuli and fear conditioning. This is the clearest material-specific effect
of this nature that we have come across.

• Subject

The subject was SB-2046, who was 22 years old at the time of the studies reported here. He is left-handed (but with standard cerebral organization, i.e., left-hemisphere speech dominance) and has a high school education. At age 3 months, he underwent partial resection of a right frontal malignant astrocytoma, which produced a right "developmental" prefrontal lesion (cf. Tranel et al., 1994).

• Neuropsychological Status

SB-2046 has a lifelong history of behavioral problems directly related to his lesion, including poor judgment and decision making, impulsiveness, impaired social conduct, and deficient personal hygiene. However, he has average to above average abilities in most cognitive domains. His intellectual abilities are average (WAIS-R verbal IQ = 94; performance IQ = 104), as are his academic achievement skills, and his memory, speech and language, and perceptual abilities are all commensurate with his intelligence. He performed defectively on some, but not all, tests of "executive functions"; for example, his performances on the Wisconsin Card Sorting Test and the Trail-making Test were normal, but he was defective on the Tower of Hanoi Test.

SM-2046 was severely impaired on a decision-making task which requires consideration of immediate and future reward and punishment (Bechara et al., 1994). His performance on this task was guided nearly entirely by immediate prospects, with disregard for long-term consequences of his decisions, even though this strategy is deleterious over the long run. The behavioral abnormality was accompanied by deficient anticipatory psychophysiological responses to response options that had been associated with immediate reward but eventual punishment. This pattern is reminiscent of that which we have reported previously in patients with prefrontal lesions (Bechara et al., 1995, 1996, 1997).

• Neuroanatomical Status and
  Psychophysiological Studies

An MRI, analyzed using standard methods (H. Damasio, 1995), showed a large area of abnormality involving much of the dorsolateral right prefrontal region. The lesion extends from the frontal pole to the anterior sector of the premotor region, although most of the premotor and all of the motor territories are spared (the patient has no neurological defects). The mesial portion of the left prefrontal lobe extends across the midline into the area of damage on the right.

The SCRs of SB-2046 were investigated in a series of special experiments, using our standard equipment and procedures.

• Responses to Emotionally Charged Stimuli

Two experiments were conducted to contrast the subject's nonverbal and verbal SCRs. In both, there were 40 stimuli, presented in random order one at a time for 2 sec each. The nonverbal experiment used pictures as stimuli, and the verbal experiment used words. There were 8 target stimuli (pictures of nudes and mutilation; taboo words) and 32 nontarget stimuli (neutral pictures or words) in each experiment.

The results are shown in Figure 9.7. A 2×2 ANOVA, with the factors of material type (pictures vs. words) and emotional type (target vs. nontarget), revealed significant main effects of both material type ($F_{1,31} = 4.53$, $p < .05$) and emotional type ($F_{1,31} = 8.91$, $p < .01$). The material-by-emotion interaction did not reach statistical significance ($p = .14$). Post-hoc Neuman-Keuls followup tests showed that for the pictures, SCRs to the target and nontarget stimuli were not different; however, for the words, SCRs to the target stimuli were significantly larger that those to the nontarget stimuli ($p < .05$). Thus, the results demonstate an interesting effect whereby the subject evidences clear discriminatory SCRs to target stimuli presented as words, but not to those presented as pictures. This dissociation is made all the more striking when one considers that the typical direction of nonverbal/verbal differences is opposite.

- Conditioning Experiments

We designed two experiments to contrast the subject's ability to acquire conditioned autonomic responses as a function of the nonverbal versus verbal nature of

RESPONSES TO EMOTIONAL STIMULI

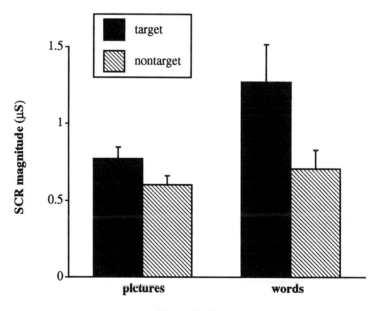

Figure 9.7. Skin conductance response (SCR) magnitudes in patient SB-2046 as a function of material type (pictures vs. words) and emotional type (target vs. nontarget). SB-2046 produced large-amplitude, discriminatory SCRs to the target (emotional) words, but not to the target pictures.

the stimulus material. Both experiments followed the format described elsewhere (Bechara et al., 1995). Briefly, there are three main phases in the procedure: habituation, conditioning, and extinction. Here, a second extinction period was added, which was the same as the first extinction period.

In one experiment, the conditioned stimuli were monochrome color slides. The blue slide served as the paired CS, conditioned with a loud noise. In the other experiment, we used neutral words as the conditioned stimuli (e.g., "frog," "fence," "barn," "land"). These words were derived from a list that has been studied extensively in previous psychophysiological experiments (Trigoboff, 1979). One of the words served as the paired CS. Otherwise, the two experiments were identical.

The results are shown in figures 9.8 and 9.9. The graphs show a striking contrast as a function of the type of stimulus material. For the colors experiment, SB-2046 failed to acquire any conditioned responses, as shown by the flat curve in figure 9.8. In contrast, his conditioning in the words experiment was entirely normal, as shown by the large-amplitude SCRs to the paired CS in the other curve of figure 9.8. These results are summarized in figure 9.9, which contrasts SCRs to the paired CS versus unpaired CS as a function of material type (colors vs. words). A two-way ANOVA revealed a significant interaction between CS type and material type ($F_{1,18} = 4.66$, $p < .05$). This outcome reflects the fact that for the colors, SB-2046 failed to acquire significant SCRs to the paired CS, but for the words, he did acquire and generate large-amplitude SCRs to the paired CS.

- Comment

These experiments demonstrate a clear and striking dissociation in the SCRs of SB-2046, which vary as a function of whether the stimulus material is nonverbal or verbal. Effects of this type have rarely been described previously; the closest examples are given by Bauer (1982), Tranel et al. (1992), and Verfaellie et al. (1991). The intriguing outcome in SB-2046 confirms that such a dissociation is possible, although interpretation of this effect in neuroanatomical terms awaits replication and extension of the current results.

Electrodermal Discrimination in Auditory Agnosia

Electrodermal activity has been used as an index of nonconscious "recognition" in patients who have lost the ability to recognize stimuli at the conscious level (Bauer, 1984; Bauer & Verfaellie, 1988; Tranel & A. R. Damasio, 1985, 1988). For instance, we found that patients with prosopagnosia, who were unable to recognize familiar faces based on measures such as self-report and multiple choice, nonetheless showed discriminatory SCRs to familiar faces (Tranel & Damasio, 1985, 1988). Recently, we had an opportunity to apply this paradigm to the investigation of a patient with a special form of auditory agnosia.

- Subject

The brain-damaged subject was X-1012, a 51-year-old, right-handed man who was a professional opera singer and professor of voice. He suffered a right temporoparietal hemorrhagic infarction a few years before the psychophysiological studies

FEAR CONDITIONING

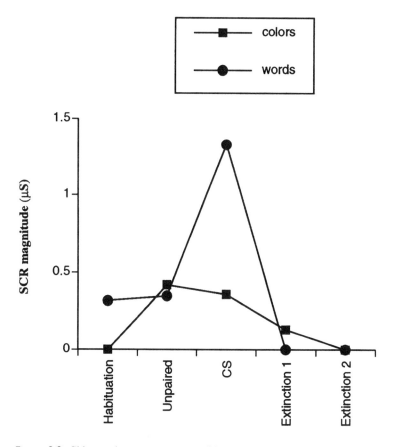

Figure 9.8. Skin conductance response (SCR) magnitudes in patient SB-2046 during fear conditioning experiments using colors or words. The patient produced normal large-amplitude SCRs to the condidtioned stimulus (CS) (middle phase on *x*-axis) in the word experiment, but not in the color experiment.

described below, which produced a mild left hemiparesis and hemihypoesthesia. Subsequently, he complained that he could no longer interpret music correctly. He had trouble recognizing pieces and performers and in judging the quality of his own voice.

Standard neuropsychological examination indicated that X-1012 had several mild nonverbal cognitive defects, in the setting of generally above-average abilities. He had superior verbal intellect (WAIS-R Verbal IQ = 125) and average nonverbal intellect (Performance IQ = 93). Mild defects in nonverbal memory were evident, but verbal memory was intact. Speech and language were normal. He complained of mild aprosodia, but this was not evident on formal assessment. Visuoperceptual

FEAR CONDITIONING

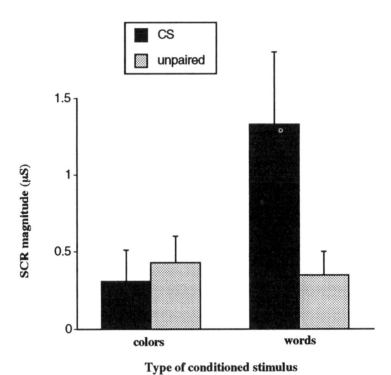

Figure 9.9. Bar graph summarizing skin conductance response (SCR) magnitudes in patient SB-2046 during fear conditioning experiments using colors (left bars) or words (right bars). He produced large-amplitude SCRs to the conditioned stimulus (CS) in the word experiment, but not in the color experiment. The graph reflects the material-specific nature of autonomic conditioning in SB-2046.

functions, attention, and executive functions were normal. In dichotic listening to word pairs, he demonstrated a complete left ear extinction.

Neuroanatomical analysis showed a posterior right-sided lesion, involving the insular cortex and white matter of the superior temporal lobe, undercutting the primary auditory cortex in Heschl's gyrus.

• Auditory Recognition and Naming

X-1012 was tested with an extensive battery of recognition and naming tests (H. Damasio et al., 1996; Tranel et al., 1997). The auditory part of the battery consists of 198 sounds drawn from various conceptual categories (e.g., animals, tools, musical instruments, vehicles). X-1012 performed defectively in the recognition component of this test (score = 143/198; >3 SDs below age-matched controls). He had particular trouble recognizing musical instruments. However, he did not have any difficulty naming the sounds that he recognized correctly.

The patient was administered a series of special experiments designed to test his ability to recognize familiar musical pieces. We selected a variety of opera segments, which were well known to X-1012 before the onset of his brain injury. Half of the segments were instrumental, and half included a singer. We tested his ability to recognize the pieces and the singers. Compared to a control subject matched for musical knowledge of the specialized type required for this task, X-1012 was severely impaired in the recognition of both instrumental and singing operatic pieces. He was even unable to recognize his own singing voice.

In short, X-1012 demonstrated a marked recognition impairment for auditory stimuli, which covered both environmental sounds and unique musical information, a profile which conforms to the designation of auditory agnosia. In this context, we conducted psychophysiological experiments aimed at determining whether the subject could demonstrate covert discrimination of the familiar music segments that he could not recognize consciously.

Psychophysiological Studies

SUBJECTS AND PROCEDURES   Three subjects were studied: X-1012; an "expert" control matched to X-1012 on musical knowledge (a voice professor at the University of Iowa); and a "naive" control who had no special experience with or knowledge of opera music (a Montana rancher). Two experiments were conducted. In each, there were 6 target stimuli (i.e., music segments with which the two expert subjects, X-1012 and the expert control, were highly familiar) and 14 nontarget stimuli (i.e., music segments selected to match the targets in overall sound characteristics, but with which the subjects had no familiarity). In the first experiment (music without voice), the music segments were instrumental; in the second (music with voice), the segments involved singing. Each segment was 8–10 sec in duration. The music segments were presented one at a time, in random order, while the subject sat quietly and listened. Skin conductance was recorded. Using the method we developed for face recognition (see Tranel & A. R. Damasio, 1988), we calculated a target SCR and nontarget SCR for each subject and for each experiment, and these constituted the dependent measures. Mann-Whitney U tests were used to compare target versus nontarget SCRs.

RESULTS   The results are presented in figures 9.10 and 9.11. The naive control, as expected, did not produce discriminatory SCRs to the target stimuli in either experiment. The expert control, in contrast, produced discriminatory large-amplitude SCRs to the target segments in both the music without voice ($p < .001$) and music with voice ($p < .05$) experiments. Thus, the target stimuli had the intended effect of serving as significant "signal stimuli" to someone expert in this music domain.

In X-1012, there were also clear discriminatory SCRs to the target stimuli. This outcome obtained for both the music without voice ($p < .05$) and music with voice ($p < .01$) experiments. Given that the target music segments in these experiments were unrecognized by the subject at the overt level, this outcome reflects a form of nonconscious recognition.

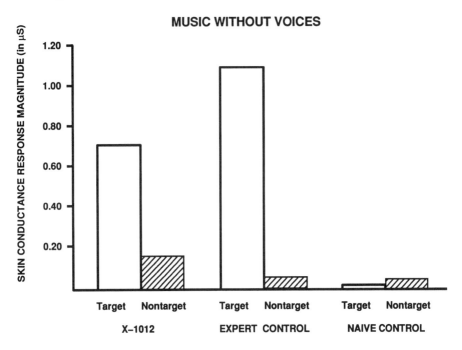

Figure 9.10. Skin conductance response (SCR) magnitudes to segments of music (without voices) in patient X-1012, expert control, and naive control. Both X-1012 and the expert control showed discriminatory, large-amplitude SCRs to the target (familiar) music segments; the naive control did not. In X-1012, who does not recognize the segments at the overt level, this electrodermal discrimination reflects "nonconscious" recognition.

• Comment

The results of these experiments indicate a clear form of nonconscious recognition in the auditory domain, which extends the phenomenon we and others have described previously in regard to visual stimuli (Bauer, 1982, 1984; Bauer & Verfaellie, 1988; Tranel & A. R. Damasio, 1985, 1988; Verfaellie et al., 1991). The results suggest that as in the case of the visual modality, it is possible for sensory association cortices to activate autonomic effectors in response to a signal stimulus, even if that stimulus is not processed in such a manner as to permit conscious recognition. As in prosopagnosia, autonomic responses (SCRs) provided a sensitive index of nonconscious recognition of familiar stimuli.

Concluding Comments

To recapitulate our work concerning the neural substrates of electrodermal activity, it is worth considering some other functional correlates of the regions identified in our studies.

    The suggestion that the anterior cingulate gyrus and adjacent supplementary

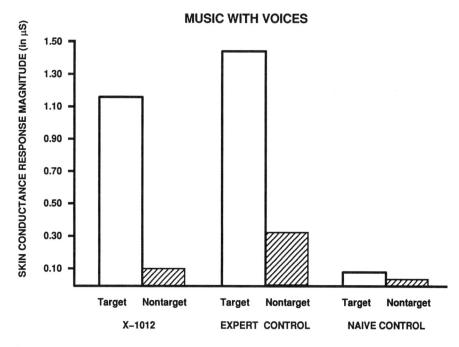

Figure 9.11. Skin conductance response (SCR) magnitudes to segments of music (with voices) in patient X-1012, expert control, and naive control. Both X-1012 and the expert control showed discriminatory, large-amplitude SCRs to the target music segments; the naive control did not. Because X-1012 does not recognize the segments at the overt level, this electrodermal discrimination reflects a form of "nonconscious" recognition.

motor area (SMA) and mesial prefrontal region may be involved in EDA is consistent with other known functional correlates and neuroanatomical relationships of this region. In an early study by Amyes and Nielsen (1955), a large series of patients with bilateral damage to the anterior cingulate gyrus was described, and the authors emphasized the development of the syndrome of "akinetic mutism" (in which patients lose their drive to move and communicate, despite intact motor systems for locomotion and speech), as well as severe autonomic disturbance. Akinetic mutism and other disturbances of basic drive and motivational capacities have also been associated with damage to the SMA (A. R. Damasio & Van Hoesen, 1983). Damasio and Van Hoesen (1983, p. 100), in fact, noted that such patients have a profound disturbance of behavior which "prevented both the normal *expression* and normal *experience* of affect." Akinetic mutism has been related to lesions of either the left or right SMA, and it is interesting that we found SCR defects with either left- or right-sided lesions in this region.

Another important aspect of our results is that the SCR impairment obtained for both basic physical and conditioned psychological stimuli, supporting the notion that the anterior cingulate gyrus is involved in EDA at a fairly basic level. This interpretation is consistent with other work showing disturbances in electrodermal habituation following bilateral cingulotomy (Cohen et al., 1994), and it is also consistent with results from functional neuroimaging studies (Fredrikson et al., 1998). From a neuroanatomical perspective, the cingulate region is considered part of the "limbic lobe," a collection of structures linked intimately to basic drive states involved in fight-or-flight, reproduction, and feeding and drinking behaviors (e.g., Van Hoesen et al., 1993; Vogt et al., 1992). Also, neurophysiological studies have shown that neurons in the cingulate gyrus respond to stimulus properties of significance and novelty (Gabriel et al., 1986). Positron emission tomography studies have demonstrated that the anterior cingulate gyrus is involved in the cortical representation of pain (Talbot et al., 1991), and in representing subjective emotional responses (Lane et al., 1997). The anterior cingulate gyrus has been shown to be important in the central regulation of other autonomic functions, such as blood pressure (Burns & Wyss, 1985).

Concerning the ventromedial frontal region, the current results are intriguing in light of work showing a special role for this region in the modulation of social conduct. In particular, this region is seen as a key area in which the social significance of external stimuli is encoded and decoded by linking those stimuli to various internal body states, especially those connected to reward and punishment (A. R. Damasio, 1994, 1996). Other theoretical formulations have also emphasized the importance of this region in linking the motivational significance of external stimuli to internal somatic states (e.g., Nauta, 1971; Rolls, 1990). Our findings suggest that the ventromedial frontal region plays a role in linking EDA to stimulus properties such as social significance and emotional value, but that it is not involved in EDA related to more basic unconditioned stimuli.

Our findings, together with those of Zoccolotti et al. (1982) and Vallar et al. (1991), indicate that the inferior parietal region on the right is important for EDA connected to stimulus properties such as emotional significance; however, this region does not appear critical for EDA connected to basic unconditioned stimuli. This outcome is consistent with the theoretical formulation of A. R. Damasio (1994), which posits that the right parietal region records information regarding "somatic memories," e.g., various visceral and motor parameters that would have been co-related as composing particular bodily states associated with particular emotions (see also Cechetto & Saper, 1990; Lang et al., 1990).

The role of the amygdala in EDA is intriguing. Although various lines of evidence suggest that the amygdala plays a major role in the central mediation of autonomic responses, several studies have not indicated a clear, or at least a necessary, role for the amygdala in the central control of EDA. In any event, the amygdala has a salient role in much emotional behavior (Adolphs et al., 1994, 1995; Cahill et al., 1996; Calder et al., 1996; Morris et al., 1996; Scott et al., 1997; Young et al., 1995, 1996). In particular, it appears to be involved in the appraisal of danger and the emotion of fear, as suggested by LeDoux (1996), A. R. Damasio (1994), and others. Consistent with this, we have recently shown that SM-046, the subject with focal bilateral amygdala lesions, is impaired in judging untrustworthiness and unapproachability in the faces of strangers (Adolphs et al., 1998). In fact, there is growing and remarkably consistent evidence that the amygdala's role in emotional processing is largely focused on aversive, negatively valenced emotions (see Tranel, 1997, for review), although this issue is clearly in need of further investigation.

Notes

1. This latency window, used in our earlier work, is one second longer than that used in the Tranel and H. Damasio (1994) study summarized in the previous section; however, we have no evidence that this difference would produce any appreciable effect on the results. In most of our recent work, we have used a 1- to 4-sec latency window.

2. The 0.05 μS threshold is more stringent than that used in some of our previous work (e.g., 0.01 μS in the Tranel & H. Damasio, 1994, study described earlier). We have found that the more lenient criterion of 0.01 μS is problematic for conditioning studies because it tends to introduce considerable noise into the operationalization of habituation. For purposes of defining defective SCR responding per se, though, as was the purpose in the Tranel and H. Damasio (1994) study, the 0.01 μS criterion was actually considered more strict.

References

Adolphs, R., Tranel, D. & Damasio, A. R. (1998). The human amygdala in social judgment. *Nature, 393*, 470–474.

Adolphs, R., Tranel, D., Damasio, H. & Damasio, A. R. (1994). Impaired recognition of emotion in facial expressions following bilateral damage to the human amygdala. *Nature, 372*, 669–672.

Adolphs, R., Tranel, D., Damasio, H. & Damasio, A. R. (1995). Fear and the human amygdala. *Journal of Neuroscience, 15*, 5879–5891.

Aggleton, J. P. (1985). A description of intra-amygdaloid connections in old world monkey. *Experimental Brain Research, 57*, 390–399.

Aggleton, J. P. (1992). The functional effects of amygdala lesions in humans: a comparison with findings from monkey. In J. P. Aggleton (Ed), *The Amygdala* (pp. 485–503). New York: Wiley-Liss.

Amyes, E. W. & Nielsen, J. M. (1955). Clinicopathologic study of vascular lesions of the anterior cingulate region. *Bulletin of the Los Angeles Neurological Societies, 20*, 112–130.

Bagshaw, M. H. & Benzies, S. (1968). Multiple measures of the orienting reaction and their dissociation after amygdalectomy in monkeys. *Experimental Neurology, 20*, 175–187.

Bagshaw, M. H., Kimble, D. P. & Pribram, K. H. (1965). The GSR of monkeys during orienting and habituation and after ablation of the amygdala, hippocampus and inferotemporal cortex. *Neuropsychologia, 3*, 111–119.

Bauer, R. M. (1982). Visual hypoemotionality as a symptom of visual-limbic disconnection in man. *Archives of Neurology, 39*, 702–708.

Bauer, R. M. (1984). Autonomic recognition of names and faces in prosopagnosia: a neuropsychological application of the Guilty Knowledge Test. *Neuropsychologia, 22*, 457–469.

Bauer, R. M. & Verfaellie, M. (1988). Electrodermal discrimination of familiar but not unfamiliar faces in prosopagnosia. *Brain and Cognition, 8*, 240–252.

Bechara, A., Damasio, A. R., Damasio, H. & Anderson, S. W. (1994). Insensitivity to future consequences following damage to human prefrontal cortex. *Cognition, 50*, 7–12.

Bechara, A., Damasio, H., Tranel, D. & Damasio, A. R. (1997). Deciding advantageously before knowing the advantageous strategy. *Science, 275*, 1293–1295.

Bechara, A., Tranel, D., Damasio, H., Adolphs, R., Rockland, C. & Damasio, A. R. (1995). Double dissociation of conditioning and declarative knowledge relative to the amygdala and hippocampus in humans. *Science, 269*, 1115–1118.

Bechara, A., Tranel, D., Damasio, H. & Damasio, A. R. (1996). Failure to respond autonomically to anticipated future outcomes following damage to prefrontal cortex. *Cerebral Cortex, 6*, 215–225.

Boucsein, W. (1992). *Electrodermal Activity*. New York: Plenum Press.

Bradley, M. M., Greenwald, M. K., Petry, M. C. & Lang, P. J. (1992). Remembering pictures: pleasure and arousal in memory. *Journal of Experimental Psychology: Learning, Memory, and Cognition, 18*, 379–390.

Burns, S. M. & Wyss, M. (1985). The involvement of the anterior cingulate cortex in blood pressure control. *Brain Research, 340*, 71–77.

Cahill, L., Babinsky, R., Markowitsch, H. J. & McGaugh, J. L. (1995). The amygdala and emotional memory. *Nature, 377*, 295–296.

Cahill, L., Haier, R. J., Fallon, J., Akire, M. T., Tang, C., Keator, D., Wu, J. & McGaugh, J. L. (1996). Amygdala activity at encoding correlated with long-term, free recall of emotional information. *Proceedings of the National Academy of Sciences, USA, 93*, 8016–8021.

Calder, A. J., Young, A. W., Rowland, D., Perrett, D. I., Hodges, J. R. & Etcoff, N. L. (1996). Facial emotion recognition after bilateral amygdala damage: differentially severe impairment of fear. *Cognitive Neuropsychology, 13*, 699–745.

Cechetto, D. F. & Saper, C. B. (1990). Role of the cerebral cortex in autonomic function. In A. D. Loewy & K. M. Spyer (Eds), *Central Regulation of Autonomic Functions* (pp. 208–223). New York: Oxford University Press.

Cohen, R. A., Kaplan, R. F., Meadows, M. E. & Wilkinson, H. (1994). Habituation and sensitization of the orienting response following bilateral anterior cingulotomy. *Neuropsychologia, 32*, 609–617.

Dallakyan, I. G., Latash, L. P. & Popova, L. T. (1970). Certain regular relationships between the expressivity of the galvanic skin response and changes of the EEG in local lesions of the limbic (rhinencephalic) structures of the human brain. *Doklady akademii nauk (SSSR), 190*, 991–999.

Damasio, A. R. (1994). *Descartes' Error: Emotion, Reason, and the Human Brain*. New York: Grosset/Putnam.

Damasio, A. R. (1996). The somatic marker hypothesis and the possible functions of the prefrontal cortex. *Philosophical Transactions of the Royal Society of London* B, *351*, 1413–1420.

Damasio, A. R., Tranel, D. & Damasio, H. (1989). Amnesia caused by herpes simplex encephalitis, infarctions in basal forebrain, Alzheimer's disease, and anoxia. In F. Boller & J. Grafman (Eds), *Handbook of Neuropsychology*, vol. 3 (pp. 149–166). Amsterdam: Elsevier.

Damasio, A. R., Tranel, D. & Damasio, H. (1990). Individuals with sociopathic behavior caused by frontal damage fail to respond autonomically to social stimuli. *Behavioural Brain Research, 41*, 81–94.

Damasio, A. R., Tranel, D. & Damasio, H. (1991). Somatic markers and the guidance of behavior: theory and preliminary testing. In H. S. Levin, H. M. Eisenberg & A. L. Benton (Eds), *Frontal Lobe Function and Dysfunction* (pp. 217–229). New York: Oxford University Press.

Damasio, A. R. & Van Hoesen, G. W. (1983). Emotional disturbances associated with focal lesions of the limbic frontal lobe. In K. Heilman & P. Satz (Eds), *Neuropsychology of Human Emotion* (pp. 85–110). New York: Guilford Press.

Damasio, H. (1995). *Human Brain Anatomy in Computerized Images*. New York: Oxford University Press.

Damasio, H. & Damasio, A. R. (1989). *Lesion Analysis in Neuropsychology*. New York: Oxford University Press.

Damasio, H. & Frank, R. (1992). Three-dimensional *in vivo* mapping of brain lesions in humans. *Archives of Neurology, 49*, 137–143.

Damasio, H., Grabowski, T. J., Tranel, D., Hichwa, R. D. & Damasio, A. R. (1996). A neural basis for lexical retrieval. *Nature, 380*, 499–505.

Davidson, R. A., Fedio, P., Smith, B. D., Aureille, E. & Martin, A. (1992). Lateralized mediation of arousal and habituation: differential bilateral electrodermal activity in unilateral temporal lobectomy patients. *Neuropsychologia, 30*, 1053–1063.

Davis, M. (1992). The role of the amygdala in conditioned fear. In J. P. Aggleton (Ed), *The Amygdala* (pp. 255–306). New York: Wiley-Liss.

Edelberg, R. (1972). The electrodermal system. In N. S. Greenfield & R. A. Sternbach (Eds), *Handbook of Psychophysiology* (pp. 367–418). New York: Holt, Rinehart and Winston.

Eslinger, P. J. & Damasio, A. R. (1985). Severe disturbance of higher cognition after bilateral frontal lobe ablation: patient EVR. *Neurology, 35*, 1731–1741.

Fowles, D. C. (1986). The eccrine system and electrodermal activity. In M. G. H. Coles, E. Donchin & S. W. Porges (Eds), *Psychophysiology: Systems, Processes and Applications* (pp. 51–96). New York: Guilford Press.

Fredrikson, M., Furmark, T., Olsson, M. T., Fischer, H., Andersson, J. & Langstrom, B. (1998). Functional neuroanatomical correlates of electrodermal activity: a positron emission tomography study. *Psychophysiology, 35*, 179–185.

Furmark, T., Fischer, H., Wik, G., Larsson, M. & Fredrikson, M. (1997). The amygdala and individual differences in human fear conditioning. *NeuroReport, 8*, 3957–3960.

Gabriel, M., Sparenborg, S. P. & Stolar, N. (1986). An executive function of the hippocampus: pathway selection for thalamic neuronal significance code. In R. L. Isaacson & K. H. Pribram (Eds), *The Hippocampus*; Vol. 4 (pp. 1–39). New York: Plenum Press.

Grueninger, W. E., Kimble, D. P., Grueninger, J. & Levine, S. (1965). GSR and corticosteroid response in monkeys with frontal ablations. *Neuropsychologia, 3*, 205–216.

Halgren, E. (1992). Emotional neurophysiology of the amygdala within the context of human cognition. In J. P. Aggleton (Ed), *The Amygdala* (pp. 191–228). New York: Wiley-Liss.

Heilman, K. M., Schwartz, H. D. & Watson, R. T. (1978). Hypoarousal in patients with the neglect syndrome and emotional indifference. *Neurology, 28*, 229–232.

Herzog, A. G. & Van Hoesen, G. W. (1976). Temporal neocortical afferent connections to the amygdala in the rhesus monkey. *Brain Research, 115*, 57–69.

Holloway, F. A. & Parsons, O. A. (1969). Unilateral brain damage and bilateral skin conductance levels in humans. *Psychophysiology, 6*, 138–148.

Hugdahl, K. (1995). *Psychophysiology: The Mind-Body Perspective*. Cambridge, MA: Harvard University Press.

Kiloh, L. G., Gye, R. S., Rushworth, R. G., Bell, D. S. & White, R. T. (1974). Stereotactic amygdaloidotomy for aggressive behaviour. *Journal of Neurology, Neurosurgery, and Psychiatry, 37*, 437–444.

Kim, J. J. & Fanselow, M. S. (1992). Modality-specific retrograde amnesia of fear. *Science, 256*, 675–677.

Kimble, D. P., Bagshaw, M. H. & Pribram, K. H. (1965). The GSR of monkeys during orienting and habituation after selective partial ablations of the cingulate and frontal cortex. *Neuropsychologia, 3*, 121–128.

LaBar, K. S., LeDoux, J. E., Spencer, D. D. & Phelps, E. A. (1995). Impaired fear conditioning following unilateral temporal lobectomy in humans. *Journal of Neuroscience, 15*, 6846–6855.

Lane, R. D., Fink, G. R., Chau, P. M. & Dolan, R. J. (1997). Neural activation during selective attention to subjective emotional responses. *NeuroReport, 8*, 3969–3972.

Lang, H., Tuovinen, T. & Valeala, P. (1964). Amygdaloid afterdischarge and galvanic skin response. *Electroencephalography and Clinical Neurophysiology, 16,* 366–374.

Lang, P. J., Bradley, M. M. & Cuthbert, B. N. (1990). Emotion, attention, and the startle reflex. *Psychological Review, 97,* 377–395.

LeDoux, J. E. (1992). Emotion and the amygdala. In J. P. Aggleton (Ed), *The Amygdala* (pp. 339–351). New York: Wiley-Liss.

LeDoux, J. E. (1994). Emotion, memory and the brain. *Scientific American, 270,* 32–39.

LeDoux, J. E. (1996). *The Emotional Brain.* New York: Simon & Schuster.

LeDoux, J. E., Cicchetti, P., Xagoraris, A., & Romanski, L. M. (1990). The lateral amygdaloid nucleus: sensory interface of the amygdala in fear conditioning. *Journal of Neuroscience, 10,* 1062–1069.

Lee, G. P., Arena, J. G., Meador, K. J., Smith, J. R., Loring, D. W. & Flanigin, H. F. (1989). Changes in autonomic responsiveness following bilateral amygdalotomy in humans. *Neuropsychiatry, Neuropsychology, and Behavioral Neurology, 1,* 119–130.

Lee, G. P., Meador, K. J., Smith, J. R., Loring, D. W. & Flanigin, H. F. (1988). Preserved crossmodal association following bilateral amygdalotomy in man. *International Journal of Neuroscience, 40,* 47–55.

Lee, G. P., Reed, M. F., Meador, K. J., Smith, J. R. & Loring, D. W. (1995). Is the amygdala crucial for cross-modal association in humans? *Neuropsychology, 9,* 236–245.

Lieblich, I. (1969). Manipulation of contrast between differential GSR responses through the use of ordered tasks of information detection. *Psychophysiology, 6,* 70–77.

Luria, A. R. (1973). The frontal lobes and the regulation of behavior. In K. H. Pribram & A. R. Luria (Eds), *Psychophysiology of the Frontal Lobes* (pp. 3–26). New York: Academic Press.

Luria, A. R. & Homskaya, E. D. (1970). Frontal lobes and the regulation of arousal processes. In D. I. Mostofsky (Ed), *Attention: Contemporary Theory and Analysis* (pp. 303–330). New York: Appleton-Century-Crofts.

Luria, A. R., Pribram, K. H. & Homskaya, E. D. (1964). An experimental analysis of the behavioral disturbance produced by a left frontal arachnoidal endothelioma (meningioma). *Neuropsychologia, 2,* 257–280.

Mangina, C. A. & Beuzeron-Mangina, J. H. (1996). Direct electrical stimulation of specific human brain structures and bilateral electrodermal activity. *International Journal of Psychophysiology, 22,* 1–8.

Markowitsch, H. J., Calabrese, P., Wurker, M., Durwen, H. F., Kessler, J., Babinsky, R., Brechtelsbauer, D., Heuser, L. & Gehlen, W. (1994). The amygdala's contribution to memory—a study on two patients with Urbach-Wiethe disease. *NeuroReport, 5,* 1349–1352.

Mefferd, R. B., Sadler, T. G. & Wieland, B. A. (1969). Physiological responses to mild heteromodal stimulation. *Psychophysiology, 6,* 186–196.

Mishkin, M. (1978). Memory in monkeys severely impaired by combined but not separate removal of amygdala and hippocampus. *Nature, 273,* 297–298.

Mishkin, M. & Murray, E. A. (1994). Stimulus recognition. *Current Opinion in Neurobiology, 4,* 200–206.

Morris, J. S., Frith, C. D., Perrett, D. I., Rowland, D., Young, A. W., Calder, A. J. & Dolan, R. J. (1996). A differential neural response in the human amygdala to fearful and happy facial expressions. *Nature, 383,* 812–815.

Morrow, L., Vrtunski, P. B., Kim, Y. & Boller, F. (1981). Arousal responses to emotional stimuli and laterality of lesion. *Neuropsychologia, 19,* 65–71.

Murray, E. A. (1990). Representational memory in nonhuman primates. In R. P. Kesner & D. S. Olton (Eds), *Neurobiology of Comparative Cognition* (pp 127–155). Hillsdale, NJ: Lawrence Erlbaum Associates.

Murray, E. A. & Gaffan, D. (1994). Removal of the amygdala plus subjacent cortex disrupts the retention of both intramodal and crossmodal associative memories in monkeys. *Behavioral Neuroscience, 108*, 494–500.

Nahm, F. K. D., Tranel, D., Damasio, H. & Damasio, A. R. (1993). Cross-modal associations and the human amygdala. *Neuropsychologia, 31*, 727–744.

Nauta, W. J. H. (1971). The problem of the frontal lobe: a reinterpretation. *Journal of Psychiatric Research, 8*, 167–187.

Öhman, A. & Soares, J. J. F. (1998). Emotional conditioning to masked stimuli: expectancies for aversive outcomes following non-recognized fear-relevant stimuli. *Journal of Experimental Psychology: General, 127*, 69–82.

Oscar-Berman, M. & Gade, A. (1979). Electrodermal measures of arousal in humans with cortical or subcortical brain damage. In H. Kimmel, E. van Olst & J. Orlebeke (Eds), *The Orienting Reflex in Humans* (pp. 665–676). Hillsdale, NJ: Lawrence Erlbaum Associates.

Phillips, R. G. & LeDoux, J. E. (1992). Differential contribution of the amygdala and hippocampus to cued and contextual fear conditioning. *Behavioral Neuroscience, 106*, 274–285.

Price, J. L. & Amaral, D. G. (1981). An autoradiographic study of the projections of the central nucleus of the monkey amygdala. *Journal of Neuroscience, 1*, 1242–1259.

Raine, A., Reynolds, G. P. & Sheard, C. (1991). Neuroanatomical correlates of skin conductance orienting in normal humans: a magnetic resonance imaging study. *Psychophysiology, 28*, 548–558.

Rolls, E. T. (1990). A theory of emotion, and its application to understanding the neural basis of emotion. *Cognition and Emotion, 4*, 161–190.

Rolls, E. T. (1992). Neurophysiology and functions of the primate amygdala. In J. P. Aggleton (Ed), *The Amygdala* (pp. 143–165). New York: Wiley-Liss.

Saper, C. B., Swanson, L. W. & Cowan, W. M. (1978). The efferent connections of the anterior hypothalamic area of the rat, cat and monkey. *Journal of Comparative Neurology, 182*, 575–599.

Schrandt, N. J., Tranel, D. & Damasio, H. (1989). The effect of focal cerebral lesions on skin conductance responses to "signal" stimuli. *Neurology, 39* (suppl. 1), 223.

Scott, S. K., Young, A. W., Calder, A. J., Hellawell, D. J., Aggleton, J. P. & Johnson, M. (1997). Impaired auditory recognition of fear and anger following bilateral amygdala lesions. *Nature, 385*, 254–257.

Talbot, J. D., Marrett, S., Evans, A. C., Meyer, E., Bushnell, M. C. & Duncan, G. H. (1991). Multiple representations of pain in human cerebral cortex. *Science, 251*, 1355–1358.

Toone, B. K., Cooke, E. & Lader, M. H. (1979). The effect of temporal lobe surgery on electrodermal activity: implications for an organic hypothesis in the aetiology of schizophrenia. *Psychological Medicine, 9*, 281–285.

Tranel, D. (1994). "Acquired sociopathy": the development of sociopathic behavior following focal brain damage. In D. C. Fowles, P. Sutker & S. H. Goodman (Eds), *Progress in Experimental Personality and Psychopathology Research*, vol. 17 (pp. 285–311). New York: Springer.

Tranel, D. (1996). The Iowa-Benton school of neuropsychological assessment. In I. Grant & K. M. Adams (Eds), *Neuropsychological Assessment of Neuropsychiatric Disorders*, 2nd ed. (pp. 81–101). New York: Oxford University Press.

Tranel, D. (1997). Emotional processing and the human amygdala. *Trends in Cognitive Sciences, 1*, 46–47.

Tranel, D., Anderson, S. W. & Benton, A. L. (1994). Development of the concept of "executive function" and its relationship to the frontal lobes. In F. Boller & J. Grafman (Eds), *Handbook of Neuropsychology*, vol. 9 (pp. 125–148). Amsterdam: Elsevier.

Tranel, D. & Damasio, A. R. (1985). Knowledge without awareness: An autonomic index of facial recognition by prosopagnosics. *Science, 228*, 1453–1454.

Tranel, D. & Damasio, A. R. (1988). Nonconscious face recognition in patients with face agnosia. *Behavioural Brain Research, 30*, 235–249.

Tranel, D. & Damasio, A. R. (1990). Defective somatic state activation following ventromedial frontal damage in humans. *Society for Neuroscience Abstracts, 16*, 27.

Tranel, D. & Damasio, A. R. (1993). The covert learning of affective valence does not require structures in hippocampal system or amygdala. *Journal of Cognitive Neuroscience, 5*, 79–88.

Tranel, D. & Damasio, H. (1989). Intact electrodermal skin conductance responses after bilateral amygdala damage. *Neuropsychologia, 27*, 381–390.

Tranel, D. & Damasio, H. (1994). Neuroanatomical correlates of electrodermal skin conductance responses. *Psychophysiology, 31*, 427–438.

Tranel, D., Damasio, H. & Damasio, A. R. (1992). Impaired feeling and autonomic activation for visual but not verbal stimuli following damage to right inferotemporal cortex. *Society for Neuroscience, 18*, 387.

Tranel, D., Damasio, H. & Damasio, A. R. (1995). Double dissociation between overt and covert face recognition. *Journal of Cognitive Neuroscience, 7*, 425–432.

Tranel, D., Damasio, H. & Damasio, A. R. (1997). A neural basis for the retrieval of conceptual knowledge. *Neuropsychologia, 35*, 1319–1327.

Tranel, D., Fowles, D. C. & Damasio, A. R. (1985). Electrodermal discrimination of familiar and unfamiliar faces: a methodology. *Psychophysiology, 22*, 403–408.

Tranel, D. & Hyman, B. T. (1990). Neuropsychological correlates of bilateral amygdala damage. *Archives of Neurology, 47*, 349–355.

Trigoboff, D. (1979). The effects of stimulus-word variables on electrodermal responding to words (Ph.D. thesis). Iowa City: University of Iowa.

Vallar, G., Bottini, G., Sterzi, R., Passerini, D. & Rusconi, M. L. (1991). Hemianesthesia, sensory neglect and defective access to conscious experience. *Neurology, 41*, 650–652.

Van Hoesen, G. W., Morecraft, R. J., Vogt, B. A. (1993). Connections of the monkey cingulate cortex. In B. A. Vogt & M. Gabriel (Eds), *The Neurobiology of Cingulate Cortex and Limbic Thalamus* (pp. 249–284). Boston: Birkhauser.

Venables, P. H. & Christie, M. J. (1973). Mechanisms and techniques. In W. F. Prokasy & D. C. Raskin (Eds), *Electrodermal Activity in Psychological Research* (pp. 1–123). New York: Academic Press.

Venables, P. H. & Christie, M. J. (1980). Electrodermal activity. In I. Martin & P. H. Venables (Eds), *Techniques in Psychophysiology* (pp. 3–67). New York: Wiley.

Verfaellie, M., Bauer, R. M. & Bowers, D. (1991). Autonomic and behavioral evidence of "implicit" memory in amnesia. *Brain and Cognition, 15*, 10–25.

Vogt, B. A., Finch, D. M. & Olson, C. R. (1992). Functional heterogeneity in cingulate cortex: the anterior executive and posterior evaluative regions. *Cerebral Cortex, 2*, 435–443.

Wang, G. H. (1964). *The Neural Control of Sweating.* Madison: University of Wisconsin Press.

Young, A. W., Aggleton, J. P., Hellawell, D. J., Johnson, M., Broks, P. & Hanley, J. R. (1995). Face processing impairments after amygdalotomy. *Brain, 118*, 15–24.

Young, A. W., Hellawell, D. J., van de Wal, C. & Johnson, M. (1996). Facial expression processing after amygdalotomy. *Neuropsychologia, 34*, 31–39.

Zoccolotti, P., Scabini, D. & Violani, C. (1982). Electrodermal responses in patients with unilateral brain damage. *Journal of Clinical Neuropsychology, 4*, 143–150.

Zola-Morgan, S., Squire, L. R., Amaral, D. G. & Suzuki, W. A. (1989). Lesions of perirhinal and parahippocampal cortex that spare the amygdala and hippocampal formation produce severe memory impairment. *Journal of Neuroscience, 9*, 4355–4370.

10

The Functional Anatomy of Innate and Acquired Fear: Perspectives from Neuroimaging

RAYMOND J. DOLAN AND JOHN S. MORRIS

Understanding the neurobiology of emotion has historically depended on studies carried out in animals or the careful documentation of patients with brain lesions that result in disorders of emotional behavior. These approaches are ultimately limited. Animal models, although informative, cannot provide adequate descriptions of phenomena as complex as human emotion whose differentiation depends on conscious experience. Likewise, inferences from patients with discrete brain insults are constrained either by the fact that lesions are seldom restricted to a single anatomical locus or their functional effects are unlikely to be bounded by anatomical locus. Physiological measures of in vivo human brain function, derived from positron emission tomography (PET) and functional magnetic resonance (fMRI), are now standard tools in cognitive neuroscience. Their ability to study the intact human brain gives them special appeal in cognitive science in general but even more so when applied in studies of human emotion where the database remains inadequate.

Neurobiological perspectives on psychological phenomena such as emotion are necessarily embedded in theoretical assumptions about how we think the brain works. Two dominant themes inform current concepts of higher brain function. One perspective, functional segregation, emphasizes that processing in discrete modules may be anatomically localized. A contrasting view is that higher brain functions are emergent properties of interactions between functionally specialized brain regions. Evidence of functional segregation within the human brain is now overwhelming. The most striking examples are derived from the impact of lesions on components of visual perception and memory function (Scoville & Milner, 1957; Zeki et al., 1991; Zihl et al., 1983). In contrast, the integrationist model derives its appeal from the likelihood that the function of even highly segregated brain regions are coordinated during normal perception and action (Roelfsema et al., 1997). A number of mechanistic accounts of how integration is realized have provided the focus for the elaboration of connectionist theories of cortical integration (Eckhorn et al., 1988; Gray et al., 1989; Singer, 1990). Indeed, recent empirical data showing parietal and striate cortex interactions, with zero time lag, during complex sensorimotor behavior point to likely mechanisms of functional integration (Roelfsema et al., 1997). Although conceptually dichotomous functional segregation and integration are amenable to a unifying framework (Tononi et al., 1994).

Perspectives on functional segregation and integration of brain function are important in providing an interpretive framework to inform data derived from functional imaging studies of emotion. In this chapter we use both perspectives in evaluating empirical data derived from functional neuroimaging experiments of innate and acquired fear responses.

Functional Imaging Approaches to the Study of Emotion

Processing Fear in the Human Face

It is generally accepted that facial emotional expressions represent innate and automatic behavior patterns determined by evolutionary selection (Darwin, 1965). Ethnological studies have identified a number of categorically distinct patterns of facial emotional expression (happiness, anger, sadness, fear, surprise, disgust) that are recognized across culture and race (Ekman, 1992). Developmental studies indicate an innate predisposition to mimic and discriminate between emotional facial expressions (Field et al., 1982; Meltzoff & Moore, 1977). Psychophysiological studies of facial mimicry in adults suggest that processing of emotional expressions is obligatory and largely independent on voluntary or conscious mediation (Ohman & Dimberg, 1978). Psychologically, facial expressions are a medium through which internal emotional states and intentions become available as external signals. In this light the face attains crucial importance in social cognition (Darwin, 1872; Ekman, 1982). Consequently, the study of face processing in the context of emotional expression represents a powerful means of accessing brain mechanisms of emotion.

How the human brain discriminates among behaviorally relevant facial expressions is unknown. One hypothesis, supported by neurobiological evidence, is that the amygdala (and related subcortical structures) has a critical neuromodulatory role in selecting among salient sensory stimuli (Friston et al., 1994; LeDoux et al., 1990; Rolls, 1994). In this respect, the most robust evidence relates to the role of the amygdala in fear processing. The amygdala's connectional architecture enables it to modulate sensory, motor, and autonomic processing that characterizes an integrated response to salient biologically stimuli. The amygdala receives direct visual projections from the thalamus, as well as highly processed sensory information from the anterior temporal lobe (Amaral & Price, 1984; Jones & Burton, 1976). It sends reciprocal projections to the same regions, as well as to earlier sensory, including visual, processing areas. Other outputs of the amygdala include projections to brain regions such as orbitofrontal cortex, anterior cingulate, ventral striatum, nucleus basalis, and brainstem nuclei, which are all implicated in emotional or evaluative functions (Amaral et al., 1992; Jones & Powell, 1970; Russchen et al., 1985b).

Animal studies implicate the amygdala in fear conditioning (LeDoux, 1993) and face perception (Rolls, 1992). Direct evidence for a similar role in humans is limited to neuropsychological studies of subjects with rare, selective amygdala lesions (Adolphs et al., 1994; Calder et al., 1996) and electrophysiological studies of epileptic patients (Halgren et al., 1978). Lesions of the amygdala can lead to selective deficits in the recognition of fearful facial expressions (Adolphs et al., 1994; Calder et al., 1996) and impaired fear conditioning (Bechara et al., 1995; LaBar et al., 1995), and direct electrical stimulation evokes fearful emotional responses (Halgren et al., 1978).

Using functional imaging (PET), we sought direct evidence for a differential neural response in the human amygdala when subjects process fearful as opposed to happy facial expressions. Our experimental approach involved measuring regional cerebral blood flow (rCBF) as an index of neural activity while subjects viewed gray-scale images of faces taken from a standard picture set of facial affect (Ekman & Friesen, 1976). These faces depicted either categories of happy or fearful expressions. Additionally, for each category of emotional expression (and for each individual face), a range of six levels of emotional intensity was produced by a computer graphical manipulation (see figure 10.1; Perrett et al., 1994).

Separate scans were acquired in each subject for each category and each intensity level of facial expression using in a 2 × 6 (category × intensity) factorial experimental design. In a single scan, 10 individual faces (from the same intensity rating of an individual emotional category) were presented for 3 sec, on a computer screen, followed by a 2-sec interval when the screen was blank. The task requirement was that, for each face, subjects make a gender classification (i.e., indicate whether the face was male or female) by pressing a left or right response button. It should be noted that no explicit recognition or categorization of emotional expression was required during the scans. Postscan debriefing confirmed that subjects were not aware that the implicit emotional variable was crucial to the experimental design.

The first experimental contrast of interest is the neural response engendered by the presentation of fearful faces versus happy faces. This categorical comparison is predicated on a perspective of functional segregation, with the experimental question being which brain region differentiates between processing of fearful or

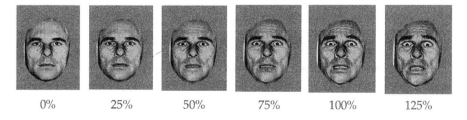

| 0% | 25% | 50% | 75% | 100% | 125% |

Figure 10.1. Graded intensities of fearful expression. Computer morphing procedures were used to shift the shape and pigmentation of a neutral prototype (0%) toward the fear prototype (100%). The 125% fear expression was created by shifting the shape of the fear prototype 25% away from neutral (i.e., increasing by 25% any differences from neutral).

happy expressions. The a priori hypothesis was that the amygdala activates during processing of fearful expressions. The prediction was confirmed by a robust activation, lateralized to the left amygdala and left periamygdaloid cortex specific to the fear condition (see Plate 1; Morris et al., 1996). There was no activation in the right amygdala, even when the significance threshold was lowered. Other areas of activation specific to the fear condition, but not predicted, involved the left cerebellum, the left cingulate gyrus, and right superior frontal gyrus). A categorical contrast of happy with fearful expressions, on the other hand, was associated with activations in the right medial temporal gyrus, right putamen, left superior parietal lobe, and the left calcarine sulcus. The critical finding in these analyses is activation of the amygdala in response to fearful faces, a finding that has subsequently been reported by others (Breiter et al., 1996).

Do Neural Responses Reflect the Intensity of Emotional Facial Expression?

The differential response in the amygdala to fearful expressions predicts that this response would be sensitive to an intensity variation. By weighting the different experimental conditions, statistical contrasts can be used to highlight brain regions sensitive to changes in emotional intensity as a function of emotional category (fearful and happy). For example, brain areas that reflected increasing fearful intensity of expression included the left pulvinar, left anterior insula, and the right anterior cingulate cortex. The left amygdala was also identified in this contrast, although at a lower level of significance. Strikingly, the majority of these regions have been previously implicated in emotional processing. In contrast, the brain regions that showed an increased neural response to increasing intensity of happy expression were different and included the bilateral striate cortex, bilateral lingual gyrus, bilateral fusiform gyri, and the right superior temporal gyrus.

In the experimental design the intensity of facial expression varied independently for each emotional category. This type of variation allowed a critical analysis of brain regions conjointly responsive to changes in category and intensity of expression. Of particular interest was whether a change in the intensity of fearful expression (relative to a change in the intensity of happy expressions) would be associated with a discriminatory neural response within the amygdala. We examined for an effect of this type by applying orthogonal contrasts involving fearful versus happy faces and a contrast that reflected varying emotional intensity (i.e., increasing activation with increasing fearfulness and decreasing activation with increasing happiness). The left amygdala was the only significant area of activation revealed by this interaction (Morris et al., 1996). Furthermore, the neural response in the left amygdala showed a monotonic increase from the most happy condition to the most fearful (Plate 1).

The Role of Amygdala in Emotional Processing of Fear in Faces

The striking component of these data is that categorical, parametric, and factorial analyses all implicated the amygdala in processing fearful facial expressions. The experimental design, in which faces were classified by gender and not by expression, suggests that this amygdala activation does not depend on explicit processing of facial expressions. In other words, the response of the amygdala appears to be obligatory, a finding supported by electrophysiological data (Halgren & Marinkovic, 1995). The unilateral response was surprising, but it parallels similar findings in a study of procaine-induced emotional states where left (but not right) amygdala rCBF correlated positively with fear and negatively with euphoria (Ketter et al., 1996). It is also consistent with a study of patients with unilateral amygdala damage which found that ratings of emotional intensity in facial expressions were significantly lower with left amygdala lesions compared to right (Adolphs et al., 1995).

The Neuromodulatory Role of the Amygdala

It has been suggested that integrated responses to threat or danger, without the necessity of higher level processing, can be mediated via the amygdala (Kling & Brothers, 1992). It is conceivable that perceiving an expression of fear in a conspecific can trigger a rapid and implicit neural response that accounts for the amygdala activation we observed in response to fearful faces. The primate amygdala receives substantial anatomical inputs from temporal visual association cortices (Aggleton et al., 1980; Iwai & Yukie, 1987) and contains neurons that respond selectively to individual faces (Perrett et al., 1982, 1992). The amygdala also has strong anatomical linkages to the autonomic nervous system (LeDoux et al., 1988). This anatomical connectivity, coupled with the selectivity of its response to stimuli of behavioural significance provides a mechanism by which the amygdala can enable integrated responses to the emotional significance of complex stimuli.

The survival value conferred by adaptive responses to danger can be expected to result in the evolutionary selection of neural mechanisms that efficiently process threatening or fear-provoking stimuli (Edelman, 1987; Friston et al., 1994; LeDoux, 1996). The amygdala's crucial role in the neural response to fearful facial expressions has already been demonstrated. However, a more general role in the neuromodulation of visual processing is suggested by its extensive anatomical connections, especially its reentrant projections to occipital cortex (Amaral & Price, 1984; Iwai & Yukie, 1987). One prediction, therefore, is that brain areas functionally connected to the amygdala will express changes in patterns of neural activity that are partly dependent on the degree of amygdala response. In view of the differential response of the amygdala to fearful and happy expressions, this prediction also entails that this neuromodulatory response should be context specific and expressed to a greater degree when subjects process fearful as opposed to happy faces.

The question of measuring functional interactions is more closely related to notions of functional integration than functional segregation. It is important to bear in mind that conventional functional imaging techniques, which depend upon perfusion mapping, have poor temporal resolution, and consequently questions of functional integration can only be addressed at slow time scales. Nevertheless, two generic approaches have been described that provide a framework within which questions concerning functional integration can be addressed (Friston et al., 1993b;

Friston et al., 1995). These approaches, based on analysis of functional and effective connectivity, are similar to those used in electrophysiological studies based on coherence analysis of multiunit recordings of separable neuronal spike trains (Gerstein & Perkel, 1969; Gerstein et al., 1989). Functional connectivity is the simplest analysis and assesses how brain activity in different brain regions, evoked by a particular cognitive task, covary as a function of time. This approach is essentially descriptive, with the resulting eigen images or spatial modes identifying brain regions that represent different systems by virtue of their functional interactions. Effective connectivity, in contrast to functional connectivity, is mechanistic in that it assesses the influence one brain region exerts on another. Moreover, effective connectivity relies on a theoretical model which may be linear or nonlinear (Friston et al., 1993a).

To test the hypothesis that the amygdala has a context-specific influence on neural activity in remote brain regions, and in particular on extrastriate cortex, the activation values in the left amygdala were grouped according to condition (i.e., happy or fearful) and used as predictor variables for activity in all other brain voxels. These regressions were then directly contrasted using statistical parametric mapping. In essence, this analysis demonstrates an aspect of the effective connectivity between the amygdala and other brain regions, where effective connectivity is defined as the influence one neural system exerts over another (Friston et al., 1993a). This influence can also can also be framed in terms of the contribution of the amygdala to other brain regions under different psychological contexts. In this analysis fear-specific changes in the influence of the amygdala on remote brain regions were significant for bilateral inferior occipital gyri, right middle temporal gyrus, brainstem, left hippocampus, right cerebellum, right fusiform gyrus, and left lingual gyrus (Morris et al., 1998). Put simply, the analysis indicates that neural responses in these brain regions are better predicted by amygdala activity during the processing of fearful as opposed to happy expressions. The category-specific nature of the inferred connectivity between the amygdala and exstrastriate cortex is illustrated graphically in figure 10.2. It can be clearly seen that the regression of extrastriate rCBF values on amygdala responses has a positive slope in the fearful condition and a negative slope in the happy condition.

The regression analysis outlined above demonstrates that the strength of the contribution of activity in the amygdala to activity in extrastriate cortex varies as a function of the facial expression being processed. This type of influence has been formulated in terms of a psychophysiological interaction, meaning a condition-specific change in the effective connectivity between brain regions (Friston et al., 1997). The analysis can be interpreted mechanistically in two ways: (1) that there is a modulation by the psychological context (i.e., viewing fearful faces) of the amygdala's contribution to extrastriate cortex activity, or (2) that there is a modulation by the amygdala of stimulus-specific activity in extrastriate cortex (i.e., responses related to fearful faces). The second interpretation appears to be more consistent with neurophysiological and neuroanatomical evidence of the amygdala's modulatory role in other brain regions. A teleological extension of this line of reasoning would suggest that under the condition of exposure to fearful faces, there is greater coherence in the response of extrastriate regions and the amygdala so as to facilitate rapid processing of stimuli that represent potential sources of threat.

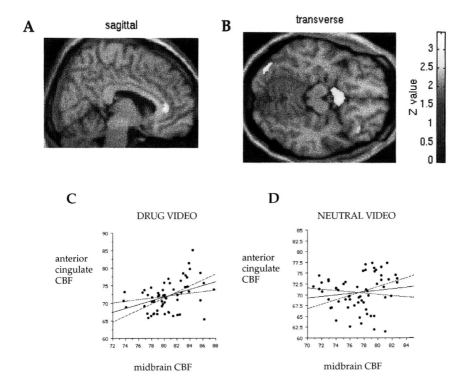

Plate 1. (A) A statistical parametric map showing activation of the left amygdala. An uncorrected p value of .01 was used as the threshold for the contrast of the fearful with the happy conditions. Views of the brain are shown for orthogonal slices at the pixel of maximal activation within the left amygdala ($x = -18$, $y = -6$, $z = -16$). The significant area of activation is displayed on the mean MRI image produced from the coregistered structural MRIs. (B) A graphical display of the regional cerebral blood flow (rCBF) values in milliliters per deciliter per minute for all conditions and all subjects at $x = -18$, $y = -6$, $x = -16$ (the pixel of maximal activation). The x-axis represents the proportion of the prototypical expression in the face stimuli, with fearful being positive (i.e., 100% = 1), and happy negative (i.e., 100% = -1). A regression line has been fitted to the data (with broken lines representing 95% confidence intervals for the gradient of the slope ($r = .514$).

transverse

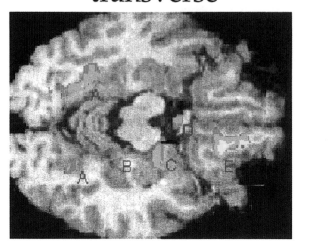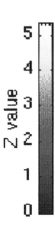

Plate 2. A statistical parametric map (SPM) of the brain regions that show a positive regression of neural activity with the right pulvinar. A, Bilateral fusiform gyri (BA19); B, right hippocampal gyrus (BA35); C, right amygdala; D, basal forebrain, in region of nucleus basalis of Meynert; E, right orbitofrontal cortex (BA11). The regions were identified by using the regional cerebral blood flow values at the pixel of maximal activation in the right pulvinar ($x = 14$, $y = -34$, $z = 4$) as a covariate of interest. A significance threshold of $p < .001$ was used. The SPM is displayed on a transverse slice of a canonical MRI at the level $z = -12$ mm.

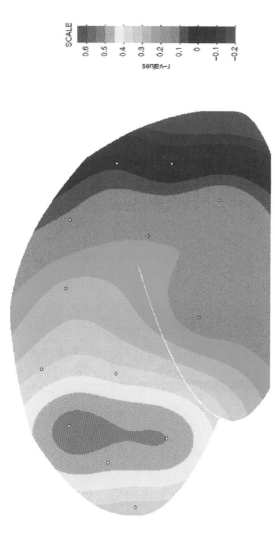

SCALE

r-values

0.6
0.5
0.4
0.3
0.2
0.1
0
-0.1
-0.2

Plate 3. Relations between electrophysiological measures of asymmetry and the difference between the standardized score on the behavioral Activation and Behavioral Inhibition Scales (BIS/BAS scales; N = 46,Carver & White, 1994). Electrophysiological data were recorded from each subject on two separate occasions separated by 6 weeks. The BIS/BAS scales were also administered on these two occasions. Data were averaged across the two time periods before performing correlations. The topographic map displays the correlations between alpha power asymmetry (log right minus log left alpha power; higher values denote greater relative left-sided activation) and the difference score between the standardized BAS minus BIS scales. After correlations were performed for each homologous region, a spline-interpo-

lated map was created. The yellow-orange end of the scale denotes positive correlations. The figure indicates that the correlation between the BAS-BIS difference score and the electrophysiology asymmetry score is highly positive in prefrontal scalp regions, denoting that subjects with greater relative left-sided activation report more relative behavioral activation compared with behavioral inhibition tendencies. The relation between asymmetric activation and the BAS-BIS difference is highly specific to the anterior scalp regions, as the correlation drops off rapidly more posteriorly. The correlation in the prefrontal region is significantly larger than the correlation in the parieto-occipital region. (From Sutton & Davidson, in press.)

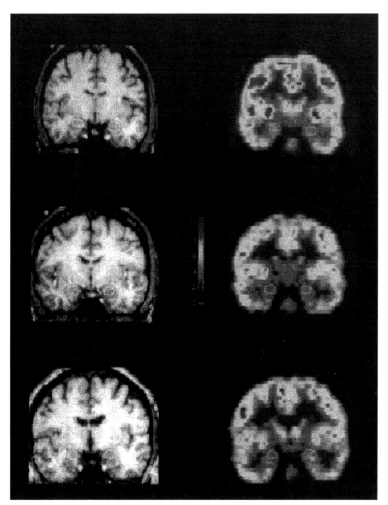

Plate 4. Illustration of PET-MRI coregistration with region of interest (ROI) drawn around the amygdala. The figure presents representative image slices that have been reformatted in the coronal orientation. The pixelated appearance of the PET images has been intentionally preserved to illustrate the effect of displaying, in the coronal orientation, images that were acquired in transaxial planes and to illustrate the high inplane resolution of the images. Each PET slice is presented side by side with the coregistered (using the Automated Image Registration algorithm; Woods et al., 1993) MRI slice for the same individual. Data for three subjects are presented. Averages of regional glucose metabolism extracted from five to eight slices as shown (slice thickness = 1.17 mm) were used to drive coregistered regional cerebral metabolic rate for glucose. Regions of interest are drawn for the left and right amygdalae in each image. PET images are from a BE Advance PET camera (inplane resolution approximately 5 mm full-width, half-maximum). Units of the PET color scale are in mg/100g/min. (From Abercrombie et al., 1998.)

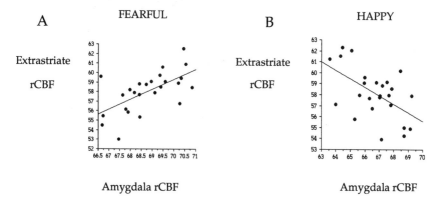

Figure 10.2. A graphical display illustrating a context-dependent interaction between left amygdala and extrastriate cortex. The regional cerebral blood flow (rCBF) values in milliliters per deciliter per minute for the voxel ($x = -14$, $y = -8$, $z = -16$) in the left amygdala and ($x = -40$, $y = -84$, $z = -4$) in the left inferior occipital gyrus are plotted against each other in (A) fearful and (B) happy conditions. Regression lines have been fitted to the data, demonstrating a positive gradient (+1.05; $r = .62$) in panel A and a negative gradient (−0.78; $r = .55$) in panel B.

Our functional neuroimaging data are entirely consistent with neurobiological data that indicate a neuromodulatory role for the amygdala. Animal studies of startle reflex potentiation have revealed that projections from the amygdala mediate modulation of brainstem activity (Davis, 1992), while the extensive amygdala efferents to visual cortex has also been interpreted as neuromodulatory in nature (Amaral & Price, 1984; Amaral et al., 1992; Iwai & Yukie, 1987). The amygdala also has strong connections with aminergic and cholinergic systems, including the nucleus basalis of Meynert, which is implicated in modulating synaptic connections (Mesulam et al., 1983). In this way the amygdala may act as part of a functional system with the basal forebrain to modulate neural activity throughout the neocortex (Mesulam et al., 1983; Russchen et al., 1985a). In this context we interpret the differential patterns of functional activity predicted by the amygdala in terms of direct and indirect neuromodulatory influences that facilitate processing of salient visual inputs of adaptive significance.

It is important to note that the type of analysis we describe provides information specifically about the amygdala's contribution to the neural processing of facial emotion and does not model the functional influence of other brain regions. Other types of network analysis, such as structural equation modeling (McIntosh et al., 1994), have been applied post hoc to neuroimaging data to model interactions between multiple brain regions and thus give a more complex account of functional neuroanatomy.

Interestingly, the extrastriate regions with the strongest functional interactions with the amygdala have also been shown to be involved in facial emotion processing in previous functional neuroimaging studies (George et al., 1995; Sergent et al., 1994). However, these regions were not identified by the categorical analyses in the present study, demonstrating that changes in covariance relationships can occur without significant differences in mean regional brain activity. Furthermore, recent neuropsychological data also provide evidence that regions of extrastriate cortex have a role in facial emotion processing (Adolphs et al., 1997). The occipital regions identified by these data are more medial to those found in our neuroimaging studies. We are not aware of any study, other the present report, which has provided evidence of the importance of extrastriate–amygdala interactions in facial emotion processing.

Functional Imaging Data from the Study of Acquired Fear

Many stimuli directly related to survival (e.g., food, sex, or pain) can be described as having innate perceptual salience, determined by evolutionarily selected value systems in the brain (Edelman, 1987; Friston et al., 1994). Fearful faces similarly have innate salience due to the threat implicit in seeing fear expressed in a conspecific. In addition to stimuli with innate salience, it is equally apparent that the biological significance of stimuli vary during the lifetime of a phenotype. In this respect it is critical for neural systems that confer value or salience to stimuli to be adaptive and flexible. The ability of an organism to confer salience to a stimulus based on prior experience would have important evolutionary advantages.

The precise neural mechanisms by which the central nervous system confers salience to environmental stimuli is uncertain. An important model in this respect is provided by classical conditioning. Classical conditioning is a simple form of associative learning in which a neutral stimulus acquires behaviorial significance (and therefore salience) through its temporal pairing with an innately salient unconditioned stimulus. This type of conditioning is manifest across the phylogenetic scale from gastropod mollusks to humans (Hawkins et al., 1983; Hodes et al., 1985). The associated plastic synaptic changes (Kandel & Schwartz, 1982) represent one of the simplest forms of value-dependent neural plasticity (Friston et al., 1994). In mammals, this plasticity of neural response appears to depend on neuromodulatory cholinergic projections, predominantly from the nucleus basalis of Meynert (Pirch et al., 1992; Hars et al., 1997).

An example of a model that provides a plausible biological account of the acquisition of salience is that of Friston et al. (1994). This model assumes the presence within the organism of evolutionarily selected regulatory systems whose activation signals behavior of value to the organism. However, organisms have to contend with unpredictable environments, and mechanisms that signal novel behaviors that enhance adaptive fitness are important. In interpreting data on acquired responses to conditioned stimuli, we relied on predictions derived from this model and its conceptual distinction between innate and acquired value. Innate salience is selected for within an evolutionary time scale and is genetically specified. Acquired value is acquired in somatic time and, to be maximally adaptive, develops over relatively brief time scales.

The specific predictions regarding the neural processes that mediate acquired value or salience involve an increase in the strength of inputs from sensorimotor processing systems, engaged by particular adaptive behaviors, to the value systems themselves. Consequently, neural patterns that antecede value-related behaviors become capable of eliciting a response in value systems. At a mechanistic level this involves an increase in the strength of afferents from sensory systems to the value systems involving neuromodulatory-mediated plasticity. A simplified depiction of this model is provided in figure 10.3.

In terms of fear conditioning to faces, the prediction we made was that acquired value (i.e., conditioned fear responses) would involve an enhancement of the connections from sensory processing regions both to the amygdala and related regions that mediate value. These other regions, according to the model, include neuromodulatory neurotransmitter systems such as cholinergic and dopaminergic systems capable of eliciting increased synaptic strength in activated networks.

Electrophysiological experiments in monkeys suggest that acquired changes in visual salience are mediated by the pulvinar nucleus of the thalamus, and neurobiological models have proposed that the pulvinar and also the thalamic reticular nucleus may be crucial in the selective processing of sensory information (Olshausen et al., 1993; Petersen et al., 1985; Posner & Petersen, 1990; Robinson & Petersen, 1992). Aversive classical conditioning, in contrast, has been shown in animals to involve the amygdala as the key structure in a neural system that includes basal forebrain, sensory thalamus, and brainstem (LeDoux et al., 1990). In humans, psychophysiological studies have identified predominantly right hemisphere involve-

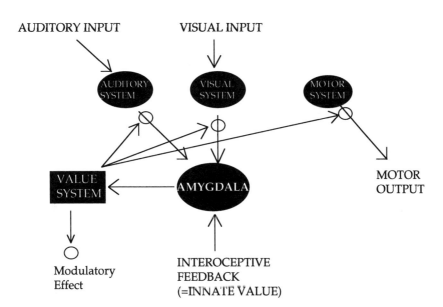

Figure 10.3. A model of value-dependent neural selection. Evolutionarily determined "value" systems in the brain, located in amygdala, basal forebrain, lateral hypothalamus, and related structures, respond to stimuli with relevance for survival (e.g., food, pain, sex). Neuromodulatory projections from the value system enhance neural activity in both sensory and motor systems to increase the likelihood of adaptive behavioral responses.

ment in aversive conditioning (Johnsen & Hugdahl, 1993). Similarly, functional imaging data indicate right-sided activations in orbitofrontal, dorsolateral prefrontal, and temporal cortices during an aversive-tone conditioning paradigm (Hugdahl et al., 1995).

We used an aversive classical conditioning paradigm to manipulate the perceptual salience of different human facial expressions (happy, fearful, and neutral) presented to volunteer human subjects during PET neuroimaging. In the period before scanning, subjects viewed a sequence of gray-scale images of faces. The sequence consisted of two different faces each repeated eight times in a pseudo-random order. Both faces in a sequence had either happy, fearful, or neutral expressions. Subjects were instructed to pay attention to the order of presentation and immediately respond "yes" if there was a consecutive repeat of a face and "no" if not. There were never more than three consecutive presentations of the same face. One face (the conditioned stimulus [CS]+) was always followed by a noise stimulus; the other face (the CS-) was always followed by silence. Subjects were warned that noises would be played during the experiment but were not informed of the conditioning contingency. Subjects were explicitly told to attend equally to all stimuli throughout the experiment.

The acquisition of neuroimaging data was timed to coincide with the end of the conditioning period. During an individual scan, 4 presentations of 1 of the preceding faces were made at 15-second intervals. No noises were played during this phase. Subjects were not informed that there were separate phases of acquisition and extinction. In six scans, the face (CS+) that had been paired with noise was presented in the extinction sequence; in the other six scans the face (CS-) explicitly unpaired with noise was presented.

In the contrast of all paired conditioned (CS+) minus all unpaired noncondi-tioned (CS-) scans, a number of brain regions, all in the right hemisphere, were significantly activated: these were the pulvinar and reticular nuclei regions of the thalamus, orbitofrontal cortex, and superior frontal gyrus (see figure 10.4). A single area showing significantly greater activation in the CS- compared to the CS+ conditions was located in the right pons.

The processing associated with the acquisition of salience should be maximally expressed when there is conflict between the innate and acquired value (i.e., fear response elicited by a happy expression). We examined for this effect by applying orthogonal contrasts in the following manner. Brain regions identified by the contrast of CS+ minus CS- conditions were subjected to a second contrast of the two different emotional categories (i.e., all happy CS+ vs. CS- minus all fearful CS+ vs. CS-). This analysis revealed a highly significant interaction in the right pulvinar between happy expressions and conditioning. This finding implies a specific effect in the pulvinar associated with the acquisition of salience.

In our theoretical model the key concept was that stimuli that acquire value or salience are defined by their ability to elicit responses in neuronal systems mediating value (e.g., amygdala, lateral hypothalamic area, and nucleus basalis); Friston et al., 1994). This implies that connections to the amygdala and nucleus basalis from sensory processing systems are selectively strengthened when stimuli acquire value. This strengthening is value dependent and depends on reinforcement by stimuli that have innate or preexisting value. In the context of our experiment the

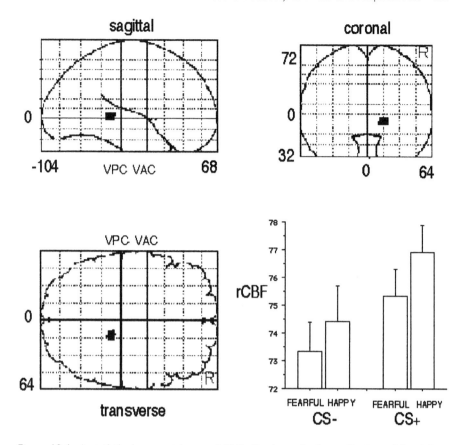

Figure 10.4. A statistical parametric map (sPM) showing selective activation of the right pulvinar, together with a graphical representation of regional cerebral blood flow (rCBF) values. The SPM is the result of two orthogonal contrasts, the first selecting brain regions with a greater response to conditioned stimulus (CS)+ compared to CS- faces, and the second selecting areas with a greater neural response to happy expressions than fearful. A threshold of $p < .01$ was used for both contrasts, giving a significance level of $p < .0001$ (uncorrected). The activation is displayed in orthogonal views of a transparent representation of the brain, showing that the right pulvinar is the only significant region. The graph displays the adjusted mean rCBF values (with bars showing 2 SEs) in milliliters per decili ter per minute at the pixel in the right pulvinar maximally activated in the orthogonal contrasts ($x = 16$, $y = -36$, $z = 0$).

aversive noise can be considered as having innate value and consequently can activate value systems. According to the model, the pairing of the CS+ faces with noise during conditioning would lead to strengthening of the connections between the associated sensory processing systems and the innate value systems. Consequently, we predicted that activity in the amygdala and nucleus basalis would be significantly correlated with thalamic activity. This model clearly implies a role for the amygdala in mediating both innate and acquired salience.

To test the above hypothesis, the activation values at the voxel of maximal activation, in the right pulvinar, were used as a covariate of interest to identify regions whose activity could be predicted by the neural response in this structure. The right amygdala, right basal forebrain in the region of the nucleus basalis of Meynert, right anterior cingulate, right orbitofrontal cortex, right hippocampal gyrus and bilateral fusiform gyri covaried positively in their response with that observed in the right pulvinar (see Plate 2).

These findings constitute remarkable empirical evidence for two neurobiological models of selective visual processing (Olshausen et al., 1993; Petersen et al., 1987). One model hypothesizes that structures within the thalamus enhance the processing of selected thalamo-cortical and cortico-thalamic signals (Olshausen et al., 1993). The other model postulates that the pulvinar nucleus of the thalamus has a controlling role in the coordination of neural processing in sensory and association cortices (Petersen et al., 1987). Evidence for the latter model includes the pulvinar's extensive reciprocal connections with visual cortical areas and other brain regions (Ungerleider et al., 1983); electrophysiological recordings in monkeys of pulvinar responses to visual salience (Robinson & Petersen, 1992); human studies showing attentional deficits with pulvinar lesions (Rafal & Posner, 1989); and functional neuroimaging experiments demonstrating pulvinar activation in a selective attention task (LaBerge & Buchsbaum, 1990). The specific responses to visual salience recorded in the pulvinar and reticular nuclei in the present study are consistent with these previous findings and provide general support for the two models. Our neuroimaging data do not have sufficient temporal or spatial resolution to test more detailed and specific predictions of each model.

Our study can be seen as providing evidence for stimulus-specific neural plasticity in the neural response of the pulvinar. We use "plasticity" here to refer to experience-dependent changes in the physiological (hemodynamic) response to stimuli. Identical stimuli and the same explicit task were used in the CS+ and CS- conditions, and the experimental design controlled for time, order, and nonspecific arousal effects. Consequently, the only difference between the CS+ and CS- conditions was the experimentally induced change in salience occurring outside the scanning window. Differential hemodynamic responses elicited by the faces were consequently experience dependent in the sense that they could only be explained by associative learning before scanning.

Interactions between emotional category and conditioning have been demonstrated in psychophysiological experiments that show a greater augmentation of startle response with aversive conditioning of pleasant pictures than with unpleasant (Hamm et al., 1993). Therefore, we predicted that the pairing of happy expressions with noise would produce larger and more significant responses than the pairing of fearful expressions with noise. This was confirmed by our results, which show a significant enhancement of value-dependent responses only in the pulvinar.

The observation that thalamic responses predict responses in subcortical structures associated with emotional learning and ascending neuromodulation is consistent with a number of empirical and theoretical lines of evidence (Friston et al., 1994). The additional observations that activity in right orbitofrontal cortex correlated negatively with responses in the pulvinar suggests this region may be involved in reversing the enhanced thalamic responses to stimulus salience. This interpretation is consistent with animal studies showing that the orbitofrontal cortex is crucially involved in the extinction of conditioned responses (Wilson & Rolls, 1990).

Although our study has shown a plasticity of thalamic response in relation to perceptual salience, it cannot determine the location of the underlying changes in synaptic strength. The finding of a correlation of activity between the pulvinar and neuromodulatory systems in the amygdala and basal forebrain suggests that this synaptic plasticity may be occurring within this system. The nucleus basalis of Meynert, which receives a significant afferent input from the amygdala, sends a strong cholinergic projection to thalamus (Russchen et al., 1985a,b). Alternatively, the synaptic changes may be occurring in cortical areas projecting to the thalamus. Future studies, using imaging techniques with higher temporal resolutions and pharmacological manipulations, may be able to address this crucial question and also further characterize the interactions among the pulvinar, reticular nucleus, neocortex, and brainstem.

A final aspects of our results that needs comment is the lateralization of activations in the amygdala across our experiments.in the respon When subjects processed innately fearful faces, activation was seen in the left amygdala. When subjects acquired, through conditioning, a fear response to previously nonfearful faces, activation was seen in the right amygdala. There is no simple explanation for these lateralized activations. One crucial difference between experiments is the fact that there is likely to be greater conscious and linguistic elaboration of stimuli when subjects process faces that are innately fearful. When faces acquire salience, the associated behavioral response is likely to be automatic and obligatory, with little need for conscious elaboration. These conjectures are entirely speculative and await experiments that explore the influence of conscious awareness and linguistic elaboration on processing of fearful stimuli.

Conclusions

In this chapter we have addressed the functional anatomy of emotion, using functional neuroimaging, from the perspective of fear. The methodological approach we adopted allowed for both segregated and integrated function during fear processing. A critical role for the amygdala has been highlighted both in terms of its overall response, its neuromodulatory effects on sensory processing, and its possible role in a form of neural plasticity that mediates the acquisition of value-dependent responses. The findings highlight the importance of studying singular instances of emotion as opposed to assuming the presence of an overall global emotional processing system.

References

Adolphs, R., Damasio, H., Tranel, D. & Damasio, A. R. (1997). Cortical systems for the recognition of emotion in facial expressions. *Journal of Neuroscience, 16*, 7678–7687.
Adolphs, R., Tranel, D., Damasio, H. & Damasio, A. (1994). Impaired recognition of emo-

tion in facial expressions following bilateral damage to the human amygdala. *Nature, 372*, 669–672.

Adolphs, R., Tranel, D., Damasio, H. & Damasio, A. R. (1995). Fear and the human amygdala. *Journal of Neuroscience, 15*, 5879–5891.

Aggleton, J. P., Burton, M. J. & Passingaham, R. E. (1980). Cortical and subcortical afferents to the amygdala in the rhesus monkey (*Macaca mulatta*). *Brain Research, 190*, 347–368.

Amaral, D. G. & Price, J. L. (1984). Amygdalo-cortical projections in the monkey (*Macaca fascicularis*). *Journal of Comparative Neurology, 230*, 465–496.

Amaral, D., Price, J. L., Pitkanen, A. & Carmichael, S. T. (1992). Anatomical organization of the primate amygdaloid complex. In J. P. Aggleton (Ed), *The Amygdala: Neurobiological Aspects of Emotion, Memory and Mental Dysfunction* (pp. 1–66). New York: Wiley-Liss.

Bechara, A., Tranel, D., Damasio, H., Adolphs, R., Rockland, C. & Damasio, A. R. (1995). Double dissociation of conditioning and declarative knowledge relative to the amygdala and hippocampus in humans. *Science, 269*, 1115–1118.

Breiter, H. C., Ectoff, N. L., Whalen, P. J., Kennedy, D. N., Rauch, S. L., Buckner, R. L., Strauss, M. M., Hyman, S. E. & Rosen, B. R. (1996). Response and habituation of the human amygdala during visual processing of facial expression. *Neuron, 2*, 875–887.

Calder, A. J., Young, A. W., Rowland, D., Perrett, D. I., Hodges, J. R. & Etcoff, N. L. (1996). Facial emotion recognition after bilateral amygdala damage: differentially severe impairment of fear. *Cognitive Neuropsychology, 13*, 699–745.

Darwin, C. (1872[1965]). *The Expression of the Emotions in Man and Animals*. Chicago: University of Chicago Press.

Davis, M. (1992). The role of amygdala in conditioned fear. In J. P. Aggleton (Ed), *The Amygdala: Neurobiological Aspects of Emotion, Memory and Mental Dysfunction* (pp. 255–306). New York: Wiley-Liss.

Eckhorn, R., Bauer, R., Jordan, W., Brosch, M., Kruse, W., Munk, M. & Reitboek, H. J. (1988). Coherent oscillations: a mechanism of feature linking in visual cortex? *Biological Cybernetics, 60*, 121–130.

Edelman, G. (1987). *The Remembered Present: A Biological Theory of Consciousness*. New York: Basic Books.

Ekman, P. (1982). *Emotion in the Human Face*. Cambridge: Cambridge University Press.

Ekman, P. (1992). Facial expression of emotion: an old controversy ad new findings. *Proceedings of the Royal Society of London B, 335*, 63–69.

Ekman, P. & Friesen, W. V. (1976). Pictures of facial affect. Palo Alto, CA: Consulting Psychologists Press.

Field, T., Woodson, R., Greenber, R. & Cohen, D. (1982). Discrimination and imitation of facial expressions in neonates. *Science, 218*, 179–181.

Friston, K. J., Buechal, C., Fink, G., Morris, J. S., Rolls, E. T. & Dolan, R. J. (1997). Psychophysiological and modulatory interactions in neuroimaging. *Neuroimage, 6*, 218–229.

Friston, K. J., Frith, C. D. & Frackowiak, R. S. J. (1993a). Time-dependent changes in effective connectivity measured with PET. *Human Brain Mapping, 1*, 69–79.

Friston, K. J., Frith, C. D., Liddle, P. & Frackowiak, R. S. J. (1993b). Functional connectivity: the prinicipal component analysis of large (PET) data sets. *Journal of Cerebral Blood Flow and Metabolism, 13*, 5–14.

Friston, K. J., Tononi, G., Reeke, G. N., Sporns, O. & Edelman, G. M. (1994). Value-dependent selection in the brain: simulation in a synthetic neural model. *Neuroscience, 30*, 77–86.

Friston, K. J., Ungerleider, L. G., Jezzard, P. & Turner, R. (1995). Characterizing modulatory interaction between areas V1 and V2 in human cortex: a new treatment of functional MRI data. *Human Brain Mapping, 2,* 211–224.

George, M. S., Ketter, T. A., Parekh, I., Horwitz, B., Herscovitch, P. & Post, R. (1995). Brain activity during transient sadness and happiness in healthy women. *American Journal of Psychiatry, 152,* 341–351.

Gerstein, G. L., Bedenbaugh, P. & Aersten, A. M. H. J. (1989). Neuronal assemblies. *Transactions of Biomedical Engineering, 36,* 4–14.

Gerstein, G. L. & Perkel, D. H. (1969). Simultaneously recorded trains of action potentials: analysis and functional interpretation. *Science, 164,* 828–830.

Gray, C. M., Konig, P., Engel, A. K. & Singer, W. (1989). Oscillatory responses in cat visual cortex exhibit inter-columnar synchronization which reflects global stimulus properties. *Nature, 338,* 334–337.

Halgren, E., Babb, T. L., Rausch, R. & Crandall, P. H. (1978). Mental phenomena evoked by electrical stimulation of the human hippocampal formation and amygdala. *Brain, 101,* 83–117.

Halgren, E. & Marinkovic, K. (1995). Neurophysiological networks integrating human emotions. In M. S. Gazzaniga (Ed), *The Cognitive Neurosciences* (pp. 1137–1380). Cambridge, MA: MIT Press.

Hamm, A. O., Greenwald, M. K., Bradley, M. M. & Lang, P. J. (1993). Emotional learning, hedonic change, and the startle probe. *Journal of Abnormal Psychology, 102,* 453–465.

Hars, B., Maho, C., Edeline, J.-M. & Hennevin, E. (1993). Basal forebrain stimulation facilitates tone-evoked responses in the auditory cortex of awake rat. *Neuroscience, 56,* 61–74.

Hawkins, R. D., Abrams, T. W., Carew, T. J. & Kandel, E. R. (1983). A cellular mechanism of classical conditioning in Aplysia: activity-dependent amplification of presynaptic facilitation. *Science, 219,* 400–405.

Hodes, R. L., Cook, E. W. & Lang, P. J. (1985). Individual differences in autonomic response: conditioned association or conditioned fear? *Psychophysiology, 22,* 545–560.

Hugdahl, K., Berardi, A., Thompson, W. L. et al. (1995). Brain mechanisms in human classical conditioning. *NeuroReport, 6,* 1723–1728.

Iwai, E. & Yukie, M. (1987). Amygdalofugal and amygdalopetal connections with modality-specific visual cortical areas in Macaques (*Macaca fuscata, M. mulatta, M. fascicularis*). *Journal of Comparative Neurology, 261,* 362–387.

Johnsen, B. H. & Hugdahl, K. (1993). Right hemisphere representation of autonomic conditioning to facial emotional expressions. *Psychophysiology, 30,* 274–278.

Jones, E. G. & Burton, H. (1976). A projection from the medial pulvinar to the amygdala in primates. *Brain Research, 104,* 142–147.

Jones, E. G. & Powell, T. P. S. (1970). An anatomical study of converging sensory pathways within the cerebral cortex of the monkey. *Brain, 93,* 793–820.

Kandel, E. R. & Schwartz, J. H. (1982). Molecular biology of learning: modulation of transmitter release. *Science, 218,* 433–443.

Ketter, T. A., Andreason, P. J., George, M. S., Lee, C., Gill, D. S., Parekh, P. I., Willis, M. W., Herscovitch, P. & Post, R. M. (1996). Anterior paralimbic mediation of procaine-induced emotional and psychosensory experience. *Archives of General Psychiatry, 53,* 59–69.

Kling, A. S. & Brothers, L. A. (1992). The amygdala and social behavior. In J. P. Aggleton (Ed), *The Amygdala: Neurobiological Aspects of Emotion, Memory and Mental Dysfunction* (pp. 353–377). New York: Wiley-Liss.

LaBar, K. S., LeDoux, J. E., Spencer, D. D. & Phelps, E. A. (1995). Impaired fear conditioning following unilateral temporal lobectomy. *Journal of Neuroscience, 15,* 6846–6855.

LaBerge, D. & Buchsbaum, M. S. (1990). Positron emission tomographic measurements of pulvinar activity during an attention task. *Journal of Neuroscience, 10*, 613–619.

LeDoux, J. E. (1993). Emotional memory systems in the brain. *Behaviour and Brain Research, 58*, 69–79.

LeDoux, J. E. (1996). *The Emotional Brain.* New York: Simon & Schuster.

LeDoux, J. E., Cicchetti, P., Xagoraris, A. & Romanski, L. M. (1990). The lateral amygdaloid nucleus: sensory interface of the amygdala in fear conditioning. *Journal of Neuroscience, 10*, 1062–1069.

LeDoux, J. E., Iwata, J., Cicchetti, P. & Reis, D. (1988). Differential projections of the central amygdaloid nucleus mediate autonomic and behavioral correlates of conditioned fear. *Journal of Neuroscience, 8*, 2517–2529.

McIntosh, A. R. & Gonzales-Lima, F. (1994). Structural equation modelling and its application to network analysis in functional brain imaging. *Human Brain Mapping, 2*, 2–22.

Meltzoff, A. N. & Moore, M. K. (1977). Imitation of facial and manual gestures by human neonates. *Science, 198*, 74–78.

Mesulam, M-M., Mufson, E. J., Levey, A. I. & Wainer, B. H. (1983). Cholinergic innervation of cortex by basal forebrain: cytochemistry and cortical connections of the septal area, diagonal band nuclei, nucleus basalis (substantia innominata) and hypothalamus in the rhesus monkey. *Journal of Comparative Neurology, 214*, 170–197.

Morris, J., Friston, K. J., Buechel, C., Frith, C. D., Young, A. W., Calder, A. J. & Dolan, R. J. (1998). A neuromodulatory role for the human amygdala in processing emotional facial expressions. *Brain, 121*, 47–57.

Morris, J., Frith, C. D., Perrett, D., Rowland, D., Young, A. W., Calder, A. J. & Dolan, R. J. (1996). A differential neural response in the human amygdala to fearful and happy facial expressions. *Nature, 383*, 812–815.

Ohman, A. & Dimberg, U. J. (1978). Facial expressions as conditioned stimuli for electrodermal responses: a case of "preparedness"? *Journal of Personality and Social Psychology, 36*, 1251–1258.

Olshausen, B. A., Anderson, C. H. & Van Essen, D. C. (1993). A neurobiological model of visual attention and invariant pattern recognition based on dynamic routing of information. *Journal of Neuroscience, 13*, 4700–4719.

Perrett, D. I., Hietanen, J. K., Oram, M. W. & Benson, P. J. (1992). Organization and functions of cells responsive to faces in the temporal cortex. *Philosophical Transactions of the Royal Society of London, 335*, 23–30.

Perrett, D., May, K. A. & Yoshikawa, S. (1994). Female shape and judgements of female attractiveness. *Nature, 368*, 239–242.

Perrett, D. I., Rolls, E. T. & Caan, W. (1982). Visual neurons responsive to faces in the monkey temporal cortex. *Experimental Brain Research, 47*, 329–342.

Petersen, S. E., Robinson, D. L. & Keys, W. (1985). Pulvinar nuclei of the behaving rhesus monkey: visual responses and their modulation. *Journal of Neurophysiology, 54*, 867–886.

Petersen, S. E., Robinson, D. L. & Morris, J. D. (1987). Contributions of the pulvinar to visual spatial attention. *Neuropsychologia, 25*, 97–105.

Pirch, J. H., Turco, K. & Rucker, H. K. (1992). A role for acetylcholine in conditioning-related responses of rat frontal cortex neurons: microiontophoretic evidence. *Brain Research, 586*, 19–26.

Posner, M. I. & Petersen, S. E. (1990). The attention system of the human brain. *Annual Review of Neurosciences, 13*, 25–42.

Rafal, R. D. & Posner, M. I. (1989). Deficits in human visual spatial attention following thalamic lesions. *Neuropsychologia, 27*, 1031–1041.

Robinson, D. L. & Petersen, S. E. (1992). The pulvinar and visual salience. *Trends in Neuroscience, 1*, 127–132.

Roelfsema, P. R., Engel, A. K., Konig, P. & Singer, W. (1997). Visuomotor integration is associated with zero time-lag synchronization among cortical areas. *Nature, 385*, 157–161.

Rolls, E. T. (1992). Neurophysiology and functions of the primate amygdala. In J. P. Aggleton (Ed), *The Amygdala: Neurobiological Aspects of Emotion, Memory and Mental Dysfunction* (pp. 143–167). New York: Wiley-Liss.

Rolls, E. T. (1995). A theory of emotion and consciousness, and its application to understanding the neural basis of emotion. In M. S. Gazzaniga (Ed), *The Cognitive Neurosciences* (pp. 1091–1106). Camgbridge, MA: MIT Press.

Russchen, F. T., Amaral, D. G. & Price, J. L. (1985a). The afferent connections of the substantia innominata in the monkey, *Macaca fascicularis*. *Journal of Comparative Neurology, 242*, 1–27.

Russchen, F. T., Bakst, I., Amaral, D. G. & Price, J. L. (1985b). The amygdalostriatal projections in the monkey. An anterograde tracing study. *Brain Research, 329*, 241–257.

Scoville, W. B. & Milner, B. (1957). Loss of recent memory after bilateral hippocampal lesions. *Journal of Neurology, Neurosurgery and Psychiatry, 20*, 11–21.

Sergent, J., Ohta, S., MacDonald, B. & Zuck, E. (1994). Segregated processing of facial identity and emotion in the human brain: a PET study. *Visual Cognition, 1*, 349–369.

Singer, W. (1990). Search for coherence: a basic principle of cortical self-organisation. *Concepts in Neuroscience, 1*, 45–54.

Tononi, G., Sporns, O. & Edelman, G. M. (1994). A measure for brain complexity: relating functional segregation and integration in the nervous system. *Proceedings of the National Academy of Science, USA, 91*, 5033–5037.

Ungerleider, L. G., Galkin, T. W. & Mishkin, M. (1983). Visuotopic organization of projections from striate cortex to inferior and lateral pulvinar in rhesus monkey. *Journal of Comparative Neurology, 217*, 137–157.

Wilson, F. A. W. & Rolls, E. T. (1990). Neuronal responses related to reinforcement in the primate basal forebrain. *Brain Research, 509*, 213–231.

Zeki, S., Watson, J. D. G., Lueck, C. J., Friston, K. J., Kennard, C. & Frackowiak, R. S. J. (1991). A direct demonstration of functional specialisation in the human visual cortex. *Journal of Neuroscience, 11*, 641–649.

Zihl, J., Von Cramon, D. & Mai, N. (1983). Selective disturbance of movement vision after bilateral brain damage. *Brain, 106*, 313–340.

11

Measuring Emotion: Behavior, Feeling, and Physiology

MARGARET M. BRADLEY AND PETER J. LANG

What are emotions? What are feelings? How can they be both central events of our experience as human beings and ephemera that seem to occur unbidden by the mind and beyond our control? Do feelings prompt behavior, or is a feeling merely the shadow of an action? Why is the expectation of pain often worse than the pain itself? Philosophers have searched for answers to such questions over centuries of thought and study. All of us wonder why emotion is sometimes so destructive, and so often the focus of mental disorder. Is a wholly rational consciousness the true ideal? Are emotions of any use?

Historically, such questions have not prompted intellectual consensus, and indeed, we may doubt that they will ever be answered in ways satisfactory to all. Emotion has many faces. Thus, the analysis offered here is frankly tentative and epistemologically incomplete. It is, however, an approach that has a good scholarly provenance; it can organize a large and diverse domain of data; it significantly encourages practical application. Emotions are viewed here from the perspective of natural science. Emotional acts and their affects are considered to be measurable biological phenomena that reflect an evolutionary inheritance. Here, we take the view that the emotions evolved from functional behaviors that facilitated the survival of individuals and species.

Emotions Are Action Dispositions

Emotions evolved from simple reflexive actions, many of which are still part of the human response repertoire. Among the most primitive and general of these responses are movements toward positive, appetitive things and movements away from negative, unpleasant things. The biologist T. C. Schneirla (1959) held that these reciprocal movements were the root-stock for all behavior. Thus, more primitive organisms—worms or mollusks—withdraw quickly from an intense energy source (e.g., a bright light or tactile stimulation); however, they readily approach weaker stimulation and ingest food that is placed in the same environment. Confronted by appropriate stimuli of aversion or appetite, insects, birds, fishes, reptiles, and mammals show analogous, stimulus-driven approach and withdrawal behavior.

In humans and other more complex organisms, elaborate neural systems support more varied responses, better facilitating adaptation to the environment. Useful behavioral modules evolved early in biological history, and many persist and are broadly shared by living organisms. For example, aggressive attack, whether in predation, sexual competition, or defense, is a highly developed survival tool that varies only in tactical detail across a host of species. Similar cross-species output patterns are found in courtship behavior, copulatory acts, and in the ways young are nurtured and protected.

Agreement is not lacking that, in human beings, these behaviors are accompanied by emotion—by reported feelings of love or sexual passion, compassion, anger, and hostility. Pertinent to the psychology of emotion, the above reports also occur in the absence of the overt behaviors with which they seem to be linked.

Inhibition and Delay

The evolution of the brain, particularly that of the cerebral cortex, has conferred on human beings a greatly increased response repertoire which can be deployed in an impressive variety of combinations. Furthermore, in ways beyond the capacity of other animals, humans have conquered time. Stimuli do not immediately and automatically evoke a limited menu of specific behaviors. In humans, responses can be delayed or seemingly inhibited entirely, or responses can be retained in storage for later use in a totally new setting. Furthermore, cues previously observed can be reviewed, reevaluated, and alternative behaviors formulated to fit changing circumstances. Finally, natural language, a system of computation and communication that appears to be unique to humans, facilitates selective control of responses and helps organizes behavior in the service of long-term goals. Thus, as species have evolved, not only has behavior become more varied, but the functional apprehension of time itself—as a dimension of behavioral organization—has expanded from a few milliseconds to the human concept of the infinite.

Language and Behavior

In young children, language and action are inseparable. That is, when linguistic skills are newly acquired a child cannot easily say one thing and do another (e.g., say "squeeze" the balloon and simultaneously release it). In Pavlov's terms, the first and second signal systems begin as one. Children soon learn, however, that power lies in separating the word from the deed (often to a parent's dismay), as the environment separately shapes these behaviors. The functional individuation of language and associated actions means that each may be expressed or modulated independently. Important for an understanding of emotion, we cannot expect emotional language (as in descriptions of inner feeling) to be wholly coordinate with the logistics or output of action.

Preparation and Physiology

Emotional acts are robust response procedures, founded on the imperatives of survival. Thus, despite the flexibility of behavior noted above, affective actions can rarely be wholly inhibited or suppressed. For example, an employee who needs his job and is unjustly berated by his employer may wisely refrain from overt counteraggression. Nevertheless, his body mobilizes for such a response: He will "stiffen the sinews and summon up the blood." Adrenaline flows and the cardiovascular system moves oxygen to the gross muscles in preparation. It is in this sense that emotions are often dispositions to action, rather than the actions themselves: when a stimulus of threat or appetite prompts the execution of an action procedure, preparatory metabolic changes occur in muscles and glands. Often in humans, however, the final step in the brain's action program, the overt response, is gated out.

The Data of Emotion

As the above discussion indicates, emotions involve multiple responses and are highly variable in their psychophysiological composition. It is helpful in organizing the measurable data to first group them into three broad output systems (Lang, 1993): (1) overt acts or functional behavioral sequences, including the defining survival actions or their variants (e.g., fight, flight, sexual approach, threat displays), as well as the modulation by emotion of other behaviors (e.g., as in stress-induced performance deficits or in mood-dependent association); (2) emotional language, including expressive communication (e.g., threat or distress cries as in many animal species, sounds of contentment or sexual passion, verbal attack), and evaluative reports (e.g., descriptions of feelings and attitudes, self-ratings); (3) physiological reactions, changes in the somatic muscles and in the viscera that are the logistic support of overt acts in emotion, of associated affective displays (e.g., facial muscle patterns, blushing), or of preparation for these responses.

This three-systems organization is, of course, an oversimplification of the myriad subsystems, response complexes, and patterns that make up even the most primitive emotional event (see table 11.1). Furthermore, it is impossible for the researcher to simultaneously consider more than a small part of this potential wealth of information. Researchers are forced to select from among these measures, and this selection inevitably constrains our interpretation of emotion in ways difficult to predict at the outset. Indeed, it is now a commonplace observation that the close covariation among response systems predicted by the traditional, subjective models of emotion does not, in fact, routinely occur. For example, if individuals are confronted by a stimulus that they reportedly fear and we measure self-rating of distress, the extent of avoidance (change in proximity to the stimulus), and autonomic arousal (heart rate or skin conductance change), the covariation among response systems seldom accounts for more than 10–15% of the variance (e.g., Lang, 1968; Mandler et al., 1961). Dramatic examples of such response discordance have been formalized in the catalogue of psychiatric symptoms; for example, alexithymia (poor verbal description of emotion; an absence of the usual reports of inner feelings) is commonly observed in psychosomatic disorders (see Nemiah et al., 1976).

TABLE 11.1. Listing of Representative Responses in Each of the Three Response Systems That Can be Measured in Emotion

Event	Description
Physiological events	
Viscera (smooth muscle and glands)	Cardiovascular system, sweat glands, tear ducts, pilo-motor response, gut motility, genitals
Facial muscle patterns	Corrugator, temporalis, masseter, zygomaticus
Other somatic muscle	Head and neck, action muscles of the limbs, overall tension (general activation of the motor pool)
Respiration	Rate, depth, variability; expired CO_2, airway resistance
Endocrine and immune systems	Antibodies; circulating epinephrine, norepinephrine, testosterone, cortisol
Brain	Bioelectric events, regional blood flow, neurochemistry (synaptic transmitter systems—dopamine, glutamate)
Language events	
Expressive language	Distress cries, prosody, changes in voice intensity and frequency
Evaluative reports	Expressed feelings, attitudes, interests
Social communications	Facilitated or disrupted communication, instrumental emotion: placating, "mobbing," verbal aggression, inhibition
Behavioral events	
Direct actions	Approach, avoidance, escape, attack, defensive reflexes, appetitive reflexes, consummation, nurturance
Task enhancements and deficits	State-mediated effects on response latency, amplitude, and organization; reflex modulation

The central challenge to theory and research in emotion continues to be a comprehension of its response diversity—the achievement of an integration that explains varying patterns of concordance and discordance among effector systems. Thus, although the emotional complex defies exhaustive measurement, it is imperative that researchers not limit themselves to the assessment of a single response (e.g., subjective report). As a bare minimum, an experiment should include a sample measure from each major system: overt acts, language, and physiology.

Measuring Emotion

A simple model of emotion measurement might conceive the database as three dimensions of a cubic space (figure 11.1). A useful theory of emotion would then specify stable intercepts within this space. That is, it would meaningfully organize the multiform structures of individual emotional states and perhaps provide rules for predicting relationships between response systems.

It is worth noting at the outset, however, some intrinsic impediments to the development of such a model. First, as previously noted, no system can be defined by a single subsystem measure. Second, the three response systems have no obvious common metric. Third, measures differ greatly in sensitivity and dynamic

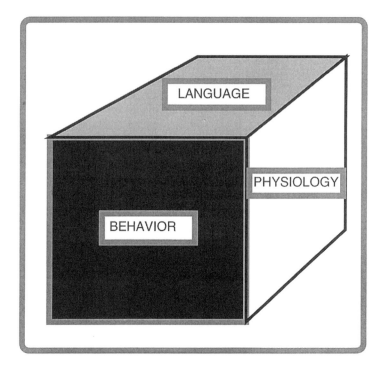

THE DATA OF EMOTION

Figure 11.1. Emotional experience seems to lie within a black box, defying external observation. Emotion's outputs, however—in behavior, language, and physiology—can be construed as the three dimensions of the box. A scientific theory could operationally define affective states as locations within this space, specified by the internal coordinates of the three data systems.

range. For example, evaluative language clearly has enormous sensitivity and extension. Words exist that make highly refined distinctions among many different affects and exquisitely grade intensity. In contrast, autonomically mediated responses (e.g., heart rate, skin conductance) are indifferent to much of language's emotional discrimination and vary little with stimulus changes that are rated in the lower range of affective intensities (Cuthbert et al., 1996; Lang et al., 1963).

Fourth, systems vary greatly in reliability, due in part to differences in sensitivity to context and stimulus modality, vulnerability to independent shaping, and characteristics of temporal integration. Thus, on the one hand, it is often easier for a therapy to modify fear behavior (i.e., avoidance of a fear object), and even associated physiological arousal, than to change verbal report of the fearful state. Effective coping may precede a change in affective experience. On the other hand, affective reports can change rapidly when such change has an independent, practical utility.

Finally, returning to the first point, each major system is actually a complex of different measurable subsystems. This has encouraged efforts at system pattern analysis, particularly when assessing physiological data. It is, for example, central in attempts to operationalize James's hypothesis that emotional experience was the perception of its physiology. In part because the body's many subsystems have their own time constants, sensitivities, and reactive ranges (and who can say which speaks to the ear of consciousness), James's idea has not found scientific proof.

The Motivational Organization of Emotion

Since the early 1960s, the concept of motivation has been somewhat neglected in psychology. Theory has been driven by the computer metaphor in which the brain is a machine for information processing and behavior is determined by output programs. Although the brain can be portrayed as a cool computational device, it is more accurately a biological organ that obeys evolutionary imperatives. Thus, motivational issues are central to any explanation of emotion.

Hebb (1949) defined motivation as factors that determine direction and vigor of behavior. Many theorists agree that this primary variance in the actions of organisms is primitively determined by survival needs. Thus, animals move toward positive stimuli and away from negative events, and, depending on strength of need states and salience of goal stimuli, the prompted behavior increases or wanes in speed and intensity of effort. These two motive features of behavior can be represented as quantifiable parameters, affective valence (positive/negative) and intensity of activation, that define a hypothetical, two-dimensional space. In principle, all actions can be represented by its x, y coordinates (e.g., see figure 11.3).

Dimensional organizations have been proposed by many theorists studying attitudes, feelings, and emotions. Thus, in the nineteenth century, Wundt (1896) proposed a dimensional model of affect as part of his mental chemistry. Osgood and co-workers (1957) later developed a dimensional theory of semantic evaluation (see also Mehrabian & Russell, 1974; Russell, 1980). Based on factor analysis of evaluative language, they determined that the largest variance was accounted for by a single factor, affective valence. Valence could be described by bipolar scales that, in aggregate, defined a continuous dimension from pleasantness (unhappy, annoyed, despairing, etc.) to unpleasantness (happy, pleased, hopeful, etc.). The fundamental role of valence in emotions received further support from studies of language categorization (Ortony et al., 1988; Shaver et al., 1987). This work showed that human knowledge about emotions is hierarchically organized and that the superordinate division is between positivity (pleasant states: love, joy) and negativity (unpleasant states: anger, sadness, fear).

Arousal was Osgood's second dimension. Although less salient than valence, it accounted for substantial variance in evaluative reactions. Bipolar scales defined this activity parameter, extending from an unaroused state (calm, relaxed, sleepy, etc.) to high arousal (excited, stimulated, wide awake, etc.).

It has been argued by some that arousal is the primary dimension of emotion. Lindsley (1951) proposed an influential "activation theory of emotion" (see also earlier formulations by Duffy, 1941, and Arnold, 1945). Lindsley's view was based in part on human electroencephalographic (EEG) studies, showing an association between alpha waves (10–13 Hz) and emotional calm (with even slower waves in sleep) and a progressive increase in frequency with increasing intensity of emotional arousal (from annoyance and anxiety to rage and panic). Other relevant data came from research with animal subjects showing that the brainstem reticular formation (Moruzzi & Magoun, 1949) modulated both EEG frequency and visceral arousal and that midbrain lesions blocked emotion, prompting lethargic, apathetic behavior.

Although the relative importance of valence and arousal is widely debated, investigators agree that these motivational parameters are the foundation of emotion. In this view, the diversity of expressed emotions developed from different tactical reactions to the context of aversive or appetitive stimulation. Thus, for example, a rat shocked on its footpads may attack a companion animal (an anger prototype) or, if alone, may become immobile, "freezing." When given an escape path, the rat may flee the field (fear prototypes). The contextual tactics of approach and withdrawal have, of course, become much more varied in humans. Nevertheless, the strategic frame of appetite and aversion remains fundamental.

It is proposed that two motive systems exist in the brain—appetitive and aversive/defensive—accounting for the primacy of the valence dimension in affective expression. These two motivational systems are associated with widespread cortical, autonomic, and behavioral activity that varies in intensity of activation. Although the tactical demands of context may variously shape affective expression, all emotions are organized around a motivational base. In this sense, we consider valence and arousal to be the strategic dimensions of the emotion world.

Motivational Systems in the Brain

We take the view that the emotions are atavars of primitive actions that evolved to ensure the survival of organisms. As already emphasized, these prototypical actions involve either approach to stimuli that are necessary to maintain or enhance individuals and species or withdrawal from dangerous and nociceptive events. Several theorists have suggested that these survival behaviors are modulated by specific neural systems that have comparable anatomical structure across the mammalian phylum.

Konorski (1967), for example, proposed that the brain has two motive systems, predicated on a classification of primary exteroceptive reflexes: (1) preservative reflexes that had to do with ingestion, copulation, nurture of progeny, and (2) protective reflexes that involved withdrawal from or rejection of noxious agents. Differentiating his views from those of Hess (1957), Konorski stressed that activation or arousal modulated both preservative and protective reactions. Furthermore, these reactions were considered to be the behavioral foundation of affects and expressed emotions. Dickinson and Dearing (1979) developed Konorski's dichotomy into two opponent motivational systems, aversive and attractive, each activated by a different, but equally wide range of unconditioned stimuli. These systems were held to have "reciprocal inhibitory connections" (p. 5) which modulate learned behavior and responses to new, unconditioned input.

Miller (1959) described a biphasic system in which strength of behavior was modulated according to distance from a goal location—the site of either appetitive or aversive reinforcement. Animal experiments indicated that strength of motivation increased with goal proximity. Miller used this approach to model conflict, considering a context in which both positive and negative reinforcers occupied the same goal location. In such situations, anxiety/arousal presumably increments, while overt action is stymied—analogous to many human affects. Importantly, arousal is not viewed here as a third system that is modulated independently, but rather as representing activation (metabolic and neural) of either the appetitive or aversive system or the co-activation of both systems (see Cacioppo & Bernston, 1994).

Neural Circuits

As already stated, the brain's appetitive and aversive motive systems are the structural foundation of valence and arousal effects. These systems consist of neural structures and their connections in subcortical or deep in primitive cortex that are directly activated by primary reinforcement. This circuitry mediates a small repertoire of reflex reactions to nociceptive and appetitive stimuli. The circuitry is plastic; it learns. Through association with primary reinforcers, new stimuli come to activate the system. Significant for the psychology of human emotion, these motivational structures have reciprocal connections to the cerebral cortex. Thus, the circuit can modulate ongoing cognitive processing, and, furthermore, stimuli that are highly processed (memories and associations) can become its inputs.

Part of the defense motive system is diagrammed in figure 11.2, as currently derived from animal experimentation (e.g., Davis, 1997; Fanselow et al., 1995; LeDoux, 1990). The output circuits shown include defensive "freezing," fight–flight, and modulation of the startle reflex and the cardiovascular system. The mediation of other related somatic and visceral reactions (facial actions, sweat gland, neurohumoral secretions) can be similarly represented. In the present view, emotions are defined as activation in a motive system and are indexed by the consequent actions. Stimuli have affective significance to the extent that they prompt a defensive or appetitive pattern.

Motivational Priming and Affective Reactions to Pictures and Sounds

The laboratory study of emotion requires stimuli that reliably evoke psychological and physiological reactions that vary systematically over the range of expressed emotions. Over the past few years, we have developed a number of such stimulus collections, including sets of color photographs (the International Affective Picture System; IAPS; Center for the Study of Emotion and Attention, 1999), digitized sounds (International Affective Digitized Sounds System; IADS; Bradley & Lang, 1999b), and verbal stimuli (Affective Norms for English Words; ANEW; Bradley & Lang, 1999a). The IAPS currently comprises more than 700 pictures for which affective norms are available for both male and female subjects (Lang et al.,

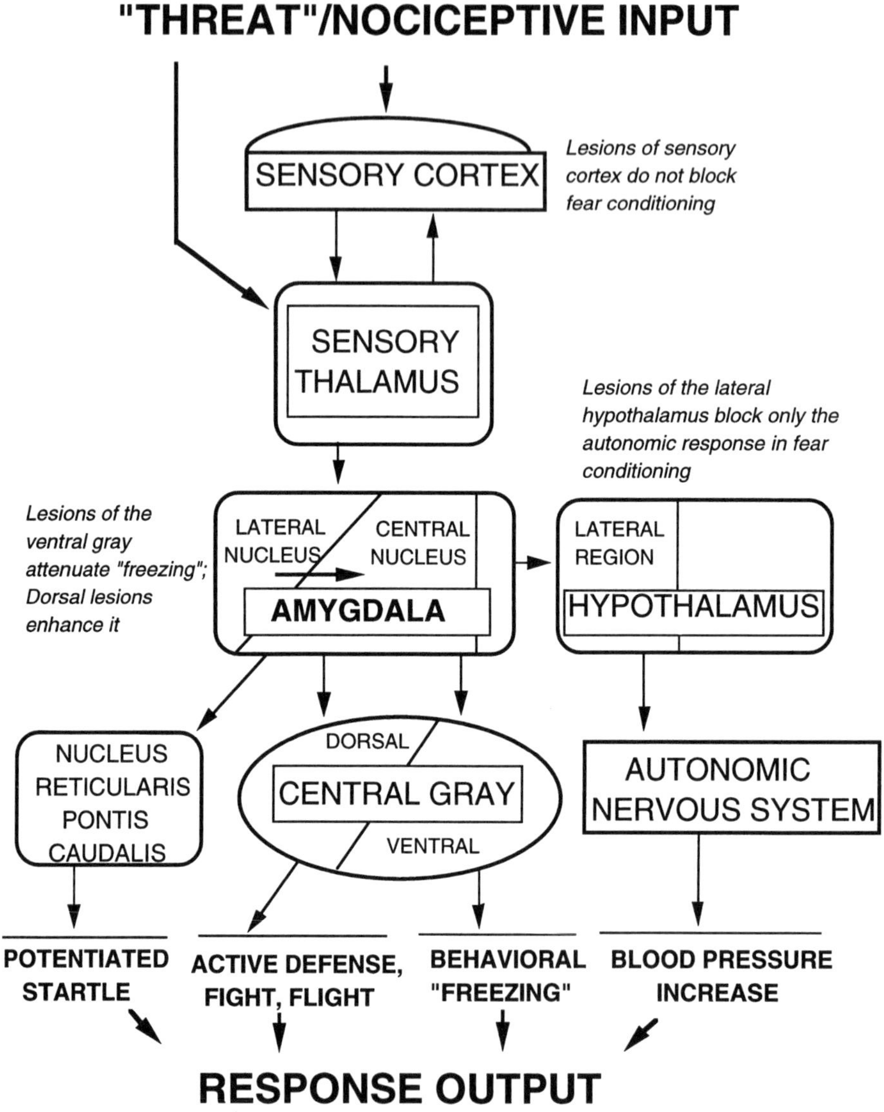

"THREAT"/NOCICEPTIVE INPUT

SENSORY CORTEX — *Lesions of sensory cortex do not block fear conditioning*

SENSORY THALAMUS

Lesions of the lateral hypothalamus block only the autonomic response in fear conditioning

Lesions of the ventral gray attenuate "freezing"; Dorsal lesions enhance it

LATERAL NUCLEUS	CENTRAL NUCLEUS
AMYGDALA	

LATERAL REGION	
HYPOTHALAMUS	

NUCLEUS RETICULARIS PONTIS CAUDALIS

DORSAL / CENTRAL GRAY / VENTRAL

AUTONOMIC NERVOUS SYSTEM

| POTENTIATED STARTLE | ACTIVE DEFENSE, FIGHT, FLIGHT | BEHAVIORAL "FREEZING" | BLOOD PRESSURE INCREASE |

RESPONSE OUTPUT

Figure 11.2. Fear stimuli proceed from sense receptor systems to the sensory cortex and/or sensory thalamus (see LeDoux, 1990) and then to the amygdala. There are three important connections efferent to the amygdala: (1) a projection from the central amygdala to the lateral hypothalamic area that mediates the autonomic components of the emotional response; (2) projections to the midbrain central gray region mediates defensive freezing and escape behaviors (see Fanselow et al., 1995); and (3) a direct projection to the nucleus reticularis pontis caudalis modulates the startle reflex (see Davis, 1989, 1997, for details).

1999); subsets of these materials have been normed in children and the elderly as well. There are approximately 120 digitized sounds currently included in the IADS, and more than 1000 verbal stimuli in ANEW, all of which similarly include affective norms for ratings of pleasure and arousal (Bradley & Lang, 1999). New materials are continuously being added to each stimulus collection. The goal is to encourage standardization, selection, and replication in emotion research within and across research sites, and, to date, hundreds of laboratories in the United States and abroad have requested these materials, currently distributed on compact disk.[1]

Affective Report

The affective norms included with each stimulus collection are acquired by asking groups of subjects to rate the pleasantness, arousal, and dominance of each stimulus, using the Self-Assessment Manikin (SAM) affective rating system devised by Lang (1980). In this system, a graphic (nonverbal) figure depicts each dimension on a continuously varying scale. SAM ranges from a smiling, happy figure to a frowning, unhappy figure when representing the valence dimension; for arousal, SAM ranges from an excited, wide-eyed figure to a relaxed, sleepy figure; for dominance, SAM ranges from a large figure (in control) to a small figure (completely controlled). In addition to a paper-and-pencil version (9-point scales), SAM also exists as a dynamic computer display on a variety of different systems, including IBM (20-point scale; Cook et al., 1987) systems. The SAM measures of pleasure and arousal correlate well with ratings on these dimensions obtained using the longer, verbal semantic differential scale (Bradley & Lang, 1994).

The photographs in the IAPS represent a wide range of semantic categories, and include pictures of babies, erotica, romantic couples, sports events, food, nature scenes, household objects, domestic and dangerous animals, guns, cemeteries, mutilated bodies, and more. In both the upper graphs in figure 11.3, each IAPS picture is located in the portion of the emotional space defined by its mean pleasure and arousal rating. The affective space for male subjects is depicted on the left and for female subjects on the right. There are several characteristic features of the resulting space. First, these materials evoke reactions across the entire range of each dimension: mean pleasure ratings for these pictures range from extremely unpleasant to extremely pleasant, and are distributed fairly evenly across the valence dimension. Similarly, a wide range of arousal levels are elicited by these materials. Second, it is clear that pleasant pictures range continuously along the arousal dimension: the upper half of emotional space has exemplars at many positions along this dimension. These data suggest that the degree of arousal is uncorrelated with the pleasantness of the slide. Pictures depicting unpleasant events tend, however, to cluster in the arousal quadrant of emotional space; there are fewer highly unpleasant items located in the calm quadrant. Finally, for items rated as neutral in valence (i.e., those occurring at or near the midline of the valence dimension), arousal ratings do not attain the high levels associated with either pleasant or unpleasant materials.

Figure 11.3 (bottom panels) shows that the distribution of stimuli in affective space is similar both for the sounds in the IADS (bottom left panel) and the words in ANEW (bottom right panel). The overall boomerang-shaped distribution for all

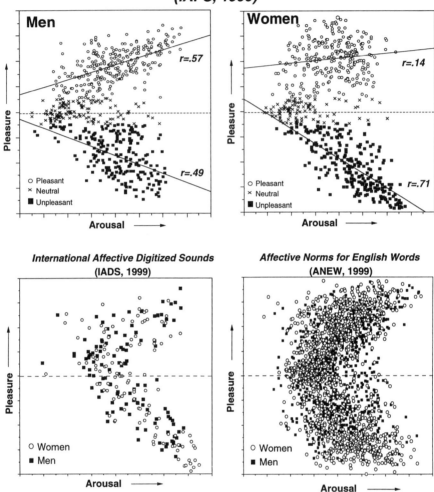

Figure 11.3. Distribution of pictures (top panels), sounds (bottom left panel), and English words (bottom right panel) currently collected in the International Affective Picture System (IAPS; Lang et al., 1999), International Affective Digitized Sounds (Bradley & Lang, 1999b), and Affective Norms for English Words (Bradley & Lang, 1999a), respectively. Each set of materials is plotted in a two-dimensional affective space, defined by mean ratings of pleasure (ordinate) and arousal (abscissa) for each stimulus. The shape of the distributions is similar in each stimulus modality, consistent with the hypothesis that emotion stems from two underlying neural systems, appetitive and defensive, that each vary in arousal. In the top panels, the a priori valence of the IAPS pictures (e.g., pleasant, neutral, and unpleasant) is indicated to highlight the fact that men and women show characteristic differences in their affective ratings (see text). Similar sex differences can be seen in the bottom panels, in which the ratings of men and women for sound and word stimuli are illustrated in each plot.

of these stimuli indicates two arms that extend from a common calm, nonaffective base toward either the high-arousal pleasant or the high-arousal unpleasant quadrant. This organization is consistent with an underlying bimotivational structure, involving two systems of appetitive and aversive motivation that each vary along a dimension of intensity or arousal.

The distribution of stimulus materials in affective space obtained in groups of subjects is not necessarily found in all individuals. There are, for example, pattern characteristics that vary with sex. As illustrated in figure 11.3 (top left panel), if only positively valent pictures are considered, ratings by men show a high correlation between increasing affective valence and increasing arousal. For women (top right panel), this relationship is somewhat weaker; the most pleasant stimuli are not rated as highly arousing. In contrast, if only unpleasant pictures are considered, women's ratings now show a high correlation between valence and arousal, whereas this covariation is less pronounced for men.

These differences in the pattern of affective reports for men and women may reflect different motive emphases in the two sexes. Men are more likely to report high pleasure for arousing adventure and sexual stimuli. On the other hand, women report stronger unpleasant reactions to pictures of threatening events or victimization. Women's ratings are consistent with a stronger protective or defensive orientation, increased fearfulness, and a primary disposition to avoid danger. To consider the extremes of this orientation, it may be this disposition that underlies the greater incidence of anxiety disorders in women than in men. Men, on the other hand, are more likely to be sensation seekers and to be sexually aggressive. To again consider extremes, men are more likely than women to be psychopaths.

The nature of the distribution also varies across the life span (figure 11.4). For young females (ages 4–7), stimuli are roughly clustered in three groups of pleasant, neutral, and unpleasant materials, with little differentiation along the arousal dimension (McManis et al., 1998). By adolescence, however, the distribution is quite similar to that obtained in the IAPS norms for female college students (figure 11.3, top right panel). For mature women (i.e., ages 50–79), the nature of the distribution has shifted dramatically, with a relatively more linear relationship between ratings of pleasure and arousal (Cuthbert et al., 1988). For the older women, if something is pleasant, it is also judged to be generally lower in arousal than for pictures rated as unpleasant. The linear relationship between pleasure and arousal found for mature adults is even more pronounced in adults who are diagnosed with an anxiety disorder, who rate pictures that are highly arousing as unpleasant in affective valence as well (Cuthbert et al., 1999).

Differences in the distribution of emotional stimuli may also reflect specific deficits in appetitive or aversive motivational systems. In a case study, we asked a patient who had undergone ablation of the right amygdala to view and rate a set of IAPS pictures (Morris et al., 1991). The resulting distribution is illustrated in figure 11.5 (left panel) and indicates that ratings of affective valence between this patient and a control sample were similar: pictures were rated as varying normally in pleasantness, with mutilations rated as extremely unpleasant, and erotica, sports, and families rated as high in pleasure. On the other hand, the distribution of arousal ratings for this patient differed dramatically from the norm: whereas pleasant materials were rated as high in arousal, unpleasant pictures were consistently rated as

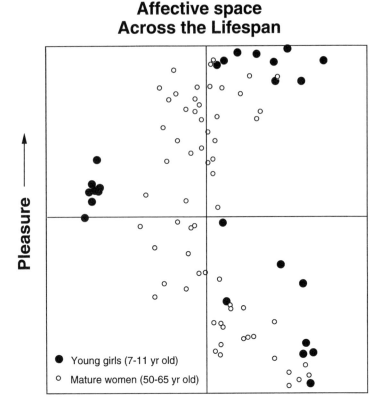

Figure 11.4. Affective ratings of emotional pictures for young girls and mature women illustrate changes across the life span. Whereas young girls find both pleasant and unpleasant pictures exciting, they do not make fine discriminations in arousal. For mature women, pictures rated as arousing tend to also be rated as unpleasant.

calm as were neutral stimuli, and the normally densely filled unpleasant–high arousal quadrant was relatively empty for this patient. This distribution was consistent with family reports that the patient was unable to respond with much urgency to aversive events following surgery, relative to before the amygdala was removed.

Psychophysiological Response

Assuming that emotion is organized by the brain's motivational systems, physiological and behavioral reactions to affective stimuli should also reflect this organization, covarying significantly with judgments of affective valence and/or arousal. To assess this hypothesis, we presented IAPS pictures to subjects in a number of different studies and measured facial muscle action (corrugator and zygomatic),

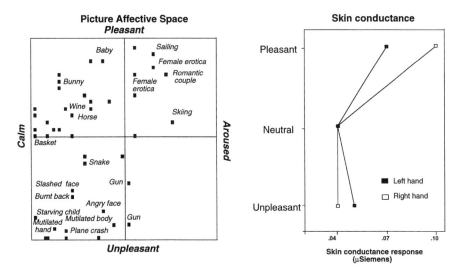

Figure 11.5. Affective ratings (left panel) and skin conductance responses (right panel) when viewing emotional pictures are depicted for a patient who had undergone a right temporal lobectomy. The distribution of pictures in affective space varies from the norm in that unpleasant pictures are consistently rated as low, rather than as high, in arousal. Consistent with these arousal ratings, electrodermal reactions when viewing unpleasant (but not pleasant) pictures are also absent for this patient.

heart rate, skin conductance, and/or electrocortical activity. We also collected post-viewing reports of pleasure and arousal and recorded the time they spent looking at each picture in a free-viewing context.

Patterns of physiological reactivity can be assessed both on the basis of the a priori groupings of pictures (i.e., determined by IAPS norms), as well as by each participant's self-reports of pleasure and arousal obtained during psychophysiological assessment sessions. In the latter method, reports of experienced pleasure and arousal are related to physiological response by ranking the picture stimuli from low to high for each subject on the basis of their own affective judgments. Then the mean activity in each physiological system is assessed at each rank, across subjects. This strategy optimizes the opportunity to observe unit changes in physiology coincident with changes in affective judgments, and provides a meaningful index of affective covariation for reports of emotion and physiological and behavioral events. Several of these relationships are described below, based on recent research (e.g., Greenwald et al., 1989; Lang et al., 1993).

- Corrugator Muscle

The corrugator muscles are responsible for a lowering and contraction of the brows, a facial action held to be an index of distress (see Ekman & Freissen, 1986; Fridlund & Izard, 1983, for a review). Thus, a significant firing of motor units in this muscle is expected when a picture (or sound) is judged to be unpleasant (even if the degree of unit activity is insufficient to produce visible brow movement). In our research, significant contraction of this muscle occurs when a picture is rated as unpleasant (see figure 11.6, top left panel). The corrugator response is modest (but still above baseline) when viewing neutral materials, and the muscle often shows relaxation below baseline activity for materials rated as highly pleasant. The dimensional correlation between valence reports and corrugator electromyographic (EMG) activity is quite high: when corrugator EMG activity is averaged over pictures ranked from most to least pleasant for each subject, a strong linear relationship is obtained between pleasure judgments and corrugator EMG activity (figure 11.7, top left panel). Moreover, more than 80% of the subjects (Lang et al., 1993) show the expected (negative) correlation between ratings of pleasure and corrugator EMG activity.

- Zygomatic Muscle

Activity of the zygomatic muscle is involved in the smile response. Zygomatic activity increases for stimuli which subjects rate as pleasant, is greatest for materials judged to be high in affective valence, and almost nonexistent for pictures rated in moderate regions of the valence dimension. For materials rated as most unpleas-

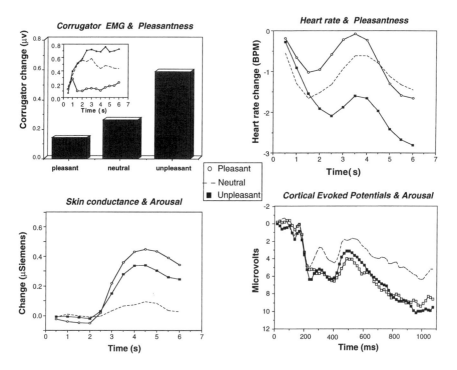

Figure 11.6. Patterns of physiological response measured as a function of the a priori valence ratings of IAPS pictures (based on normative ratings) demonstrate that facial corrugator electromyographic (EMG) activity (top left panel) and heart rate (top right panel) vary as a function of picture valence, whereas skin conductance activity (bottom left panel) and cortical evoked potentials (bottom right panel) vary with picture arousal.

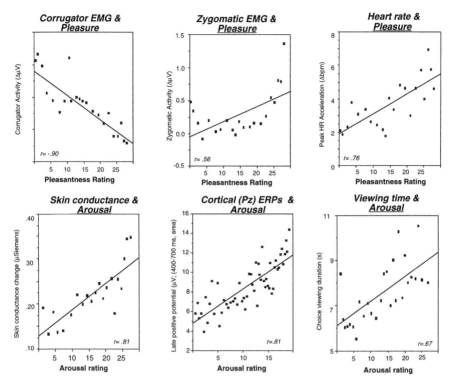

Figure 11.7. The correlation between individual's affective judgments of pleasure (top row) and arousal (bottom row) with their physiological and behavioral responses to picture stimuli. Corrugator electromyograph EMG (top left), zygomatic EMG (top middle), and heart rate (top right) each vary consistently with differences in rated pleasure. On the other hand, skin conductance (bottom left), cortical evoked potentials (bottom middle) and viewing time (bottom right) vary consistently with differences in arousal ratings. In each plot, affective judgments are rank ordered for each subject; the graphs depict the mean responses at each rank across subjects.

ant, often scenes of mutilation and death, there is a tendency for zygomatic activity to increase again. The activation of the zygomatic muscle in addition to increases in corrugator response suggests that a facial grimace may accompany perception of some aversive materials. Because of the slight increase in zygomatic EMG activity at the unpleasant end of the valence continuum (and the significant increase at the positive end), there is a reliable quadratic correlation between reports of judged pleasantness and zygomatic EMG activity, in addition to a significant linear correlation (figure 11.7, top middle panel).

Interestingly, roughly two-thirds of female subjects tend to show a relationship between zygomatic EMG activity and affective valence, whereas only a quarter of male subjects respond in this manner. This significant gender difference indicates that the expression of emotion might primarily involve different response systems in females and males, with women more facially expressive than men. Identical findings for facial EMG responses and gender were obtained by Schwartz et al. (1980) when emotional imagery, rather than picture viewing, was the foreground activity.

- Heart Rate

When viewing pictures, a classic triphasic pattern of heart rate response is obtained, with an initial deceleration (usually taken as an index of orienting, or intake), followed by an acceleratory component, and a secondary deceleration (see figure 11.6, top right panel). Affective valence contributes to the amount of initial deceleration and acceleratory activity, with unpleasant stimuli producing more initial deceleration, and pleasant stimuli producing greater peak acceleration. Klorman et al. (1975) also found greater cardiac deceleration when viewing unpleasant pictures, especially for subjects who were not highly fearful of the slide contents.

The dimensional covariation between valence and cardiac rate is modest (figure 11.7, top right panel). As an index of emotional state, cardiac rate is less straightforward than other physiological measures. During motor preparation, for example, substantial changes in heart rate can occur, even though cue stimuli are not strongly affective (Graham, 1979; Lacey & Lacey, 1970). Furthermore, the primary direction of heart rate change varies with the type of mental processing (e.g., heart rate is accelerative in recalling memory images and decelerative in orienting to external stimuli) (Lang et al., 1990). Finally, because rate is just one of several interacting variables in the cardiovascular system, such factors as posture, respiratory anomalies, and individual physical differences (body weight, fitness) all conspire to obscure affective covariation. Nonetheless, when the processing context is controlled and the subject is passive and oriented, as in the picture-viewing paradigm, group effects of affective valence are evident. There is significantly greater heart rate deceleration for unpleasant pictures, and relatively greater peak acceleration for pleasant materials, particularly during the first viewing (Bradley et al., 1993c).

- Skin Conductance

Electrodermal activity is a useful measure of arousal. It is thought to be innervated solely by the sympathetic nervous system, whose output results in a broad state of activation. Indeed, in recent studies, the amount of skin conductance activity increased linearly as ratings of arousal increased, regardless of emotional valence (see figure 11.6, lower left panel). When plotted as a function of a priori valence, a significant quadratic pattern is obtained, in which reactivity is generally higher when viewing either pleasant or unpleasant, compared to neutral materials. Winton et al. (1984) obtained similar data indicating larger skin conductance responses to slides that were rated as highly pleasant and highly unpleasant. Manning and Melchiori (1974) also observed this skin conductance pattern when the stimulus items were words that were rated as highly pleasant (e.g., sex) and highly unpleasant (e.g., violence).

That skin conductance varies consistently with reports of arousal is evident when assessing the dimensional correlation between arousal ratings and skin conductance: a significant linear relationship emerges in which unit increases in rated arousal (regardless of valence) are associated with an increase in electrodermal reactivity (see figure 11.7, lower left panel). More than 80% of the subjects in the Lang et al. (1993) study showed a positive correlation between arousal reports and conductance response. Interestingly, a larger proportion of males showed a significant correlation (46%) relative to females (16%). Thus, whereas females are more facially expressive, males are more reactive in the electrodermal system.

Figure 11.5 (right panel) illustrates skin conductance responses for patient S.L., who, as discussed earlier, rated unpleasant materials as low in arousal, unlike most normal subjects. To the extent that his reactions are concordant across response systems, one would expect to see a lack of conductivity response specifically to unpleasant pictures for this patient. This is clearly the case: whereas his responses to pleasant pictures are larger than for neutral stimuli, he fails to respond in the electrodermal system specifically for unpleasant pictures rated low in arousal. Thus, this patient not only verbally reports a lack of arousal associated with aversive picture stimulation, but a physiological index of sympathetic reactivity is also absent.

- Cortical Event-Related Potentials and
  Slow Wave Activity

When EEG activity is measured during picture viewing, specific event-related potentials and sustained positive slow wave activity are both observed in response to emotionally arousing picture stimuli, irrespective of affective valence (Crites & Cacioppo, 1996; Cuthbert et al., 1999; Palomba et al., 1997). As figure 11.6 (bottom right panel) illustrates, positive-going cortical evoked potentials starting at about 400 msec after picture presentation are larger for both pleasant or unpleasant, compared to neutral, materials, and a slow, sustained positivity is maintained until the picture is terminated. The dimensional correlation between ratings of arousal and cortical positivity (measured at its maximum between 400–700 msec) is also quite high (see figure 11.7, lower middle panel), indicating that activity measured from the cortical surface indicates that an emotional (i.e., arousing) stimulus is the focus of processing. Because emotionally evocative pictures are consistently rated as more interesting and more complex than neutral, low-arousal images (Bradley et al., 1993b; Lang et al., 1990), these cortical effects may also reflect a variation in attentional engagement that covaries with judged affective arousal.

- Summary: Affective Patterns in
  Physiological Responses

Taken together, the data reviewed above are consistent with the hypothesis that motivational variables of affective valence and arousal predominate in organizing physiological and subjective reports of affective reactions. Supporting this, factor analyses conducted on self-report, physiological, and behavioral measures have consistently produced a strong two-factor solution (e.g., Cuthbert et al., 1998; Lang et al., 1993). As table 11.2 illustrates, the first factor involves high loadings for pleasantness ratings, heart rate change, facial muscle activity, and startle reflex, consistent with the interpretation that this is a primary valence factor of appetite or aversion. A second factor involves high loadings for rated experience of arousal, viewing time, skin conductance, and cortical slow waves, which identifies an

TABLE 11.2. Factor Analyses of Measures of Emotional
Picture Processing: Sorted Loadings of Dependent
Measures on Principal Components

Measure	Factor 1 (valence)	Factor 2 (arousal)
From Lang et al. (1993)		
Valence ratings	0.86	−0.00
Corrugator muscle[a]	−0.85	0.19
Heart rate	0.79	−0.14
Zygomatic muscle[a]	0.58	0.29
Arousal ratings	0.15	0.83
Interest ratings	0.45	0.77
Viewing time	−0.27	0.76
Skin conductance	−0.37	0.74
From Cuthbert et al. (1998)		
Valence ratings	0.89	0.07
Corrugator muscle[a]	−0.83	−0.10
Heart rate	0.73	−0.02
Arousal ratings	−0.11	0.89
Cortical slow wave	−0.06	−0.79
Skin conductance	0.19	0.77

[a]Bioelectric potentials from muscles that mediate facial expression.

arousal or intensity factor. The cross-loadings for all measures are low. Thus, affects are built around motivational determinants.

• Neural Imaging: Activation of the Visual Cortex

Newer technologies for measuring brain correlates of affective processing promise to facilitate our understanding of how and where emotion is processed in the brain. Several methods of brain imaging are now available that assess regional neural activity indirectly through variations in blood flow, including positron emission tomography (PET) and functional magnetic resonance imaging (fMRI).

Using the PET method, Lane and co-workers (1997) examined regions of brain activity in a group of female subjects viewing pleasant, neutral, and unpleasant pictures from the IAPS collection. Both pleasant and unpleasant pictures prompted more activity in the thalamus and in the medial prefrontal cortex than did neutral pictures. Interestingly, large increases in activity were also obtained for unpleasant pictures in extrastriate visual cortex (e.g., Brodmann's visual areas 18 and 19) relative to neutral pictures. In contrast, pleasant pictures did not show more activity than did neutral stimuli in occipital cortex. This finding is consistent with skin conductance recordings taken coincident with the PET measurement. That is, for this sample of 10 female subjects, pleasant pictures tended to prompt less electrodermal activity than did unpleasant materials, suggesting pleasant pictures were not as emotionally arousing as were the unpleasant. For male subjects, PET activity during highly arousing pleasant pictures (e.g., erotica) clearly shows increased activity in visual occipital cortex (Lane et al., 1999).

We recently extended the exploration of brain activity during emotional picture processing to an analysis using fMRI (Lang et al., 1998). Among the advantages of using fMRI are that the method does not require insertion of a radioactive tracer into the body, it allows a faster rate of data acquisition (permitting analysis of individual pictures), and it results in more accurate spatial resolution of brain tissue activation, both within and between subjects. In our study, functional brain activity was monitored in both female ($n = 8$) and male ($n = 12$) subjects from four coronal slices in the occipital cortex. Data were collected while subjects viewed blocks of pleasant, neutral, or unpleasant pictures. The pictures were each presented for a 12-second "on" period, and signal intensities were compared to those obtained during a preceding 12-second "off" period of equal duration, in which no visual stimulus was presented.

In one analysis of functional activity during picture viewing, the number of active voxels during picture processing (compared to no visual stimulation) was calculated and expressed as a proportion of the total number of voxels in a region and averaged across subjects. Figure 11.8 (bottom panel) illustrates the pattern of functional activation that resulted: significantly more extensive activation was obtained when subjects were viewing emotional, compared to neutral, pictures. This pattern was obtained throughout the regions of the brain sampled in this study, including both the right and left hemispheres and both the anterior and posterior occipital slices.

In a second analysis, localization of differential activity was accomplished by averaging functional maps across subjects transformed into the standard Talairach-Tournoux coordinates. Whereas processing any type of picture produced activation in Brodmann's area 17 in the calcarine fissure, areas specific to processing emotional stimuli were apparent in Brodmann's areas 18 (see figure 11.8, top panel) and 19, in the fusiform gyrus, and at parietal sites. Paralleling the PET data described above (Lane et al., 1997), females showed significantly more activation (particularly in the right hemisphere) when processing unpleasant pictures than did men. Conversely, men tended to show more extensive activation when viewing pleasant pictures.

The above experiment was replicated (using the same pictures) in an apparatus that appeared physically similar to the MRI scanning context, but which had no magnetic field. This permitted easy recording of psychophysiological data. As expected, larger skin conductance responses were found for arousing emotional stimuli, regardless of valence, compared to neutral pictures. As already noted, this is a general finding for conductance (and also for the cortical slow waves in the EEG). In contrast, eye movement activity did not vary with picture content, eliminating this variable as a source of artifact in evaluating the fMRI finding of differential visual system activation in emotion.

The fMRI data suggest that emotional inputs undergo more processing than nonaffective stimuli at a relatively early stage in cortical afferent analysis. One explanation is based on research findings with animal subjects (Amaral et al., 1992), which suggests that reentrant projections from the amygdala feed back to primary visual cortex. The PET experiment results (Lane et al., 1997) are not

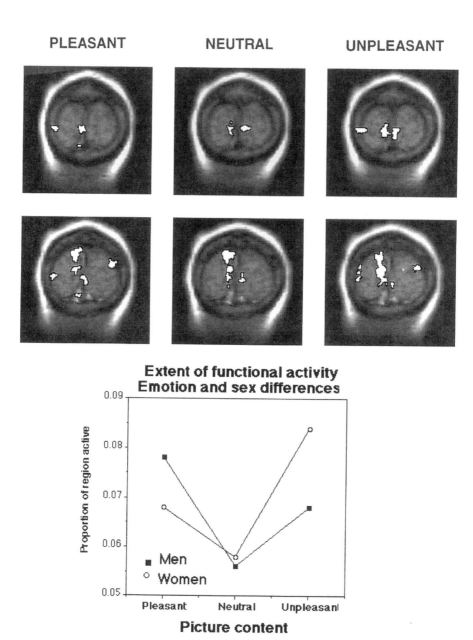

PLEASANT   **NEUTRAL**   **UNPLEASANT**

Extent of functional activity
Emotion and sex differences

Proportion of region active

■ Men
○ Women

Pleasant   Neutral   Unpleasant
Picture content

Figure 11.8. (Top) Sites of functional activity in the visual cortex during processing of pleasant (left column), neutral (center column), and unpleasant (right column) pictures, compared to no picture processing, as determined from averaging functional maps across subjects. All picture contents show activity centered on the calcarine fissure, as well as in a portion of area 18 directly above the calcarine fissure. Only emotional pictures show bi-lateral activity in the occipital gyrus. (Bottom) The extent of functional activity in occipital cortex is greater for emotionally arousing (pleasant or unpleasant) pictures compared to neutral pictures for all subjects. Women show significantly more activation for unpleasant pictures compared to men, whereas men show a tendency for more extensive activation when viewing pleasant pictures.

inconsistent with this view, in that activity temporally coincident with occipital activation was apparent in the left ventral temporal stream (which could include the amygdala). Furthermore, Irwin et al. (1996) have reported significant differences in amygdaloid activation between people viewing unpleasant, compared to neutral, IAPS pictures, supporting the hypothesis of differential amygdala activation for emotional stimuli. A second hypothesis is based on Posner's (1996) view that projections from cingulate cortex determine attentional priming of the visual area. These different anatomical hypotheses can be tested with newer fMRI methods that permit imaging of the whole brain during picture processing, in which presumed connections between neural structures can be assessed by analyzing coincident and lagged cross-correlations between regions of functional brain activity.

Emotional Priming

Emotional responses elicited during picture viewing presumably reflect the engagement of neural structures and pathways, many subcortical, in either the appetitive or aversive motivation systems. This system activation is assumed to prepare the subject for taking action appropriate to the current motivational state. During the period when motivational circuitry is active, the brain's processing operations are modulated in ways that prepare one to cope with appetitive or aversive events. Specifically, associations, representations, and action programs linked to the engaged motivational system are primed. Priming results in a higher probability that these representations will be accessed (with a concomitant greater potential output strength) than other information. Conversely, mental events and programs linked to the nonengaged system have a reduced probability and strength of activation (Lang, 1994). Thus, if the defensive motivational system is dominant (i.e., the affective state is unpleasant), responses to aversive cues are primed, and at the same time, responses to appetitive cues may be reduced or absent.

The most primitive and fundamental motivational priming is at the level of unconditioned reflexes. Thus, an independently evoked defensive reflex will be augmented when the organism is already reacting to an aversive foreground stimulus (i.e., is in an unpleasant state); this same reflex will be reduced in amplitude when the organism is processing an appetitive foreground. Both of these priming effects (potentiation and diminution of responding) are expected to be enhanced according to the level of affective drive or activation.

The startle response has proven to be a convenient defensive reflex for testing these hypotheses (see Bradley et al., 1999, for a review). Startle is a primitive reflex that serves a protective function, helping to avoid organ injury (as in the eyeblink) and acting as a behavioral interrupt (Graham, 1979), clearing processors to deal with possible threat. According to the motivational priming hypothesis, the defensive startle reflex should be of significantly greater amplitude (and faster) when the aversive motivational system is active (e.g., as in a fear state). This was first examined systematically by Brown et al. (1951), who compared reflex responses to startle probes (shots from a toy pistol) presented to rats during neutral or shock-conditioned stimuli at extinction. Results conformed to expectation: animals did indeed react more forcefully, as measured by a stabilimeter in the floor of the cage, when the startle stimuli were presented during fear-conditioned signals (see also Ross, 1961; Spence & Runquist, 1958).

The Rat Brain's Fear-Startle Circuit

Davis and his associates (e.g., Davis, 1989, 1997; Davis et al., 1987) and others (Fendt et al., 1994) have gathered considerable evidence that the brain structure mediating fear-conditioned startle potentiation is, at least in the rat, the same aversive system previously described. As Davis (1997) has shown, after stimulation of the ear by an abrupt noise, the afferent path of the startle reflex proceeds from the cochlear nucleus to the reticular formation; from there efferent connections pass through spinal neurons to the reflex effectors. This is the basic obligatory circuit, directly driven by the parameters of the input stimulus (e.g., stimulus intensity, frequency, steepness of the onset ramp).

Startle potentiation though learned fear implies that a secondary circuit modulates this primary reflex pathway. There is now overwhelming evidence that the amygdala, the key structure in aversively motivated behavior, is a critical part of this modulatory circuit (see figure 11.2). First, it has been shown that there are direct, monosynaptic projections from the amygdala to the key reticular site (i.e., to the structure in the basic circuit on which modulation of the reflex depends). Second, electrical stimulation of the amygdala (below the level for kindling) directly enhances startle reflex amplitude. Finally, and most important, lesions of the amygdala abolish fear-conditioned startle potentiation.

The Startle Reflex in Humans

In studies with human beings, rapid eye closure is one of the most reliable components of the behavioral cascade that constitutes the startle reflex. The magnitude of the blink can be measured by monitoring the orbicularis oculi muscle, using electrodes placed just beneath the lower lid.The acoustic stimulus used to evoke the blink is relatively modest—typically a 50-msec burst of white noise at around 95 decibels which, while prompting a clear blink response, rarely interferes with ongoing foreground tasks.

Many studies have now confirmed reliable potentiation of the blink response in humans following simple shock exposure or as a function of learned associations that parallel the modulatory patterns obtained with rats (e.g., Greenwald et al., 1998; Hamm et al., 1993). In brief, the blink response to a startle probe is generally larger after subjects experience electric shock and selectively larger to startle probes presented during exposure to a shock-conditioned stimulus than to probes presented during exposure to an unshocked control stimulus. These results, coupled with clinical neurological evidence linking the amygdala to aversive emotion (Aggleton, 1992), encourage the hypothesis that similar neural pathways might be responsible for potentiation effects in both rats and human beings.

Probing Emotional Perception

Startle potentiation during learned fear implies that this reflex is primed when the defensive motivational system is active. To assess reflex inhibition in the context of appetitive activation, we presented startle probes while subjects were viewing a series of pleasant, neutral, or unpleasant pictures selected from the IAPS. When startle probes are administered in this context, results have consistently conformed to the motivational priming hypothesis: As figure 11.9 (top panel) illustrates, a significant linear trend is reliably observed over judged picture valence, with the blink responses potentiated when viewing unpleasant pictures and inhibited when viewing pleasant pictures, compared to neutral picture processing (e.g., Bradley et al., 1990, 1991, 1993a,c, 1995; Cook et al., 1991; Patrick et al., 1993; Vrana et al., 1988).

Affective modulation of the startle response has proved highly replicable and seems ubiquitous. Balaban (1995) found modulation of the startle reflex even in five-month-old infants looking at angry or happy faces. Furthermore, affective modulation is not confined to visual percepts. When the foreground stimuli consist of short, six-second sound clips of various affective events (e.g., sounds of love making; babies crying; bombs bursting) and the startle probe is a visual light flash, the same affect-startle effect is obtained, suggesting that its mediation is broadly motivational and thus consistent across affective foregrounds of differing stimulus modality (Bradley & Lang, in press). The startle reflex is also modulated by affective valence when affective films (Jansen and Frijda, 1994) or odors (Erlichman et al., 1995) constitute the foreground stimuli. Finally, affective modulation of the startle reflex is obtained during picture viewing regardless of whether the startle probe is visual, acoustic, or tactile (e.g., Bradley et al., 1990; Hawk & Cook, 1997), indicating that modality-specific processes are not central in these modulatory effects.

Emotional modulation of the reflex also does not depend on novelty. It persists with the repeated presentation of either the same or different picture stimuli. That is, while there is an overall diminution of the startle reflex over blocks of trials, affective potentiation and inhibition remain even when the same pictures are repeatedly presented (see figure 11.9; Bradley et al., 1993c). Similarly, affective modulation persists when the same (or a different) set of pictures is viewed in separate experimental sessions (Bradley et al., 1995).

For picture stimuli, the startle reflex is reliably affected by affective valence as early as 500 msec after picture presentation and is maintained throughout a 6-sec viewing interval (Bradley et al., 1993a). The same temporal pattern of modulatory effects occurs regardless of whether the subject ignores or attends to the startle probe (Bradley et al., in press), suggesting that affective modulation is not secondary to modality-driven attentional processes. Interestingly, it is not necessary for the actual picture stimulus to be present. When the picture is removed from view at 500 msec, strong effects of affective valence on reflex modulation are obtained for up to 3 sec, suggesting that the startle stimulus probes processing in the "mind's eye," that is, even when the stimulus is not perceptually available (Codispoti et al., 1998).

Consistent with the motivational priming hypothesis, modulatory effects on the startle reflex also appear to increase with greater activation in each motive system. That is, probe startle potentiation is largest for unpleasant pictures that are rated most arousing, while conversely, the most arousing pleasant pictures prompt the greatest probe startle inhibition (Cuthbert et al., 1996). Figure 11.9 (bottom panel) illustrates reflex modulation for pleasant and unpleasant pictures as they

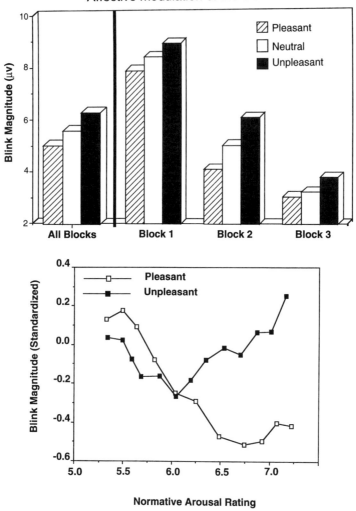

Figure 11.9. (Top) The startle reflex is clearly modulated by affective valence, with blinks elicited when viewing unpleasant pictures potentiated,
and blinks evoked when viewing pleasant pictures inhibited, compared to
neutral stimuli. Although the overall magnitude of the blink reflex decreases (i.e., habituates) with repeated presentation, affective modulation
of the startle reflex continues to occur even when the same pictures are repeatedly presented. (Bottom) Startle potentiation for unpleasant pictures increases with increases in rated arousal, and blink inhibition for pleasant
pictures increases with rated arousal, demonstrating that affective startle
modulation is strongest for intense emotional pictures.

vary in rated arousal. For pleasant pictures, startle reflex magnitude decreases progressively with increases in rated arousal. For aversive pictures, an initial reduction in blink magnitude is also suggested, with somewhat greater reflex inhibition as arousal begins to increase. Somewhat farther along the scale, however, the direction of reflex modulation is abruptly reversed: startle magnitude begins to increase, peaking for pictures judged unpleasant and highest in arousal level.

In many ways, this change in the direction of the reflex response, associated with increasing arousal of unpleasant pictures, is reminiscent of Sokolov's (1963) description of how orienting changes to defense with increasing intensity of physical stimulation after a period of oscillation between the two responses. It is also consistent with Miller's (1959) classic conflict theory (for a recent assessment, see Cacioppo & Berntson, 1994), in which behavior is assumed to be driven by activation along gradients of approach and avoidance. Modeling startle modulation from this perspective, and considering that aversive pictures are consistently judged to be more "interesting" as well as more unpleasant than neutral pictures, reflex magnitude might be expected to be inhibited up to the point of gradient intersection. That is, reflex inhibition to unpleasant stimuli of moderate arousal reflects activation related to orienting, a key feature of appetitive motivation. The abrupt change to increasing startle potentiation reflects the subsequent dominance of avoidance motivation, as stimuli become more unpleasant and threatening.

The Defense Cascade

When reflex magnitude is considered together with other measures of affective reactivity, it is clear that different response systems change in different ways as arousal increases. For instance, like normal subjects, specific phobics show potentiated startles when viewing unpleasant pictures. Startle reflexes are even more enhanced when these subjects view pictures of their own phobic objects, however (Hamm et al., 1997; Sabatinelli et al., 1996). Interestingly, the typical bradycardia obtained during unpleasant picture viewing does not characterize the response of phobic subjects to pictures of objects they fear (e.g., Cook & Turpin, 1997; Hamm et al., 1997; Klorman & Ryan, 1980; Klorman et al., 1977). Rather, when these highly fearful subjects view pictures of the phobic object, the sympathetic system dominates and the heart accelerates. Also, unlike average subjects, they quickly terminate looking in a free-viewing situation. Thus, whereas reflex potentiation to aversive materials characterizes responses for highly arousing unpleasant pictures for both normal and phobic subjects, cardiac and other behavioral measures of attentive orienting are absent when phobics process highly fearful content.

Thus, instead of a single response indicating activation of the defensive motivation system and reflected in a wholly parallel way by all measures, we instead observe a cascade of different response events, changing in different ways and at different levels, as activation increases (see Lang et al., 1997). Attentive orienting is not a response confined only to neutral or pleasant stimuli. As was noted by Lacey (1958), even very unpleasant events can evoke a physiology consistent with sustained attention. Aversive stimulus contents are not automatically "rejected"; rather, attention is allocated to processing them in detail, particularly when they first appear. On the other hand, strong aversive motivation is clearly a major factor in initiating defense.

Figure 11.10 is a diagram prompted by these considerations (Lang et al., 1997). It draws on earlier work by Tinbergen (1951), Blanchard and Blanchard (1989), and Fanselow and colleagues (e.g., Fanselow & Lester, 1988; Fanselow et al., 1995), who have proposed a three-stage continuum of defensive responding based on predator imminence. In their view, three stages of pre-encounter, peri-encounter, and circa-strike are defined on the basis of the proximity of the threatening stimulus, with circa-strike involving defensive actions taken when the threat is proximal. In figure 11.10, stages in the defensive cascade are controlled by increases in judged arousal, an analog to predator imminence. The amplitude of various measures of orienting (and defense) are shown schematically on the ordinate. It is presumed that aversively motivated attending does not fundamentally differ from appetitive orienting at lower levels of activation and involves (1) a brief, modest, parasympathetically driven heart rate deceleration that occurs in reaction to any stimulus change. This bradycardia becomes larger and more sustained as stimuli are perceived to be more arousing. (2) When stimulus arousal is low, sympathetically mediated changes in skin conductance are small and unreliable, but they increase in frequency and amplitude progressively with greater activation. (3) Regardless of the motivational system engaged, reactions to the startle probe are predominantly inhibitory when stimulus activation is not intense. This is consistent with the hypothesis of attentional resource allocation to a meaningful foreground.

Defense responding occurs later in the sequence. Clear evidence that the organism has changed to a defensive posture is first seen in the probe reflex response: when activation is high enough (the threatened nociception more imminent), the organism is defensively primed. The probe stimulus now acts as a trigger that releases a supranormal reflex reaction. The reflex motor reaction is accompanied by heart rate acceleration (Cook & Turpin, 1997) that can accompany the motor reflex potentiation. The degree of potentiation increases with greater activation until the foreground stimulus itself invokes a motivationally relevant action (fight–flight). Startle potentiation occurs primarily in the context of an increasing attentive focus and a parallel, still increasing and dominant bradycardia. Only at the highest activation level, just before action, does the vagus release the heart, giving way subsequently to a sympathetically driven acceleration that is the classical defense response. Thus, for phobic subjects, cardiac acceleration, rather than deceleration, occurs when processing pictures of their feared material because these subjects are further along in the "defense cascade" than normal subjects processing standard unpleasant pictures.

Interestingly, incarcerated psychopaths fail to show startle reflex potentiation for aversive pictures, and instead show reflex inhibition (relative to neutral pictures) when viewing either arousing pleasant or arousing unpleasant picture stimuli (Patrick et al., 1993). This finding, quite different from what is seen in the normal population or in specific phobics, is consistent with the hypothesis that unpleasant pictures are relatively less activating for these individuals, and that their reflex modulation reflects motivated attention, rather than activation of defensive responding. For psychopaths, pictures do not seem to convey the symbolic danger as

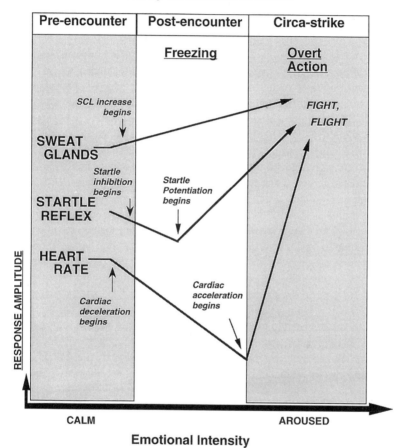

Figure 11.10. A schematic presentation of the defense response cascade underlying processing of increasingly arousing aversive stimuli. The arousal or intensity dimension is viewed here as analogous to a dimension of predator imminence that has been implicated in studies of animal fear. Stimuli presented early in the defense cascade include an initial, partial inhibition of startle probe reflexes, "freezing," immobility, "fear bradycardia," and a focused attentive set. The probability of an overt defensive action increases with increasing stimulus arousal (i.e., predator imminence). This motor disposition is reflected by an increase in potentiated startle to probe stimuli. Heart rate acceleration and a general sympathetic dominance of the autonomic system are characteristic of the period just before overt fight or flight.

with normal subjects, nor do they have the more imminent threat that prompts a phobic reaction. These nonempathic, detached people remain distanced, perhaps only at an early stage in the defense cascade, reflecting a deficit in defense motivation (e.g., Lykken, 1957; Patrick, 1994).

Summary and Conclusions

What are emotions? What are feelings? For many, the exploration of emotional perception offered here will not address the profound meaning of these questions. From the perspective of natural science, however, limited as it is by requirements of operational measurement and community observation, a functional approach was proposed here. We suggest that a fruitful experimental approach begins with the assumption that emotions have evolved from primitive actions that facilitated the survival of individuals and species. These reflexive behaviors, beginning with simple approach to appetitive stimuli and withdrawal from danger and pain, constitute the foundation of motive systems in the brain that underlie affects.

In humans, emotions are more often dispositions to action than the overt behaviors themselves. That is, the evolution of the brain has greatly increased the human repertoire of responses. Delay and inhibition are intrinsic to motivated behaviors in complex species, conferring an increased survival value. Furthermore, the development of language in humans has permitted the symbolic manipulation of events, the organization of behavioral sequences in time, and future planning. Thus, what we call emotions often exist in a behavioral hiatus and are popularly viewed as primarily mental phenomena.

We propose that emotions are better understood as behavioral complexes, organizations of responses that include three broad output systems, including (1) overt acts. Often the emotion modulates secondary behaviors (i.e., as in task deficits prompted by an unrelated stressor); (2) emotional language, which includes both expressive and evaluative responses; and (3) physiological reactions, including changes in the brain and in the somatic and visceral systems that are conceived to be the logistic support of intended action and affective display. The resulting emotional response patterns that are observed across systems have two major determinants: the practical dictates of the specific local context and the consistent emotional strategy of appetite or defense.

The organization of these three-system responses in emotion is founded on activation in two basic motive systems, appetitive and defensive. The subcortical and deep cortical structures that determine primary motivated behavior are similar across mammalian species. Animal research has helped to illuminate these neural systems and define their reflex outputs. Although emotional behavior in humans is often more complex, we have argued that the simpler underlying patterns persist. In this chapter, we have tried to illuminate these basic motivational phenomena in the context of perception. Thus, our research examines humans when processing uniquely human stimuli (primarily picture media, but also words and sounds) and indicates how the underlying motivational structure is apparent in the organization of visceral and behavioral responses, in the priming of simple reflexes, and in the reentrant processing of these symbolic representations in the sensory cortex.

Furthermore, for defensive responding, reactions in different physiological systems appear in the form of a defense cascade, mediated by increases in activation or arousal.

The motivational states elicited by these affective cues (and the somatic, cortical, and autonomic substrates of their perception) are assumed to be fundamentally similar to those occurring when organisms stop, look, and listen, sifting through the environmental buzz for cues of danger, social meaning, and incentives to appetite. In this sense, emotions share an evolutionary link to primitive neural systems (defensive and appetitive) designed to maintain and sustain life. Whereas the strategic foundation of emotion is fully described by parameters of affective valence and arousal, the tactics involved in specific affective contexts vary widely and, indeed, can comprise highly sophisticated behaviors in human subjects (see Lang et al., 1990). It is this tactical diversity of specific emotional expression, dictated by local contexts of loss, pain, anger, and so on, that has made it difficult to understand and categorize emotion. When the local context is constrained and controlled, however, as in picture viewing, clear covariation in physiological, behavioral, and expressive systems occurs as a function of affective valence and arousal, supporting the inference that these parameters are fundamental in organizing emotion.

The motivational approach to emotional perception described in this chapter has proven highly productive. The conception has inspired development of a methodology as well as stimulus materials that have extended our understanding of emotional processing. The biphasic model of emotion proposed here integrates animal and human research, can comprehend the diverse data of emotion (subjective report, behavior, and physiology), and has proved suitable to guide research in many modalities, from analyses of affective language to neural imaging. In our view, emotions are driven by subcortical and deep cortical motivation systems that are part of our evolutionary inheritance. Understanding these systems and their interaction is the primary goal of contemporary research on emotion.

Note

1. The International Affective Picture System (IAPS, 1999), International Affective Digitized Sounds (IADS, 1999) and Affective Norms for English Words (ANEW, 1999) are available on CD-ROM. The IAPS is also available as photographic slides. These stimulus sets and technical manuals can be obtained on request from the authors at the NIMH Center for the Study of Emotion and Attention, Box 100165 HSC, University of Florida, Gainesville, FL 32610-0165, USA.

References

Aggleton, J. P. (1992). *The Amygdala: Neurobiological Aspects of Emotion, Memory, and Mental Dysfunction.* New York: Wiley.
Amaral, D. G., Price, J. L., Pitkanen, A. & Carmichael, S. T. (1992). Anatomical organization of the primate amygdaloid complex. In J. P. Aggleton (Ed), *The Amygdala: Neurobiological Aspects of Emotion, Memory, and Mental Dysfunction* (pp. 1–66). New York: Wiley.

Arnold, M. B. (1945). Physiological differentiation of emotional states. *Psychological Review, 52,* 35–48.

Balaban, M. T. (1995). Affective influences on startle in five-month-old infants: reactions to facial expressions of emotion. *Child Development, 66,* 28–36.

Blanchard, R. J. & Blanchard, D. C. (1989). Attack and defense in rodents as ethoexperimental models for the study of emotion. *Progress in Neuro-Psychopharmacology and Biological Psychiatry, 13,* 3–14.

Bradley, M. M., Cuthbert, B. N. & Lang, P. J. (1990). Startle reflex modification: emotion or attention? *Psychophysiology, 27,* 513–523.

Bradley, M. M., Cuthbert, B. N. & Lang, P. J. (1991). Startle and emotion: lateral acoustic probes and the bilateral blink. *Psychophysiology, 28,* 285–295.

Bradley, M. M., Cuthbert, B. N. & Lang, P. J. (1993a). Pictures as prepulse: attention and emotion in startle modification. *Psychophysiology, 30,* 541–545.

Bradley, M. M. & Lang, P. J. (1999a). *Affective Norms for English Words (ANEW). Technical Manual and Affective Ratings.* Gainesville, FL: The Center for Research in Psychophysiology, University of Florida.

Bradley, M. M. & Lang, P. J. (1999b). *International Affective Digitized Sounds. Technical Manual and Affective Ratings.* Gainesville, FL: The Center for Research in Psychophysiology, University of Florida.

Bradley, M. M., Cuthbert, B. N. & Lang, P. J. (1999) Affect and the startle reflex. In M. E. Dawson, A. Schell & A. Boehmelt (Eds), *Startle Modification: Implications for Neuroscience, Cognitive Science and Clinical Science.* Stanford, CA: Stanford University Press.

Bradley, M. M., Gianaros, P. & Lang, P. J. (1995). As time goes by: stability of affective startle modulation [Abstract]. *Psychophysiology, 32,* 521.

Bradley, M. M., Greenwald, M. K. & Hamm, A. O. (1993b). Affective picture processing. In N. Birbaumer & A. Öhman (Eds), *The Structure of Emotion: Psychophysiological, Cognitive, and Clinical Aspects* (pp. 48–65). Toronto: Hogrefe & Huber.

Bradley, M. M. & Lang, P. J. (1994). Measuring emotion: the self-assessment manikin and the semantic differential. *Journal of Behavioral Therapy and Experimental Psychiatry, 25,* 49–59.

Bradley, M. M., Lang, P. J. & Cuthbert, B. N. (1993c). Emotion, novelty, and the startle reflex: habituation in humans. *Behavioral Neuroscience, 107,* 970–980.

Bradley, M. M. & Lang, P. J. (in press). Affective reactions to acoustic stimuli. *Psychophysiology.*

Brown, J. S., Kalish, H. I. & Farber, I. E. (1951). Conditioned fear as revealed by magnitude of startle response to an auditory stimulus. *Journal of Experimental Psychology, 32,* 317–328.

Cacioppo, J. T. & Bernston, G. G. (1994). Relationships between attitudes and evaluative space: a critical review with emphasis on the separability of positive and negative substrates. *Psychological Bulletin, 115,* 401–423.

Center for the Study of Emotion and Attention. (1999). The International Affective Picture System. Gainesville, FL: University of Florida.

Codispoti, M., Bradley, M. M., Cuthbert, B. N. & Lang, P. J. (1998). Probing the mind's eye: prepulse inhibition and affective modulation of startle for briefly presented pictures. Manuscript submitted for publication.

Cook, E. W. III, Atkinson, L. & Lang, K. G. (1987). Stimulus control and data acquisition for IBM PCs and compatibles. *Psychophysiology, 24,* 726–727.

Cook, E. W. III, Hawk, L. W. Jr., Davis, T. L. & Stevenson, V. E. (1991). Affective individual differences and startle reflex modulation. *Journal of Abnormal Psychology, 100,* 5–13.

Cook, E. & Turpin, G. (1997). Differentiating orienting, startle and defense responses: the role of affect and its implications for psychopathology. In P. J. Lang, R. F. Simons & M. T. Balaban (Eds), *Attention and Orienting: Sensory and Motivational Processes* (pp. 137–164). Hillsdale, NJ: Lawrence Erlbaum Associates.

Cuthbert, B. N., Bradley, M. M. & Lang, P. J. (1988). Psychophysiological responses to affective slides across the life span [abstract]. *Psychophysiology, 25*, 441.

Cuthbert, B. N., Bradley, M. M. & Lang, P. J. (1996). Probing picture perception: activation and emotion. *Psychophysiology, 33*, 103–111.

Cuthbert, B. N., Schupp, H. T., Bradley, M. M., Birbaumer, N. & Lang, P. J. (1999). Cortical slow waves: emotional perception and processing. Manuscript submitted for publication.

Cuthbert, B. N., Strauss, C., Drobes, D., Patrick, C. J., Bradley, M. M. & Lang, P. J. (1999). Startle and the anxiety disorders. Manuscript submitted for publication.

Crites, S. L. & Cacioppo, J. T. (1996). Electrocortical differentiation of evaluative and non-evaluative categorizations. *Psychological Science, 7*, 318–321.

Davis, M. (1989). Sensitization of the acoustic startle reflex by footshock. *Behavioral Neuroscience, 103*(3), 495–503.

Davis, M. (1997). The neurophysiological basis of acoustic startle modulation: research on fear motivation and sensory gating. In P. J. Lang, R. F. Simons & M. T. Balaban (Eds), *Attention and Orienting: Sensory and Motivational Processes* (pp. 69–96). Hillsdale, NJ: Lawrence Erlbaum Associates.

Davis, M., Hitchcock, J. & Rosen, J. (1987). Anxiety and the amygdala: pharmacological and anatomical analysis of the fear potentiated startle paradigm. In G. H. Bower (Ed), *Psychology of Learning and Motivation*, vol. 21 (pp. 263–305). New York: Academic Press.

Dickinson, A. & Dearing, M. F. (1979). Appetitive-aversive interactions and inhibitory processes. In A. Dickinson & R. A. Boakes (Eds), *Mechanisms of Learning and Motivation* (pp 203–231). Hillsdale, NJ: Lawrence Erlbaum Associates.

Duffy, E. (1941). An explanation of "emotional" phenomena without the use of the concept "emotion." *Journal of General Psychology, 25*, 283–293.

Ekman, P. & Freissen, W. V. (1986). A new pan-cultural facial expression of emotion. *Motivation and Emotion, 10*, 159–168.

Ehrlichman, H., Brown, S., Zhu, J. & Warrenburg, S. (1995). Startle reflex modulation during exposure to pleasant and unpleasant odors. *Psychophysiology, 32*, 150–154.

Fanselow, M. S., DeCola, J. P., De Oca, B. M. & Landeira-Fernandez, J. (1995). Ventral and dorsolateral regions of the midbrain periaqueductal gray (PAG) control different stages of defensive behavior: dorsolateral PAG lesions enhance the defensive freezing produced by massed and immediate shock. *Aggressive Behavior, 21*(1), 63–77.

Fanselow, M. S. & Lester, L. S. (1988). A functional behavioristic approach to aversively motivated behavior: predatory imminence as a determinant of the topography of defensive behavior. In R. C. Bolles & M. D. Beecher (Eds), *Evolution and Learning* (pp. 185–211). Hillsdale, NJ: Lawrence Erlbaum Associates.

Fendt, M., Koch, M. & Schnitzler, H. (1994). Amygdaloid noradrenaline is involved in the sensitization of the acoustic startle response in rats. *Pharmacology, Biochemistry, and Behavior, 48*, 307–314.

Fridlund, A. J. & Izard, C. E. (1983). Electromyographic studies of facial expressions of emotion and patterns of emotion. In J. T. Cacioppo & R. E. Petty (Eds), *Social Psychophysiology* (pp. 243–280). New York: Guilford Press.

Graham, F. K. (1979). Distinguishing among orienting, defense, and startle reflexes. In H. D. Kimmel, E. H. van Olst & J. F. Orlebeke (Eds), *The Orienting Reflex in Humans. An International Conference Sponsored by the Scientific Affairs Division of the North*

Atlantic Treaty Organization (pp. 137–167). Hillsdale, NJ: Lawrence Erlbaum Associates.

Greenwald, M. K., Bradley, M. M., Cuthbert, B. N. & Lang, P. J. (1998). Sensitization of the startle reflex in humans following aversive electric shock exposure. *Behavioral Neuroscience, 112*, 1069–1079.

Greenwald, M. K., Cook, E. W. III & Lang, P. J. (1989). Affective judgment and psychophysiological response: dimensional covariation in the evaluation of pictorial stimuli. *Journal of Psychophysiology, 3*, 51–64.

Hamm, A. O., Cuthbert, B. N., Globisch, J. & Vaitl, D. (1997). Fear and startle reflex: blink modulation and autonomic response patterns in animal and mutilation fearful subjects. *Psychophysiology, 34*, 97–107.

Hamm, A. O., Greenwald, M. K., Bradley, M. M. & Lang, P. J. (1993). Emotional learning, hedonic change, and the startle probe. *Journal of Abnormal Psychology, 102*, 453–465.

Hawk, L. W. & Cook, E. W. (1997). Affective modulation of tactile startle. *Psychophysiology, 34*, 23–31.

Hebb, D. O. (1949). *The Organization of Behavior: A Neuropsychological Theory*. New York: Wiley.

Hess, W. R. (1957). *The Functional Organization of the Diencephalon*. New York: Grune & Stratton.

Irwin, W., Davidson, R. J., Lowe, M. J. & Mock, Bryan J. (1996). Human amygdala activation detected with echo-planar functional magnetic resonance imaging. *NeuroReport, 7*, 1765–1769.

Jansen, D. M. & Frijda, N. (1994). Modulation of acoustic startle response by film-induced fear and sexual arousal. *Psychophysiology, 31*, 565–571.

Klorman, R. & Ryan, R. M. (1980). Heart rate, contingent negative variation, and evoked potentials during anticipation of affective stimulation. *Psychophysiology, 14*, 45–51.

Klorman, R., Weissbert, R. P. & Wiessenfeld, A. R. (1977). Individual differences in fear and autonomic reactions to affective stimulation. *Psychophysiology, 14*, 45–51.

Klorman, R., Wiesenfeld, A. & Austin, M. L. (1975). Autonomic responses to affective visual stimuli. *Psychophysiology, 12*, 553–560.

Konorski, J. (1967). *Integrative Activity of the Brain: An Interdisciplinary Approach*. Chicago: University of Chicago Press.

Lacey, J. I. (1958). Psychophysiological approaches to the evaluation of psychotherapeutic process and outcome. In E. A. Rubinstein & M. B. Perloff (Eds), *Research in Psychotherapy*. Washington, DC: National Publishing.

Lacey, J. I. & Lacey, B. C. (1970). Some autonomic-central nervous system interrelationships. In P. Black (Ed), *Physiological Correlates of Emotion* (pp. 205–227). New York: Academic Press.

Lane, R. D., Chua, P. M-L., Dolan, R. J. (1999). Common effects of emotional valence, arousal and attention on neural activation during visual processing of pictures. *Neuropsychologia, 37*(9).

Lane, R. D., Reiman, E. M., Bradley, M. M., Lang, P. J., Ahern, G. L., Davidson, R. J. & Schwartz, G. E. (1997). Neuroanatomical correlates of pleasant and unpleasant emotion. *Neuropsychologia, 35*, 1437–1444.

Lang, P. J. (1968). Fear reduction and fear behavior: problems in treating a construct. In J. M. Schlien (Ed), *Research in Psychotherapy*, vol. 3 (pp. 90–103). Washington, DC: American Psychological Association.

Lang, P. J. (1980). Behavioral treatment and bio-behavioral assessment: computer applications. In J. B. Sidowski, J. H. Johnson & T. A. Williams (Eds), *Technology in Mental Health Care Delivery Systems* (pp. 119–137). Norwood, NJ: Ablex Publishing.

Lang, P. J. (1993). The three system approach to emotion. In N. Birbaumer & A. Öhman (Eds), *The Organization of Emotion* (pp. 18–30). Toronto: Hogrefe-Huber.

Lang, P. J. (1994). The motivational organization of emotion: affect-reflex connections. In S. VanGoozen, N. E. Van de Poll & J. A. Sergeant (Eds), *Emotions: Essays on Emotion Theory* (pp. 61–93). Hillsdale, NJ: Lawrence Erlbaum Associates.

Lang, P. J., Bradley, M. M. & Cuthbert, B. N. (1990). Emotion, attention, and the startle reflex. *Psychological Review, 97*, 377–395.

Lang, P. J., Bradley, M. M. & Cuthbert, M. M. (1997). Motivated attention: affect, activation and action. In P. J. Lang, R. F. Simons & M. T. Balaban (Eds), *Attention and Orienting: Sensory and Motivational Processes*. Hillsdale, NJ: Lawrence Erlbaum Associates.

Lang, P. J., Bradley, M. M. & Cuthbert, B. N. (1999). *International Affective Picture System (IAPS): Technical Manual and Affective Ratings*. Gainesville, FL: The Center for Research in Psychophysiology, University of Florida.

Lang, P. J., Bradley, M. M., Fitzsimmons, J. R., Cuthbert, B. N., Scott, J. D., Moulder, B. & Nangia, V. (1998). Emotional arousal and activation of the visual cortex: an fMRI analysis. *Psychophysiology, 35*, 1–13.

Lang, P. J., Greenwald, M. K., Bradley, M. M. & Hamm, A. O. (1993). Looking at pictures: affective, facial, visceral, and behavioral reactions. *Psychophysiology, 30*, 261–273.

Lang, P. J., Hnatiow, M. & Geer, J. (1963). Semantic generalization of conditioned autonomic responses. *Journal of Experimental Psychology, 65*, 522–558.

LeDoux, J. E. (1990). Information flow from sensation to emotion plasticity in the neural computation of stimulus values. In M. Gabriel & J. Moore (Eds), *Learning and Computational Neuroscience: Foundations of Adaptive Networks* (pp. 3–52). Cambridge, MA: Bradford Books/MIT Press.

Lindsley, D. B. (1951). Emotion. In S. S. Stevens (Ed), *Handbook of Experimental Psychology* (pp. 473–516). New York: Wiley.

Lykken, D. T. (1957). A study of anxiety in the sociopathic personality. *Journal of Abnormal & Social Psychology, 55*, 6–10.

Mandler, G., Mandler, J. M., Kremen, I. & Sholiton, R. (1961). The response to threat: relations among verbal and physiological indices. *Psychological Monographs, 75*, no. 513.

Manning, S. K. & Melchiori, M. P. (1974). Words that upset urban college students: measured with GSRs and rating scales. *Journal of Social Psychology, 94*, 305–306.

McManis, M., Bradley, M. M., Berg, W. K., Cuthbert, B. N. & Lang, P. J. (1998). Children looking at pictures: verbal, physiological, and behavioral responses to affective pictures. Manuscript submitted for publication.

Mehrabian, A. & Russell, J. A. (1974). *An Approach to Environmental Psychology*. Cambridge, MA: MIT Press.

Miller, N. E. (1959). Liberalization of basic S-R concepts: extensions to conflict behavior, motivation and social learning. In S. Koch (Ed), *Psychology: A Study of a Science*, vol. 2 (pp. 196–292). New York: McGraw-Hill.

Morris, M., Bradley, M., Bowers, D., Lang, P. & Heilman, K. (1991). Valence-specific hypoarousal following right temporal lobectomy. *Journal of Clinical and Experimental Neuropsychology, 13*, 42. [Abstract]

Moruzzi, G. & Magoun, H. W. (1949). Brain stem reticular formation and activation of the EEG. *Electroencephalography & Clinical Neurophysiology, 1*(sup), 455–473.

Nemiah, J., Freyberger, H. & Sifneos, P. (1976). Alexithymia: a view of the psychosomatic process. In O. Hill (Ed), *Modern Trends in Psychosomatic Medicine*, vol. 3 (pp. 430–439). London: Butterworths.

Ortony, A., Clore, G. L. & Collins, A. (1988). *The Cognitive Structure of Emotions.* Cambridge: Cambridge University Press.

Osgood, C., Suci, G. & Tannenbaum, P. (1957). *The Measurement of Meaning.* Urbana: University of Illinois.

Palomba, D., Angrilli, A. & Mini, A. (1997). Visual evoked potentials, heart rate responses and memory to emotional pictorial stimuli. *International Journal of Psychophysiology, 27,* 55–67.

Patrick, C. J. (1994). Emotion and psychopathy: startling new insights. *Psychophysiology, 31,* 319–330.

Patrick, C. J., Bradley, M. M. & Lang, P. J. (1993). Emotion in the criminal psychopath: startle reflex modification. *Journal of Abnormal Psychology, 102,* 82–92.

Posner, M. I. (1996). Converging cognitive and neuroscience approaches to attention. *International Journal of Psychology, 31,* 33–40.

Ross, L. E. (1961). Conditioned fear as a function of CS-UCS and probe stimulus intervals. *Journal of Experimental Psychology, 61,* 265–273.

Russell, J. (1980). A circumplex model of affect. *Journal of Personality and Social Psychology, 39,* 1161–1178.

Sabatinelli, D., Bradley, M. M., Cuthbert, B. N. & Lang, P. J. (1996). Wait and see: aversion and activation in anticipation and perception. *Psychophysiology, 34,* S77.

Schneirla, T. (1959). An evolutionary and developmental theory of biphasic processes underlying approach and withdrawal. In M. Jones (Ed), *Nebraska Symposium on Motivation* (pp. 1–42). Lincoln: University of Nebraska Press.

Schwartz, G. E., Brown, S. L. & Ahern, G. L. (1980). Facial muscle patterning and subjective experience during affective imagery: sex differences. *Psychophysiology, 17,* 75–82.

Shaver, P., Schwartz, J., Kirson, D. & O'Connor, C. (1987). Emotion knowledge: further exploration of a prototype approach. *Journal of Personality and Social Psychology, 52,* 1061–1086.

Sokolov, Y. N. (1963). *Perception and the Conditioned Reflex* (S. W. Waydenfeld, trans). New York: Macmillan.

Spence, K. W. & Runquist, W. N. (1958). Temporal effects of conditioned fear on the eyelid reflex. *Journal of Experimental Psychology, 55,* 613–616.

Tinbergen, N. (1951). *The Study of Instincts.* New York: Oxford University Press.

Vrana, S. R., Spence, E. L. & Lang, P. J. (1988). The startle probe response: a new measure of emotion? *Journal of Abnormal Psychology, 97,* 487–491.

Winton, W. M., Putnam, L. E. & Krauss, R. M. (1984). Facial and autonomic manifestations of the dimensional structure of emotion. *Journal of Experimental Social Psychology, 20,* 195–216.

Wundt, W. (1896). *Gundriss der Psychologie* [Outlines of Psychology]. Leipzig, Germany: Entgelmann.

12

Blindsight: Implications for the Conscious Experience of Emotion

LAWRENCE WEISKRANTZ

Blindsight refers to residual visual function in the field defects caused by damage to striate cortex in primates, including both monkeys and humans. That there should be a remaining visual capacity is not, in itself, surprising because there are nine targets in the brain other than the striate cortex receiving inputs from the retina—admittedly, over much smaller pathways than the geniculo-striate pathway, but by no means trivial. Together, in fact, these pathways constitute five times as many fibers as the intact auditory nerve. It is not surprising, therefore, that animals in which the striate cortex has been removed can still carry out a range of visual discriminations. The capacity is altered both quantitatively and qualitatively, but still can be quite impressive. What *is* surprising is that humans with such damage say they do not see in their field defects. But using tests formally akin to those we must use with animals, good discriminative function can be demonstrated (Miller et al., 1980; Schilder et al., 1972; see also reviews by Weiskrantz, 1986, 1996). These tests involve routines such as forced-choice guessing between alternative unseen stimuli (e.g., their orientation, color, form, movement, presence or absence of bars on a grating used to measure acuity) or manually reaching for the unseen target, or saccading to it (Barbur et al., 1980, 1988; Blythe et al., 1986, 1987; Pöppel et al., 1973; Stoerig & Cowey, 1992; Weiskrantz, 1986; Weiskrantz et al., 1974).

Some caveats have to be mentioned at the outset. First, while subjects typically say they do not see the stimuli, they can be shown to be able to discriminate. Under particular conditions, there are some subjects who report a kind of "feeling" or "awareness" that an event has occurred, and even whether that event was moving or stationary. This occurs with stimuli that are rapidly moving or have sudden onsets and offsets. Such a reported experience must be accepted as conscious awareness, but not "seeing." I call this blindsight type 2. But with nontransient stimuli (e.g., color, orientation, with ramped onset/offset) or moving stimuli with parameters (e.g., low contrast or velocity) outside the narrow range that generate type 2 responses, discrimination may be possible in the complete absence of acknowledged awareness—blindsight type 1. Thus, wavelength can be discriminated by forced-choice guessing by some subjects who never report any experience of the color, or the bars in a grating, or its orientation. The same applies to, say, the direction of a slowly moving target, or of a low-contrast target, which can be discriminated by forced-choice guessing without any accompanying visual experience. The distinction between type 1 and type 2 offers an interesting potential entrée into the study of brain mechanisms of visual awareness, to which I turn a little later. In distinguishing between types 1 and 2, I do not wish to assert that there is not a gray area from one to the other as the parameters for each approach each other. I do think, however, for various reasons considered elsewhere (Weiskrantz, 1986, 1996), that they are categorically and functionally different. It is also fair to say that after residual function was first systematically explored, it often continued to be described in the literature as "blindsight," without distinguishing between a capacity with and without awareness. In *Blindsight* (Weiskrantz, 1986), the two varieties are evident and often contrasted in observations starting in 1974 and extending over 10 years (Weiskrantz, 1986), but they were not distinguished in explicitly categorical terms. Indeed, the distinction I have drawn between type 1 and type 2 has not been clearly drawn, or not at all, in many studies, and has not yet been drawn in animals (although I believe it could be done in principle). It is not surprising that most investigators, not to mention their subjects, prefer to work with phenomena that are actually reported as experienced (blindsight type 2), rather than forcing subjects to guess, so to speak, in the dark. (Parenthetically, with D.B., with whom the term "blindsight" was first applied, there were good practical reasons why we deliberately arranged parameters to put him in the type 1 mode; see Weiskrantz, 1986, chpt. 13).

A second caveat is that clinically there is great variation in the extent and disposition of brain damage to the occipital lobes in human subjects and also variation in the numbers of subjects in whom blindsight can be demonstrated. We know in the monkey that residual function degrades as the cortical lesion extends outside of V1 (Pasik & Pasik, 1971, 1982). This has meant that research on residual function, as in many other areas of neuropsychology, has tended to focus on a small number of suitable subjects, and especially those who are willing to endure the hours or even weeks of tedious testing. The tedium might be exacerbated when subjects are asked again and again to discriminate stimuli they cannot see. It is for such reasons that indirect, nonverbal tests have begun to be pursued (Weiskrantz, 1990), which circumvent the need to engage in arcane verbal exchanges or puzzling instructions to skeptical subjects to respond to the unseen and the indescribable. One such indirect method will be discussed later in the context of autonomic function.

There is a third caveat. The best studied subjects are those who have unilateral cortical damage and hence have a visual defect in only one-half of their fields, contralateral to the damaged hemisphere. Indeed, bilateral cases are rare and hardly investigated at all, although this is a current focus of interest. The early work in monkeys, in contrast, was with bilateral lesions. The implication is obvious: in their everyday lives, such patients can negotiate their visual worlds happily and efficiently using an intact half field of vision combined with effective head and eye movements. You would be hard pressed to pick them out—or the monkey with unilateral damage—in a crowd of normal subjects. This means that one cannot tell much from studying their general behavior in the natural environment, or even in most unnatural environments. One must obviously ensure that stimuli are directed to their field defects to draw any conclusions, although such subjects offer the valuable advantage of having a built-in control available in allowing comparisons to be made with the intact hemifield.

There is an additional limitation, which is a longitudinal one. We know that in the monkey, concerted practice in discriminating within the field defect produces a marked improvement in sensitivity for detection—it can be as much as 3 log units—and also a shrinkage of the field defect (Cowey, 1967; Mohler & Wurtz, 1977; Weiskrantz & Cowey, 1970). But such improvement occurs only with such practice, and not just with passive stimulation of the retina in the location of the field defect, which is, of course, occurring more or less continuously in the subjects' waking lives. There is evidence that such practice can also produce similar beneficial effects in humans (Kasten & Sabel, 1995; Kerkhoff et al., 1994; Zihl, 1980, 1981; Zihl & von Cramon, 1979; Zihl & Werth, 1984), but with a good half field, few humans have been subjected to the drudgery of putting the potential capacity of their blind half fields under much pressure. The blindsight subjects who have been popular candidates for repeated and intensive study by experimenters are interesting exceptions to the more general clinical situation, in which scotomata caused by visual cortex damage are typically found to be stable and persistent over years.

(A fourth and final caveat I will reserve until later for the discussion of the determination of the stimulus parameters relevant to discrimination with and without awareness.)

Caveats aside, what can one say about blindsight and the experience of emotion? Clearly, in the narrow sense we are only concerned with the experience of visually evocative events. But in the wider sense, we are interested in the general issue of how an intact capacity is or is not rendered conscious. What brain systems are involved, and how might they be organized?

Let us start with the narrow question. Does the blindsight subject respond to emotionally salient visual stimuli? And, if so, does the subject have any experience of having done so? With blindsight type I, there is no evidence available of any differential response to emotional, as opposed to neutral, events. This is not to say that it does not exist potentially. No one has looked for it. Electrodermal responses can be measured to luminant visual stimuli preceded by an auditory warning signal and are found to be larger than those to the auditory stimulus followed by "blanks" (Zihl et al., 1980), similar in this formal sense to the seminal results of Tranel and Damasio (1985) and Bauer (1984) with prosopagnosic patients for familiar versus neutral faces. And so the autonomic system responds to lights even if the subject may not see them, but given the absence of more than rudimentary form discrimination, no response to emotion-evoking visual stimuli delivered to the blind field has been reported.

One can go back to the early animal literature for a graphic description of the lack of differential overt responding to emotion-evoking versus neutral stimuli. (I use the word "neutral" for convenience; no object is wholly neutral.) Indeed, a good description was given more than 100 years ago by the Italian neurophysiologist Luigi Luciani (1884, p. 153) of monkeys with bilateral occipital ablations:

When some time has elapsed after the extirpation . . . they are able to see minute objects, what they want is the discernment of things and a right judgment concerning their properties and their nature. . . . For example, if small pieces of fig mixed with pieces of sugar, are offered to them, they are incapable of choosing by sight alone but require to take the sugar in their hand and put it in their mouths to reassure themselves. . . . The animal is not able to distinguish meat from sugar by its visual impressions only.

A closely similar type of description emerges from the accounts of Humphrey (1970, 1974) of the monkey Helen with bilateral striate cortex lesions, whom he studied for several years in a variety of free field as well as more experimentally constrained situations. Helen could avoid obstacles very skillfully in an open field, would readily pick up small bits of material scattered on the ground, but was agnosic for what they were without mouthing them. A dramatic result was obtained by Cowey, who measured the field detects of monkeys precisely in a "monkey perimeter" (Cowey, 1967; Cowey & Weiskrantz, 1963). He had shown earlier that a monkey after unilateral striate cortex removal recovered much of its fine sensitivity to brief and small light stimuli in its hemianopic field. But when a strange doll was suspended in the perimeter so as to fall entirely within the affected field, the animal continued to behave normally and ignored it altogether, although monkeys respond with loud shrieks of fear and outrage if confronted with such a doll in the normal field; indeed, Cowey's monkey refused to test when the doll was visible. Similarly, it completely ignored a highly prized banana suspended in the affected field, but grabbed it swiftly when in the normal field. The point is not that responses to emotional stimuli have been specifically damped, but that the identification of all meaningful visual stimuli, emotion arousing or not, has been removed.

If we turn to blindsight type 2, where there is some conscious awareness without seeing, we might be more hopeful of seeing evidence of a difference between emotional and neutral stimuli. But I know of no evidence that is convincing, although this issue has scarcely been examined. In the study of electrodermal responses, Zihl et al. (1980) found that moving light patches were more effective than stationary ones in eliciting responses, which suggests that type 2 stimuli were more powerful that type 1, but these authors also found reliable electrodermal responses to stationary lights, and commented that the subjects reported no awareness of these visual stimuli.

There is one particular autonomic response that has elegant precision and potential for assessing the residual capacity of the blind field—namely, the response of the pupil. With sensitive methods of measurement (Barbur et al., 1987), the pupil can be found to constrict not only in response to an increase in light energy, but also to particular properties of visual events that involve no change in light energy whatsoever. For example, the pupil constricts to the presentation of a visual grating whose mean luminance equals that of the background, and the size of pupillary constriction varies as a function of the spatial frequency and contrast (Barbur & Forsyth, 1986; Barbur & Thomson, 1987). The acuity determined by pupillometry correlates strongly with acuity as measured by conventional psychophysical methods. The pupil also responds to wavelength (Barbur et al., 1994b) and to movement. The response to gratings means that one can measure the acuity of the blind hemifield, as well as its contrast sensitivity nonverbally, and not only in adult humans but also in animals and human infants (Cocker et al., 1994).

Using this approach, Cowey, LeMare, and I have recently measured pupillary contraction as a function of spatial frequency in the blind hemifields of monkeys with a complete unilateral V1 removal. Using the same apparatus and the same testing environment, we have also measured pupillary contraction in the hemianopic field of the adult patient G.Y., who sustained V1 damage following head injury in childhood. The results for both monkeys and G.Y. reveal a narrowly tuned spatial channel in the "blind" hemifield, with a peak at about one cycle per degree, and with an acuity of approximately five to eight cycles per degree (figure 12.1). (This compares with an acuity of 25–30 cycles per degree in the intact hemifield.) Interestingly, all three curves—for two monkeys and the one human—map very closely onto the function for the same human subject, G.Y., when the gratings were used in a two-alternative forced-choice detection psychophysical experiment, as shown in the figure, with the default stimulus being the homogenous background matched in mean energy level (Barbur et al., 1994a).

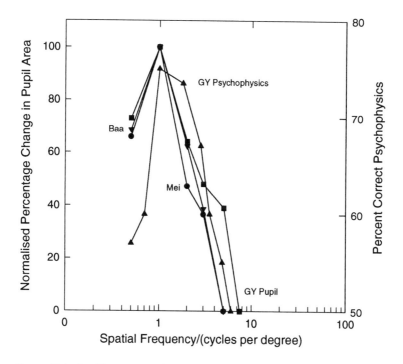

Figure 12.1. Pupillometry results for sinusoidal gratings presented in the "blind" hemifields of two monkeys (Baa, Mei) with unilateral V1 lesions, and also for G.Y. Also shown are the psychophysical results for G.Y. with gratings, labeled "GY Psychophysics", from the study by Barbur et al. (1994a). The pupillometry gratings had a contrast of 80%. All values have been normalized such that their peaks are set at 100%.

In both the psychophysical and pupillometry experiments, G.Y. reported "awareness" but not seeing (i.e., type 2 blindsight). But we did not test specifically psychophysically for type 1 at that time (e.g., by changing the slope of the onset function or the grating's contrast), and so we do not know the properties of a type 1 channel, if it exists, or whether the pupil would react for it—that is, for the future. Moreover, in the pupillometry experiments, G.Y. reported that he was aware only of the occurrence of an event (presumably, the transient onset and offset of the stimulus), but not of the grating or its structure—its bars. An important question arises as to whether the pupillary spatial frequency tuning channel remains intact when the onset and offset of the stimulus are smoothed. In any event, we have a precise verification by pupillometry of a narrow, spatially tuned visual channel available to the affected field that is independent of the integrity of V1 in monkey or human. (There is also a second channel, based on changes in energy level per se, also measured by Barbur et al., 1994a, which will not discussed here.)

It would be interesting to see whether the pupil within this narrowly tuned and robust channel would respond differentially to a frightening doll or snake or to a juicy, rewarding piece of fruit presented to the blind field of the monkey, or whatever suitable stimulus might be suggested for the human subject's hemianopic field. I suspect the answer for the monkey will be the same as already found earlier by Luciani and Humphrey, 1970, 1974, i.e., no differential response to different varieties of meaningfulness per se.

One might ask how the pupillary system comes into play. We do not know the answer to this question, except to say that a constricted pupil yields a slightly increased depth of focus, hardly of commanding evolutionary importance. Functionally, the pupillary system might be a concomitant of a detection system, to be considered in the mould of the original two-visual system hypothesis (not the more recent dorsal–ventral stream one, but the earlier subcortical vs. cortical one, e.g., as advanced by Ingle, 1967; Schneider, 1967; and Trevarthen, 1968), in which the superior colliculus was assumed to deal with questions of detection (the "whether" and the "where" of visual events) and the visual cortex with identification (the "what"). Transient events are signals of potential danger, or at least of interest, and a dedicated detection system could be expected to have evolutionary survival value and also to be ingrained at the older midbrain level. But I suspect that it is no more than that, lacking any capacity to transmit specific meaningful content. As William James (1890, p. 73) stated, "The main function [of such a system] . . . is that of sentinels which, when beams of light move over them, cry: 'Who goes there?' and calls the fovea to the spot." James was contrasting peripheral with foveal vision, but the metaphor transfers aptly to the distinction between detection and identification and correspondingly to subcortex and cortex.

The distinction between good performance without awareness, by forced-choice guessing or some indirect approach, and performance with awareness gives one an opening into a rather broader and exciting arena. If one could measure brain activity in the two different modes, both possessing demonstrably good, matched levels of performance, one might get a handle on what brain systems are associated with subjective awareness. Beyond that, the answer might generate some hypotheses that have broader application outside the realm of visual performance per se. We have compared the two directional movement modes, aware versus unaware, psychophysically (Weiskrantz et al., 1995) and compared their corresponding functional magnetic resonance brain images. We found that G.Y. was able to mimic the pathway of a moving target remarkably well, provided the velocity was high (see Weiskrantz, 1995). For these stimuli he also said that he was aware; he knew that something was moving, although he did not see anything as such. In contrast, with low velocities he appeared not to respond at all, and he said he had no awareness. The question arose, prompted by a preemptory discussion by Dennett (1991), of whether G.Y. was able nevertheless to discriminate the direction of the slowly moving targets, of which he was unaware, by pure guessing (i.e., whether there would be type 1 blindsight). To assess whether G.Y. could discriminate without any acknowledged awareness, we added two response keys, for a total of four. There were the usual two response keys for the forced-choice discrimination between the two stimulus alternatives, and there were two additional "commentary keys" (Weiskrantz et al., 1995). G.Y. was required on every trial not only to discriminate, by guessing if necessary, whether the target moved in, say, a horizontal or a nonhorizontal direction, responding accordingly on key 1 or 2, but also whether he had any awareness, responding appropriately on key 3 or 4. He was repeatedly instructed to press the "yes" key if he had any experience, no matter how feeble or whatever its character, and to press the "no" key if he had absolutely no reportable experience. Such a commentary method is a *sine qua non* for determining whether a discrimination is accompanied by acknowledged awareness. One has to go "off-line" to the discrimination per se. No degree of complexity of on-line discrimination per se will do for this purpose. Confidence ratings address the same issue, but not quite as directly. Results indicated that there was a range of conditions under which good performance could be produced for events in G.Y.'s blind field, even when he reported no awareness (figures 12.2, 12.3).

Because the binary choice between aware and unaware may have been too crude a measure, and because there might have been a small degree of conscious awareness even when our subject pressed the "no" key, we also repeated the experiment using an awareness scale, from 0 to 5+. The results were the same (Sahraie et al., submitted).

I now address the fourth caveat mentioned earlier. Replication is at the heart of scientific progress and is always of some concern. The fine tuning of visual parameters is as crucial for our kind of research as is, say, the impedance of an electrode for the electrophysiologist. A good example of the importance of parameters in residual vision is a report by Hess and Pointer (1989). These authors concluded that they could find absolutely no evidence of any residual function in the blind fields of G.Y. and two other hemianopic patients. In their study they used specially constructed, sophisticated visual stimuli bounded by Gaussian spatial and temporal envelopes, but their Gaussian parameters, one spatial and one temporal envelope, were fixed—based on values no doubt found to be useful for testing normal visual fields. When we repeated their experiment with G.Y. using Hess and Pointer's parameters, we indeed confirmed that G.Y. responded at chance. But with only a small decrease in the size of the Gaussian temporal standard deviation, of the order of 50 msec, G.Y.'s detection performance rose from chance to virtual perfection (Weiskrantz et al., 1991). The same was true if we increased the size of the stimulus. (A considerably more extreme example of inappropriate choice of

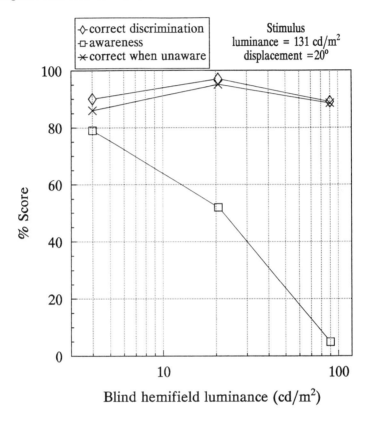

Figure 12.2. Discrimination of horizontal versus vertical movement (FR paradigm) as a function of stimulus contrast. The subject had to indicate (by guessing if necessary) whether the presented stimulus was moving horizontally or vertically by pressing the appropriate response key. He also had two commentary keys to use on every trial. "Awareness" refers to the percentage of trials on which the subject pressed the "aware" key. "Correct when unaware" refers to performance during those trials when the subject pressed the "unaware" key. The luminance of the test stimulus was held constant at 131 cd/m², and background luminance in the blind field was altered systematically, thus changing the contrast of the stimulus. (From Weiskrantz et al., 1995, with permission from the National Academy of Sciences.)

stimulus parameters for G.Y. is reviewed in Weiskrantz, 1997.) Fine details do matter.

We have replicated our commentary key type of experiment (Weiskrantz et al., 1995) on two subsequent occasions, with a comparable pattern of results for the aware versus unaware modes as the major outcome each time, although with a quantitative sensitivity change in the last replication.

A comparable dissociation between performance and awareness, in some ways even more striking, has been found in G.Y. by Kentridge et al. (1997) studying

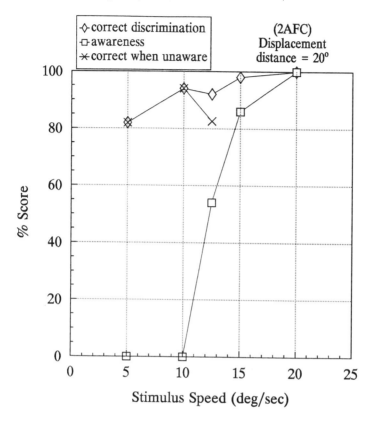

Figure 12.3. Discrimination of horizontal versus vertical movement
(two alternative forced-choice paradigm) as a function of stimulus velocity. Horizontal movement was presented in either the first or second
of two intervals selected randomly and vertical movement in the other,
and the subject's task was to indicate (by guessing if necessary) the
correct interval of horizontal presentation and also to select a commentary key after every trial. "Awareness" refers to the percentage of trials
on which the subject pressed the "aware" key. "Correct when unaware" refers to performance during those trials when the subject
pressed the "unaware" key. (From Weiskrantz et al., 1995, with permission from the National Academy of Sciences.)

visual detection with an eye tracker which stabilized the retinal position. This was
done to test the suggestion by Fendrich and colleagues (1992) that blindsight was
based on islands of intact striate cortex, revealed by isolated islands of residual
function in an otherwise "dead sea" in one of their subjects. G.Y. did not show
any such tiny visual islands, although, of course, other patients might be of the
type studied by Fendrich et al. On the same point, islands cannot be a relevant
explanation of residual function in monkeys with V1 lesions because the complete-
ness of the lesion is confirmed. The close similarity of the pupillometry results for
monkeys and humans (see figure 12.1) obviously speaks against the argument that

islands of cortex are an explanation for residual function in the human but not the monkey. But Kentridge et al. also introduced commentary keys in some variations of the Fendrich et al. detection paradigm, and conditions were found under which here, too, there was excellent detection in the absence of acknowledged awareness.

Another interesting dissociation between awareness and detection has been found by Kentridge et al. (1999) using an attention paradigm for cues and targets both located in the blind field. Again, with G.Y. positive effects can be found even with 0% awareness for targets and for cueing signal, or for the unseen target alone with an "aware" cueing signal. The pattern of results can be interpreted in terms of unconscious priming (i.e., an increase in sensitivity to a target stimulus caused by the prior presentation of the cue, without awareness of either the cue or the target).

Another example of good performance either with or without awareness, again within G.Y.'s blind field, was recently found by Cowey and Stoerig (in preparation) in a color substitution task. The subject was instructed to indicate the locus on the screen at which a change from a white to a small color patch occurred. In switches from white to blue or from white to red, there was no value of luminance of the colored stimulus that ever reduced the discriminative performance to chance. Even when G.Y. claimed it was pure guesswork, discrimination remained well above chance. As luminance differences between white and color increased, G.Y. then reported awareness, as expected (but not of color, as such, or of normal "seeing"). In contrast, with a switch from white to green, the performance did drop to chance when the white and color stimuli were of equal or near equal luminance. The result is an indication not only of differential responses to wavelength in blindsight, but also makes it clear that G.Y.'s commentary responses are not based simply on a different response criterion between aware and unaware modes, as otherwise all wavelengths should be affected similarly. And so a number of dissociations have emerged between aware and unaware modes using the commentary key paradigm either explicitly or by verbal commentary.

There may be another phenomenon of some interest concerning G.Y. He says he is becoming more aware (a greater sensitivity of type 2) than he used to be. We know from animal results, and from some human results, that sustained practice in the blind field can have marked effects in increasing sensitivity and even some shrinkage of a cortical field defect. The third time we tested G.Y., about 2 years after the original tests, his movement thresholds were lower than they were originally, although the same overall qualitative pattern obtained. We recently retested him on the Kentridge and Heywood attention/priming paradigm, and here, too, his sensitivity has increased substantially. Within the past year or so G.Y. has been tested repeatedly by more than six different groups at numerous locations in Europe and the United States, often on similar movement discriminations for which we originally demonstrated performance without awareness. G.Y.'s sensitivity may well be shifting. There may be a Heisenberg effect; repeated measurements may be changing the phenomena being measured. G.Y., like Cowey's repeatedly tested monkeys, may one day even show some shrinkage of his hemianopia. If so, that would be a gratuitously marvelous outcome of the sustained and intense efforts of visual experimenters around the world to test him, plus his own dedication to the scientific cause!

One must take the question of replicability very seriously. The reason we repeated the movement discrimination experiment the second time was that we wanted to carry out functional magnetic resonance imaging (fMRI) for the aware versus unaware modes. To do so, a new portable, battery-driven projection system had to be designed to fit into the fMRI chamber. We then had to redo the psychophysics to see if the same aware–unaware commentary key difference still obtained with the new screen and new projection equipment, with both modes generating high and matched levels of performance. At that stage it matched the performance levels previously reported (Sahraie et al., 1997). G.Y. was then scanned under each of the conditions that gave rise to the two modes. We ran a block of experiments in which velocity and contrast were varied appropriately in both the blind hemifield and the intact, seeing hemifield.

What emerged from the analysis (Sahraie et al., 1997), using a conservative thresholding procedure (Bullmore et al., 1996) is first, that in the aware mode in the affected hemifield, there was activation in right prefrontal cortex, areas 46 and 47. Area 46 also was activated with stimulation of the sighted hemifield (in which, of course, he is also aware). There was also activation of area 18 in both hemispheres. Interestingly, Blakemore and Spekreise (personal communication), after replicating our results, ran G.Y. on brain imaging for the two modes with SPECT and also found a dorsal prefrontal focus. In the unaware mode there was no dorsolateral prefrontal activation; instead, any frontal activation was in the medial and orbital regions. In the unaware mode, and only in this mode, there was activation of the superior colliculus. There was also activation of area 19 ipsilateral to the lesion, which implies that activation of such a visual cortical area is not sufficient for phenomenal visual awareness. It also appeared that the unaware mode yielded more areas of activation than the aware mode in both hemispheres. It is as though as many possible routes are being recruited as possible to try to deal discriminately with the stimuli, and there are a multitude of routes that remain possible in the absence of V1 (see Cowey and Stoerig, 1991). The emergence of increased activity of the superior colliculus in the unaware mode fits well with the important mediating role of the superior colliculus in the absence of V1, as demonstrated by Rodman et al. (1989). Its role in the recovery within a scotoma caused by V1 damage in the monkey was impressively demonstrated by Mohler and Wurtz (1977).

The finding that the ipsilateral area 18 increases its activity in the aware mode with the fMRI may well be the homologue of one of the areas, putatively V5, reported to be active in a positron emission tomography (PET) study with moving stimuli for which G.Y. also reported awareness (Barbur et al., 1993). (I have confirmed, incidentally, in a recorded interview with G.Y. that his experience in that PET experiment was one of conscious awareness, but not of "seeing"—there has been some misunderstanding of that point.) Such findings suggest that prestriate visual cortical engagement is necessary to render a discrimination aware to the subject. But it cannot be concluded that it is sufficient for visual awareness. Not only area 18 but also prefrontal areas, among others, become active in the aware mode, but not in the unaware mode, and this is also the case for visual stimulation of the sighted hemifield. Necessary but not sufficient is also consistent with Herculean experiments originating with early work by Sperry et al. (1960) and Gazzaniga (1966) and by Nakamura and Mishkin (1979, 1980, 1982, 1986). All three sets of workers asked the question whether vision is possible if all nonvisual cortex is removed in animals (cats in Sperry's case and monkeys in the others), leaving the whole constellation of visual cortices intact, including inferotemporal cortex. The result was that animals were visually unresponsive, behaviorally blind, even though single neuronal activity in V1 was still intact electrophysiologically in the monkey in the Nakamura and Mishkin preparation (Nakamura et al., 1986).

Given such considerations, what kind of neural system might be necessary for rendering a discrimination conscious? I speculate it is perhaps the very one that allows a subject to generate the commentary key response. Beyond this, it may be what is actually meant by being "aware." I find the approach of the philosopher David Rosenthal (1986, 1990, 1993), congenial on this point: he posits that consciousness of sensory events requires a further thought, a further operation. The commentary key, incidentally, is not restricted just to humans, if one means by it a method of testing a subject's "off-line" response to a discrimination. Cowey and Stoerig (1995) have done this, in effect, in the case of V1 lesions in the monkeys, producing results that are parallel those of human blindsight. That is, having confirmed that the monkeys with V1 lesions can detect targets with high reliability in their blind fields, they then showed that the animals classified these stimuli as "blanks" rather than as "lights," just as a human blindsight subject would. Wherever the system is that controls the commentary response, it has to be well outside of sensory systems as such and is probably part of a larger system that permits cognitive evaluation of the stimulus in its relevant context. The commentary key need not be verbal, and in the monkey obviously is not.

Neuropsychology is now replete with examples of intact capacities in the absence of acknowledged awareness of them by the subjects, not only in blindsight but also in other sensory systems (Rossetti et al., 1995) and also in subcomponents of such systems (Goodale et al., 1994; Heywood et al., 1991; Milner & Goodale, 1995; see reviews by McGlynn & Schacter, 1989; Schacter et al., 1988; Weiskrantz, 1991). This phenomenon can be seen in the amnesic syndrome, where it surfaced early (Warrington & Weiskrantz, 1968), in unilateral neglect (Ladavas et al., 1993; Marshall & Halligan, 1988), prosopagnosia (DeHaan et al., 1991; Tranel & Damasio, 1985; Young, 1994), dyslexia (Shallice & Saffran, 1986), and even in aphasia (Frederici, 1982; Linebarger et al., 1983; Tyler, 1988). What about in emotion? The essay by Lane and colleagues (1997) on alexithymia presents an intriguing possible parallel.

One is tempted to consider a general pattern that might apply across all systems, cognitive as well as emotional. Sensory and emotion-provoking events (which can be internally generated) have early processing demands placed on them in order for those events to be identified as such, or at least to be put in addressable form for identification. In the case of vision, for example, there has been a cascade, indeed, an avalanche, of studies concerning the complex welter of anatomical pathways involved in the various stages of visual processing, from V1 over diverging dorsal and ventral streams to parietal and inferotemporal cortex, through V1 to all the visual areas. It is within this complex that the transformation takes place from simple edge and orientation feature detection, sensitive only in small visual fields and only in one half-field retinal coordinates, to object-based coordinates, coded in categorical or prototypical form, ultimately with fields that are large and include both halves, and with broad retinal generalization. All these aspects have been the subject of intense investigation and cognitive neuroscientific analysis, imposed on the complex anatomical relationships exemplified in the well-known anatomical chart of Felleman and Van Essen (1991) and the more functional one of Young (1992). These complexities are displayed in their diagrams only for cerebral cortex, and in such analyses perhaps the subcortical targets of retinal inputs, as well as the efferent outputs from cortex to subcortical relays, fail to gain the attention they deserve.

For awareness to be associated with a discriminative act, the subject must potentially be able to acknowledge the results of such processing, and this involves a variety of different cognitive systems depending on context and also on mnemonic inputs. It may be that the activation of the commentary system generates the awareness (the activation of the system, it should be stressed, not necessarily the actual production of a commentary response as such, which can remain potential). It would seem extremely unlikely that there is just one "awareness module," whatever that might be, or indeed any module at all, or just one narrowly endowed commentary system, but a variety of networks depending on the demands and the planning of action, as well as on the response modes to be engaged. Some of these networks would be dedicated to particular kinds of events, but there is bound to be a great deal of flexible overlap of the systems involved in all varieties of awareness. Without such demands there is no need for the processing to go beyond automatic or routine levels. I have already discussed the demands that certain visual stimuli place on the subject—namely, that transient events can signal danger. Emotion-provoking events are those that entail strong reinforcing or aversive properties, the demand properties of which are obvious. An interesting example that there can be an intact but entirely and undeniably unconscious response to an aversive stimulus occurs in paraplegia: "A needle-prick causes invariably the drawing up of the limb . . . The nervous arcs of pain-nerves, broadly speaking, dominate the spinal centres . . . *where pain is, of course, non-existent*" (Sherrington, 1957, p. 257, italics added). It is interesting, to follow this digression a bit further, how rapidly young children after a fall switch from intense shrieking to happy chortling in just a matter of seconds, whereas adults—and spoiled domestic pets—will continue to preserve the painful reaction (and the pain) for much longer. The example from Sherrington is, of course, of a disconnexion between one part of the central nervous system, the spinal cord, and another, the brain. I am referring here to disconnexions that occur entirely within the brain, but perhaps in principle are no different from those between spinal cord and brain.

Emotion-provoking events are those that normally demand cognitive assessment and tactical action, and hence the condition of alexithymia is a counterintuitive one, just as all examples of disconnected awareness in clinical cases are counterintuitive. Alternatively, just as in visual processing, there might be certain advantages of economy and speed, or even of self-protection, in not wasting precious cognitive capacity by continuing to think about the event. Why bother to reflect on why a red light means "stop" or to try to conjure up the source of that piece of learning, if we can do this without thinking and continue to drive while carrying on a vigorous discussion about the nature of brain mechanisms of awareness! Beyond this, we are all familiar with the counterproductive effects of persistent rehearsal of emotional experience. One does not have to consider anything as intangible (or untestable) as active repression to know that there are positive benefits in avoiding overrehearsal of experiences that would otherwise capture the stage (even if the stage is in a non-Cartesian theatre). From this point of view, blindsight and alexithymia alike might lead to inferences about aspects of adaptive mechanisms in normal function.

These indirect benefits are slight in relation to the severe adaptive penalties that patients suffer if their processing is not amenable to conscious acknowledgment. Although some limited recovery may be possible with focused and dedicated therapeutic measures in for example, blindsight (Zihl & von Cramon, 1980), amnesia (Glisky & Schacter, 1988; Glisky et al., 1986; Wilson, 1995), and prosopagnosia (Sergent & Poncet, 1990), these are marginal crutches rather than cures. In all of the neuropsychological domains in which implicit processing has been reported in the absence of acknowledged awareness, which I believe includes virtually the whole cognitive gamut, the patients are severely handicapped in manipulating the material for which they have residual capacity. It is fortunate that the blindsight subject is typically only unilaterally damaged; if the blindness were bilateral, the handicap would be too incapacitating. No amnesic patient can survive on implicit processing alone. The amnesic patient is the only person who cannot be persuaded that he or she has an intact ability to store new information. The patient cannot compare different memories, just as a blindsight patient cannot compare a current input with the image of a past input. The aphasic patient whose patterns of reaction times are qualitatively just as sensitive to the patterns of degradation of semantic and syntactic items as those of normal subjects still cannot comprehend the material to which he or she responds so remarkably on an implicit level. Similar observations apply to prosopagnosia and unilateral neglect. The spectrum of handicaps associated with alexithymia are well reviewed by Lane et al. (1997). Being aware of a an outcome feeds back upon the process itself, elaborates it, allows comparisons with others, categorizes it, and, often to the despair of the obsessional, keeps it alive. Awareness is not just switching on a monitor. It is a condition that allows cognitive manipulation of the material, and in so doing greatly enhances and manipulates and filters that material.

The brain regions involved in vision when information progresses from the early stage of processing to the commentary stage appear to include the frontal regions, and perhaps are even predominantly frontal. What they are for other sensory systems it not known, although Young (1993), who has carried out some of the most detailed analyses of anatomical connectedness of pathways in the visual system, has forwarded a view that several sensory systems all converge on frontal-limbic regions. In regard to emotion-provoking events in humans, inputs to the amygdala, in particular, and its hypothalamic and orbito-frontal limbic partners would seem to play a role at the stage of organizing some of the components of processing (Damasio, 1994). Considering the later stages, if the parallel argument is accepted that awareness requires a commentary stage, I am less certain. Lesions of the anterior cingulate cortex (ACC) are, at least in this respect, thought to be comparable for emotional states to the kind of disconnexion from visual awareness caused by striate cortex lesions. The gamut of bodily reactions associated with emotion-evoking events still can be evoked, but the subject has blunted awareness of them. But it is not clear whether the analogy stops at that point. The striate cortex lesion effectively disconnects certain categories of visual cortical outputs from reaching the commentary system, but in principle, if not in practice, it would be possible to do the same by disconnecting all of the separate extrastriate visual outputs of V1 via the extrastriate cortical areas to which V1 is connected. What is not clear is whether the ACC lesion is the final output, comparable to the anterior inferior temporal and anterior parietal lobes in vision, say, leading to a further commentary stage. Given that there must be some interaction between emotional and other cognitive domains, one is inclined to ask whether ACC is an output of an well-integrated stage of processing, but only a stage nonetheless, rather than the final stage at which awareness of emotion can be expressed and consciously registered. At some point there must be the same ability to think consciously about emotional events as there is to think about any other kind of events and to think about them in the same context. That, at least, is what therapists think they are getting their clients to do, especially those who claim that achievement of narrative truth is the final aim. Whether it is therapeutically effective is not for us to say, but it certainly is what they succeed in getting their clients to do, and it is what most of us do well even without therapists. Reflective awareness is an umbrella that tolerates both emotional and nonemotional events and offers protection during calm cogitation about how avoid or to get out of the rain or how to progress while one while is swamped in a deluge.

References

Barbur, J. L. & Forsyth, P. M. (1986). Can the pupil response be used as a measure of the visual input associated with the geniculo-striate pathway? *Clinics in Visual Science, 1,* 107–111.

Barbur J. L., Forsyth P. M. & Findlay J. M. (1988). Human saccadic eye movements in the absence of the geniculocalcarine projection. *Brain, 111,* 63–82.

Barbur, J. L., Harlow, J. A. & Weiskrantz, L. (1994a). Spatial and temporal response properties of residual vision in a case of hemianopia. *Philosophical Transactions of the Royal Society of London, B, 343,* 157–166.

Barbur, J. L., Harlow, J. A., Sahraie, A., Stoerig, P. & Weiskrantz, L. (1994b). Responses to chromatic stimuli in the absence of V1: pupillometric and psychophysical studies. *Optical Society of America Technical Digest, 2,* 312–315.

Barbur, J. L., Ruddock, K. H. & Waterfield, V. A. (1980). Human visual responses in the absence of the geniculo-striate projection. *Brain, 103,* 905–920.

Barbur, J. L. & Thomson, W. D. (1987). Pupil response as an objective measure of visual acuity. *Ophthalmic and Physiological Optics, 7,* 425–429.

Barbur, J. L., Thomson, W. D. & Forsyth, P. M. (1987). A new system for the simultaneous measurement of pupil size and two-dimensional eye movements. *Clinics in Visual Science, 2,* 131–142.

Barbur, J. L., Watson, J. D. G., Frackowiak, R. S. J. & Zeki, S. (1993). Conscious visual perception without V1. *Brain, 116,* 1293–1302.

Bauer, R. M. (1984). Autonomic recognition of names and faces in prosopagnosia: a neuropsychological application of the guilty knowledge test. *Neuropsychologia, 22,* 457–469.

Blythe, I. M., Bromley, J. M., Kennard, C. & Ruddock, K. H. (1986). Visual discrimination of target displacement remains after damage to the striate cortex in humans. *Nature, 320,* 619–621.

Blythe, I. M., Kennard, C. & Ruddock, K. H. (1987). Residual vision in patients with retro-geniculate lesions of the visual pathways. *Brain, 110*, 887–905.

Bullmore, E. T., Rabe-Hesketh, S., Morris, R. G., Williams, S. C. R., Gregory, L., Gray, J. A. & Branner, M. J. (1996). Functional magnetic resonance imaging analysis of a large-scale neurocognitive network. *Neuroimage, 4*, 16–33.

Cocker, D., Moseley, M. J., Bissenden, J. G. & Fielder, A. R. (1994). Visual acuity and pupillary responses to spatial structure in infants. *Ophthalmic Visual Science, 35*, 2620–2625.

Cowey, A. (1967). Perimetric study of field defects in monkeys after cortical and retinal ablations. *Quarterly Journal of Experimental Psychology, 19*, 232–245.

Cowey, A. & Stoerig, P. (1991). The neurobiology of blindsight. *Trends in Neuroscience, 29*, 65–80.

Cowey, A. & Stoerig, P. (1995). Blindsight in monkeys. *Nature, 373*, 247–249.

Cowey, A. & Stoerig, P. (in preparation). Colour discrimination in the absence of V1 in monkeys and in a patient with blindsight.

Cowey, A. & Weiskrantz, L. (1963). A perimetric study of visual field defects in monkeys. *Quarterly Journal of Experimental Psychology, 15*, 91–115.

Damasio, A. (1994). *Descartes' Error*. New York: G. P. Putnam's Sons.

DeHaan, E. H. F., Young, A. W. & Newcombe, F. (1991). Covert and overt recognition in prosopagnosia. *Brain, 114*, 2575–2591.

Dennett, D. C. (1991). *Consciousness Explained*. London: Penguin Press.

Felleman, D. J. & Van Essen, D. C. (1991). Distributed hierarchical processing in the primate cerebral cortex. *Cerebral Cortex, 1*, 1–47.

Fendrich, R., Wessinger, C. M. & Gazzaniga, M. S. (1992). Residual vision in a scotoma; implications for blindsight. *Science, 258*, 1489–1491.

Frederici, A. D. (1982). Syntactic and semantic processes in aphasic deficits: the availability of prepositions. *Brain and Language, 15*, 245–258.

Gazzaniga, M. S. (1966). Visuomotor integration in split-brain monkeys with other cerebral lesions. *Experimental Neurology, 16*, 289–298.

Glisky, E. L. & Schacter, D. L. (1988). Long-term retention of computer learning by patients with memory disorders. *Neuropsychologia, 26*, 173–178.

Glisky, E. L., Schacter, D. L. & Tulving, E. (1986). Learning and retention of computer-related vocabulary in memory-impaired patients: method of vanishing cues. *Journal of Clinical and Experimental Neuropsychology, 8*, 292–312.

Goodale, M. A., Jakobson, L. S. & Keiller, J. M. (1994). Differences in the visual control of pantomimed and natural grasping movements. *Neuropsychologia, 32*, 1159–1178.

Hess, R. F. & Pointer, J. S. (1989). Spatial and temporal contrast sensitivity in hemianopia. A comparative study of the sighted and blind hemifields. *Brain, 112*, 871–894.

Heywood, C. A., Cowey, A. & Newcombe, F. (1991). Chromatic discrimination in a cortically color blind observer. *European Journal of Neuroscience, 3*, 802–912.

Humphrey, N. K. (1970). What the frog's eye tells the monkey's brain. *Brain, Behavior, and Evolution, 3*, 324–337.

Humphrey, N. K. (1974). Vision in a monkey without striate cortex: a case study. *Perception, 3*, 241–255.

Ingle, D. (1967). Two visual mechanisms underlying the behavior of fish. *Psychologie Forschung, 31*, 44–51.

James, W. (1890). *Principles of Psychology*. London: Macmillan.

Kasten, E. & Sabel, B. A. (1995). Visual field enlargement after computer training in brain-damaged patients with homonymous deficits: an open pilot trial. *Restorative Neurology and Neuroscience, 8*, 113–127.

Kentridge, R. W., Heywood, C. A. & Weiskrantz, L. (1997). Residual vision in multiple retinal locations within a scotoma: implications for blindsight. *Journal of Cognitive Neuroscience, 9*, 191–202.

Kentridge, R. W., Heywood, C. A. & Weiskrantz, L. (1999). Effects of temporal cueing on residual visual discrimination in blindsight. *Neuropsychologia, 37*, 479–483.

Kerkhoff, G., Munsinger, U. & Meier, E. (1994). Neurovisual rehabilitation in cerebral blindness. *Archive of Neurology, 51*, 474–481.

Ladavas, E., Paladini, R. & Cubelli, R. (1993). Implicit associative priming in a patient with left visual neglect. *Neuropsychologia, 31*, 1307–1320.

Lane, R. D., Ahern, G. L., Schwartz, G. E. & Kaszniak, A. W. (1997). Is alexithymia the emotional equivalent of blindsight? *Biological Psychiatry, 42*, 834–844.

Linebarger, M. C., Schwartz, M. F. & Saffran, E. M. (1983). Sensitivity to grammatical structure in so-called agrammatic aphasics. *Cognition, 13*, 361–392.

Luciani, L. (1884). On the sensorial localisations in the cortex cerebri. *Brain, 7*, 145–160.

Marshall, J. & Halligan, P. (1988). Blindsight and insight in visuo-spatial neglect. *Nature, 336*, 766–767.

McGlynn, S. & Schacter, D. L. (1989). Unawareness of deficits in neuropsychological syndromes. *Journal of Clinical and Experimental Neuropsychology, 11*, 143–205.

Miller, M., Pasik, P. & Pasik, T. (1980). Extrageniculate vision in the monkey. VII. Contrast sensitivity functions. *Journal of Neurophysiology, 43*, 1510–1526.

Milner, A. D. & Goodale, M. A. (1995). *The Visual Brain in Action.* Oxford: Oxford University Press.

Mohler, C. W. & Wurtz, R. H. (1977). Role of striate cortex and superior colliculus in visual guidance of saccadic eye movements in monkeys. *Journal of Neurophysiology, 43*, 74–94.

Nakamura, R. K. & Mishkin, M. (1979). Chronic blindness following nonvisual cortical lesions in monkeys. *Society of Neuroscience Abstracts, 5*, 800.

Nakamura, R. K. & Mishkin, M. (1980). Blindness in monkeys following non-visual cortical lesions. *Brain Research, 188*, 572–577.

Nakamura, R. K. & Mishkin, M. (1982). Chronic blindness following nonvisual lesions in monkeys: partial lesions and disconnection effects. *Society of Neuroscience Abstracts, 8*, 812.

Nakamura, R. K. & Mishkin, M. (1986). Chronic blindness following lesions of nonvisual cortex in the monkey. *Experimental Brain Research, 62*, 173–184.

Nakamura, R. K., Schein, S. J. & Desimone, R. (1986). Visual responses from cells in striate cortex of monkeys rendered chronically 'blind' by lesions of nonvisual cortex. *Experimental Brain Research, 63*, 185–190.

Paillard, J., Michel, F. & Stelmach, G. (1983). Localization without content: a tactile analogue of 'blind sight'. *Archives of Neurology, 40*, 548–551.

Pasik, P. & Pasik, T. (1971). The visual world of monkeys deprived of visual cortex: effective stimulus parameters and the importance of the accessory optic system. In T. Shipley & J. E. Dowling (Eds), *Visual Processes in Vertebrates*, Vision Research Supplement no. 3 (pp. 419–435). Oxford: Pergamon Press.

Pasik, P. & Pasik, T. (1982). Visual functions in monkeys after total removal of visual cerebral cortex. *Contributions to Sensory Physiology, 7*, 141–200.

Pöppel, E., Held, R. & Frost, D. (1973). Residual visual function after brain wounds involving the central visual pathways in man. *Nature, 243*, 295–296.

Rodman, H. T., Gross, C. G. & Albright, T. D. (1989). Afferent basis of visual response properties in area MT of the macaque. I. Effects of striate cortex removal. *Journal of Neuroscience, 9*, 2033–2050.

Rosenthal, D. (1986). Two concepts of consciousness. *Philosophical Studies, 49*, 329–359.

Rosenthal, D. (1990). *A Theory of Consciousness.* Report no. 40, Research Group on Mind and Brain. Perspectives in Theoretical Psychology and the Philosophy of Mind. Biele-feld: University of Bielefeld.

Rosenthal, D. (1993). Thinking that one thinks. In M. Davies & G. W. Humphreys (Eds), *Consciousness. Psychology and Philosophical Essays* (pp. 198–223). Oxford: Black-well.

Rossetti, Y., Rode, G. & Boisson, D. (1995). Implicit processing of somaesthetic informa-tion: a dissociation between where and how? *NeuroReport, 6,* 506–510.

Sahraie, A., Weiskrantz, L., Barbur, J. L., Simmons, A., Williams, S. C. R. & Brammer, M. J. (1997). Pattern of neuronal activity associated with conscious and unconscious processing of visual signals. *Proceedings of the National Academy of Science, USA, 94,* 9406–9411.

Schacter, D. L., McAndrews, M. P. & Moscovitch, M. (1988). Access to consciousness: dissociations between implicit and explicit knowledge in neuropsychological syn-dromes. In L. Weiskrantz (Ed), *Thought Without Language* (pp. 242–278). Oxford: Oxford University Press.

Schilder, P., Pasik, P. & Pasik, T. (1972). Extrageniculate vision in the monkey. III. Circle vs triangle and 'red vs green' discrimination. *Experimental Brain Research, 14,* 436–448.

Schneider, G. E. (1967). Contrasting visuomotor functions of tectum and cortex in the golden hamster. *Psychologie Forschung, 31,* 52–62.

Sergent, J. & Poncet, M. (1990). From covert to overt recognition of faces in a prosopag-nosic patient. *Brain, 113,* 989–1004.

Shallice, T. & Saffran, E. (1986). Lexical processing in the absence of explicit word identifi-cation: evidence from a letter-by-letter reader. *Cognitive Neuropsychology, 3,* 429–458.

Sherrington, C. C. (1957). Spinal cord. *Encyclopaedia Brittanica, 21,* 227.

Sperry, R. W., Myers, R. E. & Schrier, A. M. (1960). Perceptual capacity in the isolated visual cortex in the cat. *Quarterly Journal of Experimental Psychology, 12,* 65–71.

Stoerig, P. & Cowey, A. (1992). Wavelength sensitivity in blindsight. *Brain, 115,* 425–444.

Tranel, D. & Damasio, A. R. (1985). Knowledge without awareness: an autonomic index of facial recognition by prosopagnosics. *Science, 228,* 1453–1455.

Trevarthen, C. B. (1968). Two mechanisms of vision in primates. *Psychologie Forschung, 31,* 299–337.

Tyler, L. K. (1988). Spoken language comprehension in a fluent aphasic patient. *Cognitive Neuropsychology, 5,* 375–400.

Warrington, E. K. & Weiskrantz, L. (1968). New method of testing long-term retention with special reference to amnesic patients. *Nature, 217,* 972–974.

Weiskrantz, L. (1986). *Blindsight. A Case Study and Implications.* Oxford: Oxford Univer-sity Press.

Weiskrantz, L. (1990). Outlooks for blindsight: explicit methodologies for implicit pro-cesses. The Ferrier Lecture. *Proceedings of the Royal Society of London, B 239,* 247–278.

Weiskrantz, L. (1991). Disconnected awareness for detecting, processing& remembering in neurological patients. *Journal of the Royal Society of Medicine, 84,* 466–470.

Weiskrantz, L. (1995). Blindsight: not an island unto itself. *Current Directions in Psycho-logical Science, 4,* 146–151.

Weiskrantz, L. (1996). Blindsight revisited. *Current Opinion in Neurobiology, 6,* 215–220.

Weiskrantz, L. (1997). *Consciousness Lost and Found. A Neuropsychological Exploration.* Oxford: Oxford University Press.

Weiskrantz, L., Barbur, J. L. & Sahraie, A. (1995). Parameters affecting conscious versus unconscious visual discrimination without V1. *Proceedings of the National Academy of Science, USA, 92,* 6122–6126.

Weiskrantz, L. & Cowey, A. (1970). Filling in the scotoma: a study of residual vision after striate cortex lesions in monkeys. In E. Stellar & J. M. Sprague (Eds), *Progress in Physiological Psychology*, vol. 3 (pp. 237–260). New York: Academic Press.

Weiskrantz, L., Harlow, A. & Barbur, J. L. (1991). Factors affecting visual sensitivity in a hemianopic subject. *Brain, 114*, 2269–2282.

Wilson, B. A. (1995). Management and remediation of memory problems in brain-injured adults. In A. D. Baddeley, B. A. Wilson & F. N. Watts (Eds), *Handbook of Memory Disorders* (pp. 451–479).

Young, A. W. (1994). Conscious and unconscious recognition of familiar faces. In C. Umulta & M. Moscovitch (Eds), *Attention and Performance XV* (pp. 153–178). Cambridge, MA: MIT Press.

Young, M. P. (1992). Objective analysis of the topological organization of the primate cortical visual system. *Nature, 358*, 152–155.

Young, M. P. (1993). The organization of neural systems in the primate cerebral cortex. *Proceedings of the Royal Society of London, B, 252*, 13–18.

Zihl, J. (1980). 'Blindsight': improvement of visually guided eye movements by systematic practice in patients with cerebral blindness. *Neuropsychologia, 18*, 71–77.

Zihl, J. (1981). Recovery of visual functions in patients with cerebral blindness. *Experimental Brain Research, 44*, 159–169.

Zihl, J., Tretter, F. & Singer, W. (1980). Phasic electrodermal responses after visual stimulation in the cortically blind hemifield. *Behavioural Brain Research, 1*, 197–203.

Zihl, J. & von Cramon, D. (1979). Restitution of visual function in patients with cerebral blindness. *Journal of Neurological Neurosurgery and Psychiatry, 42*, 312–322.

Zihl, J., von Cramon, D. & Mai, N. (1983). Selective disturbance of movement vision after bilateral brain damage. *Brain, 106*, 313–340.

Zihl, J. & Werth, R. (1984). Contributions to the study of 'blindsight'—I. The role of specific practice for saccadic localization in patients with postgeniculate visual field defects. *Neuropsychologia, 22*, 13–22.

13

Unconscious Emotion: Evolutionary Perspectives, Psychophysiological Data, and Neuropsychological Mechanisms

ARNE ÖHMAN, ANDERS FLYKT, AND DANIEL LUNDQVIST

An Evolutionary Perspective on Emotion

The Function of Emotion

Emotions can be understood as action sets (e.g., Frijda, 1986; Lang, 1984) preparing the organism to act in some ways rather than in others. From this perspective, there is no clear boundary between emotion and motivation. Traditionally, motivation has been more related to action tendencies induced from internal states such as hunger, whereas emotion most often has been related to states elicited by external stimuli. A fundamental dimension in both emotion and motivation is that of approach–avoidance, ranging from a readiness to stay in a situation and engage in its potentialities to abandoning it because of the threats and dangers it implies (Lang et al., 1990). The functional advantage of these processes is that they allow for flexibility in the interaction between organism and environment. In effect, a primary function of emotion has been described as the decoupling of stimuli and responses (Scherer, 1994). Rather than the rigid stimulus–response relationship of signal stimuli and fixed action patterns described by ethologists (e.g., Tinbergen, 1951), emotions in many contexts allow flexible use of environmental support to achieve desired outcomes (e.g., Archer, 1979; Damasio, 1994). For example, when distressed, children seek the support and comfort of their parents whether by their own locomotion (crawling, walking, or running) or by vocal behavior prompting parental approach. However, the decoupling of stimulus and response is by no means absolute, because time for deliberation is not always an advantage. A predator, for example, strikes fast and hard, and the quicker defensive maneuvers are initiated by the potential prey, the better its chances to survive the encounter. Particularly in defensive circumstances, therefore, time is a critical issue, and then emotional activation and reflexive escape action may be virtually instantaneous.

Emotions are means designed to regulate behavior in relation to agendas set by biological evolution. Thus, emotion pervaded the critical ecological problems that our distant ancestors had to solve if their genes were to be represented in the next generation. These problems included finding and consuming food and drink, finding shelters, seeking protection and support from conspecifics, asserting oneself socially, satisfying curiosity, getting access to and engaging with sexual partners, caring for offspring, and avoiding and escaping life-threatening events. These are all activities structured by emotions (see Tooby & Cosmides, 1990). In a biological perspective, therefore, emotions can be understood as clever means shaped by evolution to make us want to do what our ancestors had to do successfully to pass genes on to coming generations (e.g., Öhman, 1993a, 1996).

Conceptual Implications

The evolutionary–functional perspective on the psychology of emotion shifts the emphasis from the unique phenomenology of human feeling to action tendencies and response patterns that we share with fellow inhabitants of the animal kingdom. Rather than conceptualizing emotion as a central feeling state more or less imperfectly mirrored in verbal reports, physiological responses, and expressive behavior, the evolutionary perspective views emotion as complex responses that include several partly independent components (see Öhman & Birbaumer, 1993, for a more thorough discussion of some key conceptual issues in the study of emotion). "Emotional phenomena" (Frijda, 1986) occur in situations that are significant to the person for phylogenetic or ontogenetic reasons. They are related to verbal responses implying affective appraisal and evaluation of the situation. At the behavioral level, emotional phenomena are manifested, for example, as approach or avoidance tendencies (e.g., Lang et al., 1990), expressive facial gestures (e.g., Fridlund, 1994), or noninstrumental (e.g., "overflow") characteristics of behavior (Frijda, 1986). Finally, because emotions involve often vigorous action tendencies, they recruit metabolic support from bodily mechanisms related to behavioral energetics and arousal processes, which become accessible to scientific study through psychophysiological measures (e.g., electrodermal activity and heart rate). In this perspective, the verbal, behavioral, and physiological components of emotions should not be understood as alternative avenues to unitary internal states presumably isomorphic with phenomenological experience, but as loosely coupled and dissociable components of a complex emotional response (Lang, 1993).

A Perspective on Unconscious Emotion

Conceptualizing emotion as composed of dissociable components implies that "unconscious emotion" simply is a specific case of a dissociation—evidence of physiological or behavioral emotional activation in the absence of verbal reports of emotion or emotionally relevant stimulation (Lang, 1993). From the evolutionary perspective it follows that activation of basic emotional systems is more or less independent of conscious awareness of what is going on (see LeDoux, 1996; Öhman, 1999). This is a consequence of the assumption that the evolution of emotion by far preceded the emergence of linguistically competent organisms. For humans, however, once basic emotional systems are activated, both the eliciting conditions and aspects of the emotional response are accessible in conscious experience, and conscious elaboration then is likely to shape the further fate of the emotional state, as well as its consequences for action.

Unconscious emotion becomes a serious problem only if one claims that feeling is the necessary condition of emotion, because then it implies a contradiction in terms (Clore, 1994). The notion of emotion as experience is typically part of the common-sense view that all causally important psychological events converge in consciousness before they, for instance, are channeled into action. From such a mentalistic perspective, claims of unconscious emotion break with psychological common sense and require special explanations as in the Freudian theory of the unconscious. The broader evolutionary perspective, in contrast, leads researchers to address issues such as, Which conditions determine that an episode of emotion becomes consciously accessible? What effects does this have for further emotional processing? and Does the neural circuitry differ between unconscious and conscious emotion? (See Öhman, 1999, for a more thorough theoretical analysis of unconscious emotional processes).

In this chapter we address unconscious emotion in the sense that emotion can be activated without conscious recognition of the eliciting stimulus. This may happen when an emotionally relevant stimulus, which is presented outside conscious attention, automatically redirects attention to become its focus, or when a stimulus that is prevented from reaching conscious awareness through backward masking nonetheless elicits psychophysiological responses suggesting emotional activation. In both instances we argue that an important factor determining whether the emotional stimulus becomes consciously perceived is time. In the interest of promoting rapid responding to biologically significant stimuli, perceptual and energetic processes may respond to emotional stimuli before they are consciously registered. These lines of evidence suggest that emotions can be activated independently of consciousness, much as in Zajonc's (1980) slogan that "preferences need no inferences."

Emotion and Attention

The Signal Function of Emotion

Even though the functional focus of this evolutionary perspective on emotion is on the organization of action, emotions have pervasive effects on all types of psychological processes, from perception to cognition, learning, and so on (Tooby & Cosmides, 1990). To become favorably evaluated by natural selection, the successful behavioral strategies regulated by emotions must recruit efficient action, which presupposes extraction of critical information from the environment. To this end, emotion guides attention. Indeed, many theorists agree that emotions have important "signal functions" that prompt the organism to focus attention on particular aspects of the surroundings (e.g., Folkman et al., 1979; Hamburg et al., 1975; Izard, 1979, 1991). For example, as stated by Izard (1979, p. 163), "a particular emotion sensitizes the organism to particular features of its environment . . . [and] ensures a readiness to respond to events of significance to the organism's survival and adaptation." According to Izard (1991), this sensitization function is most obviously seen in the emotion of interest, but it is also coupled to a powerful disrupt-and-reset function when unexpected stimuli are encountered, the emotional counterpart of which is surprise. The purpose of this function is to redirect the activity of the organism toward significant but unexpected stimuli.

In many respects this function of emotion is similar to that ascribed to the orienting reflex (Öhman, 1987; Sokolov, 1963). Through the automatic capture of attention by stimuli that are significant to the organism, processing of the stimulus is shifted from an automatic stimulus analysis mechanism working in parallel across the perceptual field to the capacity-limited, serial, and effortful controlled processing that has been associated with focused attention and consciousness (Öhman, 1979, 1987).

The signal function of emotion implies that we attend to different aspects of the environment when in different emotional states. When in a euphoric mood, we may concentrate attentional resources on cues signaling success, which may facilitate performance (Isen, 1993), but sometimes also incur a risk of missing task-relevant signals that call for a change in the course of action if failure is to be avoided. When in separation distress, the child's attention may be focused on sounds that indicate the return of the parents, such as car noise in the driveway, and when plagued by fear and anxiety, attention becomes biased to focus on threats in the surrounding world (Mathews, 1990; Öhman, 1993a).

The Attentional Spotlight

Focused spatial attention can be represented as a spotlight cutting through the dark to illuminate a specific object in the environment or an item in memory (e.g., Johnston & Dark, 1986). However, it is important to remember that the darkness outside the spotlight is not composed of homogeneous, empty space, but rather should be envisioned as a dark but often familiar room, which we examine by help of a focused flashlight. Thus, we typically know quite well which objects are hidden in the dark and where they are located, and we can easily focus the flashlight on the objects we need in terms of our current concerns. Even if the room were entered for the first time, we would not be at a loss, but would expect to find furniture more probably located at some locations rather than others, and as soon as the flashlight would reveal a bed, for example, hypotheses as to which other furniture were likely to be located in the presumed bedroom would be readily formulated. Furthermore, depending on the dominating current concern (e.g., finding the light switch, stealing jewelry, or escaping from the house) the flashlight would search different aspects of the room and its content.

In an analogous way, emotion regulates attention systematically to specific aspects of the environment according to both phylogenetic contingencies of the far past of our ancestors and our own more recently encountered ontogenetic contingencies. Thus, hypotheses (more or less explicitly formulated) as to where critical information may hide in the yet-to-be-explored environment are activated by the emotional state and help to shape the attentional search for critical information.

Technically speaking, stimulus-driven attention capture always interacts with the goal-driven control of attention activated by an emotional state (Yantis, 1998).

Particularly if there is time pressure involved, such as when suspecting danger (e.g., a lurking predator), directing the spotlight may be assisted by automatic routines which may use preexisting knowledge to locate potential threats anywhere in the perceptual field. In this way, the flashlight can be quickly moved to critical areas of the surroundings to promote rapidly dealing with the threat. These automatic, preattentive routines are likely to make use of superficial stimulus information to alert the attentional spotlight. Thus, they are likely to be biased toward "false positives" (reacting to a stimulus that turns out innocuous on closer examination) rather than "false negatives" (failing to react to what turns out to be a critical stimuli) because of the potential deadly cost of the latter alternative. This is just one example of what Mineka (1992) has termed "adaptive conservatism" to describe the cautiousness of animals when it comes to dealing with fear stimuli. From this functional scenario, one would postulate that there are mechanisms automatically locating significant stimuli in the surroundings by means of parallel processing perceptual systems that focus on critical information in the environment on the basis of superficial feature analyses. Thus, the conventional attentional spotlight would only come into play after this first preliminary and preattentive analysis of the stimulus array. Even though the type of division of labor between preattentive, automatic attention mechanisms and the spotlight of conscious attention that we have described here may characterize many individual emotions, it was developed in relation to the specific emotion of fear, which is the topic to which we now turn.

Fear, Anxiety, and Attention

Fear is a negative or aversive, highly activated emotional state that prompts avoidance of and escape from situations that threaten the survival or well-being of organisms. Öhman et al. (1985) analyzed fear within two important evolutionarily derived behavioral systems: a predatory defense system and a social submissiveness system. Thus, in this perspective, fear operates to bring organisms away from predators and to promote yielding in the face of dominant group members. These two types of fear have important differences (Öhman, 1986), but they also have a common core centered on avoidance. Successful avoidance of threatening situations requires perceptual systems that can locate stimuli related to threat wherever they occur in the perceptual field. Clearly, there is a premium on speed: fast identification of threat allows early activation of defenses, which may bring the potential victim out of reach of the striking predator or the moody authority figure before any damage can happen. Defined in this way, fear is an emotion associated with active coping with threats. However, if efforts to cope with the threat fail, one is left in a situation of uncertain controllability, and fear is transformed into anxiety (Epstein, 1972). Thus, fear and anxiety have a common evolutionary descent, which gives them a common core, but they also differ profoundly with respect to behavioral outlets. Fear is related to active coping (sometimes in the form of immobility or freezing), whereas anxiety takes over when the threat is resilient to coping efforts.

The evolutionary perspective implies that stimuli that have been associated with threat throughout mammalian evolution should be easily connected to fear and anxiety and that, as emotion-provoking, they should be effective attention catchers. The analyses presented by Öhman et al. (1985) suggests that evolutionary fear-relevant stimuli are likely to be found among threatening beasts and humans. Specifically, we concentrate on what may be termed the prototype of animal fears, snakes and spiders (Öhman, 1986; Öhman et al., 1985), and on an equally prototypical threatening facial gesture related to anger and dominance (Dimberg & Öhman, 1996; Öhman & Dimberg, 1984). The first hypothesis to be examined, therefore, is straightforward: evolutionary relevant threat stimuli should be very effective in capturing attention.

Automatic Attention to Facial Threat

The Face-in-the-Crowd Effect

Hansen and Hansen (1988) exposed subjects to complex matrices of visual stimuli with the task of pressing different buttons depending on whether all stimuli in a matrix were similar or whether it included a deviant stimulus. In support of the evolutionarily derived hypothesis, they reported that subjects were faster to locate a deviant angry face in a background crowd of happy faces than vice versa. This "anger superiority effect," furthermore, was reported to be unaffected by the size of the background crowd, which was taken as support for attributing it to an automatic "pop-out" effect of preattentive origin. In line with the previously developed argument, Hansen and Hansen (1988) proposed that angry faces were located by parallel processing mechanisms that automatically picked out the target, whereas the location of happy faces required a postattentive serial search. In agreement with the evolutionary scenario, this interpretation suggested that evolutionarily significant threat stimuli were automatically located in a complex visual display.

However, there are several problems with this interpretation. Most important, an error of experimental design confounded the report of the pop-out effect. Only one angry and one happy face was used, and the angry face had a characteristic shadow, which appears to account for the pop-out effect (Purcell et al., 1996). Furthermore, subjects were faster to decide that a deviant target was not present in a matrix of happy than in a matrix of angry faces. Consistent with other data (e.g., Kirouac & Doré, 1984), this finding suggests that the angry faces were harder to process than the happy ones, perhaps because happy faces are much more prevalent in the environment of the typical subject population for this type of experiment, college students (Bond & Siddle, 1996). Later reports that response latencies to angry targets were affected by location of the target in the matrix (Hampton et al., 1989) suggest that sequential search strategies were used in the search for angry targets, too. Consequently, the shorter latency for angry targets in happy crowds could be attributed to more efficient processing of the background happy faces (i.e., to postattentive rather than to preattentive mechanisms) (Hansen & Hansen, 1994). Thus, the original Hansen and Hansen (1988) data cannot be invoked as support for automatic selection of threatening stimuli.

The Face-in-the-Crowd Effect with
Schematic Facial Stimuli

Because the findings reported by Hansen and Hansen (1988) are critical for our hypothesis, we have performed a series of studies aiming at a further elucidation of the face-in-the-crowd effect while avoiding the hazards that plagued interpretation of their findings. A strategical first choice in our research was to use schematic rather than real faces. The use of real faces is complicated because it is difficult directly to control their physical features. For example, angry faces are more similar than happy faces to neutral control faces, which may explain why happy faces are often more quickly found among neutral ones than are angry faces (e.g., Byrne & Eysenck, 1995; Öhman et al., unpublished data). With schematic faces, on the other hand, threatening and nonthreatening faces can be constructed so that their physical difference from a neutral face is identical. By using schematic faces, furthermore, we should be able to determine more exactly which facial features are critical for a potential angry superiority effect.

Attempting to delineate the critical feature of threatening symbolic faces, Aronoff et al. (1988) collected threatening masks from a wide assortment of cultures and defined features that were common to most of them. Such features included static aspect of faces such as pointed ears and dynamic features such as frowning eyebrows or smiling mouths. Many of the features isolated as dynamic characteristic of facial threat by Aronoff et. (1988) conformed to findings reported from studies of schematic faces by McKelvie (1973). Specifically, McKelvie's data indicated that frowning eyebrows were critical for negative evaluation of faces and for perception of anger in a face. Based on these findings, we constructed facial stimuli in which several features such as eyebrows, mouths, eyes, and cheekbones could be independently manipulated. In a series of rating studies (Lundqvist et al., 1999) we found that these features appeared to be hierarchically structured in an affective space defined by the semantic differential dimensions of evaluation, activity, and potency. First, frowning eyebrows made faces cluster within an area of affective space that could be characterized as negatively evaluated, potent, and highly activated, whereas faces with the opposite eyebrow (i.e., raised in the middle) were clustered in a positively evaluated area of the affective space. These clusters were divided into subclusters by the mouth (happy or sad), and these subclusters, in turn, were further split depending on the shape of the eye, and so on.

On the basis of these findings, we selected threatening, nonthreatening. and neutral faces for use in the type of visual search paradigm developed by Hansen and Hansen (1988). These faces are illustrated in the sample of actual matrices shown in figure 13.1.

In the first experiment we exposed subjects to 3×3 matrices of schematic faces (see figure 13.1), of which half showed 9 identical facial expressions (neutral, threatening [angry], or nonthreatening [happy]). In the remaining half of the trials, one of the nine faces showed a deviant gesture: angry against a neutral background, happy against neutral background, angry against a happy background, happy against an angry background, and neutral against any of the expressive backgrounds. The deviant stimulus occurred equally often at all positions in the matrix.

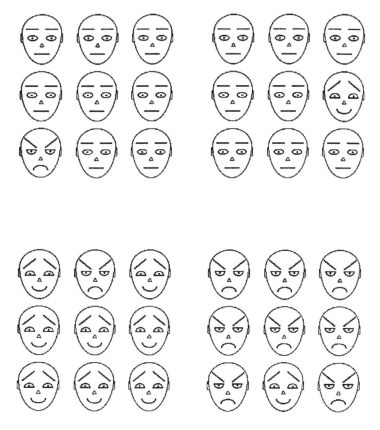

Figure 13.1. Examples of 3 × 3 matrices of schematic faces used in visual search studies. The task of the subject was to determine whether a face with a deviant expression was present in the (separately presented) 3 × 3 matrices. The two upper matrices show angry (left) and happy (right) faces against neutral background faces, and the two lower show angry against happy background (left) and happy against angry backgrounds (right). In the experiment half the matrices did not include a deviant face.

Exposure times were 1 or 2 sec. The subjects pressed one button if all faces were the same and another one it there was a deviant stimulus in the matrix.

The results (figure 13.2) showed a clear overall effect of threat in the detection time for deviant stimuli. Regardless of background condition, detection was faster for threatening (angry) than for nonthreatening (happy) stimuli. However, finding a neutral face among angry or happy faces was still faster because of the distinct physical difference between targets and distractors in this condition. The background condition interacted with exposure time. With neutral background, detection of the threatening face was faster both with 1- and 2-sec exposure. With the opposite-expression background (nonthreatening with a threatening deviant; threatening with a nonthreatening deviant), however, the faster detection of threatening

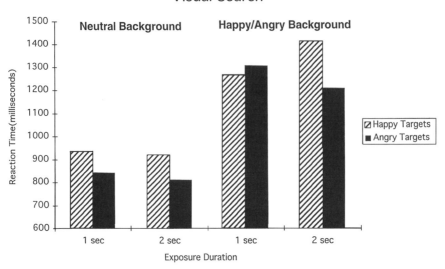

Figure 13.2. Detection latencies (reaction times) from a visual search experiment where subjects determined whether a deviant target stimulus (happy or angry) was present in matrices composed of neutral background faces or happy/angry background faces. Exposure time of the matrix was either 1 or 2 sec.

faces was evident only at the longer interval. Similar to the fast detection of neutral deviants against backgrounds of angry or happy faces, this implies that the difficulty of the perceptual discrimination was important. When discrimination was easy (i.e., when the background had horizontal features and the targets diagonal ones), 1-sec exposure was sufficient to get the anger superiority effect. However, when the perceptual discrimination was difficult (i.e., both background and targets had diagonal lines), 2-sec were needed for the anger superiority effect to emerge. This implies that the search for angry faces, although more efficient than that for happy faces, was not fully automatic. Rather, the data appear to indicate that the angry faces were quickly found against a neutral background but that the more difficult task of finding an angry face against a background of happy faces was more effort-demanding and required more time. However, even though angry and happy faces were equally discriminable from each other and from the neutral face, the detection times for angry deviants were always faster than those for happy deviants. This search asymmetry in favor of angry faces suggests that angry, but not happy, faces had a critical feature that could be preattentively located (Treisman & Souther, 1985).

There was no difference in latency to decide that a deviant stimulus was not present in matrices of threatening and nonthreatening faces, which both took significantly longer than matrices of neutral stimuli. Error rates were low and tended to be lower for threatening than for nonthreatening deviants.

These results show clearly that a threatening facial display is more rapidly detected against a background crowd of faces than are nonthreatening facial displays. None of the confounding factors that becloud interpretation of the original Hansen and Hansen findings were present in this study. Error rates were low, there was no confounding factor favoring the threat condition, and subjects were as fast to detect that a deviant stimulus was not present in a matrix of threatening faces as in matrices of nonthreatening faces. Thus, these results provide support for the hypothesis that humans in general are particularly effective in discovering threatening stimuli in their surroundings.

Potentiation of Attention to Facial Threat by Anxiety

One may wonder whether emotion is critical to the effects reported with our schematic facial stimuli. The happy and angry faces were physically similar, as both had diagonal lines for eyebrows and curved lines for mouths, and the eyes were simply inverted from one expression to the other. This made both expressions differ to the same degree from neutral faces. Nevertheless, the subjects were consistently faster in finding the angry face in the crowd, even though we know nothing about whether they actually responded emotionally to the expressions. One way to clarify this finding would be to use a subject population likely to respond emotionally to the threatening stimulus and then see whether they would be faster than normal subjects in finding a deviant threatening face. Such an experiment still remains to be done in our laboratory, but there are recent data available from other investigators starting from the premise that anxiety is associated with a generalized bias to focus attention on threatening words (e.g., MacLeod, 1991; Mathews, 1990).

First, Byrne and Eysenck (1995) examined detection latencies for real angry and happy faces against a background of neutral faces and happy faces against backgrounds of neutral or angry faces. Highly anxious subjects were faster than subjects low in anxiety to find angry faces against a background of neutral faces, whereas the two groups did not differ in latency to find happy faces against a neutral background. When the background consisted of angry faces, anxious subjects were slower to find happy faces than were nonanxious subjects, suggesting a powerful distracting effect from angry background faces. These findings suggest that high anxiety enhances the normal bias to be faster in discriminating threatening than nonthreatening stimuli.

Bradley and Mogg (1996) used normal controls and persons diagnosed with generalized anxiety disorder or depression as subjects in an attentional experiment using faces as stimuli. A trial started with 1-sec exposures of two faces with different emotional expressions side by side on a screen. Facial expressions included anger (threat), sadness, and happiness, as well as a neutral control expression. When the faces disappeared, a probe stimulus emerged, centered at the point where one of the faces had been. The probe occurred equally often after either face, and the subjects were required to press different response keys depending on the side of the face after which the probe was presented. In addition to probe reaction times, eye movements were measured to determine at which of the two pictures the subjects looked and with what latency. The results showed a bias of the generalized anxiety disorder patients to look at angry faces, with reliably shorter latencies than for other expressions. Again, threatening facial stimuli proved effective attention catchers, particularly for persons with anxiety disorder. Following Yantis (1998), it can be argued that stimulus-driven attention capture was potentiated because anxiety sensitized the setting of goal-driven attention for threatening stimuli. Emotion, therefore, appears to drive attention.

Automatic Attention to Threatening Animal Stimuli

The Snake-in-the-Grass Effect

The results reviewed in the previous section show clearly that facial stimuli implying threat are more effective than nonthreatening stimuli in capturing the attention of both normal and anxious subjects. This provides good support for the evolutionary hypothesis suggesting that fear stimuli that have followed humans through their evolution should be efficient attention capturers. From this perspective, one wonders whether similar results would be observed with other classes of evolutionarily fear-relevant stimuli such as pictures of snakes and spiders. Such studies have been performed in our laboratory (Öhman et al., 1999).

Subjects were exposed to matrices of pictures of either snakes, spiders, flowers, or mushrooms. In half of the cases all stimuli in the matrix were of the same category, whereas the other half had a stimulus from a deviant category. In support of the evolutionary hypothesis, subjects were quicker to find a deviant snake or spider among flowers and mushrooms than vice versa. This increase in speed of detection was not accompanied by more errors; to the contrary, there were fewer errors in detecting fear-relevant than fear-irrelevant deviant stimuli. Response latencies were shortest for deviant snakes among background flowers followed by spiders among mushrooms. The longest latencies were found for deviant mushrooms among background snakes and flowers among spiders. This distribution of detection latencies appears to make ecological sense. When flowers or mushrooms served as deviant stimuli, detection times were influenced by their location in the matrix. With snake and spider deviants, however, location in the matrix had no effect on detection latency, which suggests that they were automatically detected.

Furthermore, overall it took longer to detect a target in a large (3×3) than in a small (2×2) matrix, but, as indicated by the interaction between fear relevance and size of matrix, this effect was more obvious for fear-irrelevant than fear-relevant targets. In fact, separate tests showed a reliable size-of-matrix effect only for fear-irrelevant targets. Thus, attention appeared to be automatically drawn to deviant snakes and spiders, whereas a more sequential search strategy was used to locate deviant flowers and mushrooms. These results indicate that fear-relevant stimuli were picked up independently of their position in the perceptual field in a process reminiscent of a "pop-out" effect of preattentive origin.

As with the visual search studies using schematic faces as stimuli, these data cannot be accounted for in terms of the confounding factors plaguing interpretation of the original Hansen and Hansen (1988) studies (see Hansen & Hansen, 1994). Because we used categories of stimuli rather than single exemplars for each fear-relevance condition, it is unlikely that some common confounding factor for all animal stimuli could account for finding shorter latencies to them. Indeed, with our design, one cannot but wonder what stimulus features were used by the visual system to quickly extract that a critical stimulus was present in the display. Second, latencies to decide that a critical stimulus was not present were shorter for the fear-relevant than the fear-irrelevant categories, which precludes appeal to faster recognition of the fear-irrelevant stimulus as a basis for the shorter detection latency of deviant fear-relevant stimuli (cf. Hampton et al., 1989).

Snakes in the Grass: Fearful Subjects

A similar question to that raised with regard to the facial stimuli could be raised in the context of biologically fear-relevant animal stimuli: would subjects fearful of snakes or spiders show a more pronounced bias than nonfearful subjects in detecting such stimuli?

Specific-fear questionnaires were administered to a large group of students (of medicine, physical therapy, or optics), and those scoring above the 80th percentile in snake fear and below the 50th percentile in spider fear, or vice versa, were invited to participate in an experiment. A nonfearful control group, scoring below the 50th percentile in both types of fear, was also recruited. With this selection procedure, each subject could be exposed both to feared and nonfeared fear-relevant stimuli, e.g., snakes and spiders, respectively, for a specifically snake-fearful subject. All subjects were exposed to the previously described procedure for the second experiment. They had 2×2 and 3×3 matrices, half of which had only pictures of flowers, mushrooms, snakes, or spiders. The remaining half had one picture from a deviant category, i.e., snakes or spiders among flowers or mushrooms, or flowers or mushrooms among snakes or spiders.

The results replicated earlier findings in showing overall shorter reaction times to identify deviant snakes or spiders among flowers or mushrooms than vice versa. Similar to the previous experiments, matrix size had a clear effect on fear-irrelevant stimuli, whereas latencies were as fast with the 2×2 as with the 3×3 matrix for fear-relevant stimuli. Finally, and most important, fearful subjects were faster specifically in identifying their feared as opposed to their nonfeared fear-relevant stimulus (see figure 13.3) (e.g., snake-fearful subjects were faster with snakes than with spiders and vice versa). Thus, having an emotional response connected to the fear-relevant stimulus facilitated its detection.

To sum up, in these section we have described two series of studies that provide converging evidence in support of the hypothesis that evolutionarily relevant threat stimuli are highly effective in engaging attention. Indeed, because the size and complexity of the display seemed to matter less for fear-relevant than for fear-irrelevant stimuli, finding fear-relevant stimuli in a complex display appears to depend on an automatic process that does not require conscious attention. Even among normal (nonfearful, nonanxious) subjects, detecting fear-relevant stimuli among fear-irrelevant ones was faster than vice versa. This difference, however, was further enhanced in populations of subjects likely to respond emotionally to the target stimuli. Thus, subjects with generalized anxiety disorder showed a bias to direct their attention and respond faster to threatening facial displays, and subjects specifically fearful of snakes or spiders were extremely fast to discover their specific feared stimulus. These results imply that all of us share a sensitivity to identify

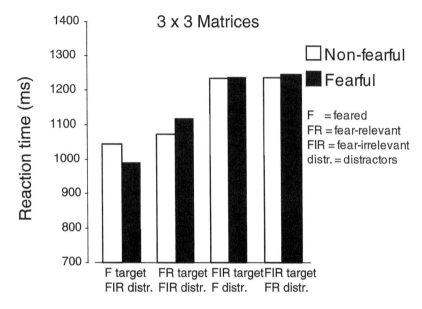

Figure 13.3. Detection latencies (reaction times) for fear-relevant (snakes, spiders) or fear-irrelevant (flowers, mushrooms) stimuli in fearful and nonfearful subjects. Fearful subjects were selected to fear either snakes or spiders but not both. The nonfearful subjects were arbitrarily allocated as controls for feared and nonfeared fear-relevant targets in the fearful subjects. Note that all subjects were faster to detect fear-relevant than fear-irrelevant stimuli and that fearful subjects were even faster to detect the specific stimuli they feared.

features of potential danger and that this general tendency becomes more obvious for persons who respond with acute fear to the stimuli.

Automatic Activation of Fear to Phobic Stimuli

Theoretical Considerations

An important question raised by the demonstration of enhanced attention to threatening stimuli concerns its consequences for emotional activation. One possibility is that we all share a preattentive bias to attend to threat and that, as a result, conscious attention is focused on the threat. This bias would be more pronounced in fearful subjects so that their attention would be more rapidly redirected. However, once attention is redirected to the threat, further responding would be dependent on conscious appraisal of the situation, so that an emotional episode is evoked only if the result of the appraisal implies that fear is justified. In other words, emotional activation would be a postattentive process. The alternative possibility is that not only attention, but also emotion, is controlled from the automatic, preattentive level, so that the attentional shift and the emotional activation would occur in parallel. Evolutionary considerations speak in favor of the latter alternative because rapid emotional activation would mobilize resources immediately to deal with the threat, which would improve the odds of surviving the encounter. There are neural mechanisms to boost this argument. LeDoux (e.g., 1996) has delineated a neural network in rodents that may route fear-related stimulus information monosynaptically via the thalamus to the amygdala, thus bypassing the slower multisynaptic pathway via the cortex to prompt early responding to threats. In this way the emotional response would be activated before the stimulus is completely processed at the cortical level.

Autonomic Responses to Phobic Stimuli

The hypothesis that fear activation does not require conscious perception of the fear-eliciting stimulus for its elicitation was tested by Öhman and Soares (1994). They made use of the consistent finding that snake- and spider-phobic subjects show elevated psychophysiological responses to visual representations of their feared object (e.g., Fredrikson, 1981; Hare & Blevings, 1975; see Sartory, 1983, for a review). For example, Globisch et al. (1999) reported that snake- or spider-fearful subjects, in contrast to normal controls, showed enhanced skin conductance responses, a heart rate acceleration as opposed to a deceleration, and a blood pressure increase to pictures of snakes or spiders as compared to neutral or positively evaluated pictures (see figure 13.4). In addition, startle probe stimuli presented after onset of the feared pictures showed substantial potentiation of the startle blink reflex (figure 13.5), indicating escape and avoidance inclinations (Lang et al., 1990) even if stimulus durations were very short (150 msec). Thus, these results document that fearful subjects show a pronounced emotional response to feared stimuli.

Backward Masking as a Method to Assure Preattentive Processing

In normal perception, preattentive and conscious information processing interact to determine what is eventually perceived. These levels are intimately interwoven, and therefore special methods are needed to tease them apart if one wants to demonstrate that emotional responding can be elicited after only a preattentive, automatic analysis of the stimulus in the absence of its conscious recognition (Öhman, 1999). One method to tease apart nonconscious automatic mechanisms of stimulus analysis from conscious appraisal of the stimulus is backward masking. With this procedure, the conscious recognition of a target stimulus is blocked by an immediately following masking stimulus. The extent to which the target stimulus is perceived is primarily dependent on the interval between the onsets of the target and the masking stimuli, the stimulus-onset asynchrony (SOA) (Esteves & Öhman, 1993). When this interval is short (say, less than 50 msec), the masking stimulus tends to completely block recognition of the target stimulus. Yet, it can be demonstrated that the target stimulus, even though it remains blocked from awareness, influences the person's behavior (see Bornstein & Pittman, 1992, for reviews). For example, Marcel (1983) demonstrated that reaction times to identify the color of

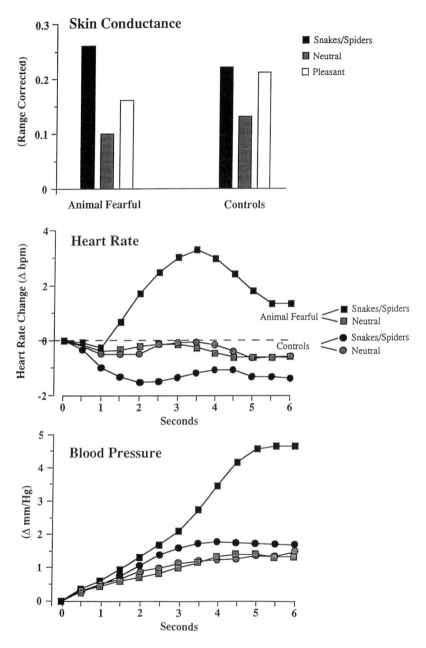

Figure 13.4. Skin conductance, heart rate, and blood pressure responses in spider- or snake-fearful and nonfearful subjects exposed to snakes/spiders, pleasant (data only shown for skin conductance), or neutral stimuli. Note the larger skin conductance responses and the pronounced heart rate acceleration and the clear blood pressure increase to the feared stimulus. (Data from Globish et al., 1999.)

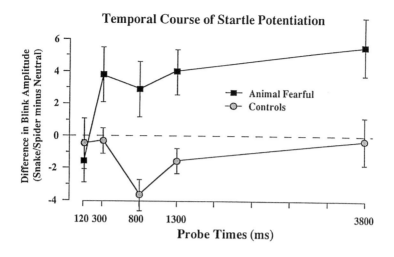

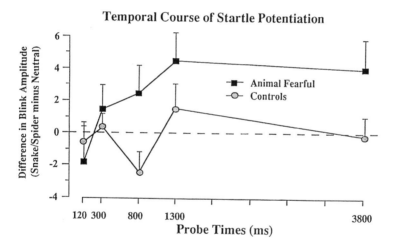

Figure 13.5. Difference in startle blink amplitude to startle probes between reflexes elicited against a background snakes/spider and neutral pictures as a function of interval between picture onset and startle probe. The upper panel shows data from 6-sec picture exposures, and the lower panel shows data from 150 msec exposures. Note the clear startle potentiation to the feared stimuli already 300 msec after their onset, and also that a very short fear-stimulus elicited a response that ran its course long after picture offset (lower panel). (Data from Globish et al., 1999.)

patches presented to subjects were affected by preceding color-words even when the words were impossible to recognize because of backward masking.

Esteves and Öhman (1993) and Öhman and Soares (1993, 1994) adapted the backward masking technique for use with emotional stimuli. As masks for common phobic objects, such as pictures of snakes and spiders, Öhman and Soares (1993, 1994) used pictures of similar objects that were cut in pieces and then randomly reassembled and rephotographed so that no central object could be discerned. Esteves and Öhman (1993) examined the effectiveness of facial pictures with a neutral emotional expression as masks for facial pictures portraying affects of anger or happiness.

A forced-choice procedure was used to determine masking effects as a function of the SOA. The subjects were exposed to long series of stimulus pairs, in which the first stimulus served as target and the second as mask. They were required to guess the nature of the target stimulus and then to state their confidence in the guess. The results showed that the subjects required an SOA of about 100 msec for confident correct recognition of the target stimulus, and there were no differences between the stimulus categories. When the SOA was 30 msec or less, the subjects both performed and felt that they performed randomly. These results were stable irrespective of whether the subjects were randomly selected nonfearful university students or classified as highly fearful or nonfearful on the basis of questionnaire data.

Phobic Responses to Masked Stimuli

Using the backward masking technique, Öhman and Soares (1994) tested the hypothesis that phobic fear can be preattentively activated and, thus, that more than shifts in attention can be achieved by automatic stimulus analyses. They selected subjects who were either highly fearful of snakes or of spiders (but not of both) as well as nonfearful controls using the previously described method.

These subjects were exposed to two stimulus series consisting of repeated presentations of pictures of snakes, spiders, flowers, and mushrooms. In the first series, these target pictures were masked by immediately following nonrecognizable pictures (cut and randomly reassembled) at an SOA producing effective masking (30 msec). In the second series, the targets were presented without masks.

Skin conductance responses (SCRs) were recorded as an index of the physiological response component of fear. In addition, the subjects were exposed to an extra series of pictures in which they were asked to rate their subjective response in terms of valence (like/dislike) activation and control.

According to skin conductance data, the subjects who were afraid of snakes showed elevated responding to snakes compared to spiders and neutral stimuli, the spider-fearful subjects showed specifically elevated responses to spiders, and the nonfearful subjects did not differentiate between the categories, regardless of masking condition. Thus, the results from the masked series were similar to those from the nonmasked series, which suggests that most of the response was preattentively recruited.

Interestingly, the psychophysiological findings were paralleled in the ratings of the subjective response to the pictures. Thus, the snake-fearful subjects rated themselves as more disliking, more activated, and less in control when exposed to the masked snakes pictures than to any other pictures. Similar results were obtained for spiders pictures in the spider-fearful subjects, whereas the nonfearful controls did not differentiate between the stimulus categories. Thus, emotional aspects of the stimulus content became available to the cognitive system even though conscious recognition was ruled out. This conforms to data from a split-brain patient described by LeDoux (1996). Even though the left hemisphere could not understand the meaning of single words presented to the right hemisphere, it could rate quite accurately the emotional tone of the words.

These results show conclusively that conscious perception of the phobic stimulus is not necessary to activate fear in phobics. Masked presentation of the phobic stimulus appeared as effective as nonmasked presentation in inducing enhanced SCRs to feared pictures. Thus, preattentive processing of a phobic stimulus is sufficient to recruit at least part of the phobic response. Not only can fear stimuli recruit attention after a mere preattentive analysis of the stimulus array, but fear and anxiety can be activated from stimuli in the environment that are too weak or too peripheral in the perceptual field to enter the focus of conscious attention. Thus, it appears that emotional activation is simultaneous with the shift of attention toward the fear-eliciting stimulus. When the stimulus information eventually is registered in consciousness, this occurs against a background of raising emotional activation, which is likely to shape the appraisal of the stimulus as an emotional one and to give the resulting fear an automatic, uncontrollable quality.

Preattentive Processes in Pavlovian Fear Conditioning

Masked Elicitation of Conditioned Responses

An important question raised by the findings reported by Öhman and Soares (1994) concerns the origin of the enhanced psychophysiological reactivity to fear stimuli shown by fearful subjects. For example, because twin studies suggest that there is a genetic component behind animal fears (Kendler et al., 1992), one possibility is that the susceptibility to respond preattentively to feared animal stimuli simply reflects genetic variance. Another possibility is that it reflects prior learning, most likely in terms of Pavlovian fear-conditioning episodes. From this latter perspective, one would expect any stimulus that had served as the conditioned stimulus (CS) for an aversive unconditioned stimulus (US) to acquire the power to elicit responses after only the preattentive analysis allowed by masked stimulus exposure. A third possibility is a combination of the other two. According to Seligman (1971), phobic fear of the type exhibited by the snake- and spider-fearful subjects examined by Öhman and Soares (1994) results from biologically prepared conditioning. As a result of evolutionary contingencies, stimuli related to recurrent survival threats in mammalian evolution were assumed to enter selectively into associations with aversive events. Consequently, common phobic objects such as snakes would easily be turned into fear stimuli because humans have a genetic readiness to form such associations, and it would seem reasonable to expect such conditioning to result in responses that, similar to phobic responses, would not require a full conscious analysis of the stimulus for their elicitation.

This hypothesis was tested by Öhman and Soares (1993). They used a differential conditioning paradigm to condition different groups of subjects to either biologically fear-relevant (snakes or spiders) or fear-irrelevant (flowers or mushrooms) stimuli. Subjects in the fear-relevant groups were shown two pictures portraying snakes and spiders, respectively. Subjects in the fear-irrelevant groups were shown pictures of flowers and mushrooms. After a few habituation trials, there was an acquisition phase where one of the stimuli was followed by an electric shock US, with a 0.5-sec interstimulus interval. This picture was designated the CS+. The other picture (e.g., a spider if the CS+ was a snake), which was never followed by the US, was designated the CS-. With this paradigm the difference in skin conductance response to the CS+ and the CS- reflects pure conditioning effects uncontaminated by sensitization, initial responding, and so on (see Öhman, 1983). In the extinction phase that terminated the experiment, the CS+ and the CS- were presented without any USs. Half the subjects conditioned to fear-relevant and fear-irrelevant stimuli, respectively, were extinguished with masked stimuli and the other half without any masks. Thus, subjects in the masked groups had both the CS+ and the CS- masked by a randomly cut and reassembled picture with a 30-msec SOA, exactly as in the experiment on fearful subjects reported by Öhman and Soares (1994).

Both the groups tested without masks during the extinction phase showed reliable differential skin conductance responding to the CS+ and the CS-, suggesting continuing conditioning effects in both groups. For the groups tested with masked CSs during extinction, however, fear relevance made a clear difference. Whereas masking completely abolished differential responding in the group conditioned to fear-irrelevant stimuli, reliable, albeit reduced, differential responding to the CS+ and the CS- remained in the group conditioned to snakes or spiders. The result for this group therefore paralleled those obtained with fearful subjects in the experiment reported by Öhman and Soares (1994).

This basic effect was closely replicated in two studies by Soares and Öhman (1993a,b), again using snakes and spiders as fear relevant stimuli, and by Esteves et al. (1994a) and Parra et al. (1997) using an angry face as the CS+.

This series of studies showed that skin conductance responses conditioned to fear-relevant stimuli (snakes/spiders or angry faces) reliably survived backward masking, whereas differential response to fear-irrelevant stimuli was abolished by this procedure. Most important from the perspective of the preparedness theory (Seligman, 1971), the effect appeared specific to particular stimulus categories, such as snakes, spiders, or angry faces. These data suggest that a perceptual mechanism of a preattentive origin contributes to the preparedness effect seen in human conditioning. It appears as if the control of responses conditioned to evolutionarily fear-relevant stimuli is easily transferred to preattentive mechanisms of response elicitation. Such a transfer of control is not seen for responses conditioned to neutral stimuli, and this difference is helpful in accounting for the differences in conditioning seen between these two stimulus classes. It is as if different types of responses were conditioned to the two types of stimuli; one more primitive and immune to cognition is conditioned to phobic stimuli, and one more advanced and cognitively governed is conditioned to neutral stimuli (see Öhman, 1993b; Öhman et al., 1978, in press).

Conditioning to Masked Stimuli

In the conditioning studies by Öhman and co-workers (Esteves et al., 1994a; Öhman & Soares, 1993; Soares & Öhman, 1993a,b), subjects were conditioned to unmasked presentations of fear-relevant or fear-irrelevant stimuli before they were tested in extinction with masked stimuli. Thus, the results demonstrate that previously conditioned responses can be elicited without conscious awareness of the eliciting stimulus. But what about learning new responses? Can autonomic responses be conditioned to stimuli that are prevented from reaching awareness by means of backward masking?

Contemporary learning theorists directed both at human (Dawson & Schell, 1985; Öhman, 1979, 1983) and animal (e.g., Wagner, 1976) learning concur that forming associations between experimental events requires the type of limited-capacity processing typically associated with consciousness (e.g., Posner & Boies, 1971). But because the preparedness theory is directed toward the ease of forming associations between specific types of events, it is somewhat consistent with this theory to expect some conditioning to masked stimuli. For example, Seligman and Hager (1972) operationalized preparedness inversely in terms of input degradation: the more degraded the input about a contingency tolerated in the forming of associations between its elements, the more prepared the association. Masking the CS, of course, can be viewed as an extreme way to degrade input about a contingency. Hence, if any stimulus should allow fear learning in spite of masking, it should be a prepared stimulus.

To test this hypothesis experimentally, normal nonfearful subjects were exposed to CS pictures consisting either of faces (angry, happy, and neutral) from the Ekman and Friesen (1976) set or pictures of snakes, spiders, flowers, and mushrooms. Emotional faces were masked by neutral ones, and for the small-animal stimuli the masking technique developed by Öhman and Soares (1993, 1994) was used. The electric shock USs were presented at an individually determined intensity level defined as "uncomfortable but not painful."

The critical experimental condition always involved an effectively masked CS (i.e., a 30-msec target stimulus immediately followed by a masking stimulus of 30 or 100 msec duration). During the acquisition phase, the masked CS+ was reinforced by the US, typically with a CS–US interval of 500 msec, whereas the masked CS- was never followed by the shock. This critical condition was compared to various control conditions. Some of the experiments included a conditioning control condition, where the target was on for 30 msec but where the mask was delayed (to 330 or 500 msec) to allow accurate identification of the target stimulus while retaining the mask as an interfering stimulus in the CS–US interval. This control condition was included to ensure that it was not the occurrence of an interfering stimulus in the CS–US interval per se, but its properties as an effective masking stimulus, that mediated the effect on conditioning. Other control conditions were designed to rule out nonassociative bases for possible conditioning effects in the preattentive conditioning groups. They involved either conditioning to masks without any preceding target stimulus or random presentations of masked CSs and individual USs.

The primary test of masked conditioning effects occurred at a series of unmasked extinction trials in which the previously masked stimuli were presented without masks, thus allowing full recognition of the CSs. If the Pavlovian conditioning contingency had been effective during acquisition training in spite of masking, differential responding to the previously masked CS+ and CS- would be expected during this unmasked extinction series. Some of the experiments also included masked test-trials during acquisition, in which the masked CS+ was presented without the US.

Esteves et al. (1994b) exposed subjects to pictures of angry and happy faces that were followed by a neutral face either after an effective (30 msec) or an ineffective (330 msec) masking interval. Conditioning subjects had an electric shock US following the masked angry face at a 500-msec CS–US interval, whereas control subjects had the shock following the neutral masks without any preceding target stimulus. In the nonmasked extinction session, skin conductance responses were larger to angry than to happy faces for subjects conditioned to masked angry faces both with effective and ineffective masking intervals, whereas no differential response was observed to angry and happy faces in subjects conditioned to the neutral masks without any preceding target stimulus. Thus, these results provided the first support for the hypothesis that Pavlovian conditioning can be demonstrated to masked fear-relevant stimuli.

In a second experiment, Esteves et al. (1994b) again examined conditioning to effectively and ineffectively masked facial stimuli in two groups that were compared to a sensitization control condition where shocks and masked facial stimuli were presented in random order to assess sensitization effects. Half the conditioning subjects had the shock following the masked angry faces, and half had the shocks following the masked happy faces. Both the groups of subjects conditioned to masked angry faces showed remaining differential response to unmasked presentations of angry and happy faces during extinction. This effect was as large in groups exposed to an effective target-mask interval as in groups exposed to a long, ineffective target-mask interval. Furthermore, the effect was observed with a masked angry but not with a masked happy CS+, and no differences between angry and happy faces were observed in groups exposed to shocks and masked pictures in random order. Thus, these data clearly support that skin conductance responses can be conditioned to nonconsciously presented CSs, provided that they are fear relevant (i.e., evolutionarily prepared to become associated with aversiveness and fear).

Öhman and Soares (1998) reported similar results using snakes and spiders as fear-relevant and flowers and mushrooms as fear-irrelevant stimuli. One group of subjects was conditioned to masked snakes or spiders as CSs+ with masked spider and snakes, respectively, serving as CSs-. Another group of subjects was conditioned to masked flowers or mushrooms in a similar differential conditioning paradigm. In all instances, the masking interval was 30 msec and the CS–US interval was 500 msec. In this experiment, the effect of the conditioning contingency was not only assessed during nonmasked extinction but also in a series of acquisition test-trials where the masked CS+ was presented without the shock unconditioned stimulus. The results from these test trials showed increasing and larger responses to the masked CS+ than to adjacent masked CSs- during the test trials provided that the stimuli were fear relevant. No such effects were observed for fear-irrelevant stimuli. In addition, as in the study by Esteves et al. (1994b), subjects conditioned to masked fear-relevant stimuli showed reliable differential response to the CS+ and the CS- when they were presented nonmasked during extinction. Such differential responding was not observed in subjects conditioned to fear-irrelevant stimuli. Thus, again, the data clearly demonstrate that electrodermal responses can be aversively conditioned to effectively masked stimuli, but only provided that the target stimulus is fear relevant.

One way of salvaging the traditional human conditioning wisdom that conditioning always requires conscious awareness of the CS–US contingency would be to argue that perceptual threshold could have been lowered as a result of repeated exposure to the masked stimuli during conditioning training. Perhaps subjects could improve their recognition of the masked stimuli as conditioning training proceeded, and for some reason this process was more obvious for fear-relevant than for fear-irrelevant stimuli. As a consequence, the subjects may also start to show differential skin conductance responses to shock-associated and non–shock-associated masked fear-relevant pictures as a correlate to expectancies of shock based on the improved recognition of the target stimuli.

Another possibility would be that the subjects were able to discriminate but not necessarily recognize the masked CS+ and the masked CS- when they were fear relevant. In this case, they would be able to predict, and thus expect, the shock, even though they would not be able to specify which masked CS presentation involved the snake and which involved the spider. Rather, they could base their expectancies on vague hunches either from some information "leaking through" the mask or, perhaps more theoretically interesting, from bodily feedback originated in the conditioned response.

To choose among these alternatives, Öhman and Soares (1998) ran three groups of subjects through an identical differential conditioning paradigm. The CS+ was either a masked snake or a masked spider, with masked spider and snakes, respectively, serving as the CS-. As usual, the masking interval was 30 msec. Rather than the short (500 msec) interstimulus interval used in previous studies, the interval between the onset of the CS and the shock was extended to 4 sec to allow subjects in one of the three groups to express their shock expectancy by rotating a knob from −100 ("sure of no shock") to 0 ("shock as likely as no shock") to +100 ("sure of shock") in the CS–US interval. Thus, this group would allow conclusions about a relationship between conscious shock expectancy and electrodermal responding. A second group was simply required to guess after each trial whether the masked stimulus had been a snake or a spider. This group provided a test of the hypothesis that recognition could improve as a function of repeated reinforced exposure to the masked stimuli. The third group had no additional task, but was only exposed to the conditioning contingency. Thus, it provided a replication of the previously used procedure and allowed assessment of whether the previous results would hold with a longer CS–US interval. In addition, this group was included to assess whether the added task would alter electrodermal responding.

All groups showed reliable differential responding both during the masked acquisition and the nonmasked extinction series. The upper panels of figure 13.6 show the skin conductance data for the group having no additional task. Again, we replicated that electrodermal responses could be conditioned to masked fear-rele-

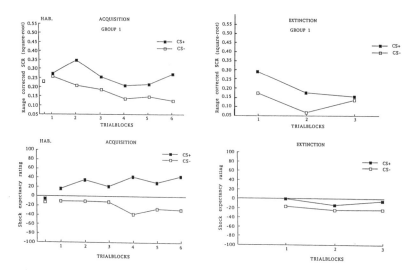

Figure 13.6. Skin conductance responses to masked presentations of a spider or snake followed by an electric shock unconditioned stimulus (CS+) and a snake or a spider not followed by shock (CS-) during acquisition (upper left panel) and extinction (upper right panel). The lower panels show shock expectancy ratings in a separate groups of subjects exposed to the same conditioning contingency. Note that the subjects showed differential expectancies even though the masking procedure effectively prevented conscious recognition of the stimuli. (Data from Öhman & Soares, 1998.)

vant stimuli. The groups required to guess whether a snake or a spider was presented performed randomly (50.5% correct) during the masked acquisition, but performed well (approximately 90% correct) during the nonmasked extinction. Thus, there was no evidence that the subjects were able to recognize the masked stimuli during acquisition. This excludes the hypothesis that subjects may have improved their recognition as a function of conditioning training. The subjects rated shock as equally unlikely after the masked CS+ and the masked CS—during the first few habituation trials where no shocks were given. Somewhat surprisingly, however, during acquisition they gradually rated shock as somewhat likely after the CS+ and as somewhat unlikely after the CS-. During extinction, when the shock and the mask were omitted, they rated shock as more unlikely after the CS- than after the CS+ (see lower panels of figure 13.6). The difference in ratings to the CS+ and the CS- was statistically reliable both during acquisition and extinction. Thus, these results indeed show that subjects had differential expectancies during the CS+ and the CS- even though they were not able consciously to recognize the stimuli. They suggest that the subjects were able to discriminate but not recognize the masked CS+ and the masked CS-. However, shock expectancy ratings were unrelated to skin conductance responses, which suggests independent control of these two response modalities.

These results provide an example of nonconscious emotional learning in the sense that subjects were able to associate aversion to a stimulus, the identity of which remained unknown because of the masking procedure. Thus, conscious discovery of the CS–US contingency is not a necessary condition for all types of human Pavlovian conditioning. However, the nonconscious learning effect was only evident for stimuli with a likely evolutionarily derived fear relevance. For neutral or positive stimuli there was no evidence of this type of nonconscious learning.

Neuropsychological Mechanisms: Some Speculations

Unconscious Elicitation of
Psychophysiological Responses

A neural circuit for fear activation and fear learning is being delineated in contemporary neuroscience (e.g., Damasio, 1994; Davis, 1992; Fanselow, 1994; LeDoux, 1990, 1992, 1996). According to this notion, information about a fear stimulus enters the brain via the classical sensory pathways and is bifurcated into parallel processing cortical and subcortical circuits at the midbrain and thalamic levels (LeDoux, 1987, 1990, 1992, 1996). In the subcortical circuit, sensory information is mediated primarily through the posterior intralaminar and geniculate nuclei of the thalamus to the lateral nucleus of the amygdala and from there it is passed on to the basolateral and then to the central nucleus of the amygdala (Fanselow, 1994; LeDoux, 1992). The cortical circuit originates in the classical sensory nuclei of the thalamus, which conveys information to primary sensory and association areas of the cortex in several parallel processing pathways (e.g., Crick, 1994; Livingston & Hubel, 1988). For example, according to Damasio et al. (1990), facial stimuli are processed as fragmented and distributed feature representations in early sensory cortices. These scattered features are integrated by time-locked activation in convergence zones resulting in face records in visual association cortices (posterior and inferior). The linking of facial components to a unique face is assumed to involve the right occipito-parietal cortex, and various other characteristics of the face are extracted in a series of steps in the temporal neocortices, in which the final representation of the face is formed. Then information is projected back to the subcortical circuit to paralimbic and limbic fields, including the hippocampus and the amygdala. Information is also conveyed to insular and prefrontal cortices, where particularly the ventromedial region of the frontal lobes is given a key role as the interface between cognition and the body (Damasio, 1994). These processing stations are interconnected by continuous feed forward and feed backward projec tions at many levels (Damasio et al., 1990), and the critical structures for verbal identification of visual input is assumed to reside in occipito-temporal and occipito-parietal regions (Tranel et al., 1995). Importantly, collateral information is projected back to the amygdala from several cortical loci and from the hippocampus (LeDoux, 1987, 1996) so that the preliminary analysis of input that reaches the amygdala via the subcortical thalamic route is more or less continuously updated by processing products from the cortical circuits. Efferent to the amygdala, a fear response is recruited via lateral hypothalamus (autonomic responses; LeDoux, 1990), the central gray of the brainstem (active skeletal defense responses via its dorsal part, and behavioral freezing via its ventral part (Fanselow, 1994), and the pons (potentiated startle via the nucleus reticularis; Davis, 1992).

Our findings from the masking studies are broadly consistent with this type of a fear network in the sense that masking may have interfered primarily with the cortical circuit, thus preventing conscious recognition of the stimuli, whereas information still could reach the amygdala via the subcortical route or via collaterals from early cortical processing to activate SCRs via hypothalamic efference. More specifically, the dissociation between autonomic responding and conscious recognition of fear stimuli reviewed above (Esteves et al., 1994a; Öhman & Soares, 1993, 1994) is conceptually similar to the dissociation between recognition failure and enhanced SCR responding to familiar faces by prosopagnosics, as reported by Bauer (1984) and by Tranel and Damasio (1985, 1988; Tranel et al., 1995). However, an important difference between the two sets of data is that the dissociation in prosopagnosics concerned identity and not the emotional expression of faces (Tranel et al., 1988). Nevertheless, the interpretation of the prosopagnosic and ventro-medial frontal cortex data advanced by Tranel et al. (1995) may apply to our findings as well. They argued that in their prosopagnosics, processing of facial information was disrupted by lesions in the occipito-temporal cortex, thus preventing conscious access to the identity of the face. However, information from visual association cortex could cascade to the frontal lobes through parietal and temporal routes to dorsolateral frontal structures and eventually to the ventromedial region, which is assumed by Damasio (1994) to be a critical relay station in activating somatic responses through the amygdala. In agreement with this interpretation, patients with lesions in the ventromedial part of the frontal cortex showed unimpaired verbal recognition of familiar faces but no evidence of enhanced SCRs to familiar as compared to unknown faces (Tranel et al., 1995).

The application of this interpretation to our data is relatively straightforward. There is evidence that the amygdala is not only sensitive to emotional facial expressions (Adolphs et al., 1995; Young et al., 1995) but, according to single-unit studies in monkeys (Ono & Nishijo, 1992), also to other types of biologically fear-relevant stimuli used in our studies, such as spiders. Thus, it could be suggested that masking disrupted processing of the visual stimuli at the occipito-parietal level, after processing of feature information is converged to face records in visual association cortices. In this way, subjects were prevented from correctly labeling the masked stimulus. However, according to PET data, the visual association cortex was activated in phobics exposed to phobic stimulation (Fredrikson et al., 1993, 1995), and perhaps processing at this level is sufficient to activate the amygdala and thence, via autonomic nuclei in the hypothalamus, the SCRs. As explained by Damasio (1994, pp. 131–132): "in order to cause a body response, one does not even need to 'recognize' the bear, or snake, or eagle as such. . . . All that is required is that early sensory cortices detect and categorize the key feature or features of a given entity (e.g., animal, object), and that structures such as the amygdala receive signals concerning their *conjunctive* presence."

The central role of the amygdala for the type of phenomena dealt with in this chapter was confirmed in a recent study by Morris et al. (1998). They conditioned subjects to one of two angry faces (the CS+ and the CS-) by pairing it with an aversive noise. With the subject placed in a PET scanner, the angry faces were presented either masked by, or masking, a neutral face to examine regional cerebral blood flow correlates of nonconscious and conscious activation of the conditioned fear response. Contrasts between the masked CS+ and CS- revealed specific activation of the right amygdala, whereas contrasts between the nonmasked CS+ and CS- showed specific activation of the left amygdala. Thus, the results confirmed that the emotional response conditioned to the CS+ was specifically mediated by the amygdala and suggested differential roles for the right and the left amygdala in nonconscious and conscious processing of the stimulus. In a subsequent study, Morris et al. (1999) reported data suggesting that nonconscious activation of the right amygdala in fact could occur independently of the visual cortices. Their results showed that the response of the amygdala correlated with activity in the superior colliculus and the pulvinar, but not with cortical sites. These findings were interpreted to suggest that the effect of masked stimuli was mediated by the subcortical visual circuitry that also mediates blindsight (see Weiskrantz, 1997).

Unconscious Conditioning and the Dissociation between
Expectancy and Recognition

So far, the interpretation in terms of a brain network has been used to understand the data on elicitation of autonomic responses (conditioned or phobic) to masked fear stimuli. But what about the data from the experiments on conditioning to masked stimuli? The fact that conditioned SCRs could be established to masked fear-relevant stimuli is consistent with the decisive role that LeDoux (1992, 1996) gives to the amygdala for fear conditioning. The central role of the amygdala for human emotional conditioning was confirmed by Bechara et al. (1995) and LaBar et al. (1995). Bechara et al. (1995) reported a double dissociation to the effect that patients with damage to the amygdala failed to show SCR conditioning (in spite of normal USs) but did acquire a cognitive understanding of conditioning situation (which CS is associated with the US, etc.). Patients with hippocampal damage, on the other hand, showed normal SCR conditioning but showed no evidence of cognitive learning.

As previously discussed, masking did not interfere with delivery of information to the amygdala, and therefore our general finding of conditioning to masked fear-relevant stimuli could be understood. It could be argued that the specificity of the effect to fear-relevant stimuli was due to direct access to the amygdala via circuits serving what Damasio (1994) called "primary emotions." However, in our masked conditioning data there was not only a dissociation between conditioned SCRs and the failure to recognize the CSs, but also a dissociation between recognition and explicit expectancies of the US (Öhman & Soares, 1998). In general, it appeared from our data that the subjects were able to discriminate between the masked CS+ and the masked CS- without being able to recognize them and that this discrimination was sufficient to goad the expectancy ratings. Conceptually similar findings were reported by Wong et al. (1994), who used slow shifts in cortical potentials to index covert expectancy for aversive outcomes after masked facial stimuli. They reported that a systematic electrocortical shift in negative direction preceded the point in time where an electric shock US had been presented during (nonmasked) training, even though the masking conditions during extinction trials effectively ruled out conscious recognition. Thus, a cortical measure that has been reliably related to expectancy and anticipation (see, e.g., Rohrbaugh & Gaillard, 1983) was elicited from nonconscious stimulation much like the masked stimuli in our experiment could elicit voluntarily controlled, overt indices of expectancy.

Weiskrantz (1997) suggested one route for understanding the dissociation between conscious recognition and expectancy reported by Öhman and Soares (1998): "stimuli of especial importance for detecting danger . . . may have an independent and older system that can have access—perhaps even privileged access—to a commentary stage independently of the visual cortices" (Weiskrantz, 1997, p. 230). Thus, subjects who were able to predict that nonrecognized stimuli were likely to be followed by shock (Öhman & Soares, 1998) may have used the "the commentary stage" (i.e., consciousness) to access information hidden from consciousness by masked stimuli independently of the visual cortices.

Conclusions

In this chapter, we have argued that humans have an evolutionarily determined readiness to let their attention be captured automatically by emotionally significant stimuli lurking in the psychological darkness outside the spotlight of conscious attention. As a result, attention is shifted to the potentially threatening event, and at the same time, autonomic responses related to emotional activation are recruited. Thus, in this way, emotional responding may be initiated unconsciously, outside the focus of attention. This is true particularly for stimuli related to survival threats in the evolutionary ecology of mammals. When associated with aversiveness through a Pavlovian conditioning procedure, such threatening stimuli acquire the power to control fear responding from an automatic level of stimulus analysis. Not only can fear responses be preattentively elicited, but the data also indicate that fear responses can be learned to nonconsciously presented stimuli that are presented followed by an aversive unconditioned stimulus in a Pavlovian contingency. However, according to the data so far available, such unconscious conditioning appears to occur only to fear-relevant stimuli deriving their fear-eliciting power from evolutionary sources. Even though subjects exposed to such a Pavlovian contingency remain unaware of the content of masked stimuli, they are able to develop systematic and veridical expectancies about which fear-relevant stimuli will be followed by the unconditioned stimulus. In general, these data can be understood in terms of the neural network model for emotional activation as proposed by Damasio and co-workers and for fear in particular as proposed by LeDoux.

References

Adolphs, R., Tranel, D., Damasio, H. & Damasio, A. R. (1995). Fear and the human amygdala. *Journal of Neuroscience, 15*, 5879–5891.
Archer, J. (1979). Behavioural aspects of fear. In W. Sluckin (Ed), *Fear in Animals and*

Man (pp. 56–85). Wokingham, Berkshire, England: Van Nostrand Reinold Company.

Aronoff, J., Barclay, A. M. & Stevenson, L. A. (1988). The recognition of threatening facial stimuli. *Journal of Personality and Social Psychology, 54*, 647–655.

Bauer, R. M. (1984). Autonomic recognition of names and faces in prosopagnosia: a neuro-psychological application of the Guilty Knowledge Test. *Neuropsychologia, 22*, 457–469.

Bechara, A., Tranel, D., Damasio, H., Adolphs, R., Rockland, C. & Damasio, A. R. (1995). Double dissociation of conditioning and declarative knowledge relative to the amygdala and hippocampus in humans. *Science, 269*, 1115–1118.

Bond, N. W. & Siddle, D. A. T. (1996). The preparedness account of social phobia: some data and alternative explanations. In R. M. Rapee (Ed), *Current Controversies in the Anxiety Disorders* (pp. 291–316). New York: Guilford Press.

Bornstein, R. F. & Pitmam, T. S. (Eds). (1992). *Perception without Awareness*. New York: Guilford Press.

Bradley, B. P. & Mogg, K. (1996). Eye movements to emotional facial expressions in clinical anxiety [abstract]. *International Journal of Psychology, 31*, 541.8.

Byrne, A. & Eysenck, M. W. (1995). Trait anxiety, anxious mood, and threat detection. *Cognition and Emotion, 6*, 549–562.

Clore, G. L. (1994). Why emotions are never unconscious. In P. Ekman & R. J. Davidson (Eds), *The Nature of Emotion. Fundamental Questions* (pp. 285–290). New York: Oxford University Press.

Crick, F. (1994). *The Astonishing Hypothesis: The Scientific Search for the Soul*. New York: Macmillan.

Damasio, A. R. (1994) *Descartes' Error. Emotion, Reason, and the Human Brain*. New York: G. P. Putnam's Sons.

Damasio, A. R., Tranel, D. & Damasio, H. (1990). Face agnosia and the neural substrates of memory. *Annual Review of Neuroscience, 13*, 89–109.

Davis, M. (1992). The role of amygdala in conditioned fear. In J. P. Aggleton (Ed), *The Amygdala: Neurobiological Aspects of Emotion, Memory, and Mental Dysfunction* (pp. 255–306). New York: Wiley-Liss.

Dawson, M. E. & Schell, A. M. (1985). Information processing and human autonomic classical conditioning. *Advances in Psychophysiology, 1*, 89–165.

Dimberg, U. & Öhman, A. (1996). Behold the wrath: Psychophysiological responses to facial stimuli. *Motivation and Emotion, 20*, 149–182.

Ekman, P. & Friesen, W. (1976). *Pictures of Facial Affect*. Palo Alto, CA: Consulting Psychologists Press.

Epstein, S. (1972). The nature of anxiety with emphasis upon its relationship to expectancy. In C. D. Spielberger (Ed), *Anxiety: Current Trends in Theory and Research* vol. II (pp. 292–338). New York: Academic Press.

Esteves, F., Dimberg, U. & Öhman, A. (1994a). Automatically elicited fear: conditioned skin conductance responses to masked facial expressions. *Cognition and Emotion, 8*, 393–413.

Esteves, F. & Öhman, A. (1993). Masking the face: recognition of emotional facial expressions as a function of the parameters of backward masking. *Scandinavian Journal of Psychology, 34*, 1–18.

Esteves, F., Parra, C., Dimberg, U. & Öhman, A. (1994b). Nonconscious associative learning: Pavlovian conditioning of skin conductance responses to masked fear-relevant facial stimuli. *Psychophysiology, 31*, 375–385.

Fanselow, M. S. (1994). Neural organization of the defensive behavior system responsible for fear. *Psychonomic Bulletin & Review, 1*, 429–438.

Folkman, S., Schaeffer, C. & Lazarus, R. S. (1979). Cognitive processes as mediators of stress and coping. In V. Hamilton & D. M. Warburton (Eds), *Human Stress and Cognition: An Information Processing Approach* (pp. 265–298). Chichester, UK: Wiley.

Fredrikson, M. (1981). Orienting and defensive responses to phobic and conditioned stimuli in phobics and normals. *Psychophysiology, 18*, 456–465.

Fredrikson, M., Wik, G., Annas, P., Ericson, K. & Stone-Elander, S. (1995). Functional neuroanatomy of visually elicited simple phobic fear: additional data and theoretical analysis. *Psychophysiology, 32*, 43–48.

Fredrikson, M., Wik, G., Greitz, T., Eriksson, L., Stone-Elander, S., Ericson, K. & Sedvall, G. (1993). Regional cerebral blood flow during experimental phobic fear. *Psychophysiology, 30*, 127–131.

Fridlund, A. J. (1994). *Human Facial Expression: An Evolutionary View*. New York: Academic Press.

Frijda, N. H. (1986). *The Emotions*. Cambridge: Cambridge University Press.

Globisch, J., Hamm, A. O., Esteves, F. & Öhman, A. (1999). Fear appears fast: temporal course of startle reflex potentiation in animal fearful subjects. *Psychophysiology, 36*, 66–75.

Hamburg, D. A., Hamburg, B. A. & Barchas, J. D. (1975). Anger and depression in perspective of behavioral biology. In L. Levi (Ed), *Emotions: Their Parameters and Measurement* (pp. 235–278). New York: Raven Press.

Hampton, C., Purcell, D. G., Bersine, L., Hansen, C. H. & Hansen, R. D. (1989). Probing "pop-out": another look at the face-in-the-crowd effect. *Bulletin of the Psychonomic Society, 27*, 563–566.

Hansen, C. H. & Hansen, R. D. (1988). Finding the face in the crowd: an anger superiority effect. *Journal of Personality and Social Psychology, 54*, 917–924.

Hansen, C. H. & Hansen, R. D. (1994). Automatic emotion: attention and facial efference. In P. M. Niedertahl & S. Kitayama (Eds), *The Heart's Eye: Emotional Influences in Perception and Attention* (pp. 217–243). San Diego, CA: Academic Press.

Hare, R. D. & Blevings, G. (1975). Defensive responses to phobic stimuli. *Biological Psychology, 3*, 1–13.

Isen, A. M. (1993). Positive affect and decision making. In M. Lewis & J. M. Haviland (Eds), *Handbook of Emotions* (pp. 261–277). New York: Guilford Press.

Izard, C. E. (1979). Emotions as motivations: an evolutionary-developmental perspective. In H. E. Howe, Jr. & R. A. Dienstbier (Eds), *Nebraska Symposium on Motivation 1978* (pp. 163–200). Lincoln: University of Nebraska Press.

Izard, C. E. (1991). *The Psychology of Emotions*. New York: Plenum Press.

James, W. (1890[1950]). *The Principles of Psychology*, vol. 1. New York: Dover.

Johnston, W. A. & Dark, V. J. (1986). Selective attention. *Annual Review of Psychology, 37*, 43–75.

Kendler, K. S., Neale, M. C., Kessler, R. C., Heath, A. C. & Eaves, L. J. (1992). The genetic epidemiology of phobias in women: the interrelationship of agoraphobia, social phobia, situational phobia and simple phobia. *Archives of General Psychiatry, 49*, 273–281.

Kirouac, G. & Doré, F. Y. (1983). Accuracy and latency of judgment of facial expressions of emotions. *Perceptual and Motor Skills, 59*, 147–150.

LaBar, K. S., LeDoux, J. E., Spencer, D. & Phelps, E. (1995). Impaired fear conditioning following unilateral temporal lobectomy in humans. *Journal of Neuroscience, 15*, 6846–6855.

Lang, P. J. (1984). Cognition in emotion: concept and action. In C. E. Izard, J. Kagan & R. B. Zajonc (Eds), *Emotion, Cognition, and Behavior* (pp. 192–228). New York: Cambridge University Press.

Lang, P. J. (1993). The three-system approach to emotion. In N. Birbaumer & A. Öhman

(Eds), *The Structure of Emotion: Psychophysiological, Cognitive and Clinical Aspects* (pp. 18–30). Seattle, WA: Hogrefe & Huber.

Lang, P. J., Bradley, M. M. & Cuthbert, B. N. (1990). Emotion, attention, and the startle reflex. *Psychological Review, 97*, 377–395.

LeDoux, J. E. (1987). Emotion. In F. Plum (Ed), *Handbook of Physiology. 1: The Nervous System*, vol. V. *Higher Functions of the Brain* (pp. 419–460). Bethesda, MD: American Physiological Society.

LeDoux, J. E. (1990). Information flow from sensation to emotion: plasticity in the neural computation of stimulus value. In M. Gabriel & J. Moore (Eds), *Learning and Computational Neuroscience. Foundations of Adaptive Networks* (pp. 3–50). Cambridge, MA: Bradford Books/MIT Press.

LeDoux, J. E. (1992). Brain mechanisms of emotion and emotional learning. *Current Opinion in Neurobiology, 2*, 191–197.

LeDoux, J. E. (1996). *The Emotional Brain: The Mysterious Underpinnings of Emotional Life*. New York: Simon & Schuster.

Livingstone, M. & Hubel, D. (1988). Segregation of form, color, movement, and depth: anatomy, physiology, and perception. *Science, 240*, 740–749.

Lundqvist, D., Esteves, F. & Öhman, A. (1999). The face of wrath: critical features for conveying facial threat. *Cognition and Emotion, 13*, in press.

MacLeod, C. (1991) Clinical anxiety and the selective encoding of threatening information. *International Review of Psychiatry, 3*, 279–292.

Marcel, A. (1983). Conscious and unconscious perception: an approach to the relations between phenomenal experience and perceptual processes. *Cognitive Psychology, 15*, 238–300.

Mathews, A. (1990). Why worry? The cognitive function of anxiety. *Behaviour Research and Therapy, 28*, 455–468.

McKelvie, S. J. (1973). The meaningfulness and meaning of schematic faces. *Perception & Psychophysics, 14*, 343–348.

Morris J. S., Öhman, A. & Dolan, R. J. (1998). Conscious and unconscious emotional learning in the human amygdala. *Nature, 393*, 467–470.

Morris, J. S., Öhman, A. & Dolan, R. J. (1999). A subcortical pathway to the right amygdala mediating "unseen" fear. *Proceedings of the National Academy of Sciences, 96*, 1680–1685.

Mineka, S. (1992). Evolutionary memories, emotional processing, and the emotional disorders. In D. Medin (Ed), *The Psychology of Learning and Motivation*, vol. 28 (pp. 161–205). New York: Academic Press.

Öhman, A. (1979). The orienting response, attention, and learning: an information processing perspective. In H. D. Kimmel, E. H. van Olst & J. F. Orlebeke (Eds), *The Orienting Reflex in Humans* (pp. 443–472). Hillsdale, NJ: Lawrence Erlbaum Associates.

Öhman, A. (1983). The orienting response during Pavlovian conditioning. In D. A. T. Siddle (Ed), *Orienting and Habituation: Perspectives in Human Research* (pp. 315–369). Chichester, UK: Wiley.

Öhman, A. (1986). Face the beast and fear the face: animal and social fears as prototypes for evolutionary analyses of emotion. *Psychophysiology, 23*, 123–145.

Öhman, A. (1987). The psychophysiology of emotion: an evolutionary-cognitive perspective. *Advances in Psychophysiology, 2*, 79–127.

Öhman, A. (1993a). Fear and anxiety as emotional phenomena: clinical phenomenology, evolutionary perspectives, and information processing mechanisms. In M. Lewis & J. M. Haviland (Eds), *Handbook of Emotions* (pp. 511–536). New York: Guilford Press.

Öhman, A. (1993b). Stimulus prepotency and fear: data and theory. In N. Birbaumer & A.

Öhman (Eds), *The Organization of Emotion: Cognitive, Clinical and Psychophysiological Perspectives* (pp. 218–239). Toronto: Hogrefe.

Öhman, A. (1996). Preferential preattentive processing of threat in anxiety: preparedness and attentional biases. In R. M. Rapee (Ed), *Current Controversies in the Anxiety Disorders* (pp. 253–290). New York: Guilford Press.

Öhman, A. (1999). Distinguishing unconscious from conscious emotional processes: methodological considerations and theoretical implications. In T. Dalgleish & M. Power (Eds), *Handbook of Cognition and Emotion* (pp. 321–352). Chichester, UK: Wiley.

Öhman, A. & Birbaumer, N. (1993). Psychophysiological and cognitive-clinical perspectives on emotion: introduction and overview. In N. Birbaumer & A. Öhman (Eds), *The Organization of Emotion: Cognitive, Clinical, and Psychophysiological Aspects* (pp. 3–17). Toronto: Hogrefe and Huber.

Öhman, A. & Dimberg, U. (1984). An evolutionary perspective on human social behavior. In W. M. Waid (Ed), *Sociophysiology*, (pp. 47–85). New York: Springer-Verlag.

Öhman, A., Dimberg, U. & Öst, L.-G. (1985). Animal and social phobias: biological constraints on learned fear responses. In S. Reiss & R. R. Bootzin (Eds), *Theoretical Issues in Behavior Therapy* (pp. 123–178). New York: Academic Press.

Öhman, A., Flykt, A. & Esteves, F. (1999). "Look out! There are snakes in the grass" on the capture of attention by fear-relevant stimuli. Manuscript submitted for publication.

Öhman, A., Fredrikson, M. & Hugdahl, K. (1978). Orienting and defensive responding in the electrodermal system: palmar-dorsal differences and recovery rate during conditioning to potentially phobic stimuli. *Psychophysiology, 15*, 93–101.

Öhman, A., Hamm, A. O. & Hugdahl, K. (in press). Cognition and the autonomic nervous system: orienting, anticipation, and conditioning. In J. T. Cacioppo, L. Tassinary & G. G. Berntson (Eds), *Handbook of Psychophysiology*. New York: Cambridge University Press.

Öhman, A. & Soares, J. J. F. (1993). On the automaticity of phobic fear: conditioned skin conductance responses to masked phobic stimuli. *Journal of Abnormal Psychology, 102*, 121–132.

Öhman, A. & Soares, J. J. F. (1994). Unconscious anxiety: phobic responses to masked stimuli. *Journal of Abnormal Psychology, 103*, 231–240.

Öhman, A. & Soares, J. J. F. (1998) Emotional conditioning to masked stimuli: expectancies for aversive outcomes following non-recognized fear-relevant stimuli. *Journal of Experimental Psychology: General, 127*, 69–82.

Ono, T. & Nishijo, H. (1992). Neurophysiological basis of the Klüver-Bucy syndrome: responses of monkey amygdaloid neurons to biological significant objects. In J. P. Aggleton (Ed), *The Amygdala: Neurobiological Aspects of Emotion, Memory, and Mental Dysfunction* (pp. 167–190). New York: Wiley-Liss.

Parra, C., Esteves, F., Flykt, A. & Öhman, A. (1997). Pavlovian conditioning to social stimuli: backward masking and the dissociation of implicit and explicit cognitive processes. *European Psychologist, 2*, 106–117.

Posner, M. I. & Boies, S. J. (1971). Components of attention. *Psychological Review, 78*, 391–408.

Purcell, D. G., Stewart, A. L. & Skov, R. (1996). It takes a confounded face to pop out of a crowd. *Perception, 25*, 1091–1108.

Rohrbaugh, J. W. & Gaillard, A. W. K. (1983). Sensory and motor aspects of the contingent negative variation. In A. W. K. Gaillard & W. Ritter (Eds), *Tutorials in ERP Research. Endogenous Components* (pp. 269–310). Amsterdam: North-Holland.

Sartory, G. (1983). The orienting response and psychopathology: anxiety and phobias. In D. Siddle (Ed), *Orienting and Habituation: Perspectives in Human Research* (pp. 449–474). Chichester, UK: Wiley.

Scherer, K. R. (1994). Emotion serves to decouple stimulus and response. In P. Ekman & R. J. Davidson (Eds), *The Nature of Emotion: Fundamental Questions* (pp. 127–130). New York: Oxford University Press.

Seligman, M. E. P. (1971). Phobias and preparedness. *Behavior Therapy, 2*, 307–320.

Seligman, M. E. P. & Hager, J. E. (Eds). (1972). *Biological Boundaries of Learning.* New York: Appleton-Century-Crofts.

Soares, J. J. F. & Öhman, A. (1993a). Backward masking and skin conductance responses after conditioning to non-feared but fear-relevant stimuli in fearful subjects. *Psychophysiology, 30*, 460–466.

Soares, J. J. F. & Öhman, A. (1993b). Preattentive processing, preparedness, and phobias: effects of instruction on conditioned electrodermal responses to masked and non-masked fear-relevant stimuli. *Behaviour Research and Therapy, 31*, 87–95.

Sokolov, E. N. (1963). *Perception and the Conditioned Reflex.* Oxford: Pergamon Press.

Tinbergen, N. (1951). *The Study of Instinct.* Oxford: Clarendon Press.

Tooby, J. & Cosmides, L. (1990). The past explains the present: emotional adaptations and the structure of ancestral environments. *Ethology and Sociobiology, 11*, 375–424.

Tranel, D. & Damasio, A. R. (1985). Knowledge without awareness: an autonomic index of facial recognition by prosopagnosics. *Science, 228*, 1453–1454.

Tranel, D. & Damasio, A. R. (1988). Non-conscious face recognition in patients with face agnosia. *Behavioural Brain Research, 30*, 235–249.

Tranel, D., Damasio, A. R. & Damasio, H. (1988). Intact recognition of facial expression, gender, and age in patients with impaired recognition of face identy. *Neurology, 38*, 690–696.

Tranel, D., Damasio, H. & Damasio, A. R. (1995). Double dissociation between overt and covert face recognition. *Journal of Cognitive Neuroscience, 7*, 425–432.

Treisman, A. & Souther, J. (1985). Search asymmetry: a diagnostic for preattentive processing of separable features. *Journal of Experimental Psychology: General, 114*, 285–310.

Wagner, A. R. (1976). Priming in STM: an information-processing mechanism for self-generated or retrieval-generated depression in performance. In T. J. Tighe & R. N. Leaton (Eds), *Habituation: Perspectives from Child Development, Animal Behavior, and Neurophysiology* (pp. 95–128). Hillsdale, NJ: Lawrence Erlbaum Associates.

Weiskrantz, L. (1997). *Consciousness Lost and Found.* Oxford: Oxford University Press.

Wong, P. S., Shevrin, H. & Williams, W. J. (1994). Conscious and nonconscious processes: an ERP index of an anticipatory response in a conditioning paradigm using visually masked stimuli. *Psychophysiology, 31*, 87–101.

Yantis, S. (1998). Control of visual attention. In H. Pashler (Ed), *Attention* (pp. 223–256). Hove, UK: Psychology Press.

Young, A. W., Aggleton, J. P., Hellawell, D. J., Johnson, M., Broks, P. & Hanley, J. R. (1995). Face processing impairments after amygdalotomy. *Brain, 118*, 15–24.

Zajonc, R. B. (1980). Feeling and thinking: preferences need no inferences. *American Psychologist, 35*, 151–175.

14

Emotional Experience: A Neurological Model

KENNETH M. HEILMAN

Cannon (1927) noted that emotions are primarily adaptive. They help prepare the organism to deal with important events. Emotions are also one of the strongest motivating forces that direct human behavior. The adaptive and motivational aspects of emotions help ensure the survival of an organism, its family, and society.

Emotions have at least two major components. There are emotional behaviors, including overt and covert. Overt behaviors are the ones we can see such as emotional faces, gestures, and words. Covert behaviors include changes in the viscera and autonomic nervous system. These overt and covert behaviors are the adaptive aspect of emotions. The second component is emotional feelings or experiences. Although these experiences are subjective, they are one of the major factors that motivate approach and avoidance behaviors. However, it is not only the direct experience of emotion that motivates behavior, but also the knowledge that certain stimuli, situations, and actions could in the future produce emotional states is a strong and important motivating factor. Although some may define moods as long-lasting emotions and suggest that they may be an epiphenomenon, moods modulate, influence, or bias perception, cognition, memory, and emotion. For example, a person in a depressed mood is able to remember sad events better than happy events and a person in an irritable mood is more likely to get angry than a person in a calm mood.

In this review I explore the neural basis of emotional experience and do not discuss moods or the psychopathology associated with mood disorders. I first briefly review the classical feedback and central theories and the more recent revisions of these theories. I then discuss a theory that attempts to explain the cortical control of different emotional experiences.

Feedback Theories

Facial Feedback Hypothesis

Darwin (1872) noted that, "He who gives violent gesture increases his rage." Darwin also believed that the means by which we express emotions are innate. If the facial expressions of emotions is innate, there should be little or no difference in emotional expression across cultures. To learn if the expression of emotions is innate, Izard (1977) and Ekman (1969) performed cross-cultural studies of facial emotional expressions and found that the same seven to nine emotional facial expressions appeared to be universal, thereby providing support for Darwin's innate hypothesis. Tomkins (1962, 1963) posited that it was the feedback of these facial emotions to the brain that induced emotional feeling. Laird (1974) experimentally manipulated facial expressions and found that patients felt emotions, thereby providing some support for the facial feedback hypothesis. However, there are many unresolved problems with the facial feedback theory of emotional experience. One of the major problems with the feedback theory is that it is, at least in part, circular. If facial feedback induces emotional experience, what produces the facial emotion? Is it not experience? Second, if facial feedback is producing emotional experience, then without producing an emotional face, one should not feel an emotional experience. In addition, when one is feeling a strong emotion, the valence of this emotion should be changed by altering one's facial expression. However, even when a person does not express facial emotions, that person may be experiencing emotions. Keeping a "stiff upper lip" may allow one to hide the emotion one is feeling from others, but it does not eliminate the experience of emotion. In addition, people cannot change their emotional experience by changing their facial expressions, and they can express one emotion while feeling another.

It is possible that voluntary facial emotions cannot alter emotional experience because the innervatory patterns of voluntary facial gestures are different from those that occur naturally. For example, when one smiles voluntarily, the corners of the lips may be pulled upward, but when someone is happy the muscles around the orbits of the eyes are also active. Whereas voluntary emotions are controlled by the cortical bulbar system, true emotion expression is controlled by a system that is still not well defined. Therefore, patients with corticospinal lesions may have difficulty making a smile on command but may smile normally when something funny happens. Some patients with basal ganglia disorders such as Parkinson's disease may show the opposite pattern (Jacobs et al., 1995). The observation that patients with pseudobulbar palsy may express strong facial emotions that they are not feeling is against the facial feedback hypothesis (Poeck, 1969). However, it is possible that these patient's brain lesions also interrupt facial feedback to the brain. Patients with Parkinson's disease and Parkinsonian symptoms may have a masklike face but often feel sad and depressed. Finally, patients with diseases of facial nerve motor units, even when damage is bilateral, do not report a change of emotional experience. However, smiles are usually associated with positive emotions and tears with sad emotions, and it remains possible because of associative learning that smiles can, in part, help induce a positive feeling and tears can induce the opposite. Therefore, it is possible, as Darwin suggested, that facial expressions may embellish emotions, but this embellishment is probably trivial.

Visceral Feedback Hypotheses

William James (1890) proposed that stimuli provoking an emotion induce changes in the viscera and autonomic nervous system and that it is the self-perception of these visceral changes that produces emotional experience. To have visceral feedback, one needs efferent and afferent systems. The autonomic nervous system has two components, the sympathetic and the parasympathetic. The descending sympathetic neurons receive projections from the hypothalamus, and the hypothalamus receives projections from many limbic and paralimbic areas including the amygdala. The most important parasympathetic nerve is the vagus, which originates in the dorsal motor nucleus situated in the brainstem and projects to visceral organs such as the heart. The amygdala not only projects to the hypothalamus but also sends direct projections to the nucleus of the solitary tract and the dorsal motor nucleus of the vagus. In this manner the amygdala may directly influence the parasympathetic system. The amygdala receives neocortical input. Whereas the amygdala may be the most important part of the limbic system to influence the autonomic nervous system and viscera, stimulation of other areas including the insula and orbitofrontal cortex can also induce autonomic and visceral changes (Kaada, 1960). These structures also receive input from the neocortex.

In regard to feedback, the major nerve that carries visceral afferent information back to the brain is the vagus. These afferents terminate in the nucleus of the solitary tract, which projects to the central nucleus of the amygdala. The central nucleus of the amygdala projects to other amygdala nuclei and the insula. The amygdala and insula, in turn, project to the temporal, parietal, and frontal lobes.

In humans the neocortex and limbic cortex play a critical role in the analysis and interpretation of various stimuli (see Heilman et al., 1993a, for review). Luria and Simernitskaya (1977) thought that the right hemisphere may be more important than the left in perceiving visceral changes. To test this postulate, Davidson and co-workers (1981) gave a variety of tapping tests to normal individuals. They found that the left hand was more influenced by heart rate than the right hand, suggesting the right hemisphere may be superior at detecting heartbeats. Unfortunately, this left-hand superiority in the detection of heartbeats has not been replicated by other investigators.

James's feedback theory was challenged by Cannon (1927), who thought that the viscera have insufficient afferent input to the brain to be important in inducing emotional experience. Using a heartbeat detection paradigm, Katkin et al. (1982) found that normal subjects can accurately detect their heartbeats. Katkin (1985) reported that the subjects who had the strongest emotional responses to negative slides were the subjects who were best able to detect their own heartbeat.

Cannon also argued that the separation of the viscera from the brain as occurs with cervical spinal cord injuries does not eliminate emotional experience. Hohmann (1966) studied patients with spinal cord injuries and found that patients with either high or low spinal cord transection did experience emotions, as predicted by Cannon, but patients with lower lesions reported stronger emotions than those with higher lesions. Higher cervical lesions would be more likely to affect the autonomic nervous system's efferent control of the viscera. Therefore, Hohmann's observations provide partial support for the visceral feedback theory.

Cannon thought that the same visceral responses occur with different emotions; therefore, feedback of these visceral responses could not account for the variety of emotions that humans experience. However, Ax (1953) and others have demonstrated that different bodily reactions are associated with different emotions.

Although many of Cannon's objections to the visceral feedback theory could be refuted, there are still observations for which the visceral feedback theory cannot account. Perhaps the most important are the observations of Marañon (1924), who injected epinephrine into subjects. Epinephrine does not cross the blood–brain barrier but does affect the autonomic nervous system and viscera, including increasing the activity of the heart. Marañon inquired as to the nature of the emotion felt by these subjects and found that injections of epinephrine were not associated with emotional experience but rather with "as if" feelings.

Schachter and Singer (1962) also injected epinephrine into experimental subjects and reported that pharmacologically induced autonomic and visceral activation did not, by itself, produce an emotion. If this activation was accompanied by an appropriate cognitive set, an emotion could be induced. Some cognitive sets may, by themselves, produce an emotion, but Schacter and Singer found that the emotion induced by a cognitive set was stronger in those subjects who received epinephrine and therefore had visceral activation.

Whereas Schachter and Singer's (1962) study suggested that visceral feedback together with centrally mediated cognition are important for emotional experience, observations in our laboratory do not entirely support the attribution theory. Recently, we attempted to test the autonomic-visceral feedback theory and to learn if, as suggested by Luria and Simernitskaya, the right hemisphere plays a dominant role in perceiving visceral changes. Using a shock anticipation paradigm in brain-lesioned subjects, we found that when compared to normal control subjects, patients with right hemisphere lesions had a reduced autonomic response. Although their autonomic response was reduced, they showed no differences in the experience of anticipatory anxiety (Slomine et al., 1995). In addition, in the clinic one can see patients who have strong emotions (such as fear) associated with medial temporal lobe or amygdala seizures. Sometimes patients become aware that they are beginning to have a seizure and the fear of having a seizure may lead to a fearful cognitive set. Autonomic and visceral changes may be associated with these partial seizures, and the patients may be aware of these changes and therefore experience fear. However, in many epileptic patients the emotional experience is often the first symptom. Therefore, in these patients the cognitive set comes after the experience rather than before the experience. The Schachter and Singer attribution theory cannot account for these observations. For additional discussion of the Schacter theory, see Reisenzein (1983).

The observations reviewed above do not preclude the possibility that visceral foodback, like facial feedback, may play some role in emotional experience. However, although these changes may be adaptive and thereby assist the organism in dealing with the stimuli that induced these emotions, feedback does not appear to play a critical role in emotional experience.

Central Theories

Diencephalic Theories

To account for emotional experience, Cannon (1927) proposed that afferent stimuli enter the brain and are transmitted from the thalamus to the hypothalamus. The hypothalamus activates the endocrine and autonomic nervous systems, and it is these systems that induce the physiological changes in the viscera. These autonomic and visceral changes are primarily adaptive and aid in the survival of the organism. Emotional experience is induced by the hypothalamus feeding back to the cortex. Recently, LeDoux and his co-workers (1990) have modified Cannon's thalamic-hypothalamic emotion circuit to include the amygdala in fear conditioning. These investigators conditioned animals by associating a noicioceptive stimulus with an auditory stimulus. Whereas ablation of the auditory thalamus and amygdala interrupted the behavioral emotional response to the conditioned stimulus, ablation of the auditory cortex did not. Therefore, LeDoux, like Cannon, does not propose a critical role for the cortex in the interpretation of stimuli. Although conditioned stimuli, similar to those used by LeDoux, may induce emotion without cortical interpretation, there is overwhelming evidence that in humans the neocortex is critical for interpreting the meaning of many stimuli, especially those stimuli that are complex and rely on past learning.

Primary and Social Emotions

Ross et al. (1994) observed that some patients undergoing selective hemispheric anesthesia (the Wada test) changed their emotional response to events that they previously recalled and that the emotional response appeared to be dependent on the hemisphere that was anesthestized. For example, in the absence of hemispheric anesthesia, one of their subjects told of an incident where he was very frightened. However, when his right hemisphere was anesthetized and he was asked to recall this incident, he stated that he felt embarrassed. Based on observations such as these, Ross et al. posited that whereas the right hemisphere is important for primary emotions such as fear, the left is important for social emotions such as embarrassment.

Cannon's diencephalic-hypothalamic theory, LeDoux's diencephalic-limbic (amygdala) theory, and Ross et al.'s left–right social–emotional theory either fail to account for how humans experience emotion in response to complex stimuli or fail to explain how humans can experience a variety of emotions.

Modular Theory

There are at least two ways the brain may mediate a variety of emotional experiences. One possibility is that the brain may contain specialized or devoted emotional systems for each emotional experience such that each emotion is uniquely mediated. Therefore, there would be a special system for fear, anger, happiness, and so on. A second possibility is that each emotion is not uniquely mediated but that the neural apparatus that mediates one emotion may not only play a role in some other emotions but may also mediate nonemotional functions.

The second or nondevoted systems postulate is consistent with the "dimensional" view of emotion. Wundt (1903) proposed that emotional experiences vary in three dimensions: quality, activity, and excitement (arousal). Osgood et al. (1957) performed factor analyses on verbal assessments of emotional judgments and found that the variance could be accounted for by three major dimensions:

valence (positive/negative, pleasant/unpleasant), arousal (calm/excited), and control (in control/out of control). Using this type of multidimensional view, one can define the different emotional experiences by using one or more of these three dimensions. For example, fear would be unpleasant, high arousal, and out of control, and sadness would be unpleasant and low arousal. Psychophysiological studies with normal subjects have partially supported this dimensional view (Greenwald et al., 1989). However, these three dimensions would not discriminate between anger and fear. Both are unpleasant or negative, high arousal, and out of control. Frijda (1987) also explored the cognitive structure of emotion and found that "action readiness" was an important component or dimension. Control as discussed by Osgood et al. (1957) and Greenwald et al. (1989) may be closely linked to both valence (e.g., negative = out of control, positive = in control) and motor activation (approach = in control, avoid = out of control). However, Frijda's research would suggest that action readiness may be the third dimension.

Therefore, we posited that the conscious experience of emotion is mediated by anatomically distributed modular networks (Heilman, 1994) and that the proposed network contains three major modules. One module determines valence (pleasant vs. unpleasant), another controls arousal, and a third mediates motor activation with approach or avoidance behaviors. In the following sections I briefly discuss the neurological basis of each of these modules.

- Valence

Goldstein (1948) reported that aphasic patients with left hemisphere lesions often appeared anxious, agitated, and sad, the "catastrophic reaction." Gainotti (1972) studied 160 patients with strokes of either the right or left hemisphere and reported that patients with left hemisphere lesions had catastrophic reactions. In contrast, Babinski (1914), Hécaen et al. (1951), and Denny-Brown et al. (1952) reported that patients with right hemisphere lesions often appeared either inappropriately indifferent or even euphoric. Gainotti (1972) also confirmed these observations. Gainotti proposed that the patient's psychological response to their own illness may account for some of the emotional asymmetries observed between patients with right and left hemisphere lesions. Whereas patients with left hemisphere deficits are aware of their deficits, patients with right hemisphere lesions may be unaware (anosognosia). However, other observations are not consistent with this reactive postulate. Terzian (1964) and Rossi and Rosadini (1967) studied the emotional reactions of patients recovering from selective hemispheric barbiturate-induced anesthesia (the Wada test). These investigators noted that whereas right carotid injections were often associated with euphoria, barbiturate injections into the left carotid artery were often associated with catastrophic reactions. Gainotti's reactive postulate could not account for these intrasubject asymmetries. The Wada test is a diagnostic test that only causes transient hemiparesis and aphasia; therefore, it is unlikely that this procedure would cause a reactive depression that occurred just in the middle of the test. In addition, we have seen right hemisphere-damaged stroke patients who are emotionally indifferent but who are aware of their deficits and do not demonstrate anosognosia or verbally explicit denial of illness.

The catastrophic–depressive reaction associated with left hemisphere lesions is seen most commonly in patients who have anterior (frontal) perisylvian lesions

(Benson, 1979; Robinson & Sztela, 1981). It is possible that the hemispheric emotional asymmetries reported by Gainotti and others may be related to emotional communication disorders associated with frontal lesions (see Heilman et al., 1993b, for a review), rather than differences in emotional experience. Although hemispheric defects of emotional expression may account for some of the behavior observations by Goldstein (1948), Babinski (1914), and Gainotti (1972), they cannot explain the results of Gasparrini et al. (1978), who administered the Minnesota Multiphasic Inventory (MMPI) to a group of left and right hemisphere-damaged patients. The left hemisphere-damaged patients were not severely aphasic, and the right and left hemisphere patients were balanced for cognitive and motor defects. The MMPI does not require emotionally intoned speech or facial expressions. The Gasparrini et al. findings using the MMPI supported the hemispheric valence hypothesis. They found that, whereas patients with left hemisphere disease showed a marked elevation of the depression scale, patients with right hemisphere disease did not. Therefore, the right–left differences in emotional behavior observed by Gainotti and others cannot be attributed to emotional expressive disorders or to the severity of the motor or cognitive deficit.

Starkstein et al. (1987) studied emotional changes associated with stroke and also found that about one-third of stroke patients had depression. They found that depression was associated with both left frontal and left caudate lesions. The closer to the frontal pole the lesion was located, the more severe was the depression. Many of the patients with left hemisphere lesions and depression were also anxious. In contrast, patients with right frontal lesions were often indifferent or even euphoric. However, not all investigators agree that after stroke there is more depression with left than right hemisphere lesions. House et al. (1990) and Milner (1974) could not replicate the emotional symmetries of prior reports.

To learn if there are discrete physiological changes of the brain associated with depression, several groups of investigators have studied patients with primary depression using functional imaging. Some of these investigations have noted a decrease of activation in the left frontal lobe as well as the left cingulate gyrus (Bench et al., 1992; Phelps et al., 1984). However, Drevets and Raichle (1992) found increased activity in the left prefrontal cortex, amygdala, basal ganglia, and thalamus. More recently, Drevets et al. (1997) found that abnormalities of the subgenual prefrontal cortex may be important in depression. Mayberg (1997) proposed that the rostral anterior cingulate gyrus that projects to both the dorsolateral and ventral frontal lobes may be important in depression.

Davidson et al. (1979) and Tucker (1981) investigated the hemispheric valence hypothesis by studying normal subjects using electrophysiological techniques and confirmed the results of the ablation studies. Unfortunately, it is not known how the right and left hemisphere may influence emotional valence. Fox and Davidson (1984) suggest that left hemisphere-mediated positive emotions are related to approach, and right hemisphere-mediated negative emotions are related to avoidance behaviors. In our laboratory we studied emotions and approach–avoidance behavior. We found that negative emotions can be associated with both approach and avoidance behaviors (Crucian et al., 1997). For example, fear and anger both have a negative valence, but fear is associated with avoidance and anger with approach. In addition, this approach–avoidance model does not explain how the two hemispheres are differently organized such that they make opposite contributions to mood, how other emotions are mediated, or the role of other areas in the brain such as the limbic system. Tucker and Williamson (1984) think that hemispheric valence asymmetries may be related to asymmetrical control of neuropharmacological systems, with the left hemisphere being more cholinergic and dopaminergic and the right hemisphere being more noradrenergic than the left hemisphere. Mayberg et al. (1988) reported that pharmacologic changes in the two hemispheres may be different after stroke. Using positron emission tomography (PET) they reported that strokes in the right hemisphere appear to increase serotonergic receptor binding and left hemisphere strokes lower serotonergic binding. The lower the serotonergic binding, the more severe the depression. Although it is well known from clinical psychiatry that neurotransmitter systems may have a profound influence on mood, the mechanism by which the pharmacological changes induce mood remain unknown. In addition, as discussed above, moods and emotions may not be synonymous and may be mediated differently. For example, drugs that are used to treat depression will not prevent someone from becoming sad. I therefore confine the remainder of this discussion to anatomic and physiological models of emotion.

• Arousal

Arousal has both behavioral and physiological components. Behaviorally, an aroused organism is awake, alert, and prepared to process stimuli. An unaroused organism is lethargic to comatose and not prepared to process stimuli. Physiologically, arousal has several definitions. In the central nervous system, arousal usually refers to the excitatory state of neurons or the propensity of neurons to discharge when appropriately activated. In functional imaging, arousal is usually measured by increases of blood flow, and electrophysiologically, it is measured by desynchronization of the EEG or by the amplitude and latency of evoked potentials. Outside the central nervous system, arousal usually refers to activation of the sympathetic nervous system and the visceral organs such as the heart.

Arousal and attention are intimately linked and appear to be mediated by a modular cortical limbic reticular network (Heilman, 1979; Mesulam, 1981; Watson et al., 1981). Here I provide an overview of this network, but for details one should refer to the original articles (or, for a review, see Heilman et al., 1993b). Much of what we know about this anatomically based network initially came from studies of monkeys and patients with discrete brain lesions. More recently, functional imaging has confirmed much of this ablation research. In humans, lesions of the inferior parietal lobe are most often associated with disorders of attention and arousal (Critchley, 1966; Heilman et al., 1983), and in monkeys temporoparietal ablations are also associated with attentional disorders (Heilman et al., 1970; Lynch, 1980). Physiological recordings from neurons in the parietal lobes of monkeys appear to support the postulate that the parietal lobe is important in attention. Unlike neurons in the primary sensory cortex, the rate of firing of these "attentional" neurons in the parietal lobe appears to be associated with the significance of the stimulus to the monkey such that relevant stimuli are associated with higher firing rates than are unimportant stimuli (see Bushnell et al., 1981; Lynch, 1980).

Sensory information projects to the thalamic relay nuclei. From the thalamus these modality-specific sensory systems project to the primary sensory cortices.

Each of these primary sensory cortices (e.g., visual, tactile, auditory) project only to their association cortices. For example, Brodmann's area 17, the primary visual cortex, projects to Brodmann's area 18. Subsequently, each of these modality-specific association areas converge upon polymodal areas such as the frontal cortex (periarcuate, prearcuate, and orbitofrontal) and both banks of the superior temporal sulcus (Pandya & Kuypers, 1969). Both of these sensory polymodal convergence areas project to the supramodal inferior parietal lobe (Mesulam et al., 1977). Whereas the determination of stimulus novelty may be mediated by modality-specific sensory association cortex, stimulus significance requires knowledge as to both the meaning of the stimulus and the motivational state of the organism. The motivational state is dependent on at least two factors: immediate biological needs and long-term goals. It has been demonstrated that portions of the limbic system together with the hypothalamus monitor the internal milieu and develop drive states. Therefore, limbic input into regions important in determining stimulus significance may provide information about immediate biological needs. Portions of the limbic system such as the cingulate gyrus project to both the inferior parietal lobe and the frontal lobe. Regarding long-term goals, the frontal lobe has been demonstrated to play a major role in goal-oriented behavior (Damasio & Anderson, 1993; Stuss & Benson, 1986). Frontal input into the attentional–arousal systems may provide information about goals that are not motivated by immediate biological needs. Studies of cortical connectivity in monkeys have demonstrated that the temporoparietal region not only has strong connections with portions of the limbic system such as the cingulate gyrus but also with the frontal cortex.

Stimulation of the mesencephalic reticular formation (MRF) in animals induces behavioral and physiological arousal (Moruzzi & Magoun, 1949). In contrast, bilateral lesions of the MRF induce coma, and unilateral lesions cause the ipsilateral hemisphere to be both behaviorally and physiologically hypoaroused (Watson et al., 1974). The polymodal and supramodal cortex discussed above not only determine stimuli significance but also modulate arousal by influencing the MRF (Segundo et al., 1955). The exact means by which these cortical areas influence the MRF and by which the MRF influences the cortex remain unknown. However, there are at least three possible mechanisms by which the MRF may influence cortical processing. Shute and Lewis (1967) describe an ascending cholinergic reticular formation. The nucleus basalis, which is in the basal forebrain, receives input from the reticular formation and has cholinergic projections to the entire cortex. These cholinergic projections appear to be important for increasing neuronal sensitivity (Sato et al., 1987). The MRF may also influence cortical activity through thalamic projections. Steriade and Glenn (1982) demonstrated that nonspecific thalamic nuclei such as the centralis lateralis and the paracentralis project to widespread cortical regions, and these thalamic nuclei can be activated by stimulation of the mesencephalic reticular formation. The third mechanism that may help account for cortical arousal involves the thalamic nucleus reticularis (NR). This thin nucleus envelops the thalamus and projects to all the sensory thalamic relay nuclei. Physiologically, NR inhibits the thalamic relay of sensory information (Scheibel & Scheibel, 1966). However, when cortical limbic networks determine a stimulus is significant or novel, corticofugal projections may inhibit the inhibitory

NR, thereby allowing the thalamic sensory nuclei to relay sensory information to the cortex (Watson et al., 1981).

The level of activity of the peripheral autonomic nervous system usually mirrors the level of arousal in the central nervous system. One means of measuring peripheral autonomic arousal is by assessing hand sweating. When the hand sweats, there is a change in resistance. To learn if there were differences in the hemispheric control of sweating, Heilman et al. (1978) studied patients with right and left hemisphere damage as well as normal controls. These subjects received nociceptive stimuli (electric shock) that was uncomfortable but not painful. The patients with right hemisphere lesions had a reduced arousal response when compared to normals and to left hemisphere-damaged controls. Other investigators reported similar findings. For example, Morrow et al. (1981) and Schrandt et al. (1989) also found that right hemisphere-damaged patients had a reduced skin response to emotional stimuli. However, when compared to normal subjects, patients with left hemisphere lesions appear to have a greater autonomic response (Heilman et al., 1978). Using changes in heart rate as a measure of arousal, Yokoyama et al. (1987) obtained similar results to those obtained using skin response. Using functional imaging, Perani et al. (1993) also found that in cases of right hemisphere stroke there is a metabolic depression of the left hemisphere. Unfortunately, results of left hemisphere-damaged control patients were not reported.

The mechanisms underlying the asymmetrical hemispheric control of arousal remain unknown. Because lesions restricted to the right hemisphere could not directly interfere with the left hemisphere's corticofugal projections to the reticular systems or the reticular system's influence on the left hemisphere, one would have to propose that the right hemisphere's control of arousal may be related to privileged communication that the right hemisphere has with the reticular activating system. Alternatively, portions of the right hemisphere may play a dominant role in computing stimulus significance. The increased arousal associated with left hemisphere lesions also remains unexplained. Perhaps the left hemisphere maintains some type of inhibitory control over the right hemisphere or over the reticular activating system.

- Motor Activation and Approach–Avoidance

Some emotions do not call for action (e.g., sadness, satisfaction), but others do (e.g., anger, fear, joy, surprise). When emotions are associated with action, this action may be toward the stimulus (approach) or away from the stimulus (avoidance) that induced the emotion. Although one would like to avoid emotions that are unpleasant and approach situations that induce pleasant emotions, when we discuss approach and avoidance, we are discussing the behavior associated with the emotion and not one's plans for structuring one's behavior in relation to the stimuli that induce these emotions. For example, whereas one would like to avoid situations that induce anger, when one becomes angry, one has a propensity to approach the stimulus that is inducing this emotion. Joy, a positive emotion, is also associated with approach behaviors.

Pribram and McGuiness (1975) use the term "activation" to denote the physiological readiness to respond to stimuli. We have posited that motor activation or motor intention is mediated by a modular network that includes portions of the cerebral cortex, basal ganglia, and limbic system (see Heilman et al., 1993b, for a detailed review). The dorsolateral frontal lobe appears to be a critical portion of this motor preparatory network (Watson et al., 1978, 1981). Physiological recordings from cells in the dorsolateral frontal lobe reveal neurons that have enhanced activity when the animal is presented with a stimulus that is meaningful and predicts movement (Goldberg & Bushnell, 1981). The dorsolateral frontal lobes receive input from the cingulate gyrus and from posterior cortical association areas. These association areas are modality specific, polymodal, and supramodal. Input from these posterior neocortical areas may provide the frontal lobes information about the stimulus, including its meaning and its spatial location. The limbic system (e.g., the cingulate gyrus, which is not only part of the Papez circuit but also receives input from Yakolov's basal lateral circuit) may provide information as to the organism's motivational state. The dorsolateral frontal lobe has nonreciprocal connections with the basal ganglia (e.g., caudate), which in turn projects to the globus pallidus, and the globus pallidus projects to the thalamus, which projects back to the frontal cortex (Alexander et al., 1986). The dorsolateral frontal lobes also have extensive connections with the nonspecific intralaminar nuclei of the thalamus (centromedian and parafasicularis). These intralaminar nuclei, which can be activated by the mesencephalic reticular system, may gate motor activation by their influence on the basal ganglia, especially the putamen, or by influencing the thalamic portion of motor circuits (ventralis lateralis pars oralis). Finally, the dorsolateral frontal lobe has strong input into the premotor areas. The observation that lesions of the dorsolateral frontal lobe, the cingulate gyrus, the basal ganglia, the intralaminar nuclei, and the ventrolateral thalamus may all cause akinesia (a failure to move in the absence of weakness) support the postulate that this system mediates motor activation.

The right hemisphere appears to play a special role in motor activation or intention. Coslett and Heilman (1987) demonstrated that right hemisphere lesions are more likely to be associated with contralateral akinesia than those of the left hemisphere. Howes and Boller (1975) measured reaction times (a measure of the time taken to initiate a response) of the hand ipsilateral to a hemispheric lesion and demonstrated that right hemisphere lesions were associated with slower reaction times than left hemisphere lesions. However, as previously discussed, this finding may be related to the important role of the right hemisphere in mediating attention and arousal. Heilman and Van Den Abell (1979) measured the reduction of reaction times of normal subjects who received warning stimuli directed to either their right or left hemisphere. Reduction of reaction times may be related to attentional–spatial cues or to preparatory motor activation. They found that, independent of the hand used, the warning stimuli delivered to the right hemisphere reduced reaction times to midline stimuli more than warning stimuli delivered to the left hemisphere. Because these cues did not contain spatial information as to where to attend, the reduction of reaction time may be related to motor activation, and these results suggest that in normal subjects the right hemisphere has a special role in motor activation.

Whereas some emotions are associated with approach behaviors (e.g., anger and joy), other emotions are associated with avoidance behaviors (e.g., fear and disgust). Unfortunately, the portions of the brain that mediate approach and avoidance behaviors have not been entirely elucidated. Denny-Brown and Chambers (1958) suggested that the frontal lobes mediate avoidance behaviors and the parietal lobes mediate approach behaviors. Denny-Brown and Chambers (1958) also suggested that approach and avoidance behaviors may be reciprocal such that a loss of one behavior may release the other behavior. Therefore, because the frontal lobes mediate avoidance behavior, frontal lobe lesions would cause inappropriate approach behaviors and because the parietal lobes mediate approach behaviors, parietal lesions would induce avoidance. In support of Denny-Brown's postulate, one can see patients with frontal lesions who demonstrate a variety of approach behaviors including manual grasp reflexes, visual grasp reflexes, rooting and sucking responses, magnetic apraxia, utilization behaviors, and defective response inhibition. Unfortunately, the specific area or areas within the frontal lobes that when damaged causes approach behaviors has not been entirely elucidated. Animals with frontal lesions show an increase in aggressive behavior. Patients with left dorsolateral frontal lesions, which, as discussed above, should induce a negative valence and increase arousal and approach behaviors, are prone to hostility and anger (Grafman et al., 1986).

Denny-Brown and Chambers (1958) demonstrated that in contrast to the manual grasp response associated with frontal lesions, patients with parietal lesions may demonstrate a palmar avoiding response. Patients with parietal lesions, especially of the right side, may not only fail to move or have a delay in moving their arms, heads, and eyes toward a part of the space that is opposite the parietal lesion, but these patients may even deviate their eyes, head, and arms toward ipsilateral hemispace. In addition, unlike patients with frontal lesions who cannot withhold their response to stimuli, patients with parietal lesions may not be able to respond to stimuli (neglect). These avoidance responses are more severe with right than with left hemisphere lesions. We have noted that patients with right parietal lesions often appear indifferent or withdrawn.

Conclusions

Although feedback does not appear to be critical in the experience of emotions, it remains possible that feedback may influence emotions. Emotions may be conditioned and use thalamic limbic (e.g., amygdala) circuits, as proposed by LeDoux. However, emotional behavior and experiences in humans are induced by complex stimuli, and the diencephalic circuit proposed by LeDoux cannot account for these experiences. The cerebral cortex of humans has complex systems that analyze stimuli, develop percepts, and interpret meaning. After meaning is derived, emotional responses are generated and emotion is experienced. The experience of emotions may be dimensional. Almost all primary emotions can be described with two or three factors, including valence, arousal, and motor activation. The determination of valence is based on whether the stimulus is beneficial (positive) or detrimental (negative) to a person's well being. Whereas the right frontal lobe appears to be important in the mediation of emotions with negative valence, the left frontal lobe may be important in the mediation of emotions with positive valence. Depending on the nature of the stimulus, some positive and some negative emotions are associated with high arousal (e.g., joy and fear) and others with low arousal (e.g., satisfaction and sadness). Whereas the right parietal lobe appears to be important in mediating arousal response, the left hemisphere appears to inhibit the arousal response. Some positive and negative emotions are associated with motor activation (e.g., anger, fear, and joy) and others are not (e.g., sadness). The frontal lobes, especially the right, appear to be important in motor activation. The motor activation associated with emotions may be either toward the eliciting stimulus (approach) or away from the stimulus (avoidance). Whereas approach behaviors may be mediated, in part, by the parietal lobes, avoidance behaviors may be mediated by the frontal lobes.

The cortical areas we have discussed above have rich interconnections. These neocortical areas also contain rich connections with the limbic system, basal ganglia, the thalamus, and the reticular system. Therefore, the anatomic modules that mediate valence, arousal, and motor activation systems are richly interconnected and form a modular network. Emotional experience may depend on the patterns of neural activation of this modular network. Future studies using ablation, functional imaging, and electrophysiological techniques are needed to test this modular hypothesis. Finally, it is well known that neurotransmitter systems play an important role in mood. However, the means by which these systems and agents influence the emotional modular systems remains to be discovered.

References

Alexander, G. E., DeLong, M. R. & Strick, P. L. (1986). Parallel organization of functionally segregated circuits linking basal ganglia and cortex. *Annual Review of Neuroscience, 9*, 357–381.

Ax, A. F. (1953). The physiological differentiation between fear and anger in humans. *Psychosomatic Medicine, 15*, 433–442.

Babinski, J. (1914). Contribution à l'étude des troubles mentaux dans l'hemisplegic organique cérébrale (anosognosie). *Review of Neurology, 27*, 845–848.

Bench, C. J., Friston, K. J., Brown, R. G., et al. (1992). The anatomy of melancholia; focal abnormalities of blood flow in major depression. *Psychological Medicine, 22*, 607–615.

Benson, D. F. (1980). Psychiatric problems in aphasia. In M. T. Sarno, O. Hook (Eds), *Aphasia Assessment and Treatment* (pp. 192–201). New York: Mason.

Bushnell, M. C., Goldberg, M. E. & Robinson, D. L. (1981). Behavioral enhancement of visual responses in monkey cerebral cortex. I. Modulation of posterior parietal cortex related to selected visual attention. *Journal of Neurophysiology, 46*, 755–772.

Cannon, W. B. (1927). The James-Lange theory of emotion: a critical examination and an alternative theory. *American Journal of Psychology, 39*, 106–124.

Coslett, H. B. & Heilman, K. M. (1987). Hemihypokinesia after right hemisphere strokes. *Brain and Cognition, 9*, 267–278.

Critchley, M. (1966). *The Parietal Lobes*. New York: Hafner.

Crucian, G., Preston, L. M., Raymer, A. M. & Heilman, K. M. (1997). Dissociation of behavioral action and emotional valence in the expression of affect. *Neurology, 48*, A352.

Damasio, A. R. & Anderson, S. W. (1993). The frontal lobes. In K. M. Heilman & E. Valenstein (Eds), *Clinical Neuropsychology*, 3rd ed. (pp. 409–460). New York: Oxford University Press.

Darwin, C. (1872). *The Expression of Emotion in Man and Animals*. London: Murray.

Davidson, R. J., Horowitz, M. E., Schwartz, G. E., et al. (1981). Lateral differences in the latency between finger tapping and heart beat. *Psychophysiology, 18*, 36–41.

Davidson, R. J., Schwartz, G. E., Saron, C., et al. (1979). Frontal versus parietal EEG asymmetry during positive and negative affect. *Psychophysiology, 16*, 202–203.

Denny-Brown, D. & Chambers, R. A. (1958). The parietal lobe and behavior. *Research Publications—Associations for Research in Nervous and Mental Disease, Proceedings of Society, 36*, 35–117.

Denny-Brown, D., Meyers, J. S. & Horenstein, S. (1952). The significance of perceptual rivalry resulting from parietal lesions. *Brain, 75*, 434–471.

Drevets, W. C. (1998). Functional neuroimaging studies of depression: the anatomy of melancholia. *Annual Review of Medicine, 49*, 341–361.

Drevets, W. C., Price, J. L., Simpson, J. R. Jr, Todd, R. D., Reich, T., Vannier, M. & Raichle, M. E. (1997). Subgenual prefrontal cortex abnormalities in mood disorders. *Nature, 386*, 824–827.

Drevets, W. C. & Raichle, M. E. (1992). Neuroanatomic circuits in depression. *Psychopharmacological Bulletin, 28*, 261–274.

Ekman, P., Sorenson, E. R. & Freisen, W. V. (1969). Pancultural elements in facial displays of emotions. *Science, 164*, 86–88.

Fox, N. A. & Davidson, R. J. (1984). Hemispheric substrates for affect: a developmental model. In N. A. Fox & R. J. Davidson (Eds), *The Psychobiology of Affective Development* (pp. 353–381). Hillsdale, NJ: Lawrence Erlbaum Associates.

Frijda, N. H. (1987). Emotion, cognitive structure, and action tendency. *Cognition and Emotion, 1*, 115–143.

Gainotti, G. (1972). Emotional behavior and hemispheric side of lesion. *Cortex, 8*, 41–55.

Gasparrini, W. G., Satz, P., Heilman, K. M., et al. (1978). Hemispheric asymmetries of affective processing as determined by the Minnesota multiphasic personality inventory. *Journal of Neurology, Neurosurgery, and Psychiatry, 41*, 470–473.

Goldberg, M. E. & Bushnell, B. C. (1981). Behavioral enhancement of visual responses in monkey cerebral cortex: II. Modulation in frontal eye fields specifically to related saccades. *Journal of Neurophysiology, 46*, 773–787.

Goldstein, K. (1948). *Language and Language Disturbances*. New York: Grune & Stratton.

Grafman, J., Vance, S. C., Weingartner, H., et al. (1986). The effects of lateralized frontal lesions on mood regulation. *Brain, 109*, 1127–1140.

Greenwald, M. K., Cook, E. W. & Lang, P. J. (1989). Affective judgment and psychophysiological response: dimensional co-variation in the evolution of pictorial stimuli. *Journal of Psychophysiology, 3*, 51–64.

Hécaen, H., Ajuriagerra, J. & de Massonet, J. (1951). Les troubles visuoconstuctifs par lesion parieto-occipitale droit. *Encephale, 40*, 122–179.

Heilman, K. M. (1979). Neglect and related disorders. In K. M. Heilman & E. Valenstein (Eds), *Clinical Neuropsychology* (pp. 268–307). New York: Oxford University Press.

Heilman, K. M. (1994). Emotion and the brain: a distributed modular network mediating emotional experience. In D. Zeidel (Ed), *Neuropsychology* (pp. 139–158). San Diego, CA: Academic Press.

Heilman, K. M., Bowers, D. & Valenstein, E. (1993a). Emotional disorders associated with neurological disease. In K. M. Heilman & E. Valenstein (Eds), *Clinical Neuropsychology*, 3rd ed. (pp. 461–497). New York: Oxford University Press.

Heilman, K. M., Pandya, D. N. & Geschwind, N. (1970). Trimodal inattention following parietal lobe ablations. *Transactions of the American Neurological Association, 95*, 259–261.

Heilman, K. M., Schwartz, H. & Watson, R. T. (1978). Hypoarousal in patients with the neglect syndrome and emotional indifference. *Neurology, 28*, 229–232.

Heilman, K. M., Valenstein, E. & Watson, R. T. (1983). Localization of neglect. In A. Kertesz (Ed), *Localization in Neurology* (pp. 471–492). New York: Academic Press.

Heilman, K. M. & Van Den Abell, T. (1979). Right hemispheric dominance for mediating cerebral activation. *Neuropsychologia 17*, 315–321.

Heilman, K. M., Watson, R. T. & Valenstein, E. (1993b). Neglect and related disorders. In K. M. Heilman & E. Valenstein (Eds), *Clinical Neuropsychology*, 3rd ed. New York: Oxford University Press.

Hohmann, G. (1966). Some effects of spinal cord lesions on experimental emotional feelings. *Psychophysiology, 3*, 143–156.

House, A., Dennis, M., Warlow, C., et al. (1990). Mood disorders after stroke and their relation to lesion location. *Brain, 113*, 1113–1129.

Howes, D. & Boller, F. (1975). Evidence for focal impairment from lesions of the right hemisphere. *Brain, 98*, 317–332.

Izard, C. E. (1977). *Human Emotions*. New York: Plenum Press.

Jacobs, D. H., Shuren, J., Bowers, D. & Heilman, K. M. (1995). Emotional facial imagery, perception and expression in Parkinson's disease. *Neurology, 45*, 1696–1702.

James, W. (1890[1950]). *The Principles of Psychology*, vol. 2. New York: Dover Publications.

Kaada, B. R. (1960). Cingulate, posterior orbital, anterior insular and temporal pole cortex. In J. Field (Ed), *Handbook of Physiology*, vol. II. *Neurophysiology* (pp. 1345–1372). Washington, DC: American Physiological Society.

Katkin, E. S. (1985). Blood, sweat and tears: individual differences in autonomic self-perception. *Psychophysiology, 22*, 125–137.

Katkin, E. S., Morrell, M. A., Goldband, S., Bernstein, G. L. & Wise, J. A. (1982). Individual differences in heartbeat discrimination. *Psychophysiology, 19*, 160–166.

Laird, J. D. (1974). Self-attribution of emotion: the effects of expressive behavior on the quality of emotional experience. *Journal of Personality and Social Psychology, 29*, 475–486.

LeDoux, J. E., Cicchetti, P., Xagoraris, A. & Romanski, L. M. (1990). The lateral amygdaloid nucleus: sensory interface of the amygdala in fear conditioning. *Journal of Neuroscience, 10*, 1062–1069.

Luria, A. R. & Simernitskaya, E. G. (1977). Interhemispheric relations and the functions of the minor hemisphere. *Neuropsychologia, 15*, 175–178.

Lynch, J. C. (1980). The functional organization of posterior parietal association cortex. *Behavioral Brain Science, 3*, 485–534.

Marañon, G. (1924). Contribution à l'étude de l'action emotive de l'adrenaline. *Revue Française d'Endocrinologie, 2*, 301–325.

Mayberg, H. S. (1997). Limbic-cortical dysregulation: a proposed model of depression. *Journal of Neuropsychiatry and Clinical Neuroscience, 9*, 471–481.

Mayberg, H. S., Robinson, R. G., Wong, D. F., Parikh, R., Bolduc, P., Price, T., Dannals, R. F., Links, J. M., Wilson, A. A., Ravert, H.T. & Wagner, H. N. Jr. (1988). PET imaging of cortical S2-serotonin receptors following stroke: lateralized changes and relationship to depression. *American Journal of Psychiatry, 145*, 937–943.

Mesulam, M. M. (1981). A cortical network for directed attention and unilateral neglect. *Annals of Neurology, 10*, 309–325.

Mesulam, M. M., Van Hesen, G. W., Pandya, D. N., et al. (1977). Limbic and sensory connections of the inferior parietal lobule (area PG) in the rhesus monkey: a study with a new method for horseradish peroxidase histochemistry. *Brain Research, 136*, 393–414.

Milner, B. (1974). Hemispheric specialization: scope and limits. In F. O. Schmitt & F. G. Worden (Eds), *The Neurosciences: Third Study Program* (pp. 75–89). Cambridge, MA: MIT Press.

Morrow, L., Vrtunski, P. B., Kim, Y., et al. (1981). Arousal responses to emotional stimuli and laterality of lesions. *Neuropsychologia, 19*, 65–71.

Moruzzi, G. & Magoun, H. W. (1949). Brainstem reticular formation and activation of the EEG. *Electroencephalography and Clinical Neurophysiology, 1*, 455–473.

Osgood, C., Suci, G. & Tannenbaum, P. (1957). *The Measure of Meaning*. Urbana: University of Illinois Press.

Pandya, D. M. & Kuypers, H. G. J. M. (1969). Cortico-cortical connections in the rhesus monkey. *Brain Research, 13*, 13–36.

Perani, D., Vallar, G., Paulesu, E., et al. (1993). Left and right hemisphere contributions to recovery from neglect after right hemisphere damage. *Neuropsychologia, 31*, 115–125.

Phelps, M. E., Mazziotta, J. C., Baxter, L., et al. (1984). Positron emission tomographic study of affective disorders: problems and strategies. *Annals of Neurology, 15*, S149–S156.

Poeck, K. (1969). Pathophysiology of emotional disorders associated with brain damage. In P. J. Vinken & G. W. Bruyn (Eds), *Handbook of Neurology*, vol. 3. New York: Elsevier.

Pribram, K. H. & McGuiness, D. (1975). Arousal, activation and effort in the control of attention. *Psychology Review, 182*, 116–149.

Reisenzein, R. (1983). The Schachter theory of emotion: two decades later. *Psychological Bulletin, 94*, 239–264.

Robinson, R. G. & Sztela, B. (1981). Mood change following left hemisphere brain injury. *Annals of Neurology, 9*, 447–453.

Ross, E. D., Homan, R. W. & Buck, R. (1994). Differential hemispheric laterlization of primary and social emotions. *Neuropsychiatry, Neuropsychology, and Behavioral Neurology, 7*, 1.

Rossi, G. S. & Rosadini, G. (1967). Experimental analysis of cerebral dominance in man. In C. Millikan & F. L. Darley (Eds), *Brain Mechanisms Underlying Speech and Language* (pp. 167–184). New York: Grune & Stratton.

Sato, H., Hata, Y., Hagihara, K., et al. (1987). Effects of cholinergic depletion on neuron activities in the cat visual cortex. *Journal of Neurophysiology, 58*, 781–794.

Schacter, S. & Singer, J. E. (1962). Cognitive, social, and physiological determinants of emotional state. *Psychology Review, 69*, 379–399.

Scheibel, M. E. & Scheibel, A. B. (1966). The organization of the nucleus reticularis thalami: a Golgi study. *Brain Research, 1*, 43–62.

Schrandt, N. J., Tranel, D. & Damasio, H. (1989). The effects of total cerebral lesions on skin conductance response to signal stimuli. *Neurology, 39S*, 223.

Segundo, J. P., Naguet, R. & Buser, P. (1955). Effects of cortical stimulation on electrocortical activity in monkeys. *Neurophysiology, 1B*, 236–245.

Shute, C. C. D. & Lewis, P. R. (1967). The ascending cholinergic reticular system, neocortical olfactory and subcortical projections. *Brain, 90*, 497–520.

Slomine, B., Bowers, D., Heilman, K. M., Bauer, R. M. & Bradley, M. (1995). Shock induced anticipatory anxiety: impact of right or left hemisphere lesions in humans. *Society for Neuroscience Abstracts, 21*, 378.2.

Starkstein, S. E., Robinson, R. G. & Price, T. R. (1987). Comparison of cortical and subcortical lesions in the production of poststroke mood disorders. *Brain, 110*, 1045–1059.

Steriade, M. & Glenn, L. (1982). Neocortical and caudate projections of intralaminar thalamic neurons and their synaptic excitation from the midbrain reticular core. *Journal of Neurophysiology, 48*, 352–370.

Stuss, D. T. & Benson, D. F. (1986). *The Frontal Lobes*. New York: Raven Press.

Terzian, H. (1964). Behavioral and EEG effects of intracarotid sodium amytal injections. *Acta Neurochirugica, 12*, 230–240.

Tomkins, S. S. (1962). *Affect, Imagery, Consciousness*, vol. 1. *The Positive Affects*. New York: Springer.

Tomkins, S. S. (1963). *Affect, Imagery, Consciousness*, vol. 2. *The Negative Affects*. New York: Springer.

Tucker, D. M. (1981). Lateral brain function, emotion and conceptualization. *Psychological Bulletin, 89*, 19–46.

Tucker, D. M. & Williamson, P. A. (1984). Asymmetric neural control in human self-regulation. *Psychology Review, 91*, 185–215.

Watson, R. T., Valenstein, E. & Heilman, K. M. (1981). Thalamic neglect: the possible role of the medical thalamus and nucleus reticularis thalami in behavior. *Archives of Neurology, 38*, 501–507.

Watson, R. T., Heilman, K. M., Miller, B. D., et al. (1974). Neglect after mesencephalic reticular formation lesions. *Neurology, 24*, 294–298.

Watson, R. T., Miller, B. D. & Heilman, K. M. (1978). Nonsensory neglect. *Annals of Neurology, 3*, 505–508.

Wundt, W. (1903). *Grundriss der Psychologie*. Stuttgart: Engelmann.

Yokoyama, K., Jennings, R., Ackles, P., et al. (1987). Lack of heart rate changes during an attention-demanding task after right hemisphere lesions. *Neurology, 37*, 624–630.

15

Neural Correlates of Conscious Emotional Experience

RICHARD D. LANE

It is now well established that people can display emotional behavior in the absence of concomitant conscious emotional experience (Öhman et al., this volume). This is one example of the known dissociations that have been observed among the experiential, expressive, and evaluative components of emotion (Lang, 1993b). These dissociations raise fundamental questions about what emotion is and why such dissociations occur. One of the key fundamental questions is whether conscious experience is a necessary component of emotion.

Some investigators (Bradley & Lang, this volume; LeDoux, 1996) have argued that the conscious experience of emotion is a red herring—a distraction from the real essence of what emotion is all about. These investigators tend to focus on the biological (central or peripheral) substrates of emotion in laboratory animals or on the biological similarity between lower animals and people. Other investigators (Clore, 1994; Damasio, 1994; Heilman, 1997) consider the conscious experience of emotion to be a core component of the emotion construct (i.e., a fundamental element in the range of phenomena that must be described and explained). Not surprisingly, these investigators tend to study the behavior of human beings including their self-reports. These differing views likely reflect the complexity of emotion and contribute to the absence of a consensus about how emotion should be defined.

Such divergent views on the essential components of emotion may derive from a fundamental philosophical issue: that it is impossible to objectively verify the nature of subjective experience. This would appear to contrast with the ability to objectively verify the accuracy of observations in the biological domain, such as activation of the amygdala or the corrugator muscles. However, Searle (1998) argues that the subjective nature of conscious experience in no way nullifies the ability to study it scientifically. He argues that the belief that conscious experience cannot be studied scientifically arises in part from the failure to distinguish between epistemology, the way we come to know something, and ontology, the actual nature of what is being studied. The fact that consciousness is a subjective, first-person phenomenon (ontology) does not prevent us from developing an objective scientific understanding of that phenomenon (epistemology). One can use objective methods to develop an increasingly accurate portrait of the phenomenon in question, as in all other scientific domains. Indeed, the study of consciousness is increasingly being recognized as a legitimate subject of scientific inquiry (Crick, 1994; Hameroff et al., 1996, 1998).

In this chapter an approach to the study of conscious emotional experience is presented, as well as results that have been obtained in the psychometric, behavioral, and functional neuroimaging domains. A framework for conceptualizing the relationship between emotional phenomena at different levels of functional organization will also be presented. Based on findings by my collaborators and I and by those of other investigators, a rudimentary neuroanatomical model is presented that addresses the distinction between implicit and explicit emotional processes. The goal is to provide a unifying framework that will potentially contribute to a theory of emotion that includes both unconscious emotional processes and conscious emotional experience.

The Levels of Emotional Awareness Construct

Resolving the question of whether conscious experience is an essential component of emotion presents forbidding conceptual barriers. How can biological and psychological aspects of emotion be placed within the same conceptual framework?

Emotions can be defined as information about the extent to which one is successful in achieving one's goals in interaction with the environment (Ortony et al., 1988). Note that this definition potentially encompasses both implicit and explicit emotional phenomenon. Implicit phenomena would include information in the form of facial expressions, gestures, and posture which convey messages to others in the environment, whereas explicit phenomena such as conscious emotional experience, somatic experience, or recall of past emotional experiences would constitute internally directed information.

Damasio (1994) points out that the advantage of conscious awareness of emotion is that it allows emotional information to be integrated with cognitive processes. If emotions were always unconscious, it would not be possible to voluntarily control emotional responses and expressions. Rather, such responses would always be based on innate motor patterns. If emotions are conscious, it is possible to think ahead, avoid, plan, and generalize to similar but unfamiliar situations. Planning ahead requires drawing on past experiences as reference points. Thus, consciousness extends time from the present into both the past and future. Conscious awareness therefore offers flexibility of response in the moment based on the particular history of an individual's unique interactions with his or her environment. This flexibility includes the capacity for emotional control. Thus, it may be that the capacity to be consciously aware of emotions is not an epiphenomenon but in fact has evolved through natural selection because it contributes to adaptational success, including survival. To the extent that this is true, specific neural correlates of experience would be anticipated. Indeed, Damasio takes exactly this position in his chapter in this volume.

To test this assertion regarding the role consciousness in emotion, one needs a method for measuring awareness of emotions. Assessment of emotional experience typically involves asking subjects to rate the intensity (Izard, 1972; Watson et al., 1988) or frequency (Larsen & Diener, 1987) of a given emotion on an ordinal scale. Although useful in certain contexts, this approach is prone to error for a variety of reasons, including other-deception, self-deception (Paulhus, 1985), or some distortion or failure in retrospective memory. Thus, measures involving emotional state are not optimal.

An alternative approach is to measure the trait ability to be aware of emotions in a way that does not rely on the accuracy of self-reports. In contrast to the position that reason and emotion oppose one another, there is increasing recognition that in the realm of stable personal attributes and characteristics, increasing cognitive sophistication and increasing emotional sophistication can be consistent with one another (Sommers, 1981). Although within-subject designs have also been used to study conscious and unconscious emotional processes with considerable success (Ladavas et al., 1993; Morris et al., 1998; Öhman et al., this volume), an advantage of a between-subject or individual differences approach is that it is potentially applicable to a variety of clinically relevant phenomena in the domains of mental and physical health (Lane & Schwartz, 1987).

How can individual differences in the capacity to be aware of emotions be conceptualized and measured? Lane and Schwartz (1987) proposed that an individual's ability to recognize and describe emotion in oneself and others, called "emotional awareness," is a cognitive skill that undergoes a developmental process similar to that described by Piaget for cognition in general. A fundamental tenet of this model is that individual differences in emotional awareness reflect variations in the degree of differentiation and integration of the schemata used to process emotional information, whether that information comes from the external world or the internal world through introspection. To the extent that awareness of emotional information is adaptive, it follows that the more information one has about one's emotional state, the greater the potential to use this information in achieving adaptational success.

Lane and Schwartz (1987) posit five "levels of emotional awareness" which share the structural characteristics of Piaget's stages of cognitive development. The five levels of emotional awareness, in ascending order, are (1) physical sensations, (2) action tendencies, (3) single emotions, (4) blends of emotion, and (5) blends of blends of emotional experience (the capacity to appreciate complexity in the experience of self and other).

These levels describe the organization of experience. They describe traits, although they may also be used to describe states. The levels are hierarchically related in that functioning at each level adds to and modifies the function of previous levels but does not eliminate them. For example, level 4 experiences should be associated with more differentiated somatic sensations (level 1) than level 2 experiences. A given emotional experience can be thought of as a construction consisting of each of the levels of experience up to and including the highest level attained.

The term "structural characteristics" refers to the degree of differentiation and integration of the cognitive schemata used to process emotional information. This is a different use of the term "structure" from that of Ortony and colleagues (Ortony et al., 1988), who use it to refer to the determinants of the specific kind of emotion activated. In the present context I use "structure" to refer to the degree of complexity of the emotional cues that can be perceived, or the nature of the cognitive processing of an emotional experience once it has been activated. The development of schemata is driven by the words or other representation mode used to describe emotion. This perspective draws on the work on symbol formation by Werner and Kaplan (1963), who maintained that things in the world become known to an observer by virtue of the way in which they are represented symbolically. Thus, the nature of conscious emotional experience, and the ability to appreciate complexity in one's own experience and that of others, is influenced by what one knows about emotion, which is based on how emotion has been represented in the past.

This position is also consistent with that of successors to Piaget such as Karmiloff-Smith (1992), who holds that cognitive development in different domains of knowledge proceeds through a process called "representational redescription." In essence, cognitive development from this theoretical perspective consists of the transformation of knowledge from implicit (procedural, sensorimotor) to explicit (conscious thought) forms through use of language (or other representation mode), which renders thought more flexible, adaptable, and creative. This viewpoint is consistent with the present hypothesis that the way language is used to describe emotion modifies what one knows about emotion and how emotion is consciously experienced.

Wine tasting can be used to illustrate this association between language and conscious awareness. Solomon (1990) compared novice and expert wine tasters in their ability to describe wines, discriminate between wines, and match written descriptions of the wines. Expert tasters used more descriptors and dimensions to describe wine than the novices. Furthermore, experts were successful in rank ordering wines based on sweetness, balance (proportion of sugar to acid), and tannin (astringency or puckeriness), while novices successfully rank-ordered wines based on sweetness only. In addition, descriptions of wines by experts were more successfully matched to the wines themselves when read by other experts than by novices. These results are consistent with the position that a given wine is experienced differently by an expert than a novice taster. The greater precision that experts demonstrate in describing wines may not just reflect their greater knowledge, but may also contribute to their more precise discriminative performance.

It is important to note that just as a person can still taste (experience) wine despite a complete lack of words to describe it, language is not necessary for conscious experience. It is known, for example, that intelligent thought is possible in prelinguistic children (Mehler & Dupoux, 1996), in adults without language, as in "linguistic isolates" who have grown up without language (Schaller, 1992), and in certain patients with aphasia and intact intellectual faculties (Ross, 1993). However, language can help to structure and establish concepts. These concepts can modify the allocation of attentional resources and thus the contents of conscious experience. Language, therefore, can enhance discriminative performance, whether it involves wine tasting or identifying emotions. To the extent that similar conceptual and attentional processes are involved, the parallels between increasing emotional and cognitive complexity can be readily understood.

The Levels of Emotional Awareness Scale: Psychometric Findings

The Levels of Emotional Awareness Scale (LEAS) is a written performance measure that asks the subject to describe his or her anticipated feelings and those of another person in each of 20 scenes described in 2–4 sentences (Lane et al., 1990). Scoring is based on specific structural criteria aimed at determining the degree of differentiation in the use of emotion words (the degree of specificity in the terms used and the range of emotions described) and the differentiation of self from other. The details of scoring are described elsewhere (Lane et al., 1990). An example of a scene from the LEAS and responses that are scored at each level is provided in table 15.1.

The scoring involves essentially no inference by raters. Thus, the LEAS can be thought of as a performance measure of the ability to put feelings into words, which, based on the theoretical considerations reviewed above, should reflect the complexity of experience. Furthermore, because the scoring system evaluates the structure of experience and not its content, subjects cannot modify their responses to enhance their score, as is the case with some self-report instruments.

To date, eight separate psychometric studies have been conducted with the LEAS. The first study in Yale undergraduates ($n = 94$) enabled us to examine the reliability of the LEAS and its correlation with other psychological tests (Lane et al., 1990). The second study involved students at Chicago Medical School (CMS) ($n = 57$) and focused on the correlation with the Levy Chimeric Faces Test (Lane

TABLE 15.1. Example of a Scene from the Levels of Emotional Awareness Scale and Responses

---

You and your best friend are in the same line of work. There is a prize given annually to the best performance of the year. The two of you work hard to win the prize. One night the winner is announced: your friend. How would you feel? How would your friend feel?

Examples of responses at each level:

0   I don't work hard to win "prizes." My friend would probably feel that the judges knew what they were doing.

1   I'd feel sick about it. It's hard for me to say what my friend would feel—it would all depend on what our relationship was like and what the prize meant to her.

2   I'd probably feel bad about it for a few days and try to figure out what went wrong. I'm sure my friend would be feeling really good.

3   We would both feel happy. Hey, you can't win 'em all!

4   I would feel depressed—the friend in this light is just like any other competitor. I would also begrudgingly feel happy for my friend and rationalize that the judges had erred. My friend would feel very gratified but would take the prize in stride to save the friendship.

5   I'd feel disappointed that I didn't win but glad that if someone else did, that person was my friend. My friend probably deserved it! My friend would feel happy and proud but slightly worried that my feelings might be hurt.

---

et al., 1995). The third study in Arizona and Minnesota ($n = 385$) established norms for the scale (Lane et al., 1996). A fourth study with University of Arizona undergraduates ($n = 215$) involved additional psychometric and psychophysiologic assessments. The fifth and sixth studies have been conducted in collaboration with Lisa Feldman Barrett at Boston College. In addition, two international studies have been conducted: a study of 331 German students (Wrana et al., 1998) and a Canadian study of 30 subjects with borderline personality disorder and 40 control subjects (Levine et al., 1997). The findings from these studies are selectively reviewed below.

The LEAS has consistently been shown to have high inter-rater reliability and internal consistency (Lane et al., 1998a). An adequate assessment of test–retest reliability of the LEAS in the general population has not been undertaken. Norms for age, sex, and socioeconomic status have been established based on the study completed in Arizona and Minnesota.

In the Yale study we administered two instruments which, like the LEAS, are cognitive–developmental measures based on Piaget's model: the Sentence Completion Test of Ego Development by Loevinger (Loevinger & Wessler, 1970; Loevinger et al., 1970) and the cognitive complexity of the description of parents by Blatt and colleagues (1979). The LEAS correlated moderately ($r = .25$, $n = 94$; $r = .26$, $n = 92$, respectively) and significantly ($p < .02$) in the predicted direction for both tests. These results support the claim that the LEAS is measuring a cognitive–developmental continuum and that the LEAS is not identical to these other measures.

A key question is whether the LEAS is simply another measure of verbal ability. In the Yale sample the LEAS correlated ($r = .38$, $n = 90$, $p < .001$) with the vocabulary subtest of the Wechsler Adult Intelligence Scale Revised (WAIS-R). In the CMS study the LEAS correlated ($r = .17$, ns) with the Shipley Institute of Living Scale (Shipley, 1940), a multiple-choice measure of verbal ability. These data suggest that verbal ability may contribute to LEAS performance. However, several studies have now been conducted demonstrating that when verbal ability is controlled, significant effects are still observed.

For example, LEAS scores in men and women could be compared in all eight studies. In three of these studies measures of verbal ability, including the WAIS vocabulary subtest and the Shipley Institute of Living Scale, were also obtained. In each study women scored higher than men on the LEAS ($p < .01$), even when controlling for verbal ability ($p < .05$) (L. F. Barrett et al., in press). Thus, the finding that women score higher than men on the LEAS is a highly stable and generalizable finding. These data suggest that on average women are more sensitive to emotional cues in themselves and others than are men. This greater sensitivity has clear advantages in the realm of interpersonal relations and problem solving, but may also contribute to the finding that women are approximately twice as likely to suffer from affective and anxiety disorders than are men (Breslau et al., 1997; Gater et al., 1998).

Barrett administered the LEAS and the Weinberger Adjustment Inventory to 63 subjects at Pennsylvania State University and 55 subjects at Boston College. In both samples the LEAS correlated significantly ($p < .05$, two-tailed) with self-restraint, one of three superordinate dimensions of the scale. The LEAS also correlated significantly with impulse control ($r = .35$, $p < .01$, two-tailed; $r = .30$, $p < .05$, two-tailed), a component of self-restraint that involves the tendency to think before acting. Self-restraint refers directly to suppression of egoistic desires in the interest of long-term goals and relations with others. This replication in independent samples indicates that greater emotional awareness is associated with greater self-reported impulse control and is consistent with the theory that functioning at higher levels of emotional awareness (levels 3–5) modulates function at lower levels (actions and action tendencies at level 2).

Evidence for the discriminant validity of the LEAS is provided by data from the Norms study and the Arizona undergraduate study. In both studies ($n = 385$ and $n = 215$, respectively) the Affect Intensity Measure (Larsen et al., 1987), a trait measure of the tendency to experience emotions intensely, did not correlate significantly with the LEAS, despite the large sample sizes. Thus, inadequate statistical power cannot explain the lack of correlation. The LEAS also does not correlate significantly with measures of negative affect, such as the Taylor Manifest Anxiety Scale and the Beck Depression Inventory. These results are consistent with the view that the LEAS measures the structure or complexity and not the intensity of affective experience.

The Levels of Emotional Awareness Scale: Behavioral Findings

Perception of Affect Task

A key assumption in this work on emotional awareness is that language promotes the development of schemata for the processing of emotional information, whether that information comes from the internal or external world. Furthermore, once the schemata are established, they should affect the processing of emotional information whether the information is verbal or nonverbal. Thus, the LEAS should correlate with the ability to recognize and categorize external emotional stimuli. Furthermore, this correlation should hold whether the external stimulus and the response are purely verbal or purely nonverbal.

These hypotheses were tested in the Norms study by use of the Perception of Affect Task (PAT), a set of four emotion-recognition tasks (35 items each) developed by Rau and Kaszniak at the University of Arizona (Rau, 1993). The first subtask consists of stimuli describing an emotional situation without the use of emotion words. For example, "The man looked at the photograph of his recently departed wife." The response involves choosing one from an array of seven terms (happy, sad, angry, afraid, disgust, neutral, surprise) to identify how the person in question was feeling. The fourth subtask is purely nonverbal. The stimuli consist of photographs of faces developed by Ekman (1982), each of which depicts an individual emotion. The response consists of selecting one from an array of seven photographs depicting emotional scenes without faces (e.g., two people standing arm-in-arm by a grave with their backs to the camera). The other two subtasks involved a verbal stimulus (sentence) and a nonverbal response (from an array of seven faces) and a nonverbal stimulus (face) and a verbal response (from an array of seven words).

Across the entire scale, the correlation between the LEAS and the PAT was highly significant ($r = .43$, $n = 385$, $p < .001$), accounting for about 18% of the variance. Furthermore, significant correlations were observed between the LEAS and each of the PAT subtasks. When dividing the sample into upper (high), middle, and lower (low) thirds on the LEAS, the high LEAS subjects scored higher on each of the PAT subtasks than the low LEAS subjects. Thus, high LEAS scores were associated with better emotion recognition no matter whether the task was purely verbal or purely nonverbal (Lane et al., 1996). Furthermore, when combining results for each of the seven emotion categories across the four subtasks (there were five stimuli of each emotion type in each subtask), the same findings for high, moderate, and low LEAS subjects were observed (Lane et al., 1998). These findings support the claim that the LEAS is (1) a measure of the schemata used to process emotional information, whether the information is verbal or nonverbal, (2) a measure of the complexity of experience, and (3) not simply a measure of verbal ability.

Levy Chimeric Faces Test

A study performed at Chicago Medical School was our first attempt to relate the LEAS to brain function. Given that the LEAS is a psychological measure of an individual difference variable, we were interested in determining whether the LEAS correlated with individual differences in an aspect of brain function associated with the processing of emotional information. We selected the right hemispheric dominance among right-handers in the perception of facial emotion, in part because it has been consistently observed and in part because there are individual differences in the degree of lateralization of this function that are not well understood (Levy et al., 1983a).

The measure of hemispheric dominance in the perception of facial emotion which we chose was the Levy Chimeric Faces Test (LCFT) (Levy et al., 1983b). This test consists of 36 chimeric or composite faces depicting a smiling half-face juxtaposed to a neutral half-face from the same subject. This composite is paired with its mirror image in a vertical array. The only difference between the two composites is whether the smile is in the left or the right visual field. The subject is asked to indicate whether the "strange picture" on the top or the bottom looks happier (figure 15.1). Other studies have shown that the right hemispheric dominance (a preference for selecting the composite with the smile in the left visual field) on this task is consistently observed no matter whether the stimuli are presented in free field in a group format, individually in a booklet format, or individually by tachistoscope. Furthermore, the right hemispheric advantage has been demonstrated using composite photographs consisting of sad as well as happy half-faces.

The LEAS correlated significantly with the degree of right hemispheric advantage in performance of the LCFT ($r = .356$, $p < .05$). Interestingly, the correlation between the degree of right hemispheric dominance and the LEAS improved ($r = .444$, $p < .003$) when restricting the sample to native English speakers (presumably because a measure completed in English is a more accurate measure of underlying schemata if completed in the subject's native language) and when controlling for

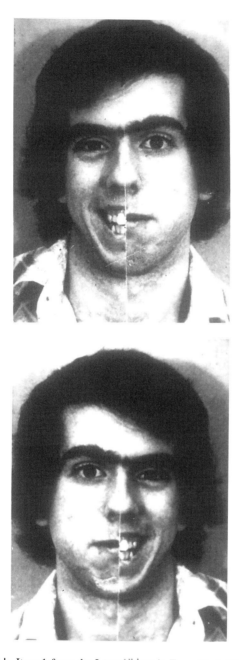

Figure 15.1. Item 1 from the Levy Chimeric Faces Task (LCFT). In this example, the top face is a normal print and the bottom face is a mirror-reversed print of the same negative. The same chimeric pair reoccurred in the test session with top and bottom positions reversed, and the same poser appears in two other pairs, but with the smile produced by the left half of his face and the neutral expression by the right half. The LCFT consists of 36 chimeric pairs generated from photographs of 9 individuals.

verbal ability using the Shipley Institute of Living Scale (Shipley, 1940). These data are consistent with the hypothesis that people who are more emotionally aware tend to preferentially use the hemisphere that is specialized for the detection of emotional cues.

Neural Correlates of Emotional Awareness

To further explore the underlying functional neuroanatomy of emotional awareness, we administered the LEAS to subjects participating in a positron emission tomography (PET) study of emotion (Lane et al., 1998a). Subjects included 12 right-handed female volunteers who were free of medical, neurological, or psychiatric abnormalities. The LEAS and other psychometric instruments were completed before PET imaging. Happiness, sadness, disgust, and three neutral control conditions were induced by film and recall of personal experiences (12 conditions). Twelve PET images of blood flow were obtained in each subject using the ECAT 951/31 scanner (Siemens, Knoxville, TN), 40 mCi intravenous bolus injections of ^{15}O-water, a 15-sec uptake period, 60-sec scans, and an interscan interval of 10 min.

To examine neural activity attributable to emotion generally, rather than to specific emotions, one can subtract the three neutral conditions from the three emotional conditions in a given stimulus modality (film or recall). This difference, which can be calculated separately for the six film and six recall conditions, identifies regions of the brain where blood flow changes specifically attributable to emotion occur. These blood flow changes, which are indicative of neural activity in that region, can then be correlated with LEAS scores to identify regions of the brain associated with emotional awareness during emotional arousal.

Findings from this covariate analysis revealed one cluster for film-induced emotion with a maximum located in the right mid-cingulate cortex (BA 23; coordinates of maximum = [16, −18, 32]; $z = 3.40$; $p < .001$, uncorrected). For recall-induced emotion, the most statistically significant cluster was located in the right anterior cingulate cortex (BA 24; coordinates of maximum = [16, 6, 30]; $z = 2.82$; $p < .005$, uncorrected). A conjunction analysis was performed next to identify areas of significant overlap between the two covariance analyses. With a height threshold of $z = 3.09$, ($p < .001$) and an extent threshold of five voxels, a single cluster was observed in the right anterior cingulate cortex (BA 24) maximal at coordinates [14, 6, 30] ($z = 3.74$, $p < .001$; $p = 9.2 \times 10^{-5}$; uncorrected). As can be observed in figure 15.2, the point of maximum change is located in white matter adjacent to the anterior cingulate cortex. Given that blood flow changes in white matter are unlikely, the imprecision in anatomical localization associated with image normalization, the extension of the area of significant change into the anterior cingulate cortex, and the absence of other gray matter structures in the immediate vicinity, the likeliest location of this cluster is the anterior cingulate cortex (Lane et al., 1998a).

The anterior cingulate cortex is a complex structure with numerous functions which are difficult to quantify or describe (Vogt et al., 1992). Traditionally the anterior cingulate cortex was thought to have a primarily affective function (Papez, 1937; Vogt et al., 1992). However, in addition to emotion, the anterior cingulate

sagittal   coronal

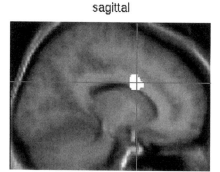   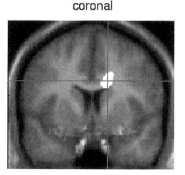

Figure 15.2. Results of the conjunction analysis demonstrating overlap of the separate associations during film and recall-induced emotion between Levels of Emotional Awareness Scale and cerebral blood flow in the dorsal anterior cingulate cortex. The cluster depicted contains 66 voxels with a maximum activation at coordinates [14, 6, 30] ($z = 3.74$, $p < .001$). These results are displayed in the sagittal and coronal planes superimposed on the average structural MRI of the 12 female subjects.

cortex is now recognized to play important roles in attention, pain, response selection, maternal behavior, vocalization, skeletomotor function, and autonomic control (Vogt & Gabriel, 1993). The multiple functions of the anterior cingulate cortex no doubt contribute to the significant changes in activation that have been observed in a variety of studies. How can these different functions be reconciled with the present findings involving emotional awareness?

One answer might be that these various functions of the anterior cingulate cortex reflect its superordinate role in executive control of attention and motor responses (Lane et al., 1998a). According to this view, emotion, pain, or other salient exteroceptive or interoceptive stimuli provide moment-to-moment guidance regarding the most suitable allocation of attentional resources for the purpose of optimizing motor responses in interaction with the environment. The conscious experience of emotion could occur concomitantly and automatically as attention gets redirected by emotion. As such, a role of the anterior cingulate cortex in the conscious experience of emotion fits well with its other functions, but suggests that this role is not exclusive to emotion. To the extent that people who are more emotionally aware attend more to internal and external emotion cues, the cognitive processing of this information can contribute to ongoing emotional development.

Attention to Emotional Experience

In his seminal work on blindsight, Weiskrantz (1986) distinguished between the fundamental constituents of a network mediating a function and the neural structures involved in commenting on or reflecting upon it. Blindsight is a condition caused by a lesion in the primary visual cortex in which patients are not consciously aware of visual stimuli but demonstrate behaviorally that the stimulus is perceived (Weiskrantz, 1986). The lessons learned from the study of blindsight patients in the aware and unaware states are potentially applicable to the understanding of the neural substrates of emotional awareness.

In his chapter in this volume, Weiskrantz raises the question of whether the dorsal anterior cingulate cortex is the final output or commentary stage at which awareness of emotion can be expressed and registered. A recent functional magnetic resonance imaging (fMRI) study of blindsight in the aware and unaware states (Sahraie et al., 1997), for example, reveals that dorsolateral prefrontal cortex is preferentially activated during visual processing in the aware state. Subsequent to this astute query by Weiskrantz, we conducted a PET study that generated new data addressing this issue.

In this study (Lane et al., 1997b) we examined the pattern of neural activation associated with attending to one's own emotional experience. We used a selective attention paradigm based on the rationale that selective attention heightens activity in those regions that mediate a particular function (Corbetta et al., 1990; Fink et al., 1996a). Thus, we reasoned that attention to one's own experience would activate those brain regions that are preferentially activated during the conscious experience of emotion. To confirm that subjects were allocating their attention as we instructed, we had them indicate on a keypad how each emotion-evoking picture made them feel. In essence, we were examining an aspect of conscious experience involving commentary on that experience.

We studied 10 healthy men as they viewed 12 picture sets, each consisting of pleasant, unpleasant, and neutral pictures from the International Affective Picture System (Lang et al., 1995). Pictures were presented for 500 msec every 3.0 sec. Twelve PET-derived measures of cerebral blood flow were obtained in each subject, one for each picture set. During half the scans subjects attended to their emotional experience (indicating on a keypad whether the picture evoked a pleasant, unpleasant, or neutral feeling); during the other half they attended to spatial location (indicating whether the scene depicted was indoors, outdoors, or indeterminate). Across subjects, picture sets were counterbalanced between the two attention conditions.

During attention to subjective emotional responses, increased neural activity was elicited in rostral anterior cingulate cortex (BA32) and medial prefrontal cortex (coordinates: [0,50,16]; $z = 6.74$, $p < .001$, corrected; figure 15.3), right temporal pole, insula, and ventral cingulate cortex (all $p < .001$, corrected). Under the same stimulus conditions when subjects attended to spatial aspects of the picture sets, activation was observed in parieto-occipital cortex bilaterally ($z = 5.71$, $p < .001$, corrected), a region known to participate in the evaluation of spatial relationships.

Our interpretation of these findings is that the rostral anterior cingulate/medial prefrontal activation may be where a representation of emotional state is established. Several lines of evidence support this view. This region is densely connected with the amygdala, orbitofrontal cortex, other sectors of the anterior cingulate cortex, and other paralimbic structures such as the insula (Price et al., 1996). It thus clearly receives information about the emotional significance of stimuli. Second, lesions in this area produce a blunting of emotional experience. For example, post-mortem studies of schizophrenic patients who underwent prefrontal leukotomy, many of whom lost the ability to experience emotion following surgery

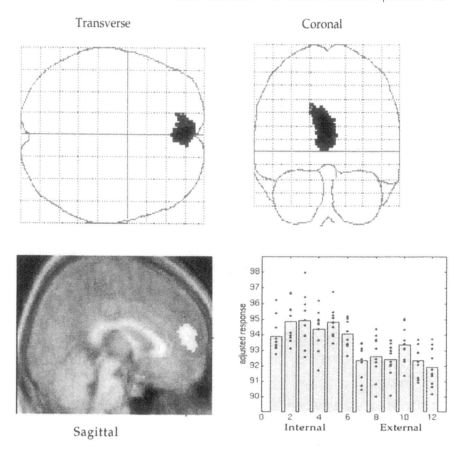

Figure 15.3. A statistical parametric map showing significant cerebral blood flow increases in anterior cingulate cortex (BA32)/medial prefrontal cortex (BA9) during selective attention to subjective emotional responses (minus activations specific to the external condition). The figures in the upper left and upper right are projection images in the transverse and coronal planes, respectively. The sagittal view in the lower left depicts the spatial distribution of the activation in the internal focus condition ($Z = 6.87$, $p < .001$, corrected) superimposed on the average structural MRI of the 10 male subjects. The figure in the lower right demonstrates blood flow values in each condition (internal, 1–6; external, 7–12)

(Hoffman, 1949), often revealed lesions in rostral anterior cingulate. Third, the neighboring dorsolateral prefrontal cortex clearly participates in working memory, keeping information on-line temporarily for use in cognitive operations (Goldman-Rakic, 1987). It is reasonable to hypothesize that a similar function may exist for interoceptive emotional information in a neighboring sector of prefrontal cortex.

Further support for this hypothesis is provided by considering the strategic location of this area. Drawing on the work of Sanides (1970) and Goldberg (1987), Tucker and colleagues (1995) proposed that frontal lobe control of motivational impulses results from an integration of ventral and dorsal corticolimbic pathways.

The ventrolateral pathway is derived from paleocortex (associated with olfactory cortex). The amygdala and orbitofrontal cortex are key structures in this pathway. This system links motor sequences to perceptual objects in a responsive manner. It restricts and monitors motivational impulses through a feedback mechanism. Lesions of orbitofrontal cortex are typically associated with disinhibition, as in the case of the patient Phineas Gage (Damasio et al., 1994). Motor planning is articulated with specific reference to the ongoing perceptual input. The mediodorsal system is derived from archicortex (associated with hipppocampus), projecting actions based on probabilistic models of the future through a feedforward mechanism. The hippocampus and anterior cingulate cortex are key structures in this system. Action is based on a preexisting model rather than ongoing feedback about the course of action in the situation. Lesions in this area are associated with apathy and indifference. Thus, there may be reactive-based and planning-based motivational systems that participate in the regulation of behavior by the frontal lobe (see also Mega et al., 1997).

The area of rostral anterior cingulate/medial prefrontal cortex that we identified appears to be precisely situated between these two systems. Clearly, a representation of current emotional state facilitates guidance of current behavior and planning future behavior. The observation that greater emotional awareness is associated with greater impulse control may be particularly relevant in this context, as impulsiveness involves a failure to consider the future in the guidance of current behavior. A lack of impulse control is certainly evident in patients with frontal lobe lesions (e.g., Phineas Gage; Damasio et al., 1994) and is consistent with the findings of Morgan and colleagues (Morgan et al., 1993) that extinction of conditioned fear is greatly prolonged with lesions of the ventromedial prefrontal cortex (but see Gewirtz et al., 1997). Cyctoarchitectural studies reveal a gradual change from caudal to rostral in laminar characteristics from limbic periallocortex toward isocortical areas in medial prefrontal cortex (Barbas & Pandya, 1989), suggesting that a rigid distinction between rostral anterior cingulate cortex and medial prefrontal cortex is misleading. The midline location is consistent with other evidence that responses generated from internal cues are associated with activation of midline structures and that responses generated from external cues are associated with activation of lateral structures (Chen et al., 1995).

The findings from this study can therefore be interpreted as follows. When attending to one's own emotional state, several brain areas are activated, including those involved in (1) establishing a representation of the emotional state (rostral anterior cingulate/medial prefrontal cortex), (2) processing visceral information (anterior insula) (Augustine, 1996), (3) performing complex visual discrimination, possibly including retrieval of emotion-laden episodic memories (right temporal pole) (Fink et al., 1996b), and (4) regulating autonomic responses (ventral cingulate) (Vogt et al., 1992).

Phenomenal versus Reflective Conscious Awareness

It is fascinating to consider the possibility that two different areas of the anterior cingulate cortex are participating in different aspects of conscious emotional experience. It is also notable that this more anterior activation in rostral anterior cingulate cortex was anticipated by Weiskrantz (this volume). What functions may be served by these two areas?

A fundamental distinction in the study of consciousness is that between primary and secondary consciousness (Farthing, 1992). Primary consciousness refers to phenomenal experience: the direct experience of an emotion, the taste of wine, or the touch of a hand. Secondary consciousness refers to cognitive operations performed on the contents of primary consciousness—for example, attending to or reflecting on the contents of phenomenal awareness. This type of consciousness has also been referred to as "metacognition" (awareness of awareness) (Jarman et al., 1995) or "reflective conscious awareness" (Farthing, 1992). It is clear that in order to engage in reflection, one must have something (e.g., a representation) to reflect upon.

It is hypothesized that the correlation between dorsal anterior cingulate cortex and level of emotional awareness reflects phenomenal awareness of emotion and that rostral anterior cingulate cortex participates in reflective awareness of emotion. It is noteworthy that Rainville and colleagues (1997) demonstrated that dorsal anterior cingulate cortex participates in the affective component of pain, entirely consistent with the first part of this formulation. It is also noteworthy that an area of medial prefrontal cortex close to that identified in our attention to emotional experience study has been implicated in the representation of the mental state of others, so-called Theory of Mind tasks (Happé et al., 1996). Given the likelihood that the capacity to establish representations of one's own emotional state in infancy is closely linked with the perception and representation of the emotional state of others, including the mother (Gergely & Watson, 1996), and given the similarity of the cognitive process involved, it is likely that the representations of one's own state and that of others are established in neighboring and interconnected regions.

Much work remains to be done to confirm these hypotheses. However, doing so could serve an integrative function. Stuss (1991a/b) has discussed how the prefrontal cortex serves a self-monitoring and regulatory function. Damasio (1994) has discussed how the sense of self may derive in part from the somatovisceral sensations associated with emotion that are integrated with the higher cognitive functions of prefrontal cortex. It will be important to explore the extent to which the rostral anterior cingulate cortex/medial prefrontal cortex serves an exclusively emotional function, or like the dorsal anterior cingulate, appears to serve a superordinate function that may be greatly influenced by, but is not necessarily exclusively dedicated to, emotion. Such a conclusion is certainly possible in light of the plasticity of higher cortical functions based on the interaction between genetics, environmental experience, and habitual modes of behavior (Elman et al., 1996). If the function of this region is not exclusively devoted to emotion, it would help to explain how emotion-related individual differences arise and contribute to an understanding of the neural substrates of unique individual personalities.

In summary, the rostral anterior cingulate/medial prefrontal cortex is hypothesized to participate in the representation of emotional experience. This structure may be essential for knowing how one is feeling, a function that is critical in the control of emotional behavior. I have discussed above the critical importance of representations in creating knowledge. The interaction between representations of emotional experience and the phenomenal experience of emotion may at least in part be mediated by the tight anatomical linkage (Price et al., 1996) between the rostral and dorsal anterior cingulate cortices. The dynamic interaction between phenomenal experience, establishing a representation of it, elaborating that representation (e.g., identifying the source of the emotional response), and integrating it with other cognitive processes are the fundamental processes involved in the cognitive elaboration of emotion addressed by the levels of emotional awareness model.

Unconscious Processing

A debate has persisted for some years between the perspectives represented by Zajonc (1984) and Lazarus (1984). At issue is whether cognitive processing is necessary before an emotional response. Zajonc and colleagues (Kunst-Wilson & Zajonc, 1980) have demonstrated that people develop preferences for stimuli to which they have been subliminally exposed but have not consciously perceived. As part of this body of work, Murphy and Zajonc (1993) have shown that subjects can accurately make crude positive or negative judgments about stimuli that are not consciously perceived, but more refined evaluations of the stimuli, such as the type of emotion depicted, are not possible in the absence of conscious awareness. This result is entirely consistent with the levels of emotional awareness model. To the extent that cognitive processing is equated with consciousness, the evidence suggests that conscious cognition is not a necessary antecedent to an emotional response.

Öhman et al. (this volume) have demonstrated autonomic responses to aversively conditioned angry faces independent of conscious recognition of the stimuli. Similar to Murphy and Zajonc, Ladavas (Ladavas et al., 1993) has shown that the presence or absence of emotional content can be accurately detected in subliminally presented pictures. Drawing on Fodor's concept of modularity (Fodor, 1983), Ladavas suggests that these and other findings support a critical distinction between modular and nonmodular emotion information processing. Modules are domain-specific computational devices that are cognitively impenetrable and generate shallow output. Cognitive penetrability (or informational encapsulation) refers to the degree to which information processing can be influenced by prior knowledge, expectations, beliefs, or other cognitive input. Ladavas argues, based on her own work and that of others, that the automatic, unconscious process of emotion-generation is cognitively impenetrable. The output of this module is crude and diffuse but becomes the substrate for further cognitive elaboration, which is highly cognitively penetrable.

A growing body of literature suggests that such a distinction may have neuroanatomical substrates. LeDoux (1996) has written widely about the distinction between the thalamo-amygdala pathway for processing exteroceptive stimuli rapidly and crudely in the absence of conscious awareness. In contrast, the neocortical-amygdala pathway provides more precise and differentiated identification of the stimulus requiring an additional 10 msec of processing time. The time savings from the crude evaluation could mean the difference between life and death and thus could have an evolutionary advantage. The neocortical processing can provide fine tuning and perhaps an alteration of the automatically generated response. These data derived from conditioning experiments in laboratory animals are consistent with Ladavas's concept of modular versus nonmodular emotional functions.

Several functional neuroimaging studies of unconscious processing of emotional stimuli have appeared in the literature. Whalen and colleagues (1998) observed bilateral amygdala activation and deactivation during the unconscious processing of fearful and happy faces, respectively, and activation of the sublenticular substantia innominata during unconscious processing of both happy and fearful faces. Morris and colleagues (Morris et al., 1998) recently extended this finding in a PET study examining neural activity during the conscious and unconscious processing of aversively conditioned angry faces. The main findings were that the right amygdala was activated during unconscious processing and the left amygdala was activated during conscious processing of the conditioned faces. These findings are consistent with the thesis that unconscious processing of emotional stimuli occurs primarily at the subcortical level. These findings are to be contrasted with the activation of paralimbic structures observed in the studies of emotional awareness and attention to emotional experience.

The Levels of Emotional Awareness Model:
Implications and Conclusions

This chapter began with a discussion of the debate about whether conscious processes are or are not a critical feature of emotion. The levels of emotional awareness model answers this question by proposing that emotional phenomena in humans at each level of functional organization are potentially associated with awareness of some type. Thus, the lowest levels of organization (e.g., the autonomic activation, level 1, and action tendencies, level 2, associated with emotional arousal), as well as the higher levels of organization (levels 3–5), are each associated with a type of conscious experience. Level 1 and 2 phenomena, viewed in isolation, would not necessarily be considered indicators of emotion, and self-report inventories of emotional experience, such as the Positive and Negative Affect Scale (PANAS) (Watson et al., 1988), do not include many terms indicative of level 1 or 2 phenomena. Thus, in the context of actual level 1 or 2 emotional responses, such inventories might falsely indicate that conscious emotional experience is not present. The levels of emotional awareness framework therefore puts conscious and unconscious processes on the same continuum, and at the same time distinguishes between types of unconscious (level 1 vs. level 2) and conscious (level 3 vs. 4 vs. 5) processes.

It is interesting to note that the major theories of emotion can be classified according to the level of processing upon which they focus. The James-Lange theory of emotion (James, 1884), which hypothesizes that somatic state is a determinant of emotional experience, is a level 1 theory. Level 2 theories, which are action oriented, include Darwin's theory that emotional displays serve adaptive functions (Darwin, 1872), or theories such as that of Lang's (1993a) that focus on appetitive/aversive motivational systems. Tomkins's theory of individual emotions (Tomkins, 1962) is a level 3 theory. Level 4 theories focus on blends of emotion, such as Izard's (1972) differential emotions theory and Ekman's (1982) theory involving patterns of emotions. Cacioppo and Berntson's (1994) theory of bivariate evaluative space, in which both positive and negative responses can occur to varying degrees in response to a stimulus, is another example of a level 4 theory. (A level 5 theory, yet to be formulated, would involve social cognition and would focus on how differentiated awareness of self and other influences social behavior and the autonomic and neuroendocrine concomitants of emotional responses.) Each theory addresses a coherent level of organization. To the extent that this is true, it is quite possible that each level of organization corresponds to an identifiable neurobiological state.

The evidence reviewed above provides the basis for a rudimentary neuroanatomical model of emotional awareness that distinguishes between implicit and explicit levels of function. Following Ladavas (Ladavas et al., 1993), levels 1 and 2 involve implicit processes that are automatic, modular, and cognitively impenetrable. It would appear that subcortical structures participate in the automatic generation of emotional responses associated with absent or diffusely undifferentiated awareness. It may be speculated that the neural substrates of level 1 include the thalamus and hypothalamus (diencephalon) and brainstem. At level 2, the sensorimotor enactive level, crude distinctions between globally positive and globally negative states can be made. Given that decorticate cats can demonstrate fear and pleasure reactions (Bard & Rioch, 1937), it is likely that the thalamus participates at this level also. The amygdala appears to be preferentially activated in association with aversive stimuli (Tranel, 1997), and the ventral striatum, including the nucleus accumbens, is preferentially activated by appetitive or reward stimuli (Koob & Goeders, 1989).

The outputs from this stage of processing are widespread. Emotions at level 2 are represented in actions such as gestures and other movements that have an either/or quality. Much evidence suggests that the basal ganglia participate in the automatic behavioral displays of emotional gestures and expression (Gray, 1995; Rolls, 1990). Orbitofrontal cortex activity appears to be associated with the perception of somatic sensations that bias behavior either toward or away from a stimulus (Damasio, 1994). This biasing process can occur without conscious awarenesss of its occurrence (Bechara et al., 1997). Orbitofrontal cortex activity affects behavior by overriding automatic processes in the amygdala and participating in extinction, among other functions (Emery & Amaral, this volume). A key tenet of this model is that structures at this level, such as the amygdala (Cahill & McGaugh, 1998; LeDoux, 1996) are essential for implicit processing and contribute to but are not sufficient for the explicit experience of discrete emotions or combinations thereof (i.e., levels 3–5).

Levels 3–5 involve explicit processes that are influenced by higher cognitive processes, including prior explicit knowledge. They are hypothesized to be mediated by the above structures and, in addition, based on the evidence presented above, by paralimbic structures, including the anterior cingulate cortex and insula, and the medial prefrontal cortex. The rostral anterior cingulate cortex/medial prefrontal cortex appears to be necessary for the representation of emotion used in conscious cognition.

The hierarchical nature of this anatomical model and the parallel hierarchical structure of the psychological model are depicted in figure 15.4. The hierarchical nature of brain structure and function has been recognized for many years. For example, Jackson (1932) described the release of lower level functions by lesions higher in the neuraxis. Yakovlev (1948) proposed three levels of nervous system function, including a primitive inner core devoted to arousal and autonomic function, surrounded by a middle layer including the limbic system and basal ganglia, and an outer layer, the most recent to emerge phylogenetically, including the neocortex and pyramidal system. This model was further elaborated by MacLean (1990) in his model of the triune brain, involving sequential evolution of the reptilian, paleomammalian, and neomammalian brains. The challenge in the years ahead will be to generate a more differentiated and specific model based on the full range of neuroscientific methods, especially functional neuroimaging. Just how cortical and subcortical structures interact to produce these different levels of function remains to be elucidated.

It may be speculated that the process of representational redescription, as described by Karmiloff-Smith (1992), is mediated at least in part by structures hypothesized to be involved in explicit processing at levels 3–5. It may be precisely because these structures are not uniquely devoted to the processing of emotion that their emotion-related functions are cognitively penetrable. Indeed, the level of emotional awareness of a given individual may be a function of the degree to which these structures are or are not devoted to processing of emotional information from the internal and external worlds.

Neuroanatomical   Psychological

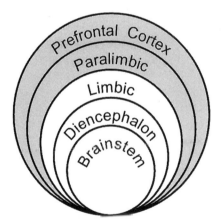
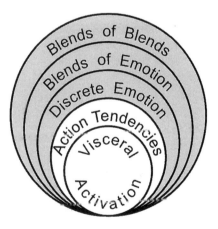

Figure 15.4. Parallels in the hierarchical organization of emotional experience and its neural substrates. The shell structure is intended to convey that each succeeding level adds to and modulates lower levels but does not replace them. Although each model contains five levels, a one-to-one correspondence between each level in the psychological and neuroanatomical models is not intended. Lower levels with white backgrounds correspond to implicit processes. Higher levels with gray backgrounds correspond to explicit processes.

Elucidating this model more fully is likely to have important clinical implications. The observation that patients with psychosomatic disorders had difficulty verbalizing feelings was the guiding clinical problem that led MacLean to expand on the Papez model of emotion (MacLean, 1949). MacLean's thesis was that interference with communication between limbic (visceral brain) and neocortical areas contributed to physical disease. The phenomenon to which MacLean referred is probably best captured currently by the clinical entity called alexithymia (Taylor et al., 1991), or "lack of words for emotion." We have argued elsewhere that alexithymia is associated with emotional arousal in the absence of conscious awareness (Lane et al., 1997a). As greater conscious awareness of emotion is theoretically associated with progressively greater regulatory control of lower level processes, the relative absence of such awareness may be associated with autonomic and neuroendocrine dysregulation (Lane et al., 1997a; Thayer & Lane, in press). The best recent evidence supporting this view comes from the observations that group psychotherapy designed to promote the awareness and expression of emotions (e.g., confronting fears directly) is associated with enhanced survival in patients with recurrent breast cancer (Spiegel et al., 1989) and malignant melanoma (Fawzy et al., 1993).

Alexithymia may be conceptualized as a failure of cognitive elaboration of modular emotion output. The challenge for the psychotherapist is to enable alexithymic individuals to make the transition from implicit to explicit processing of emotional arousal. Alexithymic patients are typically difficult to treat. If they come for treatment, they often do so at the urging of others. Successful therapy requires first educating them about the nature of their problem (Krystal, 1979). The next step is to help them overcome whatever motivational barriers exist in attending to and recognizing their own emotional experiences.

Just as wishes, expectancies, and motivational states can influence the processing of exteroceptive stimuli, a history of psychological trauma can lead to motivated inattention to one's own emotions that can result in a deficit in the capacity for conscious emotional experiences. A safe and supportive interpersonal environment is essential for success in psychotherapy. It is therefore interesting to note that post-traumatic stress disorder (PTSD) has been associated with decreased activity in the dorsal anterior cingulate relative to controls (Shin et al., 1997), and preliminary findings indicate that successful treatment of PTSD is associated with a return to normal levels of activity in this area (van der Kolk et al., 1998).

Once emotions are consciously acknowledged and experienced, the process of cognitive elaboration of emotion can then occur so that the origin and meaning of painful and distressing emotions can be understood, elaborated, and used to promote adaptive behavior. If not brought to conscious awareness, emotional distress such as anger will be translated into action and/or a peripheral physiological response that may be maladaptive. The capacity for such explicit processing of emotion may indeed modulate the activity of those structures mediating implicit emotional processes. It will be fascinating in the years ahead to explore the functional neuroanatomy of this process, the changes that occur in effective connectivity between brain regions (Buechel & Friston, 1997), and their influence on mental and physical health. Based on the concepts and data presented here, it will be important to use functional neuroimaging techniques to examine the neural mechanisms by which labeling emotions verbally modifies activity of those structures involved in the conscious experience of and conscious reflection upon one's own emotional states.

References

Augustine, J. R. (1996). Circuitry and functional aspects of the insular lobe in primates including humans. *Brain Research Reviews, 22*, 229–244.

Barbas, H. & Pandya, D. N. (1989). Architecture and intrinsic connections of the prefrontal cortex in the rhesus monkey. *Journal of Comparative Neurology, 286*, 353–375.

Bard, P. & Rioch, D. M. (1937). A study of four cats deprived of neocortex and additional parts of the forebrain. *Bulletin of the Johns Hopkins Hospital, 60*, 73–147.

Barrett, L. F., Lane, R. D., Sechrest, L. & Schwartz, G. E. (in press). Sex differences in emotional awareness. *Personality and Social Psychology Bulletin.*

Bechara, A., Tranel, D., Damasio, H. & Damasio, A. R. (1997). Deciding advantageously before knowing the advantageous strategy. *Science, 275*, 1293–1295.

Blatt, S. J., Wein, S. J., Chevron, E. & Quinlan, D. M. (1979). Parental representations and depression in normal young adults. *Journal of Abnormal Psychology, 88*, 388–397.

Breslau, N., Davis, G. C., Andreski, P., Peterson, E. L. & Schultz, L. R. (1997). Sex differences in post traumatic stress disorder. *Archives of General Psychiatry, 54*, 1044–1048.

Buechel, C. & Friston, K. J. (1997). Characterising functional integration. In R. S. J. Frackowiak, K. J. Friston, C. D. Frith, R. J. Dolan & J. C. P. Mazziotta (Eds), *Human Brain Function* (pp. 127–140). San Diego, CA: Academic Press.

Cacioppo, J. T. & Berntson, G. G. (1994). Relationship between attitudes and evaluative space: a critical review, with emphasis on the separability of positive and negative substrates. *Psychological Bulletin, 115*, 401–423.

Cahill, L. & McGaugh, J. L. (1998). Mechanisms of emotional arousal and lasting declarative memory. *Trends in Neurosciences, 21*, 294–299.

Chen, Y.-C., Thaler, D., Nixon, P. D., Stern, C. E. & Passingham, R. E. (1995). The functions of the medial premotor cortex. II. The timing and selection of learned movements. *Experimental Brain Research, 102*, 461–473.

Clore, G. L. (1994). Why emotions are felt. In P. Ekman & R. J. Davidson (Eds), *The Nature of Emotion* (pp. 103–111). New York: Oxford University Press.

Corbetta, M., Miezin, F. M., Dobmeyer, S., Shulman, G. L. & Petersen, S. E. (1990). Attentional modulation of neural processing of shape, color, and velocity in humans. *Science, 248*, 1556–1559.

Crick, F. (1994). *The Astonishing Hypothesis: The Scientific Search for the Soul.* New York: Charles Scribner's Sons.

Damasio, A. R. (1994). *Descartes' Error: Emotion, Reason, and the Human Brain.* New York: G. P. Putnam's Sons.

Damasio, H., Grabowski, T., Frank, R., Galaburda, A. M. & Damasio, A. R. (1994). The return of Phineas Gage: clues about the brain from the skull of a famous patient. *Science, 264*, 1102–1105.

Darwin, C. (1872 [1965]). *The Expression of Emotions in Man and Animals*, 2nd ed. Chicago: University of Chicago Press.

Ekman, P. (1982). *Emotion in the Human Face*, 2nd ed. New York: Cambridge University Press.

Elman, J. L., Bates, E. A., Johnson, M. H., Karmiloff-Smith, A., Parisi, D. & Plunkett, K. (1996). *Rethinking Innateness: A Connectionist Perspective on Development.* Cambridge, MA: MIT Press.

Farthing, G. W. (1992). *The Psychology of Consciousness*. Englewood Cliffs, NJ: Prentice-Hall.

Fawzy, F. I., Fawzy, N. W., Hyun, C. S., Elashoff, R., Guthrie, D., Fahey, J. L. & Morton, D. L. (1993). Malignant melanoma. Effects of an early structured psychiatric intervention, coping, and affective state on recurrence and survival 6 years later. *Archives of General Psychiatry, 50*, 681–689.

Fink, G. R., Halligan, P. W., Marshall, J. C., Frith, C. D., Frackowiak, R. S. J. & Dolan, R. J. (1996a). Where in the brain does visual attention select the forest and the trees? *Nature, 382*, 626–628.

Fink, G. R., Markowitsch, H. J., Reinkemeier, M., Bruckbauer, T., Kessler, J. & Heiss, W. D. (1996b). Cerebral representation of one's own past: neural networks involved in autobiographical memory. *Journal of Neuroscience, 16*, 4275–4282.

Fodor, J. A. (1983). *The Modularity of the Brain*. Cambridge, MA: MIT Press.

Gater, R., Tansella, M., Korten, A., Tiemens, B. G., Mavreas, V. G. & Olatawura, M. O. (1998). Sex differences in the prevalence and detection of depressive and anxiety disorders in general health care settings: report from the World Health Organization Collaborative Study on Psychological Problems in General Health Care. *Archives of General Psychiatry, 55*, 405–413.

Gergely, G. & Watson, J. S. (1996). The social biofeedback theory of parental affect-mirroring: the development of emotional self-awareness and self-control in infancy. *International Journal of Psychoanalysis, 77*, 1181–1212.

Gewirtz, J. C., Falls, W. A. & Davis, M. (1997). Normal conditioned inhibition and extinction of freezing and fear-potentiated startle following electrolytic lesions of medial prefrontal cortex in rats. *Behavioral Neuroscience, 111*, 712–726.

Goldberg, G. (1987). From intent to action: evolution and function of the premotor systems of the frontal lobe. In E. Perecman (Ed), *The Frontal Lobes Revisited* (pp. 273–306). New York: IRBN Press.

Goldman-Rakic, P. S. (1987). Circuitry of the primate prefrontal cortex and regulation of behavior by representational memory. In F. Plum (Ed), *Handbook of Physiology*, Sect. 1. *The Nervous System*, vol. 5. *Higher Functions of the Brain*, part 1 (pp. 373–417). Bethesda, MD: American Physiological Society.

Gray, J. A. (1995). A model of the limbic system and basal ganglia: applications to anxiety and schizophrenia. In M. S. Gazzaniga (Ed), *The Cognitive Neurosciences* (pp. 1165–1176). Cambridge, MA: MIT Press.

Hameroff, S. R., Kaszniak, A. W. & Scott, A. C. (1996). *Toward a Science of Consciousness: The First Tucson Discussions and Debates*. Cambridge, MA: MIT Press.

Hameroff, S. R., Kaszniak, A. W. & Scott, A. C. (1998). *Toward a Science of Consciousness II: The Second Tucson Discussions and Debates*. Cambridge, MA: MIT Press.

Happé, F., Ehlers, S., Fletcher, P., Frith, U., Johansson, M., Gillberg, C., Dolan, R., Frackowiak, R. & Frith, C. (1996). 'Theory of mind' in the brain. Evidence from a PET scan study of Asperger syndrome. *NeuroReport, 8*, 197–201.

Heilman, K. M. (1997). The neurobiology of emotional experience. *Journal of Neuropsychiatry and Clinical Neurosciences, 9*, 439–448.

Hoffman, J. L. (1949). Clinical observations concerning schizophrenic patients treated by prefrontal leukotomy. *New England Journal of Medicine, 241*, 233–236.

Izard, C. E. (1972). *Patterns of Emotions*. New York: Academic Press.

Jackson, J. H. (1932). Relations of different divisions of the central nervous system to one another and to parts of the body. In J. H. Jackson (Ed), *Selected Writings of John Hughlings Jackson* (pp. 422–443). London: Hodder and Stoughton.

James, W. (1884). What is emotion? *Mind, 4*, 118–204.

Jarman, R. F., Vavrik, J. & Walton, P. D. (1995). Metacognitive and frontal lobe processes:

at the interface of cognitive psychology and neuropsychology. *Genetic, Social, and General Psychology Monographs, 121*, 153–210.

Karmiloff-Smith, A. (1992). *Beyond Modularity: A Developmental Perspective on Cognitive Science*. Cambridge, MA: MIT Press.

Koob, G. F. & Goeders, N. E. (1989). Neuroanatomical substrates of drug self-administration. In J. M. Liebman & S. J. Cooper (Eds), *Neuropharmacological Basis of Reward* (pp. 214–263). New York: Oxford University Press.

Krystal, H. (1979). Alexithymia and psychotherapy. *American Journal of Psychotherapy, 33*, 17–31.

Kunst-Wilson, M. R. & Zajonc, R. B. (1980). Affective discrimination of stimuli that cannot be recognized. *Science, 207*, 557–558.

Ladavas, E., Cimatti, D., del Pesce, M. & Tuozzi, G. (1993). Emotional evaluation with and without conscious stimulus identification: evidence from a split-brain patient. *Cognition and Emotion, 7*, 95–114.

Lane, R. D., Ahern, G. L., Schwartz, G. E. & Kaszniak, A. W. (1997a). Is alexithymia the emotional equivalent of blindsight? *Biological Psychiatry, 42*, 834–844.

Lane, R. D., Fink, G. R., Chau, P. M. L. & Dolan, R. J. (1997b). Neural activation during selective attention to subjective emotional responses. *NeuroReport, 8*, 3969–3972.

Lane, R. D., Kevley, L. S., DuBois, M. A., Shamasundara, P. & Schwartz, G. E. (1995). Levels of emotional awareness and the degree of right hemispheric dominance in the perception of facial emotion. *Neuropsychologia, 33*, 525–528.

Lane, R. D., Quinlan, D. M., Schwartz, G. E., Walker, P. A. & Zeitlin, S. B. (1990). The Levels of Emotional Awareness Scale: a cognitive-developmental measure of emotion. *Journal of Personality Assessment, 55*, 124–134.

Lane, R. D., Reiman, E. M., Axelrod, B., Yun, L.-S., Holmes, A. & Schwartz, G. E. (1998a). Neural correlates of levels of emotional awareness: evidence of an interaction between emotion and attention in the anterior cingulate cortex. *Journal of Cognitive Neuroscience, 10*, 525–535.

Lane, R. D. & Schwartz, G. E. (1987). Levels of emotional awareness: a cognitive-developmental theory and its application to psychopathology. *American Journal of Psychiatry, 144*, 133–143.

Lane, R. D., Sechrest, L., Reidel, R. G., Weldon, V., Kaszniak, A. W. & Schwartz, G. E. (1996). Impaired verbal and nonverbal emotion recognition in alexithymia. *Psychosomatic Medicine, 58*, 203–210.

Lane, R. D., Shapiro, D. E., Sechrest, L. & Riedel, R. (1998b). Pervasive emotion recognition deficit common to alexithymia and repression. *Psychosomatic Medicine, 60*, 92.

Lang, P. J. (1993a). The motivational organization of emotion: affect-reflex connections. In S. Van Goozen, M. E. Van de Poll & J. A. Sergeant (Eds), *The Emotions: Essays on Emotion Theory* (pp. 61–93). Hillsdale, NJ: Lawrence Erlbaum Associates.

Lang, P. J. (1993b). The three-system approach to emotion. In N. Birbaumer & A. Öhman (Eds), *The Structure of Emotion: Psychophysiological, Cognitive and Clinical Aspects* (pp. 18–30). Seattle, WA: Hogrefe & Huber.

Lang, P. J., Bradley, M. M. & Cuthbert, B. N. (1995). *The International Affective Picture System (IAPS): Photographic Slides*. University of Florida: The Center for Research in Psychophysiology.

Larsen, R. J. & Diener, E. (1987). Affect intensity as an individual difference characteristic: a review. *Journal of Research in Personality, 21*, 1–39.

Lazarus, R. (1984). On the primacy of cognition. *American Psychologist, 39*, 124–126.

LeDoux, J. E. (1996). *The Emotional Brain*. New York: Simon & Schuster.

Levine, D., Marziali, E. & Hood, J. (1997). Emotion processing in borderline personality disorders. *Journal of Nervous and Mental Disease, 185*, 240–246.

Levy, J., Heller, W., Banich, M. T. & Burton, L. A. (1983a). Are variations among right-handed individuals in perceptual asymmetries caused by characteristic arousal differences between hemispheres? *Journal of Experimental Psychology: Human Perception and Performance, 9*, 329–359.

Levy, J., Heller, W., Banich, M. T. & Burton, L.A. (1983b). Asymmetry of perception in free viewing of chimeric faces. *Brain and Cognition, 2*, 404–419.

Loevinger, J. & Wessler, R. (1970). *Measuring Ego Development*, vol. I. *Construction and Use of a Sentence Completion Test*. San Francisco, CA: Jossey-Bass.

Loevinger, J., Wessler, R. & Redmore, C. (1970). *Measuring Ego Development*, vol. II. *Scoring Manual for Women and Girls*. San Francisco, CA: Jossey-Bass.

MacLean, P. D. (1949). Psychosomatic disease and the "visceral brain": recent developments bearing on the Papez theory of emotion. *Psychosomatic Medicine, 11*, 338–353.

MacLean, P. D. (1990). *The Triune Brain in Evolution: Role in Paleocerebral Functions*. New York: Plenum Press.

Mega, M. S., Cummings, J. L., Salloway, S. & Malloy, P. (1997). The limbic system: an anatomic, phylogenetic, and clinical perspective. *Journal of Neuropsychiatry and Clinical Neurosciences, 9*, 315–330.

Mehler, J. & Dupoux, E. (1996). *What Infants Know: the New Cognitive Science of Early Development*. Cambridge, MA: Blackwell.

Morgan, M. A., Romanski, L. M. & LeDoux, J. E. (1993). Extinction of emotional learning: contribution of medial prefrontal cortex. *Neuroscience Letters, 163*, 109–113.

Morris, J. S., Öhman, A. & Dolan, R. J. (1998). Unconscious processing of aversively conditioned stimuli by the human amygdala. *Nature, 393*, 467–470.

Murphy, S. T. & Zajonc, R. B. (1993). Affect, cognition and awareness: affective priming with optimal and suboptimal stimulus exposures. *Journal of Personality and Social Psychology, 64*, 723–739.

Ortony, A., Clore, G. L. & Collins, A. (1988). *The Cognitive Structure of Emotions*. New York: Cambridge University Press.

Papez, J. W. (1937). A proposed mechanism of emotion. *Archives of Neurology and Psychiatry, 38*, 725–734.

Paulhus, D. L. (1985). Self deception and impression management in test responses. In A. Angleitner & J. S. Wiggins (Eds), *Personality Assessment via Questionnaire* (pp. 143–165). New York: Springer-Verlag.

Price, J. L., Carmichael, S. T. & Drevets, W. C. (1996). Networks related to the orbital and medial prefrontal cortex; a substrate for emotional behavior? *Progress in Brain Research, 107*, 523–536.

Rainville, P., Duncan, G. H., Price, D. D., Carrier, B. & Bushnell, M. C. (1997). Pain affect encoded in human anterior cingulate but not somatosensory cortex. *Science, 277*, 968–971.

Rau, J. C. (1993). Perception of verbal and nonverbal affective stimuli in complex partial seizure disorder. *Dissertation Abstracts International B*, (Ph.D. diss., University of Arizona), *54*, 506-B.

Rolls, E. T. (1990). A theory of emotion, and its application to understanding the neural basis of emotion. *Cognition and Emotion, 4*, 161–190.

Ross, E. D. (1993). Acute agitation and other behaviors associated with Wernicke aphasia and their possible neurological bases. *Neuropsychiatry, Neuropsychology, and Behavioral Neurology, 6*, 9–18.

Sahraie, A., Weiskrantz, L., Barbur, J. L., Simmons, A., Williams, S. C. R. & Brammer, M. J. (1997). Pattern of neuronal activity associated with conscious and unconscious processing of visual signals. *Proceedings of the National Academy of Sciences USA, 94*, 9406–9411.

Sanides, F. (1970). Functional architecture of motor and sensory cortices in primates in the light of a new concept of neocortex evolution. In C. R. Noback & W. Montagna (Eds), *The Primate Brain: Advances in Primatology* (pp. 137–201). New York: Appleton-Century-Crofts.

Schaller, S. (1992). *A Man Without Words*. New York: Summit Books.

Searle, J. R. (1998). How to study consciousness scientifically. *Brain Research Reviews, 26,* 379–387.

Shin, L. M., Kosslyn, S. M., McNally, R. J., Alpert, N. M., Thompson, W. L., Rauch, S. L., Macklin, M. L. & Pitman, R. K. (1997). Visual imagery and perception in post-traumatic stress disorder: a positron emission tomographic investigation. *Archives of General Psychiatry, 54,* 233–241.

Shipley, W. (1940). A self-administering scale for measuring intellectual impairment and deterioration. *Journal of Psychology, 9,* 371–377.

Solomon, G. E. A. (1990). Psychology of novice and expert wine talk. *American Journal of Psychology, 103,* 495–517.

Sommers, S. (1981). Emotionality reconsidered: the role of cognition in emotional responsiveness. *Journal of Personality and Social Psychology, 41,* 553–561.

Spiegel, D., Bloom, J. R., Kraemer, H. C. & Gottheil, E. (1989). Effect of psychosocial treatment on survival of patients with metastatic breast cancer. *Lancet, 2,* 888–891.

Stuss, D.T. (1991a). Disturbance of self-awareness after frontal system damage. In G. P. Prigatano & D. L. Schacter (Eds), *Awareness of Deficit after Brain Injury: Clinical and Theoretical Issues* (pp. 63–83). New York: Oxford University Press.

Stuss, D. T. (1991b). Self, awareness, and the frontal lobes: a neuropsychological perspective. In J. Strauss & G. R. Goethals (Eds), *The Self: Interdisciplinary Approaches* (pp. 255–278). New York: Springer-Verlag.

Taylor, G. J., Bagby, R. M. & Parker, J. D. A. (1991). The alexithymia construct: a potential paradigm for psychosomatic medicine. *Psychosomatics, 32,* 153–164.

Thayer, J. F. & Lane, R. D. (in press). A model of neurovisceral integration in emotion regulation and dysregulation. *Journal of Affective Disorders.*

Tomkins, S. S. (1962). *Affect, Imagery, Consciousness*, vol. 1. *The Positive Affects.* New York: Springer.

Tranel, D. (1997). Emotional processing and the human amygdala. *Trends in Cognitive Sciences, 1,* 46–47.

Tucker, D. M., Luu, P. & Pribram, K. H. (1995). Social and emotional self-regulation. *Annals New York Academy of Sciences, 769,* 213–239.

van der Kolk, B. A., Burbridge, J. A. & Suzuki, J. (1997). The psychobiology of traumatic memory—Clinical implications of neuroimaging studies. *Annals New York Academy of Sciences, 821,* 99–113.

Vogt, B. A. & Gabriel, M. (1993). *Neurobiology of Cingulate Cortex and Limbic Thalamus.* Boston: Birkhauser.

Vogt, B. A., Finch, D. M. & Olson, C. R. (1992). Functional heterogeneity in cingulate cortex: the anterior executive and posterior evaluative regions. *Cerebral Cortex, 2,* 435–443.

Watson, D., Clark, L. A. & Tellegen, A. (1988). Development and validation of brief measures of positive and negative affect: the PANAS scales. *Journal of Personality and Social Psychology, 54,* 1063–1070.

Weiskrantz, L. (1986). *Blindsight.* Oxford: Oxford University Press.

Werner, H. & Kaplan, B. (1963). *Symbol Formation: An Organismic-Developmental Approach to Language and the Expression of Thought.* New York: John Wiley & Sons.

Whalen, P. J., Rauch, S. L., Etcoff, N. L., McInerney, S. C., Lee, M. B. & Jenike, M. A.

(1998). Masked presentations of emotional facial expressions modulate amygdala activity without explicit knowledge. *Journal of Neuroscience, 18*, 411–418.

Wrana, C., Thomas, W., Heindichs, G., Huber, M., Obliers, R., Koerfer, A. & Köhle, K. (1998). Levels of Emotional Awareness Scale (LEAS): ein beitrag zur empirischen überprüfung von validität und reliabilität einer deutschen fassung. Postervortrag bei der 47 Arbeitstagung des Deutschen Kollegiums für Psychosomatische Medizin, Leipzig, March 1998.

Yakovlev, P. I. (1948). Motility, behavior, and the brain. *Journal of Nervous and Mental Disease, 107*, 313–335.

Zajonc, R. B. (1984). On the primacy of affect. *American Psychologist, 39*, 117–123.

16

The Functional Neuroanatomy of Affective Style

RICHARD J. DAVIDSON

This chapter focuses on two ubiquitous features of emotion. First is the fact that emotion is valenced, with positive and negative representing a fundamental dimension along which emotion is organized. This dimension is present in virtually all systems that have been developed to classify emotion and motivation, ranging from comparative accounts that address phylogenetic origins (Shnierla, 1959) to studies of semantic structure (Osgood, 1957). The second feature of emotion that forms the core of this chapter is the striking nature of the variability among individuals in the valence and intensity of their emotional reactions to a challenging event. I have used the phrase "affective style" to refer to the broad rubric of characteristics along which individuals might differ in their reactivity to emotionally provocative events (Davidson, 1992). Differences among people in affective style appear to be associated with temperament (Kagan et al., 1988), personality (Gross et al., 1998), and vulnerability to psychopathology (Meehl, 1975). Moreover, such differences are not a unique human attribute, but appear to be present in a number of different species including rodents and nonhuman primates (e.g., Davidson et al., 1993; Kalin, 1993).

In the proceeding section of this chapter, conceptual distinctions among the various components of affective style are introduced, and methodological challenges to their study are highlighted. The third section presents a brief overview of the anatomy of two basic motivational/emotional systems: the approach and withdrawal systems. The final section considers individual differences in these basic systems and indicates how such differences might be studied. I conclude with a consideration of some of the implications of this work for the study and treatment of psychopathology.

The Subcomponents of Affective Style

Many phenomena are subsumed under the rubric of affective style. A concept featured in many discussions of affective development, affective disorders, and personality is "emotion regulation" (Thompson, 1994). Emotion regulation refers to a broad constellation of processes that serve to either amplify, attenuate, or maintain the strength of emotional reactions. Included among these processes are components of attention that regulate the extent to which an organism can be distracted from a potentially aversive stimulus (Derryberry & Reed, 1996) and the capacity for self-generated imagery to replace emotions that are unwanted with more desirable imagery scripts. Emotion regulation can be both automatic and controlled (see Wegner, 1998). Automatic emotion regulation may result from the progressive automatization of processes that initially were voluntary and controlled and have evolved to become more automatic with practice. I hold the view that regulatory processes are an intrinsic part of the landscape of emotion, and rarely does an emotion get generated in the absence of associated regulatory processes. For this reason, it is often conceptually difficult to sharply distinguish between where an emotion ends and regulation begins. Even more problematic is the methodological challenge of developing operational measures of these different components in the stream of affective behavior.

When considering the question of individual differences in affective behavior, one must specify the particular response systems in which the individual differences are being explored. It is not necessarily the case that the same pattern of individual differences will be found across response systems. Thus, for example, an individual may have a low threshold for the elicitation of the subjective experience (as reflected in self-reports) of a particular emotion but a relatively high threshold for the elicitation of a particular physiological change. It is important not to assume that individual differences in any parameter of affective responding will necessarily generalize across response systems within the same emotion. Equally important is the question of whether individual differences associated with the generation of a particular emotion will necessarily generalize to other emotions. For example, are those individuals who are behaviorally expressive in response to a fear challenge also likely to show comparably high levels of expressivity in response to positive incentives? Although systematic research on this question is still required, initial evidence suggests that at least certain aspects of affective style may be emotion specific, or at least valence specific (e.g., Wheeler et al., 1993).

In addition to emotion regulation, there are also likely intrinsic differences in certain components of emotional responding. There are likely individual differences in the threshold for eliciting components of a particular emotion, given a stimulus of a certain intensity. For example, some individuals are likely to produce facial signs of disgust upon presentation of a particular intensity of noxious stimulus, whereas other individuals may require a more intense stimulus for the elicitation of the same response at a comparable intensity. This suggestion implies that dose–response functions may reliably differ across individuals. Unfortunately, systematic studies of this kind have not been performed, in part because of the difficulty of creating stimuli that are graded in intensity and designed to elicit the same emotion. In the olfactory and gustatory modalities, there are possibilities of creating stimuli that differ systematically in the concentration of a disgust-producing component and then obtaining psychophysical threshold functions that would reveal such individual differences. However, the production of such intensity-graded stimuli in other modalities will likely be more complicated, though with the development of large, normatively rated complex stimulus sets, this may be possible. An example is the International Affective Picture System (Lang et al., 1995). This set includes a large number of visual stimuli that have been rated on valence and arousal dimensions and that comprise locations throughout this two-dimensional space. The density of stimulus exemplars at all levels within this space allow for the possibility of selecting stimuli that are graded in intensity for the sort of dose–response studies described above.

There are also likely to be individual differences in the peak or amplitude of the response. Upon presentation of a series of graded stimuli that differ in intensity, the maximum amplitude in a certain system (e.g., intensity of a facial contraction; change in heart rate) is likely to differ systematically across subjects. Some individuals will respond with a larger amplitude peak compared with others. Again, such individual differences may be quite specific to particular systems and will not necessarily generalize across systems, even within the same emotion. Thus, the individual who is in the tail of the distribution in heart rate response to a fearful stimulus will not necessarily be in the tail of the distribution in facial response.

Another parameter likely to differ systematically across individuals is the rise time to peak. Some individuals will rise quickly in a certain response system, whereas others will rise more slowly. There may be an association between the peak of the response and the rise time to the peak within certain systems for particular emotions. Thus, it may be the case that for anger-related emotion, those individuals with higher peak vocal responses also show a faster rise time, but to the best of my knowledge, there are no systematic data related to such differences.

Finally, another component of intrinsic differences across individuals is the recovery time. Following perturbation in a particular system, some individuals recover quickly and others recover slowly. For example, after a fear-provoking encounter, some individuals show a persisting heart rate elevation that might last for minutes, whereas other individuals show a comparable peak and rise time but recover much more quickly. Of course, as with other parameters, there are likely to be differences in recovery time across different response systems. Some individuals may recover rapidly in their expressive behavior, while recovering slowly in certain autonomic channels. The potential significance of such dissociations has not been systematically examined.

The specific parameters of individual differences that are delineated above describe "affective chronometry," the temporal dynamics of affective responding (see Davidson, 1998). Little is known about the factors that govern these individual differences and the extent to which such differences are specific to particular emotion response systems or the extent to which they generalize across emotions (e.g., is the heart rate recovery following fear similar to that following disgust?). Moreover, the general issue of the extent to which these different parameters that have been identified are orthogonal or correlated features of emotional responding is an empirical question that has yet to be answered. For reasons that I hope to make clear below, affective chronometry is a particularly important feature of affective style and is likely to play a key role in determining vulnerability to psychopathology. It is also a feature of affective style that is methodologically tractable and can yield to experimental study of its neural substrates.

Affective style is critical in understanding the continuity between normal and abnormal functioning and in the prediction of psychopathology and the delineation of vulnerability. On the opposite side of the spectrum, such individual differences in affective style will also feature centrally in any comprehensive theory of resilience. The fact that some individuals reside "off the diagonal" and appear to maintain high levels of psychological well-being despite their exposure to objective life adversity is likely related to their affective style (Ryff & Singer, 1998). Some of these implications will be discussed at the end of this chapter. I first consider some of the neural substrates of two fundamental emotion systems. This provides the foundation for a consideration of individual differences in these systems and the neural circuitry responsible for such differences.

The Anatomy of Approach and Withdrawal

Although the focus of my empirical research has been on measures of prefrontal brain activity, it must be emphasized at the outset that the circuit instantiating emotion in the human brain is complex and involves many interrelated structures. Few empirical studies using modern neuroimaging procedures that afford a high degree of spatial resolution have yet been performed (see George et al., 1995; Paradiso et al., 1997, for examples; see Davidson & Irwin, 1999b, for review). Therefore, hypotheses about the set of structures that participate in the production of emotion must necessarily be speculative and based to a large extent on the information available from the animal literature (e.g., LeDoux, 1987, 1996) and from theoretical accounts of the processes involved in human emotion.

Based on the available strands of theory and evidence, numerous scientists have proposed two basic circuits, each mediating different forms of motivation and emotion (see, e.g., Davidson, 1995; Gray, 1994; Lang et al., 1990). The approach system facilitates appetitive behavior and generates certain types of positive affect that are approach related (e.g., enthusiasm, pride; see Depue & Collins, in press, for review). This form of positive affect is usually generated in the context of moving toward a desired goal (see Lazarus, 1991; Stein & Trabasso, 1992, for theoretical accounts of emotion that place a premium on goal states). The representation of a goal state in working memory is hypothesized to be implemented in dorsolateral prefrontal cortex. The medial and orbital prefrontal cortices seem to play important roles in maintaining representations of behavioral-reinforcement contingencies in working memory (Thorpe et al., 1983). In addition, output from the medial prefrontal cortex to nucleus accumbens (NA) neurons modulates the transfer of motivationally relevant information through the NA (Kalivas et al., 1993). The basal ganglia are hypothesized to be involved in the expression of the abstract goal in action plans and in the anticipation of reward (Schultz et al., 1995a,b). The NA, particularly the caudomedial shell region of the NA, is a major convergence zone for motivationally relevant information from a myriad of limbic structures. Cells in this region of the NA increase their firing rate during reward expectation (see Schultz et al., 1995a). There are probably other structures involved in this circuit which depend on a number of factors including the nature of the stimuli signaling appetitive information, the extent to which the behavioral-reinforcement contingency is novel or overlearned, and the nature of the anticipated behavioral response.

It should be noted that the activation of this approach system is hypothesized to be associated with one particular form of positive affect and not all forms of such emotion. It is specifically predicted to be associated with pregoal attainment positive affect, that form of positive affect elicited as an organism moves closer toward an appetitive goal. Postgoal attainment positive affect represents another form of positive emotion that is not expected to be associated with activation of this circuit (see Davidson, 1994, for a more extended discussion of this distinction). This latter type of positive affect may be phenomenologically experienced as contentment and is expected to occur when the prefrontal cortex goes off-line after a desired goal has been achieved. Cells in the NA have also been shown to decrease their firing rate during postgoal consummatory behavior (e.g., Henriksen & Giacchino, 1993).

Lawful individual differences can enter into many different stages of the approach system. Such individual differences will be considered in detail below. For the moment, it is important to underscore two issues. One is that there are individual differences in the tonic level of activation of the approach system, which alters an individual's propensity to experience approach-related positive affect. Second, there are likely to be individual differences in the capacity to shift between pre- and postgoal attainment positive affect and in the ratio between these two forms of positive affect. Upon reaching a desired goal, some individuals will immediately replace the just-achieved goal with a new desired goal, and so will have little opportunity to experience postgoal attainment positive affect or contentment. There may be an optimal balance between these two forms of positive affect, though this issue has never been studied.

There appears to be a second system concerned with the neural implementation of withdrawal. This system facilitates the withdrawal of an individual from sources of aversive stimulation and generates certain forms of negative affect that are withdrawal related. Both fear and disgust are associated with increasing the distance between the organism and a source of aversive stimulation. From invasive animal studies and human neuroimaging studies, it appears that the amygdala is critically involved in this system (e.g., LeDoux, 1987, 1996). Using functional magnetic resonance imaging (fMRI), we have recently demonstrated for the first time activation in the human amygdala in response to aversive pictures compared with neutral control pictures (Irwin et al., 1996). In addition, the temporal polar region also appears to be activated during withdrawal-related emotion (e.g., Reiman et al., 1989). These effects, at least in humans, appear to be more pronounced on the right side of the brain (see Davidson, 1992, 1993, for reviews). In the human electrophysiological studies, the right frontal region is also activated during withdrawal-related negative affective states (e.g., Davidson et al., 1990b). At present it is not entirely clear whether this EEG change reflects activation at a frontal site or whether the activity recorded from the frontal scalp region is volume conducted from other cortical loci. The resolution of this uncertainty must await additional studies using positron emission tomography (PET) or fMRI, which have sufficient spatial resolution to differentiate among different anterior cortical regions.

In addition to the temporal polar region, the amygdala, and possibly the prefrontal cortex, it is also likely that the basal ganglia and hypothalamus are involved in the motor and autonomic components, respectively, of withdrawal-related negative affect (see Smith et al., 1990). As with the approach system, there are lawful individual differences that may arise at many stages of processing in the withdrawal system. Activation differences in particular parts of the circuit will alter specific components of the withdrawal system that then may feedback and accentuate activation in other regions of the circuit. Evidence in support of individual differences at both cortical and subcortical levels in this circuit are described in the next section.

The nature of the relation between these two hypothesized affect systems also remains to be delineated. The emotion literature is replete with different proposals regarding the interrelations among different forms of positive and negative affect. Some theorists have proposed a single bivalent dimension that ranges from unpleasant to pleasant affect, with a second dimension that reflects arousal (e.g., Russell, 1980). Other theorists have suggested that affect space is best described by two orthogonal positive and negative dimensions (e.g., Watson & Tellegen, 1985). Still other workers have suggested that the degree of orthogonality between positive and negative affect depends on the temporal frame of analysis (Diener & Emmons, 1984). This formulation holds that when assessed in the moment, positive and negative affect are reciprocally related, but when examined over a longer time frame (e.g., dispositional affect), they are orthogonal. It must be emphasized that these analyses of the relation between positive and negative affect are all based exclusively on measures of self-report, and therefore their generalizability to other measures of affect are uncertain. However, based on new data described below, a growing corpus of data does indeed indicate that one function of positive affect is to inhibit concurrent negative affect.

Affective Style: Individual Differences in Activation of Approach and Withdrawal Circuitry

This section presents a brief overview of recent work from my laboratory designed to examine individual differences in measures of prefrontal activation and their relation to different aspects of emotion, affective style, and related biological constructs. These findings will be used to address the question of what underlying constituents of affective style such individual differences in prefrontal activation actually reflect.

In both infants (Davidson & Fox, 1989) and adults (Davidson & Tomarken, 1989), we noticed that there were large individual differences in baseline electrophysiological measures of prefrontal activation and that such individual variation was associated with differences in aspects of affective reactivity. In infants, Davidson and Fox (1989) reported that 10-month-old babies who cried in response to maternal separation were more likely to have less left-side and greater right-side prefrontal activation during a preceding resting baseline compared with those infants who did not cry in response to this challenge. In adults, we first noted that the phasic influence of positive and negative emotion elicitors (e.g., film clips) on measures of prefrontal activation asymmetry appeared to be superimposed upon more tonic individual differences in the direction and absolute magnitude of asymmetry (Davidson & Tomarken, 1989).

During our initial explorations of this phenomenon, we needed to determine if baseline electrophysiological measures of prefrontal asymmetry were reliable and stable over time and thus could be used as a traitlike measure. Tomarken et al. (1992) recorded baseline brain electrical activity from 90 normal subjects on 2 occasions separately by approximately 3 weeks. At each testing session, brain activity was recorded during eight 1-min trials, four with eyes open and four with eyes closed, presented in counterbalanced order. The data were visually scored to remove artifact and then Fourier transformed. Our focus was on power in the alpha band (8–13 Hz), though we extracted power in all frequency bands (see Davidson et al., 1990a, for a discussion of power in different frequency bands and their relation to activation). We computed coefficient alpha as a measure of internal consistency reliability from the data for each session. The coefficient alphas were quite high, with all values exceeding .85, indicating that the electrophysiological measures of asymmetric activation indeed showed excellent internal consistency reliability. The test–retest reliability was adequate, with intraclass correlations ranging from .65 to .75 depending on the specific sites and methods of analysis. The major finding from this study was the demonstration that measures of activation asymmetry based on power in the alpha band from prefrontal scalp electrodes showed both high internal consistency reliability and acceptable test–retest reliability to be considered a traitlike index.

The large sample size in the reliability study discussed above enabled us to select a small group of extreme left and extreme right-frontally activated subjects for MR scans to determine if there were any gross morphometric differences in anatomical structure between these subgroups. None of our measures of regional volumetric asymmetry revealed any difference between the groups (Davidson et al., unpublished observations). These findings suggest that whatever differences exist between subjects with extreme left versus right prefrontal activation, they are likely functional and not structural.

On the basis of our prior data and theory, we reasoned that extreme left and extreme right frontally activated subjects would show systematic differences in dispositional positive and negative affect. We administered the trait version of the Positive and Negative Affect Scales (PANAS; Watson et al., 1988) to examine this question and found that the left-frontally activated subjects reported more positive and less negative affect than their right-frontally activated counterparts (Tomarken et al., 1992; see figure 16.1). More recently (Sutton & Davidson, 1997), we showed that scores on a self-report measure designed to operationalize Gray's concepts of behavioral inhibition and behavioral activation (the BIS/BAS scales; Carver & White, 1994) were even more strongly predicted by electrophysiological measures of prefrontal asymmetry than were scores on the PANAS scales (see Plate 3). Subjects with greater left-sided prefrontal activation reported more relative BAS to BIS activity compared with subjects exhibiting more right-sided prefrontal activation.

We also hypothesized that our measures of prefrontal asymmetry would predict reactivity to experimental elicitors of emotion. The model we have developed

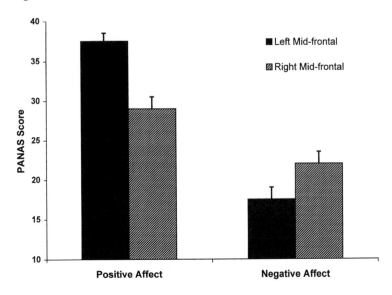

Figure 16.1. Dispositional positive and negative affect (from scores on the Positive and Negative Affect Scales [PANAS]-General Affect Scales) in subjects who were classified as extreme and stable left-frontally active ($n = 14$) and extreme and stable right-frontally active ($n = 13$) on the basis of electrophysiological measures of baseline activation asymmetries on two occasions separated by 3 weeks. (From Tomarken et al., 1992.)

over the past several years (see Davidson, 1992, 1994, 1995, for background) features individual differences in prefrontal activation asymmetry as a reflection of a diathesis which modulates reactivity to emotionally significant events. According to this model, individuals who differ in prefrontal asymmetry should respond differently to an elicitor of positive or negative emotion, even when baseline mood is partialed out. We performed an experiment to examine this question (Wheeler et al., 1993). We presented short film clips designed to elicit positive or negative emotion. Brain electrical activity was recorded before the presentation of the film clips. Just after the clips were presented, subjects were asked to rate their emotional experience during the preceding film clip. In addition, subjects completed scales that were designed to reflect their mood at baseline. We found that individual differences in prefrontal asymmetry predicted the emotional response to the films even after measures of baseline mood were statistically removed. Those individuals with more left-sided prefrontal activation at baseline reported more positive affect to the positive film clips, and those with more right-sided prefrontal activation reported more negative affect to the negative film clips. These findings support the idea that individual differences in electrophysiological measures of prefrontal activation asymmetry mark some aspect of vulnerability to positive and negative emotion elicitors. The fact that such relations were obtained after the statistical removal of baseline mood indicates that any difference between left and right frontally activated subjects in baseline mood cannot account for the prediction of film-elicited emotion effects that were observed.

In another study (Davidson et al., in preparation), we examined relations between individual differences in prefrontal activation asymmetry and the emotion-modulated startle. In this study, we presented pictures from the International Affective Picture System (Lang et al., 1995) while acoustic startle probes were presented and the EMG-measured blink response from the orbicularis oculi muscle region was recorded (see Sutton et al., 1997, for basic methods). Startle probes were presented both during the 6-sec slide exposure as well as 500-msec after the offset of the pictures, on separate trials.[1] We interpreted startle magnitude during picture exposure as providing an index related to the peak of emotional response, while startle magnitude after the offset of the pictures was taken to reflect the recovery from emotional challenge. Used in this way, startle probe methods can potentially provide new information on the time course of emotional responding. We expected that individual differences during actual picture presentation would be less pronounced than individual differences after picture presentation because an acute emotional stimulus is likely to pull for a normative response across subjects, yet individuals are likely to differ dramatically in the time to recover. Similarly, we predicted that individual differences in prefrontal asymmetry would account for more variance in predicting magnitude of recovery (i.e., startle magnitude poststimulus) than in predicting startle magnitude during the stimulus based on the hypothesized role of the prefrontal cortex in affective working memory (see Davidson & Irwin, 1999b for discussion). Our findings were consistent with our predictions and indicated that subjects with greater right-side prefrontal activation show a larger blink magnitude after the offset of the negative stimuli when the variance in blink magnitude during the negative stimulus was partialed out. Measures of prefrontal asymmetry did not reliably predict startle magnitude during picture presentation. The findings from this study are consistent with our hypothesis and indicate that individual differences in prefrontal asymmetry are associated with the time course of affective responding, particularly the recovery following emotional challenge.

In addition to the studies described above using self-report and psychophysiological measures of emotion, we have also examined relations between individual differences in electrophysiological measures of prefrontal asymmetry and other biological indices, which in turn have been related to differential reactivity to stressful events. Two recent examples from our laboratory include measures of immune function and cortisol. In the case of the former, we examined differences between left and right prefrontally activated subjects in natural killer cell (NK) activity because declines in NK activity have been reported in response to stressful, negative events (Kiecolt-Glaser & Glaser, 1991). We predicted that subjects with right prefrontal activation would exhibit lower NK activity compared with their left-activated counterparts because the former type of subject has been found to report more dispositional negative affect, to show higher relative BIS activity, and to respond more intensely to negative emotional stimuli. We found that right-frontally activated subjects indeed had lower levels of NK activity compared to their left-frontally activated counterparts (Kang et al., 1991; see Davidson, Coe, Dolski & Donzella, 1999 for replication and extension).

In collaboration with Kalin, our laboratory has been studying similar individual differences in scalp-recorded measures of prefrontal activation asymmetry in rhesus monkeys (Davidson et al., 1992, 1993). Recently, we obtained measures of brain electrical activity from a large sample of rhesus monkeys ($n = 50$) (Kalin et al., 1998). EEG measures were recorded during periods of manual restraint. A subsample of 15 of these monkeys were tested on 2 occasions 4 months apart. We found that the test–retest correlation for measures of prefrontal asymmetry was .62, suggesting similar stability of this metric in monkeys and humans. In the group of 50 animals, we also obtained measures of plasma cortisol during the early morning. We hypothesized that if individual differences in prefrontal asymmetry were associated with dispositional affective style, such differences should be correlated with cortisol because individual differences in baseline cortisol have been related to various aspects of trait-related stressful behavior and psychopathology (see, e.g., Gold et al., 1988). We found that animals with right-side prefrontal activation had higher levels of baseline cortisol than their left-frontally activated counterparts (see figure 16.2). Moreover, when blood samples were collected 2 years after our initial testing, animals classified as showing extreme right-sided prefrontal activation at age one year had significantly higher baseline cortisol levels when they were three years of age compared with animals who were classified at age one year as displaying extreme left-side prefrontal activation. These findings indicate that individual differences in prefrontal asymmetry are present in nonhuman primates and that such differences predict biological measures that are related to affective style.

In addition to individual differences in prefrontal activation asymmetry, we have also been examining individual differences in several aspects of amygdala

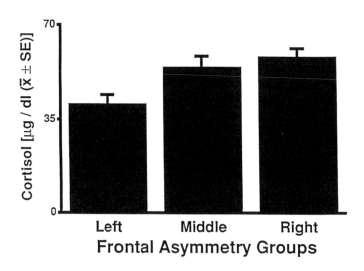

Figure 16.2. Basal morning plasma cortisol from 1-year-old rhesus monkeys classified as left ($n = 12$), middle ($n = 16$), or right ($n = 11$) frontally activated based on electrophysiological measurements. (From Kalin et al., 1998.)

function and their relation to affective style. While there is now a burgeoning literature on the anatomy and function of the amygdala (see Aggleton, 1993, for review), relatively little research has been conducted in intact humans, owing in large measure to the difficulty in imaging function in a structure that is relatively small (the adult human amygdala is approximately 1 cm in volume). However, from what is known from both the animal and human studies, it appears that the amygdala plays an important role in assigning affective significance, particularly of negative valence, to both sensory and cognitive input (see LeDoux, 1992, for review). Using PET to measure regional blood flow, several groups have reported increased blood flow in the amygdala in response to both behavioral (e.g., Schneider et al., 1995) and pharmacological (e.g., Ketterer et al., 1996) elicitors of negative affect. We have recently reported activation in the human amygdala using fMRI in response to aversive pictures (Irwin et al., 1996). Several other groups have also detected activation of the human amygdala with fMRI in response to aversive conditioning, fearful facial expressions, and other negative stimuli (see review by Davidson & Irwin, 1999a). These studies suggest that activation in the human amygdala occurs in response to a broad range of elicitors of negative affect.

To assess tonic individual differences in amygdala activation, we used PET with flourodeoxyglucose (FDG) as a tracer. For this particular study, we chose to use FDG-PET because it reflects activity integrated over approximately 30 min and is thus well-suited to examine traitlike differences in brain function. We examined individual differences in glucose metabolic rate in the amygdala and its relation to dispositional negative affect in depressed subjects (Abercrombie et al., 1998). We acquired a resting FDG-PET scan as well as a structural MR scan for each subject. The structural MR scans are used for anatomical localization by coregistering the two image sets. Thus, for each subject, we used an automated algorithm to fit the MR scan to the PET image.

Regions of interest (ROIs) were then drawn on each subject's MR scan to outline the amygdala in each hemisphere. These ROIs were drawn on coronal sections of subjects' MR images, and the ROIs were then automatically transferred to the co-registered PET images. Glucose metabolism in the left and right amygdala ROIs were then extracted. The interrater reliability for the extracted glucose metabolic rate is highly significant, with intraclass correlations between two independent raters $\geq.97$. Plate 4 illustrates ROIs drawn around the amygdala on MR scans of three subjects and the associated coregistered PET images from the same subjects. We found that subjects with greater glucose metabolism in both the right and left amygdala report greater dispositional negative affect on the PANAS scale (see figure 16.3). These findings indicate that individual differences in resting glucose metabolism in the amygdala are present and that they predict dispositional negative affect among depressed subjects.

Recently, in normal subjects, we examined the relation between the MR signal change in the amygdala in response to negative versus neutral pictures detected with fMRI and scores on the PANAS general negative affect scale. We found that subjects with greater MR signal change in the right amygdala in response to negative versus neutral pictures also reported more dispositional negative affect ($r = .75$; Irwin et al., 1997).

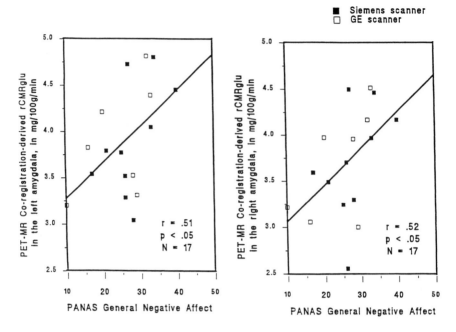

Figure 16.3. Scatter plot of correlations between dispositional negative affect assessed with the Positive and Negative Affect Scales (PANAS)-General Negative Affect Scale and PET MRI-coregistration-derived regional glucose metabolism in the left and right amygdalas for all subjects ($n = 17$). Subjects were tested on two different PET cameras. Those tested in a Siemens CTI 933/04 PET camera are represented by closed squares and those tested in the GE Advance are represented by open squares.

Implications and Conclusions

Earlier in this chapter, the constituents of affective style were described. I considered individual differences in threshold, peak amplitude, rise time to peak, and recovery time. Together these constitute parameters of affective chronometry and dictate important features of the time course of affective responding. After describing the functional neuroanatomy of the approach and withdrawal systems, I discussed individual differences in prefrontal activation asymmetry and activation in the amygdala and their relation to affective style described. In light of this information, I now turn to an important question that lies at the heart of much of this research: what do individual differences in prefrontal asymmetry reflect?

On the basis of findings from several new studies in my laboratory, I suggest that at least one important component of what prefrontal cortex "does" in affective responding is modulate the time course of emotional responding, particularly recovery time. There are several facts critical to making this claim. First, there are extensive reciprocal connections between amygdala and prefrontal cortex, particularly the medial and orbital zones of prefrontal cortex (Amaral et al., 1992). The glutamatergic efferents from prefrontal cortex likely synapse on γ-aminobutyric acid neurons (Amaral et al., 1992) and thus provide an important inhibitory input to the amygdala.

Second, LeDoux and his colleagues (Morgan et al., 1993; but see Gewirtz et al., 1997) demonstrated in rats that lesions of medial prefrontal cortex dramatically prolong the maintenance of a conditioned aversive response. In other words, animals with medial prefrontal lesions retain aversive associations for a much longer duration of time than normal animals. These findings imply that the medial prefrontal cortex normally inhibits the amygdala as an active component of extinction. In the absence of this normal inhibition, the amygdala remains unchecked and continues to maintain the learned aversive response.

Third, data from my laboratory cited above indicate that individual differences in prefrontal activation asymmetry significantly predict the magnitude of the post-stimulus startle after removal of the variance attributable to startle magnitude during the presentation of the emotional picture. In particular, left prefrontal activation appears to facilitate two processes simultaneously. First, orbitofrontal prefrontal cortex maintains representations of behavioral-reinforcement contingencies in working memory (Thorpe et al., 1983). Second, medial prefrontal cortex inhibits the amygdala. In this way, the time course of negative affect may be shortened, while the time course of positive affect may be accentuated.

And finally, new findings using PET indicate that in normal subjects, glucose metabolism in left medial and lateral prefrontal cortex is strongly reciprocally associated with glucose metabolic rate in the amygdala (Abercrombie et al., 1996). Thus, subjects with greater left-side prefrontal metabolism have lower metabolic activity in their amygdala. These findings are consistent with the lesion study of LeDoux (Morgan et al., 1993) and colleagues and imply that prefrontal cortex plays an important role in modulating activity in the amygdala. At the same time, left prefrontal cortex is also likely to play a role in the maintenance of reinforcement-related behavioral approach. Perhaps the damping of negative affect and shortening of its time course facilitates the maintenance of approach-related positive affect.

The questions featured in this chapter are more tractable now than ever before. With the advent of echoplanar methods for rapid fMRI, sufficient data can be collected within individuals to examine functional connections among regions hypothesized to constitute important elements of the approach and withdrawal circuits discussed above. Individual differences in different aspects of these systems can then be studied with greater precision. The fMRI methods also lend themselves to address questions related to affective chronometry. In particular, we can calculate the decay of MR signal intensity after the offset of an aversive stimulus to provide an index of the rapidity of recovery from activation in select brain regions. Positron emission tomography methods using new radio-ligands that permit quantification of receptor density for specific neurotransmitters in different brain regions are yielding new insights directly relevant to questions about affective style (see, e.g., Farde et al., 1997). Traitlike differences in affective style are likely reflected in relatively stable differences in characteristics of the underlying neurochemical systems. Using PET to examine such individual differences promises to provide important links between neurochemical and neuroanatomical approaches to understanding the biological bases of affective style.

Affective neuroscience seeks to understand the underlying proximal neural substrates of elementary constituents of emotional processing. In this chapter, I have provided a model of the functional neuroanatomy of approach and withdrawal motivational/emotional systems and illustrated the many varieties of individual differences that might occur in these systems. Research on prefrontal asymmetries associated with affective style was used to illustrate the potential promise of some initial approaches to the study of these questions. Modern neuroimaging methods used in conjunction with theoretically sophisticated models of emotion offer great promise in advancing our understanding of the basic mechanisms giving rise to affective style and affective psychopathology.

Note

1. In this initial study on the recovery function assessed with startle probe measures, we had only a single poststimulus probe at 500 msec after the offset of the picture. Readers may be surprised that the interval between the offset of the picture and the presentation of the probe was so short. However, it should be noted that these emotional pictures are not particularly intense and so the lingering effects of emotion after the presentation of such pictures is likely not to last very long in most individuals. Future studies will probe further out after the offset of the picture. Because at most only a single probe can be presented for each picture so that habituation effects are minimized, each new probe position requires a substantial increase in the overall number of pictures presented. There is a finite limit to the number of pictures contained in the International Affective Picture System. Even more important, we have found that it is critical to keep the picture viewing period to well under 1 hr to minimize fatigue and boredom.

Acknowledgments

Portions of this chapter appeared in Davidson (1998). The research reported in this chapter was supported in part by NIMH grants MH43454, MH40747, Research Scientist Award K05-MH00875, and P50-MH52354 to the Wisconsin Center for Affective Science (R. J. Davidson, director), by a NARSAD Established Investigator Award, and by a grant from the John D. and Catherine T. MacArthur Foundation. I thank the many individuals in my laboratories who have contributed to this research over the years, including Andy Tomarken, Steve Sutton, Wil Irwin, Heather Abercrombie, Jeff Henriques, Chris Larson, Stacey Schaefer, Terry Ward, Darren Dottl, Isa Dolski, as well as the many collaborators outside my laboratory too numerous to name.

References

Abercrombie, H. C., Schaefer, S. M., Larson, C. L., Oakes, T. R., Holden, J. E., Perlman, S. B., Turski, P. A., Krahn, D. D., Benca, R. M. & Davidson, R. J. (1998). Metabolic rate in the amygdala predicts negative affect in depressed patients. *NeuroReport, 9,* 3301–3307.

Abercrombie, H. C., Schaefer, S. M., Larson, C. L., Ward, R. T., Holden, J. F., Turski, P. A., Perlman, S. B. & Davidson, R. J. (1996). Medial prefrontal and amygdalar glucose metabolism in depressed and control subjects: an FDG-PET study. *Psychophysiology, 33,* S17.

Aggleton, J. P. (1993). The contribution of the amygdala to normal and abnormal emotional states. *Trends in Neuroscience, 16*, 328–333.

Amaral, D. G., Price, J. L., Pitkanen, A. & Carmichael, S. T. (1992). Anatomical organization of the primate amygdaloid complex. In J. P. Aggleton (Ed), *The Amygdala: Neurobiological Aspects of Emotion, Memory and Mental Dysfunction* (pp. 1–66). New York: Wiley-Liss.

Carver, C. S. & White, T. L. (1994). Behavioral inhibition, behavioral activation and affective responses to impending reward and punishment: the BIS/BAS scales. *Journal of Personality and Social Psychology, 67*, 319–333.

Davidson, R. J. (1992). Emotion and affective style: hemispheric substrates. *Psychological Science, 3*, 39–43.

Davidson, R. J. (1993). Cerebral asymmetry and emotion: conceptual and methodological conundrums. *Cognition and Emotion, 7*, 115–138.

Davidson, R. J. (1994). Asymmetric brain function, affective style and psychopathology: the role of early experience and plasticity. *Development and Psychopathology, 6*, 741–758.

Davidson, R. J. (1995). Cerebral asymmetry, emotion and affective style. In R. J. Davidson & K. Hugdahl (Eds), *Brain Asymmetry* (pp. 361–387). Cambridge, MA: MIT Press.

Davidson, R. J. (1998). Affective style and affective disorders: perspectives from affective neuroscience. *Cognition and Emotion, 12*, 307–330.

Davidson, R. J., Chapman, J. P., Chapman, L. P. & Henriques, J. B. (1990a). Asymmetrical brain electrical activity discriminates between psychometrically-matched verbal and spatial cognitive tasks. *Psychophysiology, 27*, 528–543.

Davidson, R. J., Coe, C. C., Dolski, I. & Donzella, B. (1999). Individual differences in prefrontal activation asymmetry predict natural killer cell activity at rest and in response to challenge. *Brain, Behavior and Immunity, 13*, 93–108.

Davidson, R. J., Dolski, I., Larson, C. & Sutton, S. K. (in preparation). Electrophysiological measures of prefrontal asymmetry predict recovery of emotion-modulated startle.

Davidson, R. J., Ekman, P., Saron, C., Senulis, J. & Friesen, W. V. (1990b). Approach/ withdrawal and cerebral asymmetry: Emotional expression and brain physiology, I. *Journal of Personality and Social Psychology, 58*, 330–341.

Davidson, R. J. & Fox, N. A. (1989). Frontal brain asymmetry predicts infants' response to maternal separation. *Journal of Abnormal Psychology, 98*, 127–131.

Davidson, R. J. & Irwin, W. (1999a). Functional MRI in the Study of Emotion. In C. Moonen & P. A. Bandettini (Eds), *Medical Radiology—Diagnostic Imaging and Radiation Oncology: Functional MRI* (pp. 487–499). Heidelberg, Germany: Springer.

Davidson, R. J. & Irwin, W. (1999b). The functional neuroanatomy of emotion and affective style. *Trends in Cognitive Science, 3*, 11–21.

Davidson, R. J., Kalin, N. H. & Shelton, S. E. (1992). Lateralized effects of diazepam on frontal brain electrical asymmetries in rhesus monkeys. *Biological Psychiatry, 32*, 438–451.

Davidson, R. J., Kalin, N. H. & Shelton, S. E. (1993). Lateralized response to diazepam predicts temperamental style in rhesus monkeys. *Behavioral Neuroscience, 107*, 1106–1110.

Davidson, R. J. & Tomarken, A. J. (1989). Laterality and emotion: an electrophysiological approach. In F. Boller & J. Grafman (Eds), *Handbook of Neuropsychology* (pp. 419–441). Amsterdam: Elsevier.

Depue, R. A. & Collins, P. F. (in press). Neurobiology of the structure of personality: dopamine, incentive motivation and extroversion. *Behavioral and Brain Sciences*.

Derryberry, D. & Reed, M. A. (1996). Regulatory processes and the development of cognitive representations. *Development and Psychopathology, 8*, 215–234.

Diener, V. E. & Emmons, R. A. (1984). The independence of positive and negative affect. *Journal of Personality and Social Psychology, 47*, 1105–1117.

Farde, L., Gustavsson, J. P. & Jönsson, E. (1997). D2 dopamine receptors and personality. *Nature, 385*, 590.

George, M. S., Ketter, T. A., Parekh, P. I., Horwitz, B., Herscovitch, P. & Post, R. M. (1995). Brain activity during transient sadness and happiness in healthy women. *American Journal of Psychiatry, 152*, 341–351.

Gewirtz, J. C., Falls, W. A. & Davis, M. (1997). Normal conditioned inhibition and extinction of freezing and fear-potentiated startle following electrolytic lesions of medical prefrontal cortex in rats. *Behavioral Neuroscience, 111*, 712–726.

Gold, P. W., Goodwin, F. K. & Chrousos, G. P. (1988). Clinical and biochemical manifestations of depression: relation to the neurobiology of stress. *New England Journal of Medicine, 314*, 348–353.

Gray, J. A. (1994). Three fundamental emotion systems. In P. Ekman & R. J. Davidson (Eds), *The Nature of Emotion: Fundamental Questions* (pp. 243–247). New York: Oxford University Press.

Gross, J. J., Sutton, S. K. & Ketelaar, T. V. (1998). Relations between affect and personality: support for the affect-level and affective-reactivity views. *Personality and Social Psychology Bulletin, 24*, 279–288.

Henriksen, S. J. & Giacchino, J. (1993). Functional characteristics of nucleus accumbens neurons: evidence obtained from *in vivo* electrophysiological recordings. In P. W. Kalivas & C. D. Barnes (Eds), *Limbic Motor Circuits and Neuropsychiatry* (pp. 101–124). Boca Raton, FL: CRC Press.

Irwin, W., Davidson, R. J., Lowe, M. J., Mock, B. J., Sorenson, J. A. & Turski, P. A. (1996). Human amygdala activation detected with echo-planar functional magnetic resonance imaging. *NeuroReport, 7*, 1765–1769.

Irwin, W., Mock, B. J., Sutton, S. K., Orendi, J. L., Sorenson, J. A., Turski, P. A., Kalin, N. H. & Davidson, R. J. (1997). Postive and negative affective responses: neural circuitry revealed using functional magnetic resonance imaging. *Society for Neuroscience Abstracts, 23*, 1318.

Kagan, J., Reznick, J. S. & Snidman, N. (1988). Biological bases of childhood shyness. *Science, 240*, 167–171.

Kalin, N. H. (1993). The neurobiology of fear. *Scientific American, 268*, 94–107.

Kalin, N. H., Larson, C., Shelton, S. E. & Davidson, R. J. (1998). Asymmetric frontal brain activity, cortisol, and behavior associated with fearful temperament in Rhesus monkeys. *Behavioral Neuroscience, 112*, 286–292.

Kalivas, P. W., Churchill, L. & Klitenick, M. A. (1993). The circuitry mediating the translation of motivational stimuli into adaptive motor responses. In P. W. Kalivas & C. D. Barnes (Eds), *Limbic Motor Circuits and Neuropsychiatry* (pp. 237–287). Boca Raton, FL: CRC Press.

Kang, D. H., Davidson, R. J., Coe, C. L., Wheeler, R. W., Tomarken, A. J. & Ershler, W. B. (1991). Frontal brain asymmetry and immune function. *Behavioral Neuroscience, 105*, 860–869.

Ketterer, T. A., Andreason, P. J., George, M. S., Lee, C., Gill, D. S., Parekh, P. I., Willis, M. W., Herscovitch, P. & Post, R. M. (1996). Anterior paralimbic mediation of procaine-induced emotional and psychosensory experiences. *Archives of General Psychiatry, 53*, 59–69.

Kiecolt-Glaser, J. K. & Glaser, R. (1991). Stress and immune function in humans. In R. Ader, D. L. Felten & N. Cohen (Eds), *Psychoneuroimmunology*, 2nd ed. (pp. 849–867). San Diego, CA: Academic Press.

Lang, P. J. Bradley, M. M. & Cuthbert, B. N. (1995). *International Affective Picture System*

(IAPS): Technical Manual and Affective Ratings. Gainsville, FL: The Center for Research in Psychophysiology, University of Florida.

Lang, P. J., Bradley, M. M. & Cuthbert, B. N. (1990). Emotion, attention and the startle reflex. *Psychological Review, 97,* 377–398.

Lazarus, R. S. (1991). *Emotion and Adaptation.* Oxford: Oxford University Press.

LeDoux, J. E. (1996). *The Emotional Brain.* New York: Simon & Schuster.

LeDoux, J. E. (1992). Emotion and the amygdala. In J. P. Aggleton (Ed), *The Amygdala: Neurobiological Aspects of Emotion, Memory and Mental Dysfunction* (pp. 339–352). New York: Wiley-Liss.

LeDoux, J. E. (1987). Emotion. In V. B. Mountcastle (Ed), *Handbook of Physiology,* sect. 1: *The Nervous System,* vol. V. *Higher Functions of the Brain* (pp. 419–459). Bethesda, MD: American Physiological Society.

Meehl, P. E. (1975). Hedonic capacity: some conjectures. *Bulletin of the Menninger Clinic, 39,* 295–307.

Morgan, M. A., Romanski, L. & LeDoux, J. E. (1993). Extinction of emotional learning: contribution of medial prefrontal cortex. *Neuroscience Letters, 163,* 109–113.

Osgood, C. E., Suci, G. J. & Tannenbaum, P. H. (1957). *The Measurement of Meaning.* Urbana: University of Illinois Press.

Paradiso, S., Robinson, R. G., Andreasen, N. C., Downhill, J. E., Davidson, R. J., Kirchner, P. T., Watkins, G. L., Boles, L. L. & Hichwa, R. D. (1997). Emotional activation of limbic circuitry in elderly and normal subjects in a PET study. *American Journal of Psychiatry, 154,* 382–389.

Reiman, E. M., Fusselman, M. J. L., Fox, B. J. & Raichle, M. E. (1989). Neuroanatomical correlates of anticipatory anxiety. *Science, 243,* 1071–1074.

Russell, J. A. (1980). A circumplex model of emotion. *Journal of Personality and Social Psychology, 39,* 1161–1178.

Ryff, C. D. & Singer, B. (1998). The contours of positive human health. *Psychological Inquiry, 9,* 1–28.

Schneider, F., Gur, R. E., Mozley, L. H., Smith, R. J., Mozley, P. D., Censitis, D. M., Alavi, A. & Gur, R. C. (1995). Mood effects on limbic blood flow correlate with emotional self-rating: a PET study with oxygen-15 labeled water. *Psychiatric Research: Neuroimaging, 61,* 265–283.

Schneirla, T. C. (1959). An evolutionary and developmental theory of biphasic processes underlying approach and withdrawal. In M. R. Jones (Ed), *Nebraska Symposium on Motivation* (pp. 1–42). Lincoln: University of Nebraska Press.

Schultz, W., Apicella, P., Romo, R. & Scarnati, E. (1995a). Context-dependent activity in primate striatum reflecting past and future behavioral events. In J. C. Houk, J. L. Davis & D. G. Beiser (Eds), *Models of Information Processing in the Basal Ganglia* (pp. 11–28). Cambridge, MA: MIT Press.

Schultz, W., Romo, R., Ljungberg, T., Mirenowicz, J., Hollerman, J. R. & Dickinson, A. (1995b). Reward-related signals carried by dopamine neurons. In J. C. Houk, J. L. Davis & D. G. Beiser (Eds), *Models of Information Processing in the Basal Ganglia* (pp. 233–248). Cambridge, MA: MIT Press.

Smith, O. A., DeVita, T. L. & Astley, C. A. (1990). Neurons controlling cardiovascular responses to emotion are located in lateral hypothalamus-perifornical region. *American Journal of Physiology, 259,* R943–R954.

Stein, N. L. & Trabasso, T. (1992). The organization of emotional experience: creating links among emotion, thinking, language and intentional action. *Cognition and Emotion, 6,* 225–244.

Sutton, S. K. & Davidson, R. J. (1997). Prefrontal brain asymmetry: a biological substrate of the behavioral approach and inhibition systems. *Psychological Science, 8,* 204–210.

Sutton, S. K., Davidson, R. J., Donzella, B., Irwin, W. & Dottl, D. A. (1997). Manipulating affective state using extended picture presentation. *Psychophysiology, 34*, 217–226.

Thompson, R. A. (1994). Emotion regulation: a theme in search of definition. In N. A. Fox (Ed), *The Development of Emotion Regulation: Biological and Behavioral Aspects* (pp. 25–52). Monographs of the Society for Research in Child Development, 59 (serial no. 240).

Thorpe, S., Rolls, E. & Maddison, S. (1983). The orbitofrontal cortex: neuronal activity in the behaving monkey. *Experimental Brain Research, 49*, 93–113.

Tomarken, A. J., Davidson, R. J., Wheeler, R. E. & Doss, R. C. (1992). Individual differences in anterior brain asymmetry and fundamental dimensions of emotion. *Journal of Personality and Social Psychology, 62*, 676–687.

Watson, D., Clark, L. A. & Tellegen, A. (1988). Developmental and validation of brief measures of positive and negative affect: the PANAS scales. *Journal of Personality and Social Psychology, 54*, 1063–1070.

Watson, D. & Tellegen, A. (1985). Toward a consensual structure of mood. *Psychological Bulletin, 98*, 219–235.

Wegner, D. M. & Bargh, J. A. (1998). Control and automaticity in social life. In D. Gilbert, S. T. Fisk & G. Lindzey (Eds), *Handbook of Social Psychology*, 4th ed. (pp. 446–496). Boston, MA: McGraw-Hill.

Wheeler, R. E., Davidson, R. J. & Tomarken, A. J. (1993). Frontal brain asymmetry and emotional reactivity: a biological substrate of affective style. *Psychophysiology, 30*, 82–89.

Woods, R. P., Mazziotta, J. C. & Cherry, S. R. (1993). MRI-PET registration with automated algorithm. *Journal of Computer Assisted Tomography, 17*, 536–546.

17

Positron Emission Tomography in the Study of Emotion, Anxiety, and Anxiety Disorders

ERIC M. REIMAN, RICHARD D. LANE, GEOFFREY L. AHERN,
GARY E. SCHWARTZ, AND RICHARD J. DAVIDSON

This chapter reviews six studies in which we used positron emission tomography (PET) measurements of regional cerebral blood flow (CBF), a marker of local neuronal activity, to investigate regions of the brain that participate in emotion, anxiety, and anxiety disorders. Along the way, we consider how these brain regions are related to different kinds of emotional stimuli, different types of emotion, emotional valence, and different forms of emotional pathology.

These studies were designed to generate intense emotions and emotional syndromes in the laboratory setting, acquire subjective and psychophysiologic measurements of the emotional state, and control for nonspecific aspects of the emotion-generating task. Intravenous bolus injections of ^{15}O-water were used to make multiple 40- to 60-sec scans during each imaging session, thus permitting us to acquire data during a brief and potentially uncomfortable behavioral state and use each individual as his or her own control. In all cases, the subjects were fully informed about the potential risks and discomfort involved in the study, provided their written consent, and were studied under guidelines approved by the human subjects committee of the responsible institution.

In most cases, brain mapping algorithms were used to normalize regional data for the variation in whole-brain measurements, transform each person's PET image into the coordinates of a standard brain atlas, compute statistical maps of state-dependent increases in regional CBF, and superimpose these maps onto an average of the subject's magnetic resonance images (MRIs); these algorithms permitted us to distinguish subtle state-dependent CBF increases from noise, compare data from different subjects, and compare findings from different studies. Our original brain mapping algorithm (Fox et al., 1988) was developed in direct response to challenges raised in our PET study of panic disorder. Procedures were recently developed, tested, and when possible used to address the potentially confounding effects of temporalis muscle activity, residual radiotracer activity in the internal carotid arteries, and partial-volume averaging (image blurring) on CBF measurements in the anterior temporal lobes (Chen et al., 1995; Reiman, 1996).

Externally and Internally Generated Emotions

We begin with a study in which we used PET measurements of regional CBF to investigate regions of the brain that are involved in normal human emotion, how these regions are related to the nature of the emotional stimulus, and how these regions are related to different types of emotion (Lane et al., 1997a; Reiman et al., 1997). Twelve neurologically and psychiatrically healthy females were studied as they alternated between emotion-generating and emotionally neutral control tasks. For six scans, silent film clips extensively studied by Davidson and his colleagues (Tomarken et al., 1990) were used for the external generation of three subjectively, facially, and electrophysiologically well-characterized and relatively pure target emotions, happiness, sadness, and disgust, and for the generation of three emotionally neutral conditions intended to control for potentially confounding features of the emotion-generating film task, such as visual stimulation and eye movements. For six additional scans, autobiographic scripts of recent experiences were used for the internal generation of the same three target emotions and for the generation of three emotionally neutral conditions intended to control for potentially confounding effects of the emotion-generating recall task, such as recall memory and visual imagery. During each scan, psychophysiological measurements were acquired (e.g., quantitative electroencephalographic measures of brain activity, electromyographic measurements of facial muscle activity, electro-oculographic measurements of eye movement, and electrocardiographic measurements of heart rate); a hidden camera was used to record facial expressions (Ekman & Friesen, 1982), but the quality of the videotapes turned out to be unsatisfactory for blind ratings of facial affect. Immediately following each scan, subjects rated their experience of seven emotions (happiness, sadness, disgust, interest, amusement, fear, and anger) on separate visual analogue scales. The sequence of scans was arranged to address potential order effects. In comparison to the control tasks, there were significant increases in subjective ratings of the relevant target emotion during the emotion-generating film tasks and recall tasks. If anything, the increases related to recall-generated emotions were slightly greater than those related to film-generated emotions.

Which brain regions participate in the emotional response to a complex visual stimulus (in this case, silent film clips)? Film-generated emotion was distinguished from the emotionally neutral film tasks by significant, symmetrical CBF increases in the vicinity of occipitotemporal and anterior temporal cortex, amygdala, medial prefrontal cortex, thalamus, hypothalamus, midbrain, and lateral cerebellum (Reiman et al., 1997). The CBF increases in anterior temporal regions were unrelated to the potentially confounding effects of temporalis muscle activity or residual radiotracer activity in the internal carotid arteries (Chen et al., 1995; Reiman et al., 1997).

Which brain regions participate in the emotional response to a cognitive stimulus (in this case, the recollection of recent experiences)? Like film-generated emotion, recall-generated emotion was distinguished from its own emotionally neutral condition by significant CBF increases in the vicinity of medial prefrontal cortex and thalamus; it was also associated with CBF increases in the vicinity of anterior insular cortex and in regions that appear to reflect the combined effects of temporalis muscle activity and partial volume averaging (Reiman, 1996; Reiman et al., 1997). Post-hoc analyses revealed significantly increased CBF in the anterior insular region during recall-generated sadness, and this increase was significantly greater than that associated with recall-generated happiness (Reiman et al., 1997).

How are the brain regions that participate in emotion related to the nature of the emotional stimulus? To address this question with greater statistical power, we directly compared the CBF increases related to film-generated emotion to the CBF increases related to recall-generated emotion. Film-generated emotion was distinguished from recall-generated emotion by significantly greater, symmetrical CBF increases in the vicinity of occipitotemporoparietal cortex, anterior temporal cortex, amygdala, hippocampal formation, hypothalamus, and the lateral cerebellum (Reiman et al., 1997). Although recall-generated emotion was not distinguished from film-generated emotion by any significant increases in regional CBF, post-hoc analysis revealed that recall-generated sadness was distinguished from film-generated sadness by significantly greater CBF increases in the anterior insular region (Lane et al., 1997a; Reiman, 1996; Reiman et al., 1997).

Visual association areas in occipitotemporal cortex could be involved in the evaluation procedure that invests complex visual stimuli (or certain aspects of these visual stimuli) with emotional significance. Although the anterior temporal cortex, hippocampal formation, and amygdala have long been thought to participate in the generation of emotion (LeDoux, 1987), our findings suggest that these heteromodal sensory association areas (Mesulam, 1986) are preferentially involved in the evaluation procedure that invests exteroceptive sensory stimuli with emotional significance. In contrast, findings from this study and others, noted below, suggest that the anterior insular region is preferentially involved in the evaluation procedure that invests potentially distressing thoughts or bodily sensations with negative emotional significance.

Finally, how are the implicated brain regions related to different types of emotion? Some of our findings are summarized here; additional findings are described in our original report (Lane et al., 1997a). Film- and recall-generated happiness, sadness, and disgust were all associated with increased CBF in the medial prefrontal and thalamic regions, suggesting that these regions participate in aspects of emotion that are unrelated to the nature of the emotional stimulus or the type of emotion (Lane et al., 1997a). Film-generated happiness, sadness, and disgust were associated with significantly increased CBF in the vicinity of occipitotemporal and anterior temporal cortex, suggesting that these regions participate in aspects of externally generated emotion that are independent of the particular type of emotion (Lane et al., 1997a). As previously noted, recall-generated sadness was associated with significantly increased CBF in the anterior insular region. Sadness and disgust, our two negative emotions, were each associated with significant CBF increases in the vicinity of the midbrain and cerebellar vermis—increases we also find in normal and pathological forms of anxiety (Reiman, 1996; Reiman et al., 1989b). Our findings concerning the neuroanatomical correlates of discrete emotions should be interpreted with caution because large increases in the ratings of each target emotion were associated with smaller increases in the ratings of other emotions.

Positive and Negative Emotion

In a complementary study, we used PET measurements of regional CBF and the International Affective Picture System developed and extensively studied by Lang and his colleagues (1995) to investigate regions of the brain involved in normal human emotion and this time consider how these regions are related to emotional valence (i.e., the extent to which emotion is pleasant or unpleasant) (Lane et al., 1997b). Twelve neurologically and psychiatrically healthy females had 12 scans as they alternated between watching sets of emotionally positive color pictures, emotionally negative color pictures, and a small eye-fixation cross-hair. During each scan, electromyography was used to record corrugator muscle activity (a measure of negative emotion; Lang et al., 1995) and zygomatic muscle activity (a measure of positive emotion; Lang et al., 1995), and electrodermal activity was used to provide a measure of physiologic arousal. Immediately following each scan, subjects rated their emotional valence and arousal using well-established rating scales (Lane et al., 1997b). The sequence of scans was arranged to address potential order effects.

Picture-generated positive emotion was distinguished from picture-generated neutral emotion by significantly increased CBF in the vicinity of the thalamus, hypothalamus, midbrain, and medial prefrontal cortex. Like picture-generated positive emotion, picture-generated negative emotion was distinguished from picture-generated neutral emotion by significantly increased CBF in the vicinity of the thalamus, hypothalamus, midbrain, and medial prefrontal cortex. In addition, picture-generated negative emotion was distinguished from both picture-generated neutral and positive emotions by significantly increased CBF in occipitotemporal cortex, lateral cerebellum, and the left amygdala, hippocampal formation, and parahippocampal gyrus. Increases in the vicinity of anterolateral temporal and inferolateral frontal regions appeared to be at least partly related to the combined effects of temporalis muscle activity and partial volume averaging (Lane et al., 1997b). We postulate that sensory association areas are preferentially involved in evaluative, attentional, or other aspects of the response to stimuli that are emotionally unpleasant and potentially threatening (Reiman, 1996).

Normal Anticipatory Anxiety

First in St. Louis (Reiman et al., 1989a) and subsequently in Arizona (Reiman, 1996), PET measurements of regional CBF were used to investigate regions of the brain involved in normal anticipatory anxiety. In St. Louis, eight neurologically and psychiatrically healthy subjects were studied before, during, and after the prospect of receiving an electric shock. The shock was administered just after the completion of the second 1-min scan; it was brief and well tolerated, and it preserved the investigators' credibility for the remainder of the study. In addition, the subjects were studied during a fist opening-and-closing task, another baseline task, and a tonic fist-clenching task in an attempt to address the neuroanatomical correlates of movement and muscle tension. Anticipation of shock was associated with large and significant increases in subjective ratings of anxiety, heart rate, and nonspecific fluctuations in electrodermal activity (Reiman et al., 1989a).

Anticipatory anxiety was distinguished from each of the baseline conditions by significant increases in the vicinity of anterior temporal cortex (Reiman et al., 1989a). However, subsequent studies in Montreal (Benkelfat et al., 1995) and St. Louis (Drevets et al., 1989) raised the possibility that these increases could be at least partly related to the combined effects of temporalis muscle activity of partial volume averaging. The St. Louis studies of normal anticipatory anxiety and lactate-induced panic attacks did not acquire MRIs in any of the subjects; like other PET studies conducted at the time, they excluded data from outside the brain to normal-ize local brain measurements for the whole-brain variations.

In Arizona, we repeated the study in a larger subject group and acquired MRIs for each subject (as we as we did in our Arizona studies of emotion, social phobic, and specific phobic anxiety). We also developed, tested, and applied techniques that address the potentially confounding effects of temporalis muscle activity, inter-nal carotid artery activity, and partial volume averaging on blood flow changes observed in the anterior temporal lobes (Reiman, 1996). Fourteen neurologically and psychiatrically healthy females were studied before, during, and after the pros-pect of receiving an electric shock. In addition, they were studied during a jaw-clenching task that produces robust increases in temporalis and masseter muscle activity, another baseline task, and a voluntary hyperventilation task that sought to address the potentially confounding effects of hyperventilation-induced hypocapnia on regional measurements. In each case, the subjects rested quietly in the supine position with their eyes closed; electrodes were placed on both hands for adminis-tration of the electric shock. Anticipation shock was associated with large and significant increases in subjective ratings of anxiety and heart rate (Reiman, 1996).

We first investigated the relationship between the blood flow increases related to jaw clenching, anticipatory anxiety, and (using data from another study [Chen et al., 1995]) residual radiotracer activity in the internal carotid arteries. Jaw clenching was associated with large, significant bilateral blood flow increases that extended medially from temporalis muscle into anterolateral temporal and infero-lateral frontal areas due to partial volume averaging and extended superiorly into sensorimotor areas that participate in jaw movement. Anticipatory anxiety was as-sociated with significant bilateral blood flow increases in the vicinity of temporalis muscle, anterolateral temporal, and inferolateral frontal areas that overlapped the increases associated with jaw clenching (but were smaller in magnitude and spa-tially less extensive); it was also associated with significantly increased CBF in the vicinity of anterior insular cortex. Internal carotid artery activity extended into anteromedial temporal and posterior orbitofrontal regions, but did not overlap the blood flow increases observed during anticipatory anxiety (Chen et al., 1995; Rei-man, 1996).

Although the procedure that corrects for the potentially confounding effects of temporalis muscle activity prevents us from investigating CBF increases in anterolateral temporal and inferolateral frontal regions, it improves our ability to detect CBF increases in the rest of the brain. Using this procedure, normal anticipatory anxiety was associated with significantly increased CBF bilaterally in the vicinity of anterior insular, temporoparietal, and lateral prefrontal cortex, caudate, right anterior temporal cortex, thalamus, and a region that includes anterior cingulate and medial prefrontal cortex, and by significant trends in the cerebellar vermis and midbrain. Based on these findings, we believe that the blood flow increases in anterior temporal cortex partly reflect the combined effects of temporalis muscle activity and partial volume averaging (even though electromyography failed to indicate appreciable increases in temporalis muscle activity) and partly reflect increased activity in anterior temporal cortex (Reiman, 1996).

We postulate that (1) anterior insular regions serve in part as internal alarm centers; (2) anterior temporal regions serve in part as external alarm centers (perhaps in this case representing an attempt to monitor exteroceptive sensory stimuli); (3) the anterior cingulate/medial prefrontal region participates in the conscious experience of, attentional response to, or behavioral response to the anxiety-provoking situation; (4) the cerebellar vermis participates in the behavioral response to the anxiety-provoking situation (e.g., facial expressions of anxiety, muscle tension, readiness to respond, or restraint from fleeing the situation) or cognitive features of anxiety that remain to be elucidated; (5) that the temporoparietal regions participate in spatial orientation or auditory vigilance to the threatening situation; (6) the lateral prefrontal regions participate in the process of deciding how to respond to the threatening situation, and (7) the thalamus and caudate participate in a basal ganglia-thalamic-frontal circuit that participates in the integrated expressions of anxiety (Reiman, 1996). Of course, our findings need to be replicated in an independent study and our hypotheses need to be tested using potentially complementary research strategies.

In the study described above, we investigated the brain regions that participate in normal anticipatory anxiety—normal because it is tolerable, does not interfere with the individual's ability to cope with the anxiety-provoking situation, and even mobilizes the person to respond to the threatening situation. In the studies described below, we investigated brain regions that participate in pathological forms of anxiety: anxiety disorders that are associated with intolerable distress and typically interfere with the individual's ability to cope with the anxiety-provoking situation (although they endured it during the course of the PET study). Among other questions, we wished to consider the neural processes that participate in both pathological and normal forms of anxiety and those that distinguish pathological from normal forms of anxiety.

Panic Disorder

PET and lactate infusion were used to investigate regions of the brain involved in the predisposition to, elicitation, and prevention of panic attacks in patients with panic disorder (Klein et al., 1992; Reiman, 1987, 1990; Reiman et al., 1984, 1986, 1989b). Lactate infusion precipitates a panic attack in many patients with panic disorder, but rarely does so in normal controls (Reiman, 1987). When antipanic treatments block naturally occurring panic attacks, they also block the attacks induced by lactate (Reiman, 1987). We used PET to study patients with panic disorder and normal controls before and during lactate infusion. Many of the patients were treated with alprazolam for several weeks and then restudied.

We initially compared CBF measurements acquired in the nonpanic state before lactate infusion. Patients who were predisposed to lactate-induced panic had an abnormal asymmetry (right > left) in a preselected region of interest in the posterior parahippocampal gyrus (Reiman et al., 1984). We then extended our analysis of the parahippocampal region to larger subject groups. In the nonpanic state before infusion, patients who were predisposed to lactate-induced panic had an abnormal asymmetry (right > left) of parahippocampal CBF, blood volume, and oxygen metabolism; they also had abnormally increased oxygen metabolism in the whole brain (Reiman et al., 1986). The asymmetry appeared to reflect increased measurements in the right rather than decreased measurements in the left. The asymmetry was unchanged during lactate-induced panic (Reiman et al., 1989b) and was not corrected by alprazolam treatment (Klein et al., 1992).

Because brain-mapping algorithms have not yet been established for between-group comparisons, (in particular, algorithms that adjust individual images for their shape as well as their size and orientation) we are not yet sure if the abnormality is centered in the preselected posterior parahippocampal region of interest or extends into this region from a neighboring structure (e.g., medial occipitotemporal cortex or midbrain), and we cannot yet address the possibility of additional abnormalities in unexplored regions (Klein et al., 1992; Reiman, 1987). Using a brain-mapping algorithm not yet established for between-group comparisons (one that adjusts brain images for their size and orientation, but not their shape), patients with panic disorder who were predisposed to lactate-induced panic had abnormally increased CBF in a right-sided region that included the posterior parahippocampal gyrus, occipitotemporal cortex, and midbrain. Patients with panic disorder who were not predisposed to lactate-induced panic had abnormally increased CBF in the same region bilaterally.

Next, we considered the increases in regional CBF associated with lactate infusion. Lactate-induced panic was associated with significantly increased blood flow bilaterally in the vicinity of anterior temporal cortex, anterior insular cortex, and the superior colliculi (midbrain structures) and in the left anterior cerebellar vermis (Reiman et al., 1989b). In retrospect, the blood flow increases observed in the vicinity of anterior temporal cortex, though slightly more medial than those observed during normal anticipatory anxiety, could be at least partly related to the combined effects of temporalis muscle activity and partial volume averaging (Benkelfat et al., 1995; Drevets et al., 1989). Lactate infusion was not associated with significant increases in regional CBF in the nonpanicking patients or control subjects (Reiman et al., 1989b).

Although lactate infusion was associated with significantly increased whole-brain CBF in nonpanicking patients and controls, it was not associated with increased CBF in the panicking patients (Reiman, 1990). The lactate-induced increase in whole-brain CBF could reflect the effects of hemodilution or the development of a central acidosis. The absence of a lactate-induced increase in whole-brain CBF could reflect the effects of hyperventilation or a potential reduction in the permeability · surface area product for water (PSw). The PSw, a measure of blood–brain barrier permeability to small molecules such as water, is an end-organ product of the central adrenergic system which is increased by antidepressants shown to block panic attacks (Reiman, 1987).

Finally, we considered the effects of alprazolam treatment on parahippocampal and whole-brain measurements. As previously noted, alprazolam treatment did not correct the regional abnormality (Klein et al., 1992). As previously shown with acute benzodiazepine administration, continuation treatment with alprazolam was associated with a significant reduction in whole-brain CBF (Klein et al., 1992).

Our findings led us to propose the following model to account for the predisposition to, elicitation, medication treatment, and nonmedication treatment of panic attacks in patients with panic disorder (Reiman, 1991). We postulate that a regional abnormality, present in the nonpanic state, is involved in the predisposition to panic attacks. We postulate that the abnormal region responds to a normally innocuous triggering event by sending a message to alarm centers involved in the elaboration of a panic attack. The normally innocuous triggering event might include an increase in central adrenergic activity, a decrease in central nervous system pH, certain somatic sensations, or some other process that remain to be determined. The alarm centers could reside in anterior insular and possibly anterior temporal regions (Reiman, 1996). We suggest that the regional abnormality distinguishes panic disorder from normal forms of anxiety, but we also suggest that the same alarm centers participate in the elaboration of panic attacks and normal anticipatory anxiety—a false alarm in one case, a survival-enhancing alarm in the other. Finally, we postulate that antipanic medications exert their effects by interfering with the normally innocuous triggering event (e.g., by decreasing central adrenergic activity) and that cognitive-behavioral therapy exerts its effects downstream, by increasing resistance to false alarms. Until our hypotheses are tested, we are mindful of H. L. Mencken's admonition that "for every complex problem, there is a solution which is simple, neat, and wrong!"

Social Phobic Anxiety

We used PET measurements of regional CBF to investigate regions of the brain involved in social phobic anxiety (Reiman, 1996). Seven patients with social phobia, generalized type, were studied before, during, and after the elicitation of social phobic anxiety. During all three scans, the patients sang the alphabet song with their eyes closed. During the first and third scans, they understood that there were no observers in the scanning room. During the second scan, they understood there were several observers in the scanning room monitoring their performance. In addition, the patients were studied during a jaw-clenching task, a voluntary hyperventilation task, and a nonspeaking baseline condition. The public speaking condition was distinguished from the private speaking condition by significantly higher subjective ratings of anxiety and heart rate; in turn, the private speaking condition was distinguished from the nonspeaking baseline condition by significantly higher subjective ratings of anxiety and heart rate.

The public and private singing conditions were each distinguished from the nonspeaking baseline condition by significantly increased CBF in the vicinity of auditory areas in the superior temporal gyrus, sensorimotor areas, anterior insular cortex, a region that includes posterior cingulate gyrus and precuneus, caudate, thalamus, cerebellar vermis, and midbrain (Reiman, 1996). Some of these regions appear to participate in the singing task itself, some appear to participate in monitoring the patients' own performance, and some appear to be participate in the social phobic anxiety that was present during both speaking conditions.

After addressing the potentially confounding effects of activity in temporalis muscle activity and radiotracer activity in the internal carotid arteries, the public speaking condition was distinguished from the private speaking condition by significantly increased CBF in the vicinity of auditory, motor mouth, and other sensorimotor areas, a region that includes the supplementary motor area and mid-cingulate cortex, a region that includes the posterior cingulate gyrus and precuneus, lateral prefrontal cortex, anterior temporal cortex, the thalamus, and the midbrain, and by significant trends in the vicinity of a region that includes anterior cingulate and medial prefrontal cortex, the hippocampus, amygdala, hypothalamus, and the cerebellar vermis (Reiman, 1996). Some of the brain regions thus implicated in social phobic anxiety appear to participate in vigilance to the sound of the patients' own voice, some appear to participate in effortful vocalization, and others appear to participate in the mental operations that participate in several forms of anxiety.

Once a brain-mapping algorithm is established for between-group comparisons, we will consider the possibility that the patients have one or more abnormalities in the nonspeaking, nonanxious baseline state—abnormalities that could predispose them to become anxious in social phobic situations. Although our sample size is small, we will also consider the brain regions that were selectively affected by several weeks of treatment with the investigational medication brofaromine, a reversible inhibitor of monoamine oxidase A.

Specific Phobic Anxiety

Finally, we used PET to study a form of anxiety that could be repeatedly elicited. Although not considered here, the acquisition of multiple images in the same subject during the same experimental and baseline state could permit us to characterize state-dependent changes in regional CBF in each individual person, thus localizing these changes with greater precision. Four patients with a snake phobia each had 16 scans over 2 imaging sessions as they alternated between exposure to a live 4-foot-long royal python and a stuffed stocking, similar to the snake in size and shape, that controlled for visual stimulation (Reiman, 1996). (The snake and stuffed stocking were coiled around the horizontal bar of a periscopic, ceiling-mounted trapeze hanging above the supine patient. To minimize psychophysiological habituation, the horizontal bar was lowered closer to the patient's body and repositioned closer to the patient's face after each even-numbered scan. Patients who wished to be treated after the scanning sessions improved dramatically following additional exposures to the same snake. By the end of the treatment, they could even wear the snake around their necks!

Using the 64 images acquired in the 4 patients and removing the large blood flow increases extending from temporalis muscle into anterolateral temporal cortex, snake-phobic anxiety was associated with significant CBF increases in the vicinity of occipital visual association areas, a region that includes anterior cingulate and medial prefrontal cortex, anterior insular cortex, motor cortex, supplementary motor area, thalamus, caudate, midbrain, cerebellar vermis, and lateral cerebellum, and by significant trends in the hippocampal formation and parahippocampal gyrus (Reiman, 1996). The visual association areas could participate in vigilance to and evaluation of the emotionally threatening visual stimulus. The anterior cingulate/ medial prefrontal region (also implicated in our Arizona studies of anticipatory anxiety and social phobic anxiety) could participate in the conscious experience of emotion, the attentional or behavioral response to the anxiety-provoking situation, the inhibition of excessive emotion, or the process of monitoring the individual's emotional state to make a personally relevant decision. The anterior insular region could serve as an internal alarm center, alerting the individual to potentially distressing interoceptive stimuli such as the sensation of heart pounding. The motor areas, supplementary motor area, and cerebellar regions could participate in the patients' readiness to flee from the threatening situation or in their restraint from fleeing. The thalamus and caudate could participate in a basal ganglia-thalamic-frontal circuit involved in the integrated behavioral or cognitive response to the frightening situation. The parahippocampal and hippocampal regions could serve as external alarm centers, alerting the individual to the threatening exteroceptive sensory stimulus or provide the spatial context for the frightening situation. Failure to detect CBF increases in the vicinity of the amygdala could reflect limitations in statistical power, an attenuation of these increases by the combined effects of reduced residual radiotracer activity in the internal carotid arteries and partial volume averaging, or an insignificant increase in local neuronal activity. By excluding the large blood flow increases centered in temporalis muscle and extending into neighboring brain regions, we were unable to explore CBF increases in anterolateral temporal cortex.

Overview

Reflecting on these six studies of normal and pathological emotions, we are struck by some common themes. In this section, we consider a few of these themes and their possible implications.

Limbic areas (i.e., hippocampal formation and amygdala) and paralimbic areas (anterior temporal cortex and the parahippocampal gyrus) in the anterior temporal lobe have long been postulated to participate in emotion (LeDoux, 1987; Mesulam, 1986). Based on our findings, we suggest that these regions are preferentially involved in the response to exteroceptive sensory stimuli and less involved in the emotional response to cognitive (and perhaps interoceptive sensory) stimuli. We postulate that these regions, which receive projections from multimodal sensory association areas (Mesulam, 1986), participate in the evaluation procedure that invests simple and complex exteroceptive sensory stimuli with emotional significance. We suggest that these regions (and perhaps other regions in relevant sensory association areas) serve as external alarm centers, alerting the individual about outside dangers.

In contrast, a region in the vicinity of anterior insular cortex (another paralimbic area; LeDoux, 1987; Mesulam, 1986) appears to be preferentially involved in the emotional response to potentially distressing cognitive stimuli, interoceptive sensory stimuli, and body sensations. Perhaps this region has received less attention than limbic areas in studies that investigate the neural substrates of emotion in laboratory animals because it is difficult to elicit an emotional response in the absence of an exteroceptive sensory stimulus. We have now observed CBF increases in the anterior insular region during recall-generated sadness (Lane et al., 1997a), normal anticipatory anxiety (Reiman, 1996), lactate-induced panic (Reiman et al., 1989b), the perception of temperature and pain (Bushnell et al., 1995), and the luteal phase of the normal menstrual cycle (Reiman et al., 1996). Based on these and other studies, we postulate that the anterior insular region participates in the evaluation procedure that invests potentially distressing thoughts and body sensations with negative emotional significance. Among other things, this region may serve as an internal alarm center, alerting the individual about potential dangers inside the body.

The thalamus appears to participate in aspects of emotion that are unrelated to the type of emotion, emotional valence, or the nature of the emotional stimulus (Lane et al., 1997a,b; Reiman et al., 1997). Limitations in anatomical localization and spatial resolution prevent us from relating the increases in thalamic CBF to particular thalamic nuclei, particular basal ganglia-thalamic-frontal circuits, or particular aspects of emotion, anxiety, and anxiety syndromes. Based on Cannon and Bard's classic studies of sham rage (see LeDoux, 1987), we postulate that the increases observed in anterior thalamus participate in some fashion in the integrated expression of emotion.

Like the thalamus, medial prefrontal cortex (Brodmann's area 9) appears to participate in aspects of emotion that are unrelated to the type of emotion, emotional valence, or the nature of the emotional stimulus (Lane et al., 1997a,b; Reiman et al., 1997). We postulate that this region participates in the conscious experience of emotion, inhibition of potentially excessive emotion, or the process of monitoring one's own emotional state to make personally relevant decisions. Kihlstrom (1987) suggests that "the difference that makes for consciousness" is the connection between perceptual or cognitive processes and an integrated representation of the self that resides in working memory. If, like dorsolateral prefrontal cortex (Goldman-Rakic, 1987), the medial prefrontal region is involved in working memory, it could participate in the conscious experience of emotion. Because medial prefrontal lesions prolong the time it takes to extinguish conditioned fear in laboratory rats (Morgan et al., 1993), because medial prefrontal lesions can be associated with socially inappropriate expressions of emotion in brain-injured patients (Damasio et al., 1994), and because medial prefrontal activity was found to be inversely related to amygdala activity in patients with major depressive disorder (Davidson, 1996), the medial prefrontal cortex could participate in the inhibition of excessive expressions of emotion. Finally, studies of Phineas Gage and other patients with medial prefrontal damage suggest that this region monitors the person's emotional state to make personally relevant decisions (Damasio et al., 1994). Our studies suggest that the behavioral changes observed in these patients may be related to lesions in a medial prefrontal region dorsal to the ventromedial prefrontal region highlighted by Damasio and colleagues.

In addition to these regions, we find that modality-specific sensory association areas, a region including anterior cingulate and medial prefrontal cortex (ventral to the medial prefrontal region noted above), the caudate, the cerebellar vermis, and a midbrain region participate in normal and pathological forms of anxiety (Reiman, 1996). As previously noted, we postulate that the anterior cingulate/medial prefrontal region participates in the conscious experience of, attentional response to, or behavioral response to emotionally distressing circumstances such as anxiety and pain, that the cerebellar vermis participates in the behavioral response to the distressing situation (i.e., facial expressions of anxiety, muscle tension, readiness to respond, or restraint from fleeing the situation) or cognitive aspects of anxiety that remain to be determined, and that thalamic and caudate regions are components in a basal ganglia-thalamic-frontal circuit (Alexander et al., 1986) that somehow participates in the integrated expression of anxiety.

How do pathological and normal forms of anxiety differ, how are they alike, and how do therapeutic interventions exert their beneficial effects? As indicated in our model of panic disorder, we propose that one or more regional abnormalities participate in the predisposition to pathological forms of anxiety. We suggest that these abnormalities respond to a normally innocuous triggering event (e.g., a neurochemical change, hormonal change, particular interoceptive sensory stimulus, or particular exteroceptive sensory stimulus) by sending a message to a common pathway that participates in pathological and normal forms of anxiety by sending a message to additional neuronal systems that participate in the vigilance to, monitoring, and readiness to respond to the threatening situation, and by sending a message to neuronal systems that attempt to inhibit or compensate for potentially excessive emotion.

We suggest that such features as an anxiety disorder's natural history, gender distribution, and treatment might have more to do with alterations in the normally innocuous processes that participate in the initiation and elaboration of anxiety than the regional abnormalities themselves. For instance, age of onset of panic disorder (typically the late teens to early thirties), natural history (e.g., the emergence of panic attacks in situations patients have come to fear), and gender distribution (i.e., greater frequency in females) might have more to do with normally innocuous age-, stress-, or gender-dependent variations in noradrenergic activity than with age-, stress-, or gender-dependent alterations in the abnormality that predisposes patients to panic.

Although it remains possible that treatments exert their therapeutic effects by correcting the underlying abnormality, it appears at least as likely that they compensate for the abnormality by affecting other processes (Reiman, 1991). Just as β-adrenergic blocking agents compensate for rather than correct coronary ischemia by modulating normal physiological processes in patients with angina, psychiatric treatments might compensate for the underlying abnormality by modulating normal physiological processes in patients with anxiety and other psychiatric disorders.

Although the long list of brain regions implicated in normal and pathological forms of anxiety might appear daunting, it makes an important point. We should reject the phrenologist's view that complex behaviors such as emotion can be localized to a single brain center. Instead, we should consider how the multiple mental operations and the spatially distributed brain processes that subserve them work in concert to produce a multi-faceted emotional response (Reiman, 1996).

Limitations

In this chapter, we have considered the CBF increases observed in our own PET studies of emotion, anxiety, and anxiety disorders. We did not discuss findings from the elegant PET studies of emotion (e.g., George et al., 1995; Mayberg et al., 1995; Pardo et al., 1993), anxiety (Benkelfat et al., 1995; Wik et al., 1993), and anxiety disorders (e.g., Baxter et al., 1987, 1992; Benkalfat et al., 1990; Buchsbaum et al., 1987; McGuire et al., 1994; Mountz et al., 1989; Nordahl et al., 1989, 1990; Rauch et al., 1994, 1995, 1996; Swedo et al., 1989, 1992; Wik et al., 1993) performed in other laboratories; we did not consider how PET could help characterize the neurochemical processes that underlie the observed changes in neuronal activity; we did not consider the potentially complementary role of other imaging techniques, such as structural magnetic resonance imaging (e.g., Bremner et al., 1995), magnetic resonance spectroscopy (Dager et al., 1994, 1995; Keshavan et al., 1991), and functional magnetic resonance imaging (Bandettini & Wong, 1997; Davidson et al., 1993; Kalin, 1996); and we did not consider how PET complements other research strategies (e.g., neural tract tracing; lesioning; stimulation; unit recording; cognitive approaches; developmental approaches; pharmacological challenge; treatment studies; transcranial magnetic stimulation; and other kinds of brain imaging studies) that could be performed in laboratory animals, patients with selective brain injuries, patients with psychiatric disorders, and normal volunteers (Reiman, 1988). In addition, we did not consider potentially important hemispheric asymmetries (Davidson, 1995), for which we have modified our brain-mapping algorithms to directly compare regional CBF changes in one hemisphere to those in the other. Finally, we did not consider potentially important decreases in regional CBF, some of which could be related to selective inattention to less relevant sensory modalities, emotional repression, and the disinhibition of normally repressed emotions.

Reductions in cerebral activity could play an important role in the generation of emotion. Confirming the original discovery by Goltz more than 100 years ago, Cannon and Bard found that the cerebral cortex is unnecessary for the expression of emotions such as fear and rage (see LeDoux, 1987). Surgical removal of the cerebral cortex, above the level of the hypothalamus and caudoventral thalamus, caused cats and dogs to exhibit what the investigators called "sham rage," an unprovoked and integrated emotional response with behavioral, autonomic, and endocrine components. Their findings suggest that the cerebral cortex serves to inhibit unbridled expressions of emotion. It remains to be determined which cortical structures participate in emotional inhibition, which structures, if any, need to be "turned off" for the disinhibition of emotion, and how the deactivation of such structures might lead efferent pathways to participate in the generation of emotion.

Like any research methodology, PET has several limitations that prevent researchers from using it exclusively to characterize the neuronal pathways causally related to the dissectable components of emotion and anxiety. Limitations in anatomical standardization (necessary for comparing data between subjects) and spatial resolution (i.e., the ability to distinguish measurements that are close together) make it difficult to specify the structures (e.g., particular thalamic nuclei, insular cortex vs. claustrum, etc.) responsible for the observed increases in regional CBF. Limitations in temporal resolution (i.e., the time required to acquire an image) prevent us from characterizing the sequence in which the implicated regions are activated. Although PET studies provide information about the brain regions that are selectively affected during an emotional response, lesion studies are required to determine if the implicated regions are necessary or sufficient for particular aspects of the response. Because increases in regional CBF appear to reflect the activity of terminal neuronal fields (including those from local interneurons and afferent projections arising from other sites), lesion studies may be necessary to specify the neuronal projections responsible for these increases. Finally, in some cases, failure to detect significant increases in regional CBF could be related to limitations in the contrast resolution of PET (i.e., the ability to distinguish subtle measurements from noise), spatial resolution, and statistical power, changes in the pattern rather than the overall level of neuronal activity, and heterogeneity in different subjects' responses to a particular emotion-eliciting situation. For all these reasons, negative findings should be interpreted with caution, positive findings should interpreted in the form of testable hypotheses and replicated, and PET should be used in a manner that complements other research strategies.

Of course, other research methods have their own limitations (Reiman, 1988). For instance, limitations of experimental animal studies include neuroanatomical differences among species, the problem of making inferences about an animal's experiential state on the basis of observed behaviors, the restricted range of emotions that can be studied, difficulties in studying cognitively elicited emotions, and limitations in the ability to study certain emotional disorders. Studies of brain-injured patients have their own limitations, such as difficulties in determining the extent to which emotional alterations are related to local neuronal effects, effects on fibers of passage, or indirect effects on other neuronal systems and problems in generalizing findings to normal emotions and emotional disorders.

Complementary research methods are needed to fully characterize the neuronal systems involved in normal and pathological human emotions and the potentially dissectable cognitive components to which they are related (Reiman, 1988), and standardized procedures for the elicitation and measurement of emotion are needed to bridge existing gaps among studies of emotion in nonhuman species, brain-injured patients, patients with emotional disorders, and normal volunteers. Potentially complementary research methods include, but are not limited to, the use of neural-tract tracing techniques in nonhuman and, eventually, human brains; psychophysiologic, multiunit recording and brain imaging studies of laboratory animals with selective brain lesions; psychophysiologic and brain imaging studies of patients with selective brain injuries; psychophysiologic and brain imaging studies of patients with emotional disorders; and psychophysiologic and brain imaging studies of normal volunteers. We suggest that PET and other functional brain-mapping techniques have a critical role to play in this endeavor.

In conclusion, when used in conjunction with other research strategies, PET promises to help determine how multiple mental operations and the spatially distributed brain processes that subserve them work in concert to produce multifaceted emotions and how they conspire to produce emotional disorders.

Acknowledgments

We thank the other investigators and staff members who contributed to the six PET studies reviewed in this chapter. This work was supported in part by research grants from the Robert S. Flinn Biomedical Research Enrichment Initiative, the McDonnell-Pew Program in Cognitive Neuroscience, and NIMH Research Scientist Development Awards MH-00972 and MH-00875.

References

Alexander, G. E., Delong, M. R. & Strick, P. L. (1986). Parallel organisation of functionally segregated circuits linking basal ganglia and cortex. *Annual Review of Neuroscience, 9*, 357–381.

Bandettini, P. A. & Wong, E. C. (1997). Magnetic resonance imaging of human brain function: principles, practicalities, and possibilities. *Neurosurgery Clinics of North America, 8*, 345–371.

Baxter, L. R., Phelps, M. E. & Mazziotta, J. C. (1987). Local cerebral glucose metabolic rates in obsessive-compulsive disorder. *Archives of General Psychiatry, 44*, 211–218.

Baxter, L. R., Schwartz, J. M. & Bergman, K. S. (1992). Caudate glucose metabolic rate changes with both drug and behaviour therapy for obsessive-compulsive disorder. *Archives of General Psychiatry, 49*, 681–689.

Benkelfat, C., Bradwejn, J., Meyer, E., Ellenbogen, B. A., Milot, S., Gjedde, A. & Evans, A. (1995). Functional neuroanatomy of CCK_4-induced anxiety in normal healthy volunteers. *American Journal of Psychiatry, 152*, 8.

Benkelfat, C., Nordahl, T. E. & Semple, W. E. (1990). Local cerebral glucose metabolic rates in obsessive-compulsive disorder. *Archives of General Psychiatry, 47*, 840–848.

Bremner, J. D., Randall, P., Scott, T. M., Bronen, R. A., Seibyl, J. P., Southwick, S. M., Delaney, R. C., McCarthy, G., Charney, D. S. & Innis, R. B. (1995). MRI-based measurement of hippocampal volume in patients with combat-related posttraumatic stress disorder. *American Journal of Psychiatry, 152*, 973–981.

Buchsbaum, M. S., Wu, J., Haler, R., Hazlett, E., Ball, R., Katz, M., Socolski, K., Lagunas-Solar, M. & Lanager, D. (1987). Positron emission tomography assessment of effects of benzodiazepines on regional glucose metabolic rate in patients with anxiety disorder. *Life Science, 40*, 2393–2400.

Bushnell, M. C., Craig, A. D., Reiman, E. M., Yun, L. S. & Evans, A. (1995). Cerebral activation in the human brain by pain, temperature, and the illusion of pain. Presented at the Annual Meeting of the Society of Neuroscience, 1995, San Diego, CA.

Chen, K., Reiman, E. M., Lawson, M., Yun, L. S., Bandy, D. & Palant, A. (1995). Methods for the correction of vascular artifacts in PET ^{15}O-water brain mapping studies. *IEEE Transactions in Nuclear Science, 42*, 2173–2179.

Dager, S. R., Marro, K. I., Richards, T. L. & Metzger, G. D. (1994). Preliminary application of magnetic resonance spectroscopy to investigate lactate-induced panic. *American Journal of Psychiatry, 151*, 57–63.

Dager, S. R., Strauss, W. L., Marro, K. I., Richards, T. L., Metzger, G. D. & Artru, A. A.

(1995). Proton magnetic resonance spectroscopy investigation of hyperventilation in subjects with panic disorder and comparison subjects. *American Journal of Psychiatry, 152*, 666–672.

Damasio, H., Grabowski, T., Frank, R., Galaburda, A. & Damasio, A. (1994). The return of Phineas Gage: clues about the brain from the skull of a famous patient. *Science, 264*, 1102–1105.

Davidson, R. J. (1995). Cerebral asymmetry, emotion, and affective style. In R. J. Davidson & K. Hugdahl (Eds), *Brain Asymmetry* (pp. 361–387). Cambridge, MA: MIT Press.

Davidson, R. J. (1996). Cortical and subcortical substrates of affective style. Presented at the Annual Meeting of the World Congress of Psychiatry, August 1996, Madrid, Spain.

Davidson, J. R. T., Krishnan, K. R. R., Charles, H. C., Boyko, O., Potts, N. L. S., Ford, S. M. & Patterson, L. (1993). Magnetic resonance spectroscopy in social phobia: preliminary findings. *Journal of Clinical Psychology, 54*, 19–25.

Drevets, W., Videen, T., MacLeod, A., Haller, J. & Raichle, M. (1989). PET images of blood flow changes during anxiety: correction. *Science, 256*, 1696.

Ekman, P. & Friesen, W. V. (1982). Measuring facial movement with the facial action coding system. In P. Ekman (Ed), *Emotion in the Human Face* (pp. 178–211). Cambridge: Cambridge University Press.

Fox, P. T., Mintun, M. A., Reiman, E. M. & Raichle, M. E. (1988). Enhanced detection of focal brain responses using intersubject averaging and distribution analysis of subtracted PET images. *Journal of Cerebral Blood Flow and Metabolism, 8*, 642–653.

George, M. S., Kektter, T. A., Pareh, A., Horowitz, B., Hersovitch, P. & Post, R. M. (1995). Brain activity during transient sadness and happiness in healthy women. *American Journal of Psychiatry, 152*, 341–351.

Goldman-Rakic, P. S. (1987). Circuitry of primate prefrontal cortex and regulation of behavior by representational memory. In F. Plum & V. B. Mountcastle (Eds), *Handbook of Physiology, the Nervous System V. Higher Cortical Functions of the Brain* (pp. 373–417). Bethesda, MD: American Physiological Society.

Kalin, N. (1996). Effects of venlafaxine on functional brain activity in patients with depression. Presented at the Annual Meeting of the World Congress of Psychiatry, August 1996, Madrid, Spain.

Keshavan, M. S., Kapur, S. & Pettegrew, J. W. (1991). Magnetic resonance spectroscopy in psychiatry: potential, pitfalls, and promise. *American Journal of Psychiatry, 148*, 976–985.

Kihlstrom, J. F. (1987). The cognitive unconscious. *Science, 237*, 1444–1452.

Klein, D. F., Uhde, T. W., Hollander, E., Stein, M. B., Baxter, L. R., Cameron, O., Curtis, G., Drevets, W., Dager, S. R., Gorman, J. M., Hoehn-Saric, R., Meldelson, W. B. & Zohar, J. (1992). Panic and anxiety: metabolic and autonomic features. Presented at the annual meeting of the American College of Neuropsychopharmacology.

Lane, R. D., Reiman, E. M., Ahern, G. L., Schwartz, G. E., Davidson, R. J., Axelrod, B., Yun, L., Blocher, N. & Friston, K. (1997a). Neuroanatomical correlates of happiness, sadness, and disgust. *American Journal of Psychiatry, 154*, 926–933.

Lane, R. D., Reiman, E. M., Bradley, M. M., Lang, P. J., Ahern, G. L. & Schwartz, G. E. (1997b). Neuroanatomical correlates of pleasant and unpleasant emotion. *Neuropsychologia, 35*, 1437–1444.

Lang, P. J., Bradley, M. M. & Cuthbert, B. N. (1995). *The International Affective Picture System (IAPS): Photographic Slides*. Gainesville: The Center for Research in Psychophysiology, University of Florida.

LeDoux, J. E. (1987). Emotion. In F. Plum & V. B. Mountcastle (Eds), *Handbook of Physiology, The Nervous System V. Higher Cortical Functions of the Brain*, vol. 5, Section 1 (pp. 419–459). Bethesda, MD: American Physiological Society.

Mayberg, H. S., Liotti, M., Jerabek, P. A., Martin, C. C., Fox, P. T. (1995). Induced sadness: a PET model of depression. *Human Brain Mapping, 3*(suppl 1), 396.

McGuire, P. K., Bench, C. J., Frith, C. D., Marks, I. M., Frackowiak, R. S. J. & Dolan, R. J. (1994). Functional anatomy of obsessive-compulsive phenomena. *British Journal of Psychiatry, 164*, 459–468.

Mesulam, M.-M. (1986). *Principles of Behavioral Neurology.* Philadelphia, PA: F. A. Davis.

Morgan, M., Romanski, L. & LeDoux, J. (1993). Extinction of emotional learning: contribution of medial prefrontal cortex. *Neuroscience Letters, 163*, 109–113.

Mountz, J. M., Modell, J. G., Wilson, M. W., Curtis, G. C., Lee, M. A., Schmaltz, S. & Kuhl, D. E. (1989). Positron emission tomographic evaluation of cerebral blood flow during state anxiety in simple phobia. *Archives of General Psychiatry, 46*, 501–504.

Nordahl, T. E., Benkelfat, C. & Semple, W. E. (1989). Cerebral glucose rates in obsessive-compulsive disorder. *Neuropsychopharmacology, 2*, 23–28.

Nordahl, T. E., Semple, W. E., Gross, M., et al. (1990). Cerebral glucose metabolic differences in patients with panic disorder. *Neuropsychopharmacology, 3*, 261–273.

Pardo, J. V., Park, P. J. & Raichle, M. E. (1993). Neural correlates of self-induced dysphoria. *American Journal of Psychiatry, 150*, 713–719.

Rauch, S. L., Jenike, M. A., Alpert, N. M., Baer, L., Breiter, H. C. R., Savage, C. R. & Fischman, A. J. (1995). Regional cerebral blood flow measured during symptom provocation in obsessive-compulsive disorder using oxygen 15-labeled carbon dioxide and positron emission tomography. *Archives of General Psychiatry, 51*, 62–70.

Rauch, S. L., Savage, C. R., Alpert, N. M., Miguel, E. C., Baer, L., Breiter, H. C., Fischman, A. J., Manzo, P. A., Moretti, C. & Jenike, M. A. (1994). A positron emission tomographic study of simple phobic symptom provocation. *Archives of General Psychiatry, 52*, 20–28.

Rauch, S. L., van der Kolk, B. A., Fisler, R. E., Alpert, N. M., Orr, S. P., Savage, C. R., Fischman, A. J., Jenike, M. A. & Pitman, R. K. (1996). A symptom provocation study of posttraumatic stress disorder using positron emission tomography and script-drive imagery. *Archives of General Psychiatry, 53*, 380–387.

Reiman, E. M. (1987). The study of panic disorder using positron emission tomography. *Psychiatric Developments, 1*, 63–78.

Reiman, E. M. (1988). The quest to establish the neural substrates of anxiety. *Psychiatric Clinics of North America, 11*, 295–307.

Reiman, E. M. (1990). PET, panic disorder, and normal anticipatory anxiety. In Ballenger, J. C. (Ed), *Neurobiology of Panic Disorder.* New York: Wiley-Liss.

Reiman, E. M. (1991). Contributions to the development and treatment of panic disorder: towards a piece of mind and brain. In B. D. Beitman & G. Klerman (Eds), *Integrating Pharmacotherapy and Psychotherapy* (pp. 423–434). Washington, DC: American Psychiatric Press.

Reiman, E. M. (1996). PET studies of anxiety, emotion, and their disorders. Presented at the Annual Meeting of the World Congress of Psychiatry, August 1996, Madrid, Spain.

Reiman, E. M., Armstrong, S. M., Matt, K. S. & Mattox, J. H. (1996). The application of positron emission tomography to the study of the normal menstrual cycle. *Human Reproduction, 11*, 2799–2805.

Reiman, E. M., Butler, F. K., Raichle, M. E., Herscovich, P., Robins, E., Fox, P. & Perlmutter, J. (1986). The application of positron emission tomography to the study of panic disorder. *American Journal of Psychiatry, 143*, 469–477.

Reiman, E. M., Fusselman, M. J., Fox, P. T. & Raichle, M. E. (1989a). Neuroanatomical correlates of anticipatory anxiety. *Science, 243*, 1071–1074.

Reiman, E. M., Lane, R. D., Ahern, G. L., Schwartz, G. E., Davidson, R. J. & Axelrod, B.

(1997). Neuroanatomical correlates of externally and internally generated human emotion. *American Journal of Psychiatry, 154*, 918–925.

Reiman, E. M., Mintun, M. A., Raichle, M. E., Robins, E., Price, J. L., Fusselman, M., Fox, P. T. & Hackman, K. (1989b). Neuroanatomical correlates of a lactate-induced anxiety attack. *Archives of General Psychiatry, 46*, 493–500.

Reiman, E. M., Raichle, M. E., Butler, F. K., Herscovich, P. & Robins, E. (1984). A focal brain abnormality in panic disorder, a severe form of anxiety. *Nature, 310*, 683–685.

Swedo, S. E., Pietrini, P. & Leonard, H. L. (1992). Cerebral glucose metabolism in childhood-onset obsessive-compulsive disorder. Revisualization during pharmacotherapy. *Archives of General Psychiatry, 49*, 690–694.

Swedo, S. E., Schapiro, M. & Grady C. (1989). Cerebral glucose metabolism in childhood-onset obsessive-compulsive disorder. *Archives of General Psychiatry, 46*, 518–522.

Tomarken, A. J., Davidson, R. J. & Henriques, J. B. (1990). Resting frontal brain asymmetry predicts affective responses to films. *Journal of Personality and Social Psychology, 59*, 791–801.

Wik, G., Fredrikson, M., Ericson, K., Eriksson, L., Stone-Elander, S. & Greitz, T. (1993). A functional cerebral response to frightening visual stimulation. *Psychiatry Research: Neuroimaging, 50*, 15–24.

Epilogue

The Future of Emotion Research from the Perspective of Cognitive Neuroscience

RICHARD D. LANE, LYNN NADEL, AND ALFRED W. KASZNIAK

In Chapter 1 we discussed the value of studying emotion from the perspective of cognitive neuroscience. In closing, we will draw on some of the themes from previous chapters to provide our view of how a cognitive neuroscientific approach can be useful in future emotion research.

A Cognitive Neuroscientific Approach to Emotion Research Is Not Restrictive

At the time of this writing there is considerable debate within the field of emotion research regarding the fundamental organization of emotion. For example, several authors (Ekman, 1994), including contributors to this volume (Dolan and Morris, LeDoux), hold that separate neural networks exist for each discrete emotion. There is a growing literature on the neural substrates of fear, and recent data (Sprengelmeyer, Young, Calder et al., 1996) is emerging regarding separate neural substrates of disgust. An alternative view, which is also well represented in this volume (Bradley and Lang), is that emotion is fundamentally organized along dimensions consisting of valence (appetitive and aversive emotions) and arousal. While a circumplex model can accommodate both perspectives, this debate will likely be resolved by elucidation of the neuroanatomical substrates of the phenomena in question. In a recent volume Griffiths (1997) argues that the field of emotion research needs to be clear about what emotion is and what it is not and should aim to carve nature at its joint. This viewpoint dovetails perfectly with the goal of identifying the fundamental neural circuitry underlying emotion.

Questions such as how a basic mental function such as emotion is organized are not new to cognitive neuroscience. The field of memory research serves as a good example. Lively debate still exists regarding how best to classify the various phenomena that can be considered part of memory. There is also some uncertainty regarding the definition of the precise boundary that can be used to determine whether learning has or has not occurred. Nevertheless, great strides have been made in understanding memory by use of the family of methods embraced within the field of cognitive neuroscience.

Our point in Chapter 1 was that emotion is best studied as if it were another cognitive phenomenon. Thus, questions such as the fundamental organization of emotion fit well into the cognitive neuroscience research program and do not limit it in any way. Methods and strategies used to answer questions about emotion can be enriched by the approaches taken in other domains of cognitive neuroscience, such as memory.

Implicit and Explicit Processes

The two predominant themes addressed in this book are the evaluation of emotional significance and the conscious experience of emotion. The chapters addressing the functions of the amygdala may be grouped with the former issue. These themes echo the distinction between implicit and explicit processes found in many areas of cognitive neuroscience, such as memory, language, perception, and motor control. As discussed in several chapters in this book (LeDoux, Öhman, Bradley and Lang, Lane, Weiskrantz), the process whereby emotional significance is computed and behavioral responses are generated often proceeds outside of conscious awareness. Several authors (de Gelder, Heilman, Lane) made reference to modules, which in this context reflects the view that the process of emotion generation is implicit, automatic, and cognitively impenetrable. By contrast, explicit emotion processes, which are highly cognitively penetrable, include the conscious experience of emotion and those conscious cognitive processes that contribute to the generation and regulation of emotion. Based on findings in other areas of cognitive neuroscience, the distinction between implicit and explicit processes is likely to map onto distinguishable neuroanatomical substrates (Gazzaniga, Ivry & Mangun, 1998). Given the debate about "what emotions really are," the distinction between cognitively penetrable and impenetrable processes may be useful in the search to determine how emotion is fundamentally organized.

Usefulness of a Developmental Perspective

One of the challenges confronting emotion research is the enormous variability that can be observed between individuals in their emotional behavior. This topic was addressed from the standpoint of emotional style in the chapter by Davidson. Such variability should not be surprising, in that emotion may exist to enable organisms to learn from their immediate experience and thus go beyond simple innate stimulus-response reflexes (Scherer, 1994).

Modern theorists hold that cognitive development consists of the transformation of knowledge from implicit to explicit representations (Karmiloff-Smith, 1992). Similarly, as discussed in the chapter by Lane, emotional development may consist of the transformation of automatic, modular, implicit responses to emotional responses, states, and abilities that are under conscious control. In combination with innate variability in temperament, individual differences in this developmental process may well contribute to the variability in emotional behavior evident between adults. The process by which this occurs, and the ways in which emotional development can go awry, will be important areas of neuroscientific investigation in the future.

A particularly important area for future research is that of "emotional learning." People learn scripts or blueprints for relationships during childhood that affect their emotional reactions, capacity for intimacy and love, and ability to maintain their emotional equilibrium in the face of stress or adversity. Patterns that get established early in life may be difficult to change in adulthood. There are hints of the processes involved in the findings of conditioned fear (LeDoux, Dolan and Morris), but this work, while extremely important, is only the beginning. An enormous amount remains to be learned about how such patterns get established, why they are so resistant to change or extinction, and how therapeutic change can be brought about as efficiently as possible. Neural network models of the process of emotional learning have been proposed (Friston, Tononi, Reeke, Jr. et al., 1994) that can guide hypothesis testing.

Another key area is that of empathy. The capacity for emotional self-awareness and empathy are closely related. It has been proposed that successful social adaptation requires the ability to maintain awareness of the needs of others while also paying due attention to one's own needs and goals (Baddeley, Della Sala, Papagno, & Spinnler, 1997). Learning the details of how such skills develop or fail to develop, and creating effective intervention methods to improve function in this area, could potentially have an important impact on the sense of well-being on an individual level or the eradication of prejudice and discrimination on a broader social scale.

Methods

One of the fundamental principles of cognitive neuroscience is that no single methodology will be adequate. The methods discussed in this book will likely be well represented in future research.

Studies of the future will likely be geared to address *how* specific brain areas execute their functions rather than identifying *where* in the brain these functions are instantiated. It is likely that functional magnetic resonance imaging will play a major role in future research in healthy people and patient groups. Such studies are likely to be combined with pharmacological probes to identify the neurochemical mediators of region-specific effects. Behavioral studies of patients with well-characterized lesions will continue to be important in complementing neuroimaging findings. It is also likely that parallel paradigms for nonhuman primates and people will be developed, permitting more fine-grained analysis of anatomical connections and genetic variability in interaction with environmental inputs.

Greater emphasis should be placed on plasticity of function as a result of environmental inputs either alone or in interaction with genetic variables. Longitudinal studies before and after interventions designed to promote emotional learning or empathy are likely to be particularly fruitful. Knowledge regarding developmental processes and plasticity will also be advanced by the use of high resolution, non-invasive methods for studying functional neuroanatomy in children.

Conclusion

This book has sought to bring together diverse strands of investigation, including neuroanatomical studies in rats and nonhuman primates, neuropsychological, neurological, and psychiatric investigations, studies in psychophysiology and experimental psychology, and functional brain imaging studies. A major goal has been to document current understanding of how emotion is instantiated in the brain. We also hope that we have contributed to progress in determining whether emotion should be studied in its own right, or, as we believe, can best be considered as one among many domains to be studied within a cognitive neuroscientific framework.

References

Baddeley, A., Della Sala, S., Papagno, C., & Spinnler, H. (1997). Dual-task performance in dysexecutive and nondysexecutive patients with a frontal lesion. *Neuropsychology, 11*(2), 187–194.

Ekman, P. (1994). All emotions are basic. In P. Ekman & R. J. Davidson (Eds.), *The Nature of Emotion: Fundamental Questions* (pp. 15–19). New York: Oxford University Press.

Friston, K. J., Tononi, G., Reeke, G. N., Jr., Sporns, O., & Edelman, G. M. (1994). Value-dependent selection in the brain: Simulation in a synthetic neural model. *Neuroscience, 59*(2), 229–243.

Gazzaniga, M. S., Ivry, R. B., & Mangun, G. R. (1998). *Cognitive Neuroscience: The Biology of the Mind.* New York: W. W. Norton and Company.

Griffiths, P. E. (1997). *What Emotions Really Are: The Problem of Psychological Categories.* Chicago: University of Chicago Press.

Karmiloff-Smith, A. (1992). *Beyond Modularity: A Developmental Perspective on Cognitive Science.* Cambridge, MA: MIT Press.

Scherer, K. R. (1994). Emotion serves to decouple stimulus and response. In P. Ekman & R. J. Davidson (Eds.), *The Nature of Emotion: Fundamental Questions* (pp. 127–130). New York: Oxford University Press.

Sprengelmeyer, R., Young, A. W., Calder, A. J., Karnat, A., Lange, H., Hömberg, V., Perrett, D. I., & Rowland, D. (1996). Loss of disgust: Perception of faces and emotions in Huntington's disease. *Brain, 119*, 1647–1665.

Index

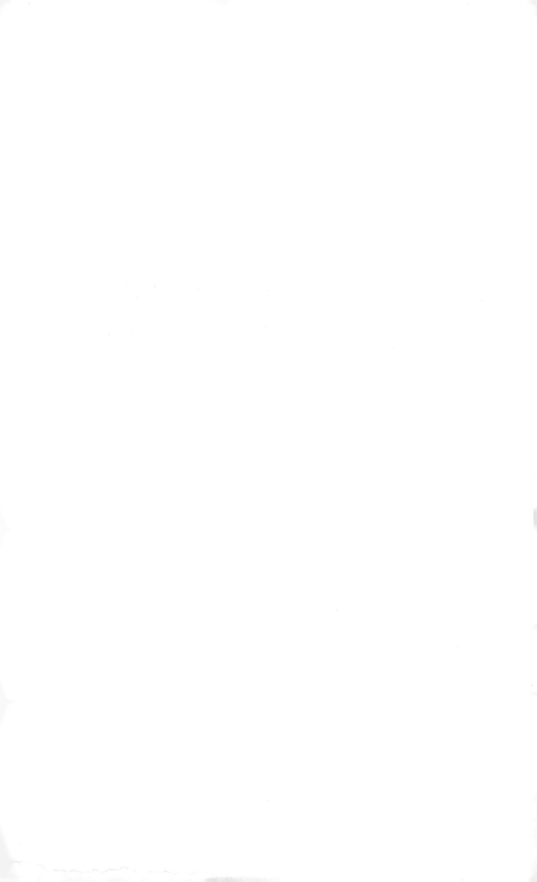